# The *Yoga* Tradition

With many blessings, peace, light —

Georg

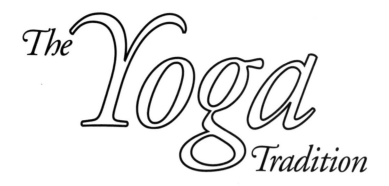

# The Yoga Tradition

## Its History, Literature, Philosophy and Practice

GEORG FEUERSTEIN, PH.D.

*Foreword by Ken Wilber*

HOHM PRESS

Prescott, Arizona

Cover design: Kim Johansen
Design and Layout: Visual Perspectives, Phoenix, Arizona

Library of Congress Cataloguing in Publication Data:
Feuerstein, Georg.
    The yoga tradition / Georg Feuerstein: foreword by Ken Wilber.
        p.   cm.
    Includes bibliographical references and index.
    ISBN: 0-934252-88-2 (cloth)      ISBN: 0-934252-83-1 (alk. paper)
    1. Yoga.   I. Title.
B132.T6F489   1998                                                    98-23466
181'.45—dc21                                                          CIP

HOHM PRESS
PO Box 2501
Prescott, Arizona 86302
800-381-2700
http://www.booknotes.com/hohm/

# Select other books by Georg Feuerstein

*The Shambhala Encyclopedia of Yoga* (Shambhala)

*The Shambhala Guide to Yoga* (Shambhala)

*Teachings of Yoga* (Shambhala)

*Tantra: The Path of Ecstasy* (Shambhala)

*The Yoga-Sûtra of Patanjali* (Inner Traditions International)

*The Essence of Yoga* (Inner Traditions International)
[coauthored with Jeanine Miller]

*Lucid Waking* (Inner Traditions International)

*Wholeness or Transcendence?* (Larson Publications)

*Sacred Paths* (Larson Publications)

*The Mystery of Light* (Integral Publishing)

*The Bhagavad-Gîtâ: Its Philosophy and Cultural Setting* (Quest Books)

*In Search of the Cradle of Civilization* (Quest Books)
[coauthored with Subhash Kak and David Frawley]

*Voices on the Threshold of Tomorrow* (Quest Books)
[coedited with Trisha Lamb Feuerstein]

*Living Yoga* (J. P. Tarcher and *Yoga Journal*)
[coedited with Stephan Bodian]

These books can be ordered from their respective publishers or from
Yoga Research Center, P.O. Box 1386, Lower Lake, CA 9545

# CONTENTS

## PART ONE: FOUNDATIONS

# PART TWO: PRE-CLASSICAL YOGA

# PART FIVE: POWER AND TRANSCENDENCE IN TANTRISM

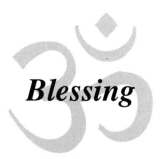

# *Blessing*

**by Sri Satguru Subramuniyaswami**
*Jagadacharya of the Nandinatha Sampradaya's*
*Kailasa Parampara Guru Mahasannidhanam*

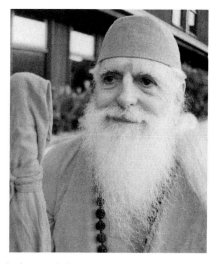

This book, *The Yoga Tradition*, is a mature rendering of Yoga, unlike other books in that, without submitting to the pitfalls of exclusivity, it preserves a deeply Hindu perspective. It outlines the end of the path as well as the path itself. While others see in Yoga a thousand techniques to be practiced and perfected toward a lofty spiritual attainment, Dr. Feuerstein intuits the Indian *rishis'* revelation that it is not something we do but something we become and are. Yoga without the yogi's all-comprehending consciousness is like the sun without heat and light. As the subject matter in this book is documented according to tradition—remembering that tradition is the best of the past that has been preserved—we can assure ourselves that the advice and guidance here has been most useful to our forefathers, theirs, and the many generations that preceded them for thousands of years.

We are most happy to give blessings from this and inner worlds to Georg Feuerstein for a long life, that he may enjoy the four *purushârthas*, "human goals," of *dharma*, wealth, pleasure, and liberation as a fulfillment of his personal quest.

xi

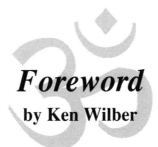

# *Foreword*
## by Ken Wilber

Author of *The Spectrum of Consciousness; The Atman Project; Up From Eden; A Sociable God; No Boundary; Grace and Grit; A Brief History of Everything; Sex, Ecology, Spirituality;* etc.

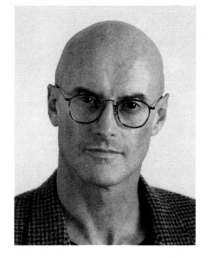

It is a great pleasure, indeed honor, to write this Foreword. I have been a fan of Georg Feuerstein ever since I read his classic *The Essence of Yoga*. His subsequent works simply reinforced my belief that in Georg Feuerstein we have a scholar-practitioner of the first magnitude, an extremely important and valuable voice for the perennial philosophy, and arguably the foremost authority on Yoga today.

In the East, as well as in the West, there tend to be two rather different approaches to spirituality—that of the scholar and that of the practitioner. The scholar tends to be abstract, and studies world religions as one might study bugs or rocks or fossils—merely another field for the detached intellect. The idea of actually practicing a spiritual or contemplative discipline rarely seems to dawn on the scholar. Indeed, to practice what one is studying is held to interfere with one's "objectivity"—one has become a believer and therefore nonobjective.

Practitioners, on the other hand, although admirably engaged in an actual discipline, tend to be very uninformed about all the various facets of their tradition. They may be naive about the cultural trappings of their particular path, or about its actual historical origins, or about how much of their path is essential truth and how much is simply cultural baggage.

Rare, indeed, to find a scholar who is also a practitioner. But when it comes to writing a book on Yoga, this combination is absolutely essential. A treatise on Yoga can be trusted neither to the scholars nor the practitioners alone. There is an immense amount of information that must be mastered in order to write about Yoga, and therefore a scholar is needed. But Yoga itself is born in the fire of direct experience. It must be engaged, and lived, and practiced. It must come from the head, but equally from the heart. And this very rare combination is exactly what Georg Feuerstein brings to this remarkable topic.

The essence of Yoga is very simple: It means *yoking* or *joining*. When Jesus said, "My yoke is easy," he meant "My Yoga is easy." Whether East or West, Yoga is the technique of joining or uniting the individual soul with absolute Spirit. It is a means of liberation. And it is therefore fiery, hot, intense, ecstatic. It will take you far beyond yourself; some say it will take you to infinity.

Therefore, choose your guides carefully. The book you now hold in your hands is, without a doubt, the finest overall explanation of Yoga currently available, a book destined to become a classic. And for a simple reason: It comes from both the head and the heart, from impeccable scholarship and dedicated practice. In this sense, it is much more perceptive and accurate than the works of, say, Eliade or Campbell.

Enter now the world of Yoga, which is said to lead from suffering to release, from agony to ecstasy, from time to eternity, from death to immortality. And know that on this extraordinary tour, you are indeed in good hands.

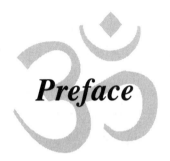

# *Preface*

My first encounter with India's spiritual heritage occurred on my fourteenth birthday when I was given a copy, in German, of Paul Brunton's *A Search in Secret India*. I have since come to regard Brunton—or "PB" as his students came to call him—as one of the finest Western mystics of this century. He certainly ranks among the pioneers of the East-West dialogue, and his writings have been widely influential. Brunton, who died in 1971, still has much to teach those of us who are walking on the razor-edged path. Apart from his books, the posthumously published sixteen volumes of his *Notebooks* are a veritable treasure chest for spiritual seekers.

I still vividly remember the yearning I experienced when reading about Brunton's remarkable encounter with Sri Ramana Maharshi, the great sage of Tiruvannamalai in South India, whose spontaneous and effortless enlightenment at the age of sixteen became an archetypal symbol for me. I dreamed of abandoning school, which I found utterly boring, to follow in the footsteps of

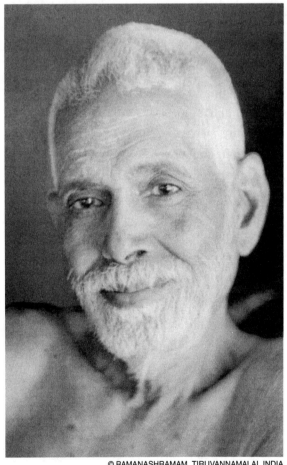

*Ramana Maharshi*

the great saints and Self-realizers of India. My concerned and well-meaning parents had a different idea.

So it was not until 1965, when I was eighteen, that I encountered the spirit of India more concretely in the person of a Hindu swami who was making headlines in Europe for his astounding physical feats. He was able to bear the weight of a steamroller on his chest, pull a loaded wagon with his long hair, and stop his pulse at will. While I was duly impressed by these spectacular abilities, they fascinated me far less than the secret behind all this physical prowess. I sensed that the mind, or consciousness, was the key not only to such astonishing abilities but, more importantly, to lasting happiness.

I felt mysteriously attracted to this latter-day miracle worker with an impressive physique and a great deal of charisma. I found a way of making contact with him and ended up as his disciple. In the year I spent with him at his hermitage in the Black Forest, Germany, I learned a great deal about Hatha-Yoga, but more about the need for self-discipline and persistence. In the middle of winter, my teacher had me move into a sparsely furnished room without carpet or wallpaper and with a broken window that I was not to repair. In the early morning, I was expected to break the ice in the well and wash myself outdoors. I quickly learned that in order to keep warm and well, I had to stay active and do a lot of breathing. It was all rather exhilarating.

Step by step I learned about the teacher-disciple relationship, which involves trust, love, and the constant willingness to be tested and go beyond one's imagined limitations. I benefited from the wonderful opportunity for self-transcendence this kind of circumstance presents. But in due course I also experienced its drawbacks. For I discovered that my teacher not only was an accomplished master of Hatha-Yoga, but he also used his charisma and paranormal powers to manipulate others. So long as enlightenment is not attained, the ego is not transcended, and there is the ever-present possibility of abusing one's yogic abilities for egoic purposes rather than for the spiritual upliftment of others.

When I tried to break loose from that close-knit relationship, I learned another invaluable lesson: Psychic powers are a reality to be reckoned with, and some teachers will use them to hold their disciples. Although I had severed my external ties to my teacher, he continued to influence my life through psychic means, which proved most disturbing.

Fortunately, I never suffered the terrible agonies of a fully awakened but misconducted life force (*kundalinî*), as described by Pandit Gopi Krishna. It was he who made the *kundalinî* a household name among Western spiritual seekers. Nevertheless, I experienced firsthand some of the disturbing side effects of a *kundalinî* that had been tampered with, particularly states of dissociation from the body. It took many years, and the benign help of another spiritual personage, before the link was finally broken and I could get on with my life. Even though the experience had been rewarding overall, it left me disappointed, and for a good many years I steered clear of any Eastern teachers.

In the meantime I had developed an interest in learning Sanskrit and studying the great religious and philosophical writings of the Hindus in the original. I channeled my frustrated spiritual impulse into a professional career in Indology. I regarded my studies and writing as a form of Karma-Yoga, of self-transcending action, and I also pursued in my daily life the great ideal of "witnessing," which is central to Jnâna-Yoga.

Periodically I dabbled with this or that yogic technique and meditative practice, and even taught Hatha-Yoga for a few years in the evenings and on weekends. However, not until 1980 did I again make a more decisive spiritual gesture. A series of life crises brought the spiritual impulse to the fore, freeing up my attention to ponder the great question *Who am I?* more seriously. I began to look for a competent teacher and a supportive environment.

Since 1966 I have enjoyed the spiritual friendship of Irina Tweedie, a Sufi master in England whose invaluable diary, *Daughter of Fire*, was published in 1986. During my spiritual crisis, I deepened that relationship, and she helped me immensely in those days of reorientation. Thanks to her I experienced my first real spiritual breakthroughs. Also, unbeknownst to me, she groomed me for a much greater spiritual adventure.

In 1982 I had my first meeting with the American-born adept Da Free John (born Franklin Jones, now Adi Da), whose early writings, especially *The Knee of Listening*, had both stimulated me intellectually and touched me deeply at the emotional level. This time around, with fifteen years' worth of learning behind me, it was rather more difficult to follow my intuition and entrust myself to the spiritual process under the guidance of a teacher. To make matters worse, Da Free John fitted none of the stereotypes I had come to associate with spiritual teachers. He was not a mild-mannered, gentle sage but, as he himself put it, a "wild character" and a "fire."

Yet, despite all my many misgivings about this larger-than-life teacher, I knew I should avail myself of his guidance. I both dreaded and felt excited about the prospect of having the artificial boundaries of my personality scrutinized and challenged by an adept who is well known for his uncompromising approach. As it turned out, my discipleship was exceedingly challenging but enormously beneficial, confronting me with aspects of myself that I had been able to ignore before.

In 1986, my discipleship came to a close when I felt that I had learned whatever lessons I was capable of learning from that teacher and that it was time to move on. I could no longer negotiate the inner conflict I was feeling about his controversial teaching approach, and did not wish to lose the benefit I had gained in the preceding years of my discipleship. In my book *Holy Madness*, first published in 1990, I have analyzed in great detail the crazy-wisdom method of teaching favored by Da Free John and several other contemporary adepts. Despite my serious concerns about the crazy-wisdom approach to teaching and my intellectual and moral differences with Da Free John, I remain grateful to him for having given me the opportunity for deepening my self-understanding.

In 1993, my spiritual life took a new turn. After many years of walking the spiritual path on my own, I met Lama Segyu Choepel (Shakya Zangpo), who has served as my mentor on the spiritual path. He is an initiate not only of Vajrayâna · Buddhism but also of Brazilian shamanism. Through his friendship and expert guidance I have been steadily discovering new levels of the spiritual process, but especially the living dimension of the Buddhist *bodhisattva* ideal. It might seem strange that after so many years of considering and practicing various aspects of Hindu Yoga I should now be engaged in a Buddhist *sâdhanâ*. But this strangeness evaporates when we adopt a long-range spiritual perspective, realizing that we are the product of all our past volitions, not merely the volitions of the present life. Moreover, Hinduism and Buddhism have many concepts and practices in common, which in the case of some of the medieval *siddhas* even makes it difficult to determine whether they were Hindus or Buddhists. Apart from this, as the nineteenth-century saint Sri Ramakrishna so ably demonstrated, if we follow any of the great spiritual paths to the end, we encounter the same spiritual truths and, ultimately, Reality or Truth itself.

I accepted long ago that spiritual life is a never-ending path of discovery that continues until we draw our last breath, and beyond. It is wonderful to know that for the dedicated aspirant there is always timely help in taking the next step. In my own life, I have received such help in bountiful measure, though often in unexpected form.

I felt it necessary to begin this volume with a brief autobiographical note, because even the most "objective" treatment is shot through with personal qualities: I approach the history, philosophy, and psychology of Yoga not as an antiquarian but as someone who has the deepest appreciation for India's spiritual genius honed in the course of many millennia. I have witnessed some of its effectiveness in my own person and in others who are spiritually more adept than I.

I am, clearly, in basic sympathy with the spiritual traditions of India, which are authentic efforts at transcending the self. My practical experience of them encourages me to assume that their fundamental insights are genuine and worthy of serious consideration. I further maintain that anyone who wishes to disclaim any of these insights or goals must do so on the basis of personal experience and experimentation rather than from mere theory. To put it simply, a person who has experienced the ecstatic state (*samâdhi*) cannot possibly call into question its intrinsic value and desirability. The experience of blissful ease in the nondual state of consciousness, wherein all sharp differences between beings and things are "outshined" (to use Da Free John's felicitous phrase), inevitably changes how we look at the whole spiritual enterprise and the world's sacred traditions, not to mention how we view everyone and everything else.

At the same time, I have come to appreciate that such higher states of consciousness, though extraordinary accomplishments, are not inherently more significant than our everyday awareness. Any experience is useful as long as it facilitates our spiritual awakening, but only enlightenment—which is not merely a transitory state of mind—is of unique significance because it reveals Reality as such. Prior to enlightenment, what matters is how we use the perspective gained in uncommon states in our daily relationship with others and life in general. As my elder son said to me when he was twenty-two years of age: It all boils down to whether we love or we don't. I wish I had arrived at this pristine insight when I was his age!

The fulcrum of spiritual life is self-transcendence as a constant orientation. As I understand it, self-transcendence is not merely the pursuit of altered states of consciousness. It also implies a constant willingness to be transformed and, in Meister Eckehart's sense, to be "superformed" by the larger Reality whose existence and benignity are revealed to us in the meditative and ecstatic condition.

This volume is the distillate of nearly three decades of scholarly and practical preoccupation with the tradition of Yoga. It has grown out of my earlier and long out-of-print *Textbook of Yoga*, published in 1975 by Rider & Co., London. I borrowed three months' time from my postgraduate research at Durham University to write that book in the summer of 1974. Even though the volume was well received, I was from the beginning diffident about its many shortcomings, which I saw perhaps more clearly than most readers. Ever since then, I had been waiting for an opportunity to revise and expand the text, and then it became apparent that a completely new book was called for. Thus, when Jeremy Tarcher expressed an interest in a comprehensive handbook on Yoga, I jumped at the opportunity and wrote an entirely new and substantially larger book, which was published in 1989 under the title *Yoga: The Technology of Ecstasy.*

The present volume is a thoroughly revised and greatly enlarged edition of that work. The changes made in the text are so substantial that a new title seemed justifiable. In addition to revising the existing text, I have more than doubled the number of pages, primarily through inclusion of my English renderings of major Sanskrit scriptures on Yoga, including complete translations of the *Yoga-Sûtra* of Patanjali, the *Shiva-Sûtra* of Vasugupta, the *Bhakti-Sûtra* of Nârada, the *Amrita-Nâda-Bindu-Upanishad*, the *Amrita-Bindu-Upanishad*, the *Advaya-Târaka-Upanishad*, the *Kshurikâ-Upanishad*, the *Dakshinamûrti-Stotra*, the *Mahâyâna-Vimshaka* of Nâgârjuna, the *Prajnâ-Pâramitâ-Hridaya-Sûtra,* and the hitherto untranslated *Goraksha-Paddhati*. There are also many renderings of sections of other significant Yoga scriptures, including Haribhadra Sûri's *Yoga-Drishti-Samuccaya*, ably translated by Christopher Chapple. In addition, I have added a new section on the adepts of Maharashtra and a whole new chapter on Yoga in Sikhism.

The objective of this volume is to give the lay reader a systematic and comprehensive introduction to the many-faceted phenomenon of Indian spirituality, especially in its Hindu variety, while at the same time summarizing in broad outlines what scholarship has discovered about the evolution of Yoga thus far. This presentation will enable the reader to grasp and appreciate not only the astonishing complexity of Yoga but also its intricate relationship to other aspects of India's complex culture. Inevitably I have had to deal with some rather involved ideas that will be foreign to those who have no background in philosophy, especially Eastern thought. I have tried, however, to introduce such ideas in as graduated a fashion as possible, without at the same time watering anything down.

The first few chapters are intended to provide an overview, and the subsequent chapters basically follow a roughly chronological order. Thus I begin with a discussion of yogic elements in the early Indian civilization as we know it from the archaeological digs at towns like Harappa and Mohenjo Daro and also from a careful study of the archaic *Rig-Veda*. This is followed by a treatment of Yoga in the early *Upanishads* (a particular genre of esoteric Hindu literature), the epic literature (including the *Bhagavad-Gîtâ*), the later *Upanishads*, the *Yoga-Sûtra* and its commentaries, and then the diversified forms of Yoga in the Post-Classical Era. The historical review ends with Tantra and Hatha-Yoga. I have refrained from a discussion of modern manifestations of Yoga, as this would have rendered the present volume prohibitively large.

For the benefit of the nonspecialist, I have appended a short glossary of key terms and a chronology beginning with the earliest known human presence on the Indian subcontinent in 250,000 B.C. and ending with India's independence in 1947.

The emphasis throughout this work is on comprehensiveness and intelligibility. While I did my best to give each facet of Yoga a fair hearing, in accord with its significance in the overall

> "Yoga is said to be the unification of the web of dualities."
>
> – *Yoga-Bîja* (84)
>
> "Yoga is the union of the individual psyche with the transcendental Self."
>
> – *Yoga-Yâjnavalkya* (1.44)

picture, I could treat many issues only to a certain depth given the scope and purpose of this volume. My other publications and the works of other scholars can help to fill in some of the gaps. I want to emphasize, however, that our knowledge of the Yoga tradition is incomplete, and in some cases pitifully so. This is particularly true of Tantra-Yoga, which has developed an elaborate esoteric technology and symbolism that is barely intelligible to those who have not been initiated. Readers wishing to pursue this particular tradition might want to study my book *Tantra: The Path of Ecstasy*, which offers an introduction to Hindu Tantrism.

While this volume is specifically geared toward a lay readership, I believe that its efficiency as an orientational tool also extends to specialists in the history of religion, intellectual history, theology, the study of consciousness, and transpersonal psychology. Obviously, it was not possible to proffer detailed treatments of all the different aspects of the Yoga tradition, but I have endeavored to make my portrayal as balanced as possible.

I am hoping that this book will particularly be useful to Yoga teachers and also serve as a reliable reference work for Yoga teacher training programs around the world. In order to make this volume more accessible, I plan to write a *Study Guide* for it in consultation with several teachers who have agreed to help optimize its didactic value.

Writing *The Yoga Tradition* has been both a challenging and a rewarding experience, because I was able to integrate materials that had been gestating in me for very many years and also because I was obliged to make my ideas as intelligible as possible, which always benefits the writer as well. To what degree I have succeeded in meeting this challenge of integration and clear presentation will be determined by my readers. I hope that they will find this book as enjoyable to read as I have found it to write.

Namas te
*Georg Feuerstein*

## Note:

The Sanskrit texts reflect the gender bias of traditional Vedic and Hindu society. For the sake of fidelity I have preserved their preference for masculine pronouns in all translations. In my own statements, however, I have tried to take modern sensibilities into account as much as possible by using the third person plural ("they," "them") or by using both masculine and feminine pronouns. One exception to the latter is my use—for simplicity's sake—of the term "*yogin*," which technically refers only to a male practitioner, but which should be assumed by the reader to also include the female practitioner (*yoginî*) in most contexts.

# *Acknowledgments*

Many individuals—friends, colleagues, and teachers—have contributed to the making of this volume. I am beholden to all of them.

The person who encouraged me the most in the early stages of my writing career, possibly without suspecting it, is Dr. Daniel Brostoff, a former editor-in-chief of Rider & Co., London. He adopted my first four books, when I was still struggling with the English language and publishing etiquette. Unfortunately, I have lost contact with him. Wherever you are, Daniel, I am greatly in your debt.

In my research I have particularly benefited from the fine scholarly works of J. W. Hauer and Mircea Eliade, two giants of Yoga research who are unfortunately no longer among us. The vast scholarship of the late Dr. Ram Shankar Bhattacharya of Varanasi, India, has also been an inspiration. More than any other researcher known to me, he was sensitive to the fact that scholars engaged in Yoga research need to be informed by Yoga practice. His always prompt and informed advice has been invaluable.

Another person whose intellectual labors have inspired me for the past two decades is my friend Jeanine Miller. In her own field of Vedic studies, she also seeks to combine scholarship with spiritual sensitivity. I have drawn on her pioneering works for my treatment of Yoga in ancient Vedic times. In this connection, I would also like to acknowledge the numerous favors and the illuminating research of my friends David Frawley and Subhash Kak, both of whom have done much to rectify our picture of ancient India. I had the pleasure of coauthoring with them *In Search of the Cradle of Civilization*. The first edition of *The Yoga Tradition* owed much to the enthusiasm and fine editing of Dan Joy. At that time I also received much-appreciated practical help from my friends Claudia Bourbeau and Stacey Koontz.

Many of the illustrations in the present volume were expertly created by James Rhea who, responding to my earlier writings, volunteered his artistic skills. I am most grateful to him both for his beautiful drawings and his moral support.

I thank Margo Gal, too, for several fine drawings of Hindu Goddesses; they certainly add to the value of this volume.

I would also like to record my gratitude to Stephan Bodian, the former editor of *Yoga Journal*, for having given me the opportunity over a period of seven or eight years to exercise my skills in writing for a nonacademic audience.

I am also beholden to Satguru Sivaya Subramuniyaswami for his blessing and kind words about this book. They mean a lot to me, coming as they do from a Westerner who has completely assimilated the Hindu tradition in thought and practice and who now serves as a luminous example not only to Western practitioners of Hinduism but even to native Indians themselves.

A heartfelt thank-you goes to Ken Wilber for his complimentary foreword. My gratitude extends to him for his many seminal works that have stimulated my own thinking over the years.

His great gift for synthesis has been both inspiration and encouragement.

For the past five years, I have received ample moral and spiritual nurturance from Lama Segyu Choepel, whose heart and mind are big enough to see the truth beyond historical categories and conceptual differences. My indebtedness to him is profound.

This new revised and expanded edition owes its existence to the keen vision of Lee Lozowick, who, through Hohm Press, allowed me to develop the best possible book despite the cost incurred in producing such a massive volume. I am also very grateful to Regina Sara Ryan, Nancy Lewis and the rest of the editorial team of Hohm Press for their enthusiasm and support, as well as Tori Bushert for her exemplary patience with the demanding typesetting of this work.

Finally, I wish to record my gratitude to, and love for, Trisha. She has been my traveling companion on the spiritual path since 1982. Her kindnesses throughout the day are numerous and her patience and steadfastness are exemplary. She did much to get the 1,100-page manuscript ready for the publisher. Whatever shortcomings remain are due to me.

# *Note on the Transliteration and Pronunciation of Sanskrit Words*

For the convenience of the lay reader, I have used a simplified transliteration of Sanskrit expressions throughout this volume, and each term is explained at its first occurrence. The expert will easily recognize the technical terms and can supply the correct diacritical marks. I also have translated most titles of the Sanskrit texts mentioned. Those left untranslated either defied translation or have meanings that are obvious from the context.

In the case of Sanskrit compounds, I have for the lay reader's convenience deviated from general practice by separating individual words by means of hyphens. Thus instead of writing *Yoga-tattvopani-shad* or *Yogacûdâmanyupanishad*, I have chosen to use the more intelligible transliteration *Yoga-Tattva-Upanishad* and *Yoga-Cûdâmani-Upanishad* respectively. In the latter name, the term *mani* ("jewel") is used in its grammatical stem form instead of its modified form *many*, required when the Sanskrit letter "i" is followed by a vowel. In the case of proper names, such as Vâcaspati Mishra, Vijnâna Bhikshu, or Abhinava Gupta, I have chosen to split the compounds in two, again for readability.

In translated passages, parentheses are used around Sanskrit equivalents, while square brackets are used for explanatory words or phrases that are not found in the Sanskrit original. To give an example: "Now [commences] the exposition (*anushâsana*) of Yoga" (*atha yoga-anushâsanam–Yoga-Sûtra* 1.1). Here the word "commences" is not found in the Sanskrit text but is certainly implied. The term *anushâsana* is the Sanskrit equivalent of "exposition" and hence is placed in parentheses rather than square brackets. Strictly speaking, the article "the" preceding "exposition" is also not found in the Sanskrit text but it is less interpretative than "commences" and therefore is not placed in brackets.

xxiii

| **Academic Transliteration** | **Simplified Transliteration** |
| (as used in most scholarly works on the subject) | (as used in the present work) |

**(I) Vowels**

| a, ā, i, ī, u, ū, ṛ, ṝ, ḷ | a, â, i, î, u, û, ri, li |
| e, ai, o, au | e, ai, o, au |

**(II) Consonants**

| Gutturals: k, kh, g, gh, ṅ | k, kh, g, gh, n |
| Palatals: c, ch, j, jh, ñ | c, ch, j, jh, n |
| Cerebrals: ṭ, ṭh, ḍ, ḍh, ṇ | t, th, d, dh, n |
| Dentals: t, th, d, dh, n | t, th, d, dh, n |
| Labials: p, ph, b, bh, m | p, ph, b, bh, m |
| Semivowels: y, r, l, v | y, r, l, v |
| Spirants: ś, ṣ, s, h | s, sh, sh, h |
| Visarga: ḥ | h |
| Anusvara: ṃ | m |

# Pronunciation

All the vowels are pronounced in an open manner, similar to the Italian vowel sounds; the vowels *ā, ī, ū* and the rare *ṝ* (not used in this book), as well as the diphthongs *e, ai, o,* and *au* are long; the not too common *ṛ*, as in *ṛgveda*, is pronounced similar to the *r* in "pretty," but in simplified transliteration it is rendered as *ri* and can be pronounced that way (hence the spelling *Rig-Veda* in this book); all aspirated consonants, like *kh, gh, ch, jh*, etc., are pronounced with a distinctly discernible aspiration, e.g., *kh* as in "ink-horn," *th* as in "hot-house," etc.; thus *hatha* in *hatha-yoga* is pronounced *hat-ha* and not as the *th* in *heath*; *ṅ* sounds like *ng* in "king," and *ñ*, as in the name Patañjali, sounds like the *n* in "punch"; the palatals *c* and *j* sound like *ch* in "church" and *j* in "join" respectively; thus *cakra* is pronounced "tshakra" rather than "shakra," as many Westerners mispronounce it; cerebrals are articulated with the tongue curled back against the roof of the mouth; *s* sounds like *s* in "sin"; *ṣ* like *sh* in "shun," and *ś* is pronounced midway between the two, whereas *v* is pronounced like *v* in "very"; the *anusvāra* (*ṃ*), as in the mantric seed syllables *oṃ* and *hūṃ*, is a nasalized sound that is pronounced somewhat like the *n* in the French word *bon*; the *visarga* (*ḥ*) is a hard *h* followed by a short echo of the preceding vowel, e.g., *yogaḥ* (in this book transliterated as *yogah*) is pronounced *yogaḥ[a]* and *bhaktiḥ* is pronounced *bhaktiḥ[i]*.

"Among thousands of men scarcely one strives for perfection."

—*Bhagavad-Gîtâ* 7.3

# *Introduction*

# THE IMPULSE TOWARD TRANSCENDENCE

## *I. REACHING BEYOND THE EGO-PERSONALITY*

The desire to transcend the human condition, to go beyond our ordinary consciousness and personality, is a deeply rooted impulse that is as old as self-aware humanity. We can see it at work in the magically charged cave paintings of Southern Europe and, earlier still, in the Stone Age burials of the Middle East. In both cases, the desire to connect with a larger reality is expressed. We also encounter that desire in the animistic beliefs and rites of archaic Shamanism, and we see its flowering in the religious traditions of the neolithic age—in the Indus-Sarasvatî civilization, and in Sumer, Egypt, and China.

But nowhere on Earth has the impulse toward transcendence found more consistent and creative expression than on the Indian peninsula. The civilization of India has spawned an almost overwhelming variety of spiritual beliefs, practices, and approaches. These are all targeted at a

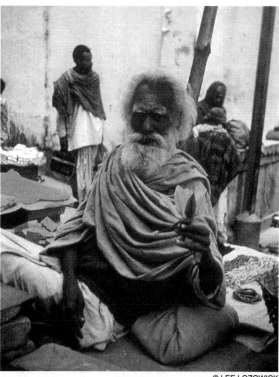

© LEE LOZOWICK

*Hindu sâdhu*

XXV

dimension of reality that far eclipses our individual human lives and the orderly cosmos of our human perception and imagination. That dimension has variously been called God, the Supreme Being, the Absolute, the (transcendental) Self, the Spirit, the Unconditional, and the Eternal.

Diverse thinkers, mystics, and sages—not only of India but from around the world—have given us a plethora of images or explanations of the ultimate Reality and its relation to the manifest universe. All, however, are in agreement that God, or the Self, transcends both language and the mind. With few exceptions, they are also unanimous in making three related claims, namely that the Ultimate:

1. is *single*—that is, an undivided Whole complete in itself, outside which nothing else exists;

2. is of a higher degree of *reality* than the world of multiplicity reflected to us through our senses; and

3. is our highest good (*nihshreyasa;* Latin: *summum bonum*), that is, the *most desirable* of all possible values.

Additionally, many mystics claim that the ultimate Reality is utterly blissful. This bliss is not merely the absence of pain or discomfort, nor is it a brain-dependent state. It is beyond pain and pleasure, which *are* states of the nervous system. This goes hand in hand with the insistence of mystics that their realization of the transcendental Identity is not an experience, as ordinarily understood. Such adepts simply *are* that Reality. Therefore, in connection with this highest accomplishment on the spiritual path I prefer to speak of God- or Self-*realization* as opposed to mystical *experience*. Other terms used are "enlightenment" and "liberation."

India's spirituality, which goes by the name of Yoga, is undoubtedly the most versatile in the world. In fact, it is hard to think of any metaphysical problem or solution that has not already been thought of by the sages and pundits of ancient or medieval India. The "sacred technicians" of India have experienced and analyzed the entire spectrum of psychospiritual possibilities—from paranormal states to the unitive consciousness of temporary God-realization to permanent enlightenment (known as *sahaja-samâdhi,* or "spontaneous ecstasy").

The methods and lifestyles developed by the Indian philosophical and spiritual geniuses over a period of at least five millennia all have one and the same purpose: to help us break through the habit patterns of our ordinary consciousness and to realize our identity (or at least union) with the perennial Reality. India's great traditions of psychospiritual growth understand themselves as paths of liberation. Their goal is to liberate us from our conventional conditioning and hence also free us from suffering, because suffering is a product of our unconscious conditioning. In other words, they are avenues to God-realization, or Self-realization, which is an utterly blissful condition.

God, in this sense, is not the Creator God of deistic religions like Judaism, Islam, and Christianity. Rather, God is the transcendental totality of existence, which in the nondualist schools of Hinduism is referred to as *brahman,* or "Absolute." That Absolute is regarded as the essential nature, the transcendental Self, underlying the human personality. Hence, when the unconscious conditioning by which we experience ourselves as independent, isolated egos is removed, we realize that at the core of our being we are all that same One. And this singular Reality is considered the ultimate destination of human evolution. As the modern *yogin*-philosopher Sri Aurobindo put it:

We speak of the evolution of Life in Matter, the evolution of Mind in Matter; but evolution is a word which merely states the phenomenon without explaining it. For there seems to be no reason why Life should evolve out of material elements or Mind out of living form, unless we accept the Vedantic[1] solution that Life is already involved in Matter and Mind in Life because in essence Matter is a form of veiled Life, Life a form of veiled Consciousness. And then there seems to be little objection to a farther step in the series and the admission that mental consciousness may itself be only a form and a veil of higher states which are beyond Mind. In that case, the unconquerable impulse of man towards God, Light, Bliss, Freedom, Immortality presents itself in its right place in the chain as simply the imperative impulse by which Nature is seeking to evolve beyond Mind, and appears to be as natural, true and just as the impulse towards Life which she has planted in certain forms of Matter or the impulse towards Mind which she has planted in certain forms of Life . . . Man himself may well be a thinking and living laboratory in whom and with whose conscious co-operation she wills to work out the superman, the god. Or shall we not say, rather, to manifest God?[2]

The idea that the impulse toward transcendence is a primary and omnipresent, if mostly hidden, force in our lives has been vocalized by a number of eminent transpersonal psychologists, notably Ken Wilber. He speaks of this force as the "Atman project":

Development is evolution; evolution is transcendence; . . . and transcendence has as its final goal Atman, or ultimate Unity Consciousness in only God. All drives are a subset of that Drive, all wants a subset of that Want, all pushes a subset of that Pull—and that whole movement is what we call the Atman project: the drive of God towards God, Buddha towards Buddha, Brahman towards Brahman, but carried out initially through the intermediary of the human psyche, with results that range from ecstatic to catastrophic.[3]

The impulse toward transcendence is thus intrinsic to human life. It manifests itself not only in humanity's religio-spiritual search but also in the aspirations of science, technology, philosophy, theology, and art. This may not always be obvious, especially in those areas that, like contemporary science, are anxious to deny any associations with metaphysical thought, and instead pay homage to the twin idols of skepticism and objectivity. Nevertheless, as perceptive critics of the scientific enterprise have pointed out, in its passionate quest for knowledge and meaning, science is merely usurping the supreme place that was once accorded to religion and theology.

Today, the metaphysical roots of science are rendered visible especially by quantum physics, which undermines the materialistic ideology that has been the creed of many, if not most, scientists for the past two hundred years. In fact, avant-garde physicists like David Bohm and Fred Alan Wolf have formulated broad quantum-physical interpretations of reality that converge in many respects with traditional Eastern ideas about the structure of the world: The universe is a single and ultimately unimaginable sea of energy ("quantum foam") in which differentiated forms—things—

appear and disappear, possibly for all eternity. Gary Zukav writes:

> Quantum mechanics, for example, shows us that we are not as separate from the rest of the world as we once thought. Particle physics shows us that the "rest of the world" does not sit idly "out there." It is a sparkling realm of continual creation, transformation, and annihilation. The ideas of the new physics, when wholly grasped, can produce extraordinary experiences. The study of relativity theory, for example, can produce the remarkable experience that space and time are only mental constructions![4]

It is clear from the work of such creative scientists as those mentioned above that science, like every other human endeavor, harbors within itself the impulse toward transcendence. Rightly, John Lilly called science a "simulation of God."[5] What Lilly meant by this phrase is this: We humans try to describe and understand ourselves and the world that apparently surrounds us. In doing so, we create models of reality and programs by which we can maneuver in our conceptualized, simulated worlds. All the while, however, we are pushed—or pulled—to reach beyond our models and programming, beyond our mind.

If we look upon science and technology as forms of the same impulse toward transcendence that has motivated India's sages to explore the inner universe of consciousness, we can see many things in a radically new perspective. We need not necessarily regard science and technology as *perversions* of the spiritual impulse, but rather as *unconscious expressions* of it. No moral judgment is implied here, and we can simply set about introducing a more comprehensive and self-critical awareness into the scientific and technological enterprise. In this way, we can hope to transform what has become a runaway obsession of the left brain into an authentic and legitimate pursuit in service of the whole human being and the whole of humankind.

In Rabindranath Tagore's delightful work *Gitanjali*, there is a line that sums up our modern attitude, which is one of dilemma: "Freedom is all I want, but to hope for it I feel ashamed."[6] We feel ashamed and awkward because we feel that the pursuit of spiritual freedom, or ecstasy, belongs to a bygone age, a lost worldview. But this is only a half-truth. While certain conceptions and approaches to spiritual freedom are clearly antiquated, freedom itself and its pursuit is as important and relevant today as it has ever been. The desire to be free is a timeless urge and concern. We want freedom, or abiding happiness, but we seldom acknowledge this deep-seated wish. It remains on the level of an unconscious program, secretly motivating us in all our undertakings—from scientific and technological ingenuity to artistic creativity, to religious fervor, to sports, to sexuality, to socializing, and, alas, also to drug and alcohol addiction. We seek to be fulfilled, made whole or happy by all these pursuits. Of course, we find that whatever happiness or freedom we gain is frustratingly ephemeral, and we take this as an incentive to continue our ritual quest for self-fulfillment by seeking further stimulation.

Today, however, we can take encouragement from the new vision embodied in quantum physics and transpersonal psychology, and boldly raise this urge to the level of a conscious need. In that event, the unrivaled wisdom of the liberation teachings of India and the Far East will assume a new significance for us, and the present-day encounter between East and West can fulfill itself.

## II. TECHNOLOGIES OF EAST AND WEST

Material technology has changed human life and the face of our home planet more than any other cultural force, but its gifts to humanity have not always proven to be benign. Since the 1970s the public attitude toward technology, and indirectly toward science, has become increasingly ambivalent. In the words of Colin Norman, an editor of *Science* magazine, technology is "the God that limps."[7] It is a God that thrives on reason but suffers from a dearth of wisdom. The consequences of a technology that is destitute of balanced judgment need no spelling out; they are everywhere apparent in our planet's ecology.

A different attitude prevails in the "counter"-technology of India, which is essentially a matter of wisdom and personal growth. It has evolved over millennia on the rich humus of hard-won inner experience, psychospiritual maturation, and nonordinary states of consciousness, and the supreme condition of Self-realization itself. The discoveries and accomplishments of the Indian spiritual virtuosos are at least as remarkable as electric motors, computers, space flight, organ transplants, or gene splicing. Their practical teachings can indeed be considered a type of technology that seeks to achieve control over the inner universe, the environment of consciousness.

Psychospiritual technology is applied knowledge and wisdom that is geared toward serving the larger evolutionary destiny of humankind by fostering the psychospiritual maturation of the individual. It avoids the danger of runaway technology by placing at its center a deep concern not merely for what is *possible* but for what is *necessary*. It is thus an ethical technology that views the human individual as a multidimensional and, above all, *self-transcending* being. It is, by definition, a technology that revolves around human wholeness. In the last analysis, psychospiritual technology is not even anthropocentric but theocentric, having Reality itself as its final reference point. If technology is, in the words of physicist Freeman J. Dyson, "a gift of God,"[8] then psychotechnology is a way to God. The former technology can, if used rightly, liberate us from economic want and social distress. The latter can, if applied wisely, free us from the psychic proclivity of living as self-encapsulated beings at odds with ourselves and the world.

Psychospiritual technology is more than applied knowledge and wisdom. It is also an instrument of knowledge, insofar as its use opens

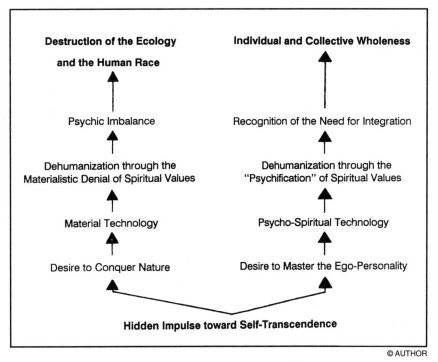

Destruction of the Ecology and the Human Race

↑

Psychic Imbalance

↑

Dehumanization through the Materialistic Denial of Spiritual Values

↑

Material Technology

↑

Desire to Conquer Nature

Individual and Collective Wholeness

↑

Recognition of the Need for Integration

↑

Dehumanization through the "Psychification" of Spiritual Values

↑

Psycho-Spiritual Technology

↑

Desire to Master the Ego-Personality

Hidden Impulse toward Self-Transcendence

© AUTHOR

*Two kinds of technology and their possibilities*

up new vistas of self-understanding, including the higher dimensions of the world that form the reaches of inner space.

The Indian liberation teachings—the great Yogas of Hinduism, Buddhism, Jainism, and Sikhism—clearly represent an invaluable resource for contemporary humankind. We have barely scratched the surface of what they have to offer us. It is obvious, however, that in order to find our way out of the tunnel of materialistic scientism, we require more than knowledge, information, statistics, mathematical formulas, sociopolitical programs, or technological solutions. We are in need of wisdom. And what better way is there to rejuvenate our hearts and restore the wholeness of our being than on the wisdom of the East, especially the great lucid insights and realizations of the Indian seers, sages, mystics, and holy folk?

## III. REALITY AND MODELS OF REALITY

It is important to remember that India's spiritual technology is also based on *models* of reality only. The ultimate realization, known as enlightenment or God-realization, is in the last analysis ineffable: It transcends thought and speech. Hence, the moment the God- or Self-realized adept opens his or her mouth to speak about the nature of that realization, he or she must resort to metaphors, images, and models—and models are intrinsically limited in their capacity to communicate that indivisible condition.

In some respects, the models proposed in the consciousness disciplines of the East have greater fidelity to reality. The reason for this is that the yogic models have been forged by a more comprehensive sensitivity. The *yogins* use means of cognition whose existence is barely

acknowledged by Western scientists, such as clairvoyance and higher states of identification with the object of contemplation, which are called *samādhi*. In other words, Yoga operates with a more sophisticated theory of knowledge (epistemology) and theory of being (ontology), recognizing levels or dimensions of existence that most scientists do not even suspect exist. At the same time, however, those traditional spiritual models are not as rigorously formulated as their modern Western counterparts. They are more intuitive-hortatory than analytical-descriptive. Manifestly, each approach has its distinct field of application and usefulness, and both can learn from each other.

The reigning paradigm of Western science is Newtonian materialistic dualism, which affirms that there are real subjects (observers) confronting real objects "out there." This view has of late been challenged by quantum physics, which suggests that there is no reality that is entirely divorced from the observer. India's psychospiritual technology has likewise been subject to a ruling paradigm, which can be described as *verticalism*: Reality is thought to be realizable by inverting attention and then manipulating the inwardly focused consciousness to ascend into ever-higher states in the inner hierarchy of experience until everything is transcended. Thus, the typical motto of Indian Yoga is "in, up, and out."

This vertical model of spirituality is founded in archaic mythical imagery, which pictures Reality in polar opposition to conditional existence: Heaven above, Earth below. As the contemporary adept Da Free John (Adi Da) has shown, this model is a conceptual representation of the human nervous system. As he put it succinctly:

> The key to mystical language and
> religious metaphor is not theology or

cosmology but anatomy. All the religious and cosmological language of mysticism is metaphorical. And the metaphors are symbols for anatomical features of the higher functional structures of the human individual.

Those who enter deeply into the mystical dimension of experience soon discover that the cosmic design they expected to find in their inward path of ascent to God is in fact simply the design of their own anatomical or psychophysical structures. Indeed, this is the secret divulged to initiates of mystical schools.[9]

More recently, Joe Nigro Sansonese explored the somatic origins of myth in his important but not widely enough known work *The Body of Myth*. He defined myths succinctly as "culture-laden descriptions of samâdhi."[10] As he explained, each meditation takes the *yogin* or *yoginî* deep into the body, putting him or her in touch with this or that organ. This somatic journey is then externalized in mythic utterances. There is much truth to Sansonese's statement, but it is not the entire truth. Some states of consciousness go beyond proprioception, beyond the body, and it is precisely these states that the Yoga adepts seek to cultivate. Enlightenment or liberation itself is definitely a body-transcending condition. Here the entire universe becomes a "body" for the liberated being.

The most severe limitation of the verticalist paradigm is that it involves an understanding of spiritual life as a progressive inward journey from unenlightenment to enlightenment. This gives rise to the misconception that Reality is to be found within, away from the world, and that, consequently, to renounce the world means to abandon it.

It is to the credit of India's adepts that this paradigm did not remain unchallenged. For instance, in Tantra, which straddles both Hinduism and Buddhism, a different understanding of spirituality is present. As will be elaborated in Chapter 17, Tantra is founded in the radical assumption that if Reality is anywhere, it must be everywhere and not merely inside the human psyche. The great dictum of Tantrism is that the transcendental Reality and the conditional world are coessential—*nirvâna* equals *samsâra*. In other words, transcendental ecstasy and sensory pleasure are not finally incompatible. Upon enlightenment, pleasure reveals itself to be ecstasy. In the unenlightened state, pleasure is simply a substitute for the ecstasy that is its abiding ground. This insight has led to a philosophy of integration between spiritual concerns and material existence, which is particularly relevant today.

## IV. YOGA AND THE MODERN WEST

In our struggle for self-understanding and psychospiritual growth, we can benefit immensely from a liberal exposure to India's spiritual legacy. We need not, of course, become converts to any path, or accept yogic ideas and practices without questioning. C. G. Jung's warning that we should not attempt to transplant Eastern teachings into the West rings true at a certain level; mere imitation definitely does more harm than good.[11] The reason is that if we adopt ideas and lifestyles without truly assimilating them emotionally and intellectually, we run the risk of living inauthentic lives. In other words, our role-playing gets the better of us. Yet, Jung was overly pessimistic about people's ability to sift the wheat from the chaff, or to learn and grow whole even from their negative experiences.

Moreover, his insistence that Westerners differ radically in their psychic constitution from Easterners is plainly incorrect. There are indeed psychological differences between the Eastern and the Western branches of the human family—differences that are readily apparent to seasoned travelers and those who cross the cultural divide between "East" and "West" or "North" and "South" in order to do business. These differences are, admittedly, even considerable when we compare ancient Easterners and contemporary Westerners, but they are not radical or unbridgeable.

Here we must remember that with the possible exception of a few isolated tribal peoples, humanity has shared the same structures of consciousness ever since what the German philosopher-psychiatrist Karl Jaspers has called the "axial age," the great transformative period around the middle of the first millennium B.C.E. During the axial age, the world of antiquity went beyond the mythopoeic form of thought characteristic of earlier ages. Pioneering spirits like Socrates, Gautama the Buddha, Mahâvîra, Lao Tzu, and Confucius embodied a new cognitive style, showing a clear preference for thinking in more strictly rational terms rather than in predominantly mythological metaphors.[12] Hence we can resonate with the ancient teachings of Yoga, even though they are the product of a personality type and culture that did not yet suffer from the excessive growth of left-brained thought, or abstract intellection, which is the hallmark of our own epoch.[13]

The dialogue between East and West is one of the most significant events of our century. If, as Jung confidently asserted, the West should create its own Yoga in the centuries to come, it will not be on the foundations of Christianity alone, which was his contention, but rather on the new global foundations laid as a result of that dialogue between the two halves of planetary humankind. At any rate, it is important to understand that this dialogue is necessarily a *personal* matter, which occurs on the stage of each individual's heart and mind. That means we—you and I—must initiate and nurture it. This undertaking is an enormous challenge and obligation, but also an unparalleled opportunity for assisting the "Atman project" as it moves us toward our own awakening in the larger Reality.

*Part One*

# FOUNDATIONS

"The face of Truth is covered with a golden disk.

Remove it, O Pûshan, so that I who adhere

to the [divine] law may behold It."

—*Îsha-Upanishad* (15)

"Yoga is collectedness (*samâdhâna*)."

—Shankara's *Yoga-Sûtra-Bhâshya-Vivarana* (1.1)

# Chapter 1

# BUILDING BLOCKS

## I. THE ESSENCE OF YOGA

Yoga is a spectacularly multifaceted phenomenon, and as such it is very difficult to define because there are exceptions to every conceivable rule. What all branches and schools of Yoga have in common, however, is that they are concerned with a state of being, or consciousness, that is truly extraordinary. One ancient Yoga scripture, Vyâsa's *Yoga-Bhâshya* (1.1), captures this essential orientation in the following equation: "Yoga is ecstasy."

In this Sanskrit text the word used for "ecstasy" is *samâdhi*. Vyâsa's definition has caused his commentators and modern scholars no end of difficulties, because how can *samâdhi*, as he

योगः समाधिः ॥

*Yogah samâdhih*

insists, be a stable quality of consciousness (*citta*) when consciousness is seen to change constantly? We can only understand this peculiar notion when we relate it to the idea that the transcendental Self, the *purusha*, is forever in the condition of ecstasy, and that this condition remains always the same regardless of the changing moods and qualities of the human mind.[1] Be that as it may, Vyâsa's use of the term *samâdhi* in this context clearly has overtones of the ecstatic state that is the hallmark of the yogic path.

The term *samâdhi* is of crucial importance in Yoga and will be encountered again and again in this volume. Therefore it seems appropriate to explain it more carefully at the outset. Sanskrit, the language in which most Yoga scriptures are written, is particularly suited for philosophical and psychological discourse. It allows the concise expression of nuances in thought that in English often require several terms. The word *samâdhi*, for instance, is composed of the prefixes *sam* (similar to the Latin *syn*) and *â*, followed by the verbal root *dhâ* ("to place, put") in its modified form *dhi*. The literal meaning of the term is thus "placing, putting together."

What is put together, or unified, is the conscious subject and its mental object or objects. *Samâdhi* is both the *technique* of unifying consciousness and the resulting *state* of ecstatic union with the object

3

of contemplation. Christian mystics speak of this condition as the "mystical union" (*unio mystica*). As the world-renowned historian of religion Mircea Eliade observed, *samâdhi* is really "enstasy" rather than "ecstasy."[2] The Greek-derived word "ecstasy" means to stand (*stasis*) outside (*ex*) the ordinary self, whereas *samâdhi* signifies one's standing (*stasis*) in (*en*) the Self, the transcendental Essence of the personality. But both interpretations are correct, because we can only abide in and as the Self (*âtman* or *purusha*) when we transcend the ego-self (*ahamkâra*). Yoga, then, is the technology of ecstasy, or self-transcendence. How this ecstatic condition is interpreted and what means are employed for its realization differ, as we will see, from school to school.

The Sanskrit term *yoga* is most frequently interpreted as the "union" of the individual self (*jîva-âtman*) with the supreme Self (*parama-âtman*).[3] This succinct definition is at home in Vedânta, the dominant branch of Hindu philosophy, which also greatly influenced the majority of Yoga schools. Vedânta proper originated with the ancient esoteric scriptures known as the *Upanishads*, which first taught the "inner ritual" of meditation upon, and absorption into, the unitary Ground of all existence.[4] However, nondualist metaphysics is foreshadowed in the archaic hymns of the *Vedas* (see the diagram in Chapter 5, mapping out the sacred literature of Hinduism).

According to Vedânta, the individual self is alienated from its transcendental Ground, the supreme Self (*parama-âtman*), or Absolute (*brahman*). How this alienation is understood differs from school to school. Some regard the finite self, together with the phenomenal universe, as merely illusory or a superimposition on Reality; others consider it to be quite real but caught in the "dis-ease" (*duhkha*) of estrangement from the ultimate Reality. Because of these differing

notions about the true existential status of the individual self, there are also a variety of interpretations of the nature of its re-union with the transcendental Reality. Some schools of thought even deny that there can be such a re-union, because we are never separated from the Ground, and our discovery of this fact is more a kind of remembering our eternal status as the ever-blissful transcendental Self.

While the notion of union makes some sense within the tradition of Vedânta, it is not representative of all forms of Yoga. It is valid in regard to the earlier (Pre-Classical) schools of Yoga and also applies to the later (Post-Classical) schools of Yoga, which subscribe to a type of Vedântic nondualist philosophy. However, the metaphor of union does not at all fit the system of Classical Yoga, as formulated by Patanjali in the second century C.E. In Patanjali's *Yoga-Sûtra*, the basic scripture of Classical Yoga, there is no mention of a union with the transcendental Reality as the ultimate target of the yogic endeavor. Given Patanjali's dualist metaphysics, which strictly separates the transcendental Self from Nature (*prakriti*) and its products, this would not even make any sense.

One of Patanjali's aphorisms (2.44) merely refers to a coming in "contact" (*samprayoga*) with one's "chosen deity" (*ishta-devatâ*) as a result of intense self-study. This chosen deity is not the Absolute itself but a specific deity of the Hindu pantheon, like Shiva, Vishnu, Krishna, or the Goddesses Durgâ and Kâlî.[5] The *yogin*, in other words, may have a vision of his adopted *representation* of the transcendental Reality, just as a devout Christian may have a visionary encounter with his or her favorite patron saint. No more is implied in that aphorism.

Patanjali (in *Yoga-Sûtra* 1.2) defines Yoga simply as "the restriction of the whirls of consciousness" (*citta-vritti-nirodha*). That is to say,

Yoga is the focusing of attention to whatever object is being contemplated to the exclusion of all others. Ultimately, attention must be focused on and merged with the transcendental Self. This is not merely a matter of preventing thoughts from arising. It is a whole-body focusing in which one's entire being is quieted. As is clear from a study of the *Yoga-Sûtra*, the terms *citta* and *vritti* are part of Patanjali's technical vocabulary and therefore have fairly precise meanings. We learn, for instance, that the process of restriction reaches far deeper than the verbal mind, because in the end one's entire conditional personality must be held in a state of balance and transparency. We can readily appreciate the difficulty of this undertaking when we try to stop the conveyor belt of our own thoughts even for thirty seconds.

Patanjali explains that when this psychomental stoppage has been accomplished, the transcendental Witness-Consciousness shines forth. This Witness-Consciousness, or "Seer" (*drashtri*), is the pure Awareness (*cit*) that abides eternally beyond the senses and the mind, uninterruptedly apperceiving all the contents of consciousness. All schools of Hinduism agree that the ultimate Reality is not a condition of stonelike stupor but of superconsciousness.

This assertion is not mere speculation but is based on the actual realization of thousands of Yoga adepts, and their great discovery is corroborated by the testimony of mystics in other parts of the world. The immutable Essence, or Spirit, is Being-Consciousness. All else is, according to Patanjali's philosophy, insentient matter that pertains to the realm of Nature, the counter-pole to the Witness-Consciousness.

Classical Yoga avows a strict dualism between Spirit (*purusha*) and matter (*prakriti*), which is reminiscent of Gnosticism, the esoteric movement that rivaled Christianity and flourished in the Mediterranean around the same time that Patanjali composed his aphorisms. On the strength of this uncompromising dualism, King Bhoja of the eleventh century C.E., who wrote a commentary on the *Yoga-Sûtra*, was able to propose that *yoga* really means *viyoga*, or "separation": The basic technique of Classical Yoga, argued King Bhoja, is the *yogin*'s "discernment" (*viveka*) between the transcendental Self and the "nonself" (*anâtman*), which is the entire psychophysical personality, belonging to the realm of matter.

Having understood this all-important distinction between Spirit and mind, the *yogin* next attempts to withdraw, step by step, from that which he has recognized as not constituting his essential nature, namely from the body-mind in its entirety. This gradual separation from the phenomenal reality is completed when the *yogin* has recovered his true Identity, the transcendental Witness-Consciousness.

Interestingly, this procedure is adopted even in the nondualist schools of Yoga and Vedânta, where it is known as "annulment" (*apavâda*). It is the method of *neti-neti* ("not thus, not thus"), as invented by the sages whose innovative teachings are recorded in the ancient *Upanishads*. This method consists in a progressive withdrawal of attention from the various aspects of psychophysical existence, thereby leading to a gradual dismantling of the false sense of identity with a particular body-mind-ego. This approach is illustrated strikingly in the *Nirvâna-Shatka*, a well-known didactic poem ascribed to Shankara, who lived in the late eighth century C.E. and is widely recognized as the greatest authority on nondualist Vedânta:

> *Om.* I am not reason, intuition (*buddhi*), egoity (*ahamkâra*), or memory. Neither am I hearing, tasting, smelling, or sight; neither ether nor earth; fire or air. I am

Shiva, in the form of Consciousness-Bliss. I am Shiva. (vs. 1)

This describes the *via negativa* of Hindu spirituality. At the same time it affords a good example for the alternative, and often complementary, method recommended by the authorities of Vedânta: Rather than "dismembering" himself or herself, the *yogin* or *yoginî* presumes fundamental identity with the transcendental Being-Consciousness. Thus, he or she affirms "I am the Absolute" (*aham brahma-asmi*, written *aham brahmâsmi*) or, as in the above-quoted text, "I am Shiva" (*shivo'ham*). Shiva is here not a personal deity but the Absolute itself. This affirmative procedure is extolled in the *Tejo-Bindu-Upanishad* (3.1–43), in which God Shiva himself at some length instructs the sage Kumâra in the highest spiritual realization. Here is an excerpt of Shiva's ecstatic confession-instruction:

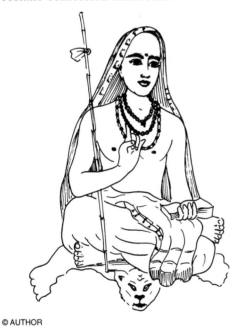

© AUTHOR

*Shankara, the great preceptor of Vedânta*

I am the supreme Absolute. I am supreme Bliss. I am of the form of unique Knowledge. I am unique and transcendental. (3.1)

I am of the form of unique tranquillity. I am made of unique Awareness (*cit*). I am of the form of unique eternity. I am everlasting. (3.2)

I am of the form of unique Being (*sattva*). Having relinquished the I, I am. I am of the essence of That which is devoid of all. I am made of the space of Awareness. (3.3)

I am of the form of the unique "Fourth" (*turya*).[6] I am the unique [Reality] transcending the Fourth. I am ever of the form of Consciousness (*caitanya*). (3.4)

We may assume that Shankara composed the above-cited *Nirvâna-Shatka* in the ecstatic or enlightened disposition. He was not in an "altered" state of consciousness, nor was he simply making a pious declaration. He was also not merely submerged in the condition of unqualified ecstasy (*nirvikalpa-samâdhi*), for in that condition no body-awareness and therefore no speech is possible. Rather, he spoke *as* that singular Being-Consciousness. His enlightenment was not a momentary flash but a permanent plateau realization. He spoke as an enlightened or liberated adept, a self-transcender of the highest order.

Liberation (*mukti*, *moksha*) is the continuous ecstatic enjoyment of the transcendental Self. It is the *raison d'être* of all authentic Yoga. The technology of Yoga fulfills itself in its own transcendence. For liberation is not a technique but a way of being in the world without being of it. After climbing to the topmost rung on the ladder of Yoga, accomplished *yogins* kick off the ladder and abandon themselves to the infinite play of Reality.

## II. WHAT'S IN A NAME? —THE TERM YOGA

Our world, the sages of ancient India tell us, is but a wonderfully bewitching collage of "name" (*nâma*) and "form" (*rûpa*). In this they anticipated contemporary philosophy. Reality is a continuum that we ourselves divide up into a multitude of discrete phenomena, and we do so by means

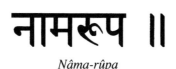

*Nâma-rûpa*

of language. Our naming of things in a way creates them. Our words reify, or "thingify," reality. For the most part, this is of practical usefulness when we want to find our way about in our rather complex universe. However, it can also be a handicap, because our words may set up barriers that block understanding and stifle love. Nevertheless, so long as we remember that words are not identical with the reality they are meant to denote, they can be useful.

Thus, it seems appropriate enough to start this section by inquiring into the meaning of the word *yoga*. In its technical sense, *yoga* refers to that enormous body of spiritual values, attitudes, precepts, and techniques that have been developed in India over at least five millennia and that may be regarded as the very foundation of the ancient Indian civilization. *Yoga* is thus the generic name for the various Indian paths of ecstatic self-transcendence, or the methodical transmutation of consciousness to the point of liberation from the spell of the ego-personality. It is the psychospiritual technology specific to the great civilization of India.

By way of extension, the word *yoga* has also been applied to those traditions that have been directly or indirectly inspired by the Indian sources, such as Tibetan Yoga (=Vajrayâna Buddhism), Japanese Yoga (=Zen), and Chinese Yoga (=Ch'an). It is, however, somewhat misleading to speak of Jewish Yoga, Christian Yoga, or Egyptian Yoga unless the word *yoga* is employed as a straightforward substitute for "mysticism" or "spirituality." Both Jewish and Christian mysticism have sprung up largely independent of the Indian spiritual adventure, and only in this century has there been some attempt to utilize yogic ideas and practices within the Judeo-Christian tradition.[7] While there are intriguing parallels between Vedic spirituality and Egyptian religious beliefs, practices, and symbols, Egypt's spirituality bears the unique stamp of the genius of the Nilotic peoples.

In a more restricted sense, the term *yoga* stands for the system of Classical Yoga, as propounded by Patanjali in the early post-Christian era. It is counted among the six great traditions or "viewpoints" (*darshana*) of Hinduism. The other five orthodox traditions are Nyâya, Vaisheshika, Sâmkhya, Mîmâmsâ, and Vedânta. The relationship of the Yoga tradition to these systems is treated in Chapter 3.

It should also be noted that, at times, the term *yoga* is used in the Sanskrit scriptures to denote the actual goal of Yoga. Thus, in the *Maitrâyanîya-Upanishad* (6.28), a pre-Christian scripture, the word refers to the realization of the transcendental Self. In the *Tattva-Vaishâradî* (3.9) and in the *Amrita-Nâda-Bindu-Upanishad* (23), the word *yoga* is employed to signify the temporary state of ecstasy (*samâdhi*). In some rare contexts, as in the *Mahâbhârata* (12.293.30), the word is also used to refer to the adherent of the Yoga tradition. This term, as well as the cognate *yauga*, can also refer to the follower of the Nyâya and Vaisheshika traditions.

The term *yoga* is frequently used in the Sanskrit literature. It is already employed in many ways in the ancient *Rig-Veda*, which is to the pious Hindu what the Old Testament is to the

Christian. The *Rig-Veda* is a collection of archaic hymns, some of which were probably composed in the fourth and fifth millennium B.C.E. The word *yoga* is etymologically derived from the verbal root *yuj*, meaning "to bind together" or "to yoke," and can have many connotations, such as "union," "conjunction of stars," "grammatical rule," "endeavor," "occupation," "team," "equipment," "means," "trick," "magic," "aggregate," "sum," and so on. It is related to English *yoke*, French *joug*, German *Joch*, Greek *zugos*, Latin *iugum*, Russion *igo*, Spanish *yugo*, and Swedish *ok*.

As mentioned before, in the *Yoga-Bhâshya* (1.1), the oldest extant commentary on the *Yoga-Sûtra*, Vyâsa proffers the equation "Yoga is ecstasy." He thus indicates precisely what kind of "yoking" is implied, namely the harnessing of attention, or consciousness, to the point of reaching the ecstatic condition (*samâdhi*) in which the mechanics of the mind are at least temporarily transcended.

In the ninth century C.E., Vâcaspati Mishra composed a scholarly subcommentary on Patanjali's aphorisms, which he entitled *Tattva-Vaishâradî*. At the beginning of his work, Vâcaspati Mishra notes that the term *yoga* should be derived from the root *yuja* (in the sense of "concentration") and not from *yuji* (in the sense of "conjunction"). Perhaps he felt called to make this comment because, as we have seen, in the nondualist tradition of Vedânta, the term *yoga* is frequently explained as the union (*samyoga*) between the individual self and the transcendental Self. This definition does not strictly apply to Classical Yoga, which is dualist, distinguishing as it does between the transcendental Self and multiform Nature.

In the *Mahâbhârata* (14.43.24), the distinguishing mark of Yoga is said to be "activity" (*pravritti*). This reminds one of the definition in the *Bhagavad-Gîtâ* (2.50), the Hindu equivalent of the New Testament, according to which "Yoga is skill in action" (*yogah karmasu kaushalam*). This means that *yogins* or *yoginîs* perform their allotted work and discharge their obligations without hankering for any reward. This attitude is further explained in Chapter 2.

The *Bhagavad-Gîtâ* (2.48) also defines *yoga* as "equanimity" (*samatva*). This Sanskrit word *samatva* means literally "sameness" or "evenness" and has all kinds of overtones, including "balance" and "harmony." Essentially it is the attitude of looking dispassionately at life and being unruffled by its ups and downs.

Thus *yoga* is a word that can apply to a multitude of things, and when reading the Yoga scriptures it is good to bear this flexibility in mind.

## III. DEGREES OF SELF-TRANSCENDENCE— THE PRACTITIONER (YOGIN OR YOGINÎ)

The word *yogin* (nominative: *yogî*) is derived from the same verbal root as *yoga*, namely *yuj*, and denotes the practitioner of Yoga, who may be a novice, an advanced student, or even a full-fledged, God- or Self-realized adept.

# योगिन् । योगी । योगिनी ॥
*Yogin, yogî, yoginî*

A female practitioner is called *yoginî*. This word is also applied to the female partner in the ritual sexuality (*maithunâ*) of certain schools of Tantra, as explained in Chapter 17. The term *yoginî* also can refer to a member of the group of sixty-four female deities particularly associated with Tantra, who are regarded as manifestations of the universal creative energy (*shakti*). The cult of the sixty-four *yoginîs* dates back to the sixth or seventh century C.E.[8]

The term *yogin* is generally loosely applied to all spiritual practitioners, but sometimes a distinction is made, for instance, between the *yogin* and the *samnyâsin* ("renouncer"), or between the *yogin* (as a practitioner of a particular discipline) and the *jnânin* ("gnostic"), who purports to follow no ideology or method, but lives on the basis of spontaneous spiritual understanding, or intuition. For example, in the *Mândûkya-Kârikâ* (3.39), an authoritative work on Advaita Vedânta, we find the following stanza:

> The intangible Yoga (*asparsha-yoga*) [of nondualism] is difficult to realize by all *yogins*. The *yogins* are afraid of it, perceiving fear in [that which is really of the essence of] fearlessness.

Here the author Gaudapâda, who was the teacher of Shankara's teacher, distinguishes between *yogins* and those who have realized the intangible, nondual Reality, that is, the *jnânins*. The distinction is somewhat idiosyncratic, because there are also realized adepts among the followers of Yoga. But then, what is in a name? Gaudapâda simply wanted to establish the superiority of the *jnânins*, free of self and fear, over those who anxiously strive to realize God, not understanding that their very search is their stumbling block. For as long as there is a goal, there is also a seeker—and thus an ego-personality trapped in the condition of unenlightenment.

The spiritual maturation of the *yogin* is thought to take place in a series of distinct phases, or stages (*bhûmi*). In the third chapter of the *Jîvan-Mukti-Viveka* ("Discernment about Living Liberation"), the medieval scholar and Yoga practitioner Vidyâranya speaks of two classes of *yogins*; those who have transcended the self and those who have not—a simple and effective classification. The famous Vedânta philosopher Vijnâna Bhikshu, who lived in the sixteenth century, distinguishes in his *Yoga-Sâra-Samgraha* ("Compendium on the Essence of Yoga") between the following grades:

1. *ârurukshu* — one who is desirous of spiritual life
2. *yunjana* — one who is actually practicing
3. *yoga-ârûdha* — one who has ascended in Yoga; also called *yukta* ("yoked one") or *sthita-prajnâ* ("one of steady wisdom")

The *Bhagavad-Gîtâ*, undoubtedly the most popular work on Yoga, characterizes the aspirant (*ârurukshu* and *yunjana*) and the adept (*yoga-ârûdha*) in these words:

> For the sage who desires to ascend in Yoga, action is stated to be the means. For him who has ascended in Yoga, serenity (*shama*) is said to be the means. (6.3)

> When he does not cling to the sense-objects or to deeds and has renounced all desires, then he is called "one who has ascended in Yoga." (6.4)

> When he has controlled the mind and is established in the Self (*âtman*) only, devoid of all desires, then he is said to be a "yoked one" (*yukta*). (6.18)

The perfected *yogin* of "steady wisdom"—*sthita-prajnâ*—is described in the *Bhagavad-Gîtâ* (2.56) as follows:

He whose mind is not affected in sorrow and is free from desire in pleasure and who is without attachment, fear, or anger—he is called a sage of "steady insight" *(sthita-dhi)*.

In the literature of the vast spiritual movement of medieval India known as Tantra, or Tantrism, a distinction is made between the "realizing aspirant" *(sâdhaka)* and the "perfected one" *(siddha)*—or adept—who has attained emancipation or perfection *(siddhi)*, the pinnacle of the "path to Realization" *(sâdhana)*. Other classifications are employed in the various *Purânas* (popular quasi-religious encyclopedias) and *Âgamas* and *Samhitâs* (sectarian works of encyclopedic scope), as well as in the scriptures of Hatha-Yoga, the "forceful" Yoga of physical discipline. Furthermore, the great religious traditions of Buddhism and Jainism, which have incorporated and contributed to the development of Yoga, also have their own scales of spiritual achievement and adeptship.

An interesting fourfold division is found in the *Yoga-Bhâshya* (3.51). The legendary author, Vyâsa, makes these distinctions:

1. *prathama-kalpika* — the neophyte in the first stage
2. *mâdhu-bhûmika* — "he who is in the delightful [lit. 'honey'] stage"
3. *prajnâ-jyotis* — "he who has attained the light *(jyotis)* of wisdom"
4. *atikrânta-bhâvanîya* — "he who is about to transcend [all of conditioned existence]"

Vyâsa (*Yoga-Bhâshya* 3.51) sheds some light on these four degrees of spiritual attainment. He explains:

The first is the practitioner *(abhyâsin)* for whom the light is just dawning. The second has "truth-bearing" transcendental wisdom. The third is he who has subjugated the elements and sense-organs and who has developed means for securing all that has been and is yet to be cultivated . . . While the fourth, who has passed beyond that which may be cultivated, has as his sole aim the resolution *(pratisarga)* of the mind [into the primordial matrix of Nature, whereupon the Self shines forth in its original purity.]

The last stage of transcendence leads directly to the realization of the supreme goal of Classical Yoga—"aloneness" *(kaivalya)*, in the sense of actualizing the transcendental Self *(purusha)*, the eternal Essence of the human being, beyond the ever-changing dimension of the cosmos. *Kaivalya* is the highest degree of spiritual perfection and the consummation of the life of the *yogin* who follows the path taught by Patanjali.

In his *Yoga-Bhâshya* (1.21), Vyâsa also explains that there are nine classes of *yogins*, according to the intensity *(samvega)* of their quest, which may be mediocre, average, or extremely vehement. Vâcaspati Mishra elucidates that the degree of intensity depends on previously acquired subliminal impressions *(vâsanâ)* as well as on invisible (karmic) influences, called *adrishta* (lit. "unseen"). In other words, our commitment to Yoga practice is not entirely a matter of conscious decision. The depth of our attraction to God, or the transcendental Self, is not subject to our will but is preconditioned by our karmic past: Our actions and intentions in past lives determine our future state of being (e.g., our genetic makeup, social circumstance, and therefore to some degree our psychosocial personality). This explains why sometimes our best intentions on the spiritual path are foiled, especially at the beginning of our practice, and why we must continue to persist in disciplining ourselves.

A frequent synonym of *yogin* is *yoga-vid*, meaning "knower of Yoga," which is widely employed particularly in the literature of Hatha-Yoga. The advanced practitioner is sometimes referred to as a *yukta*, or "yoked one," whereas the novice is occasionally known as a *yoga-yuj*, "one joined in Yoga." The perfected *yogin* is often styled "king of Yoga" (*yoga-râj*) and "lord of *yogins*" (*yoga-indra*, written *yogendra*).

The term "yogist" is of modern coinage and describes the Western enthusiast, who is primarily interested in the physical aspect of Yoga—especially the postures (*âsana*)—rather than in Yoga as a spiritual discipline of Self-realization.

## IV. GUIDING LIGHT —THE TEACHER

As Mircea Eliade pointed out in his well-known study on Yoga, "What characterizes Yoga is not only its practical side, but also its initiatory structure."[9] Yoga, like all forms of esotericism, presupposes the guidance of an initiate, a master who has firsthand experience of the phenomena and realizations of the yogic path. Ideally, he or she should have reached the ultimate spiritual destination of all yogic endeavor—enlightenment (*bodha, bodhi*), or liberation (*moksha*). Thus, contrary to the "pop" Yoga espoused by a large number of Westerners, authentic Yoga is never a do-it-yourself enterprise. "One does not learn Yoga by oneself," observed Eliade.[10] Rather, Yoga involves, as do all other traditional Indian

systems, an actual pupilage during which a master imparts his or her secrets to the worthy disciple or devotee. And those secrets are not exhausted by the kind of knowledge that can be expressed in words or printed in books.

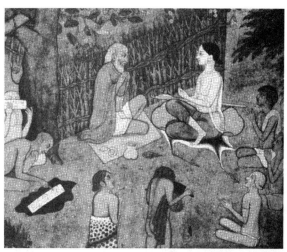

*A guru with a group of disciples*

Much of what the teacher (*guru*) imparts to the disciple falls under the category of spiritual transmission (*sancâra*). Such transmission, in which the *guru* literally empowers the student through a transference of "energy" or "consciousness" (corresponding to the "Holy Spirit" of Christian baptism), is the fulcrum of the initiatory process of Yoga. By means of it, the practitioner is blessed in his or her struggle for transcendental realization. As a result, the initiated *yogin* or *yoginî* experiences the necessary conversion or "turn-about" (*parâvritti*) that is crucial to the spiritual process: He or she begins to find the Real, or the Self beyond the ego, more attractive than the numerous possibilities of worldly experience. The basis for that attraction is a tacit intuition of the Self, which grows stronger in the course of practice.

The initiatory nature of Yoga is expressed in a variety of symbols, the most striking being that of birth. In the *Atharva-Veda* ("Atharvan's Knowledge"), one of the four Vedic *Samhitâs*, we find this verse:

Initiation takes place in that the teacher carries the pupil in himself as it were, as the mother [bears] the embryo in her body. After the three days of the [initiation] ceremony, the disciple is born. (11.5.3)

A similar archaic "gynecological" metaphor is used, more than four millennia later, in the Buddhist *Hevajra-Tantra* (2.4.61–62):

The school is said to be the body. The monastery is called the womb. Through freedom from attachment, one is in the womb. The yellow robe is the membrane [around the embryo]. And the preceptor is one's mother. The salutation is the head-first position (*mastaka-anjali*). Discipleship is one's worldly experience. And recitation of *mantras* is the [notion of] "I."

Through the teacher's grace (*prasâda* or *kripâ*), the deserving disciple is initiated into the great "alternative" of existence—the reality of the Spirit, or transcendental Being-Consciousness-Bliss. Therefore, it is important that the teacher should be a fully realized master, or adept (*siddha*). Only then is the practitioner assured of complete passage across the "ocean of phenomenal existence" (*samsâra-sâgara*). For, as the *Shiva-Purâna* (7.2.15.38) observes, if a preceptor is merely nominal, so is the "liberation" he or she will bestow on the disciple.

The initiatory teacher/disciple system dates back to the early Vedic period (4500–2500 B.C.E.), where a young boy would spend his youth and adolescence in the home of a teacher of the sacred scriptures, the repository of the epoch's deepest wisdom and finest knowledge. Study of the *Vedas* was the sacred duty of all "twice-born" (*dvija*) members of society—i.e., the *brâhmana* or priestly estate, the *kshatriya* or military estate, and the *vaishya* or agricultural estate. The *shûdra* or servile estate was excluded from this time-honored tradition, though exceptions were occasionally made for unusual individuals. The Vedic lore was transmitted to him by word of mouth and had to be carefully memorized. It was the teacher's obligation to guide the student in his study and understanding of the wisdom of the *Vedas* and to look after his welfare.

The student, in return for the teacher's guidance and paternal supervision, was expected to honor and obey the *guru* as he would his own father and to invest considerable energy in diligent study (*svâdhyâya*) and service (*sevâ*) to the teacher's household. In the *Shiva-Samhitâ* (3.13), a late medieval Hatha-Yoga text, this ideal is expressed as follows:

There is no doubt that the *guru* is father; the *guru* is mother; the *guru* is God. Therefore he should be served by all in deed, speech, and thought.

Much of the contact between teacher and pupil was strictly formalized. For the disciple it included the daily rituals of begging for "alms" (*bhiksha*)[11] and the ceremonial offering to the *guru* of fuel sticks for the sacred fire. The student was expected to stay with his teacher until the completion of his course of study. Those who, like so many Western acolytes, wandered from teacher to teacher were derogatorily called "crows at a sacred place" (*tîrtha-kâka*).[12]

Apart from the actual study of the sacred tradition, the disciple's foremost obligation was to live a chaste life (*brahmacarya*)—hence the general appellation of *brahmacârin* for the student. The term means literally "one whose conduct is brahmic," that is, one who behaves in consonance with the rules laid down for a priest (*brahma* = *brâhmana*), or whose behavior imitates the condition of the Absolute (*brahman*), which is asexual. Chastity was considered imperative for a moral life and for the cultivation of the life force (*prâna*) in the body-mind, aiding concentration, memory, and health. The institutionalized relationship between teacher and disciple is known as the *guru-kula* or "teacher's household" system. Its rationale is given in the ancient *Taittirîya-Upanishad* (3.1.1), one of the earliest scriptures of its genre, thus:

> The teacher is the first letter [of the alphabet]. The student is the last letter. Knowledge is the meeting-place. Instruction is the link.

Fortunate was the student who found a teacher who not only was well versed in the scriptures but also had realized their esoteric import. Out of this emerged the equation of the *guru* with scriptural authority. Both scripture and teacher came to be regarded as having revelatory and liberating power. The teacher is traditionally regarded as an embodiment of the living Truth that is indicated in the sacred texts. The ancient Vedic system of *guru-kula* continued to be the traditional model of education in India.

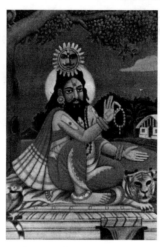

*Yâjnavalkya, a modern representation*

The *Upanishads*, the esoteric works on nondualist Vedânta, have preserved examples of some of the more profound teacher/disciple relationships, in which the excellence of wisdom and God-realization, not merely intellectual knowledge, was pursued. The enlightened master, having fulfilled the scriptural revelation, is uniquely equipped to prepare others for the same realization. One of the most touching relationships was that between the mighty sage Yâjnavalkya (c. 1500 B.C.E.) and his wife Maitreyî. His teachings are remembered in the *Brihad-Âranyaka-Upanishad* (e.g., 2.4.1ff.; 4.5.1ff.). He was married to two women, but whereas Kâtyâyanî "only possessed womanly knowledge" (4.5.1), Maitreyî was thirsting for spiritual knowledge, desiring to know the path to immortality. Before renouncing the world, Yâjnavalkya made sure to instruct Maitreyî in the secrets of Upanishadic Yoga. He told her:

> Verily, not for the husband's sake is a husband dear, but a husband is dear for the sake of the Self (*âtman*). Verily, not for the wife's sake is a wife dear, but a wife is dear for the sake of the Self. Verily, not for the sons' sake are sons dear, but the sons are dear for the sake of the Self. Verily, not for the sake of wealth is wealth dear, but wealth is dear for the sake of the Self . . . Verily, O Maitreyî, it is the Self that should be seen, heard, considered, and contemplated. Verily, by seeing, hearing, considering, and knowing the Self, all this is known. (2.4.5)

Yâjnavalkya instructed Maitreyî at length and she finally admitted to being bewildered by his discourse, whereupon the sage replied:

> For sure, I am not saying anything bewildering. This is sufficient for knowledge. (2.4.13)

Very much later, the *Shiva-Samhitâ* (3.11) states:

[Only] knowledge imparted by way of the teacher's mouth is productive; otherwise it is fruitless, weak, and causes much affliction.

# गुरु । आचार्य । उपाध्याय ॥

*Guru, âcârya, upâdhyâa*

Hinduism distinguishes between different types of teachers, who ideally belong to the *brâhmana* estate: the *guru* ("weighty one"), the *âcârya* ("preceptor," who performs the ceremony of investiture, or *upanâyana*, with the sacred thread worn by all "twice-born," and who also conveys to the student the appropriate rules of conduct, or *âcâra*), the *upâdhyâya* ("tutor," who teaches a portion of the sacred lore for a fee), the *adhvanka* ("mentor," from *adhvan* meaning "road" or "travel"), the *prâdhyâpaka* ("seasoned instructor," who may instruct other teachers), the *prâcârya* ("senior preceptor"), the *râja-guru* ("royal teacher"), and the *loka-guru* ("world teacher")—all of whom embody a particular teaching role and spiritual status. There is even a generic term for the various kinds of teacher, namely *pravaktri*, or "communicator."

The God-realized teacher grants "divine knowledge" (*divya-jnâna*), as the *Yoga-Shikhâ-Upanishad* (5.53) puts it. It is knowledge that springs from enlightenment and attracts to enlightenment. The *Advaya-Târaka-Upanishad* (16) gives an esoteric explanation of the word *guru*, deriving it from the syllable *gu* (indicating "darkness") and *ru* (indicating "dispeller"). Thus the *guru* is one who dispels the disciple's spiritual benightedness.

Of all the teachers, God-realized adepts are even today given a special place in Hindu society, for they alone are capable of initiating the spiritual seeker into the supreme "knowledge of the Absolute" (*brahma-vidyâ*). They alone are

*sad-gurus*—"teachers of the Real" or "true teachers." Here, the Sanskrit word *sat* (changed to *sad* for euphonic reasons) connotes both "real" and "true." These teachers are celebrated as potent agents of grace. As the *Shiva-Samhitâ* (3.14) states: "By the teacher's grace, everything auspicious for oneself is obtained." And the *Hatha-Yoga-Pradîpikâ* (4.9) affirms that without a true teacher's compassion (*karunâ*), the state of transcendental spontaneity (*sahaja*) is difficult to attain.

Because of his or her spiritual realization, the *guru* is considered to be an embodiment (*vigraha*) of the Divine itself. "The *guru* alone is Hari [=Vishnu] incarnate," announces the *Brahma-Vidyâ-Upanishad* (31). The teacher is not *a* specific deity but the all-encompassing Divine, here named Hari. This "deification" of the God-realized master must not be misunderstood. He or she is not God in any exclusive sense, but rather is coessential with the transcendental Reality. That is to say, he or she has abrogated the ordinary person's misidentification with a particular body-mind and abides purely as the transcendental Identity of all beings and things. There is no trace of egoity in the truly enlightened being, for the ego has been replaced by the Self. The body-mind and personality continue for their allotted time, but the enlightened being is no longer implicated by his or her automaticities. The unenlightened individual, by contrast, believes himself or herself to be a particular "entity," or individuated consciousness, somehow lodged within a body and associated with, possibly even driven by, a particular personality complex. This fatal illusion is gracefully shattered at the moment of enlightenment.

In the *Kula-Arnava-Tantra*, God Shiva, addressing his divine spouse Devî, has this to say about realized masters as opposed to ordinary teachers:

There are many *gurus,* like lamps in house after house, but hard to find, O Devî, is the *guru* who lights up all like the sun. (13.104)

There are many *gurus* who are proficient in the *Vedas* [revealed sacred knowledge] and the *Shâstras* [textbooks], but hard to find, O Devî, is the *guru* who has attained to the supreme Truth. (13. 105)

There are many *gurus* on Earth who give what is other than the Self, but hard to find in all the worlds, O Devî, is the *guru* who reveals the Self. (13.106)

Many are the *gurus* who rob the disciple of his wealth, but rare is the *guru* who removes the afflictions of the disciple. (13.108)

He is a [true] *guru* by whose very contact there flows the supreme Bliss (*ânanda*). The intelligent man should choose such a one as his *guru* and none other. (13.110)

In the same chapter, the *Kula-Arnava-Tantra* (13.126f.) also speaks of six types of *gurus*, who are classified according to their function:

1. *preraka* — the "impeller," who stimulates interest in the would-be devotee, leading to his or her initiation (also called *codaka* in the *Brahma-Vidyâ-Upanishad* 51)

2. *sûcaka* — the "indicator," who points out the form of spiritual discipline (*sâdhana*) for which the initiate is qualified

3. *vâcaka* — the "explainer," who expounds the spiritual process and its objective

4. *darshaka* — the "revealer," who shows the details of the process

5. *shikshaka* — the "teacher," who instructs in the actual spiritual discipline

6. *bodhaka* — the "illuminator," who, as the texts has it, "lights up in the disciple the lamp of mental and spiritual knowledge."

There are many other functional types of *gurus*, and in his translation of the *Kula-Arnava-Tantra*, the Yoga scholar M. P. Pandit mentions no fewer than twelve.[13] But it is always the God-realized master who is extolled in the Yoga scriptures above all others.

## SOURCE READING 1

# *Dakshinamûrti-Stotra*

The *Dakshinamûrti-Stotra* ("Hymn to Dakshinamûrti") is probably an authentic work of Shankara, the great exponent of Advaita Vedânta. The hymn, which reflects the devotional side of this intellectual giant, is addressed to Dakshinamûrti in the form of Shankara's teacher. Dakshinamûrti ("South-Facing") is another name for God Shiva. This curious name is traditionally explained by the legend that Shiva always sat facing the south while teaching the masters of yore (who were of course facing north). As art historian Stella Kramrisch informs us, in the South Indian temples of the worshippers of both Vishnu and Shiva the iconographic image of Dakshinamûrti is enshrined in a niche on the south wall of the main sanctuary.[14]

Interestingly, the word *dakshina* has the double meaning of "south" and "gift." Thus, the name also plays on Dakshinamûrti's gift of esoteric knowledge or ultimate gnosis. This poetic prayer epitomizes the traditional ideal of recognizing (and worshiping) in one's God-realized master the Divine itself.

He who sees the universe, which appears as if external through [the agency of] illusion (*mâyâ*), as contained within himself, just as in a dream, and who witnesses His own immutable Self in the moment of Awakening—to Him, the blessed Dakshinamûrti, in the form of [my] blessed teacher, this obeisance [is made]. (1)

He who, like a great *yogin* or like a magician, conjures by His own will this universe, which is [in reality] formless like the germ of a seed but is subsequently fashioned through illusion, differentiated through the diversity of space and time—to Him, the blessed Dakshinamûrti, in the form of [my] blessed teacher, this obeisance [is made]. (2)

He whose manifestation, which is of the essence of Reality (*sat*), appears as the object of notions of unreality (*asat*), who directly illumines those who have resorted to Vedic maxims such as "You are That" (*tat tvam asi*), and through direct perception

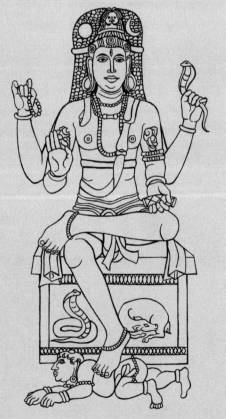

© JAMES RHEA

*Dakshinamûrti*

of whom there is no return to the ocean of [conditioned] existence—to Him, the blessed Dakshinamûrti, in the form of [my] blessed teacher, this obeisance [is made]. (3)

He whose wisdom vibrates outside, [mediated] through the eyes and the other sense gates, like the bright light of a big lamp laced in the belly of an urn with different holes—I know Him after whose radiance shines this entire universe. To Him, the blessed Dakshinamûrti, in the form of [my] blessed teacher, this obeisance [is made]. (4)

He who destroys the great delusion (*vyâmoha*), fashioned by the play of the power of illusion (*mâyâ*) of those who consider themselves the body, or the life force (*prâna*), or the senses, or the fickle mind, or the void, or who through error unhesitatingly declare themselves to be a woman, [a man], a child, blind, or stupid—to Him, the blessed Dakshinamûrti, in the form of [my] blessed teacher, this obeisance [is made]. (5)

The Male (*pumâms*)[15] who, upon the withdrawal of the senses which resembles an eclipse of the sun or the moon, [enters] deep sleep and thus becomes pure Being, but, who owing to the covering of illusion, upon waking [merely] remembers to have slept—to Him, the blessed Dakshinamûrti, in the form of [my] blessed teacher, this obeisance [is made]. (6)

He who through auspicious gestures (*mudrâ*) reveals to His worshipers His own Self, which manifests inwardly as the "I," past and present, in all states [of consciousness] such as childhood or wakefulness—to Him, the blessed Dakshinamûrti, in the form of [my] blessed teacher, this obeisance [is made]. (7)

The Man (*purusha*)[16] who, whirled about by illusion, sees in the dream or the waking [state] the universe differentiated by the relationship into owner and owned, or teacher and pupil, or father and son, etc.—to Him, the blessed Dakshinamûrti, in the form of [my] blessed teacher, this obeisance [is made]. (8)

He whose eightfold form—earth, water, fire, air, ether, sun, moon, and man—manifests as this [universe], consisting of mobile and immobile [things], and other than which supreme Lord there exists naught for those who ponder [the matter deeply]—to Him, the blessed Dakshinamûrti, in the form of [my] blessed teacher, this obeisance [is made]. (9)

Because the "All-Selfhood" (*sarva-âtmatva*)[17] has been made evident in this hymn, therefore by hearing it, by reflecting and contemplating on its meaning, and by reciting it, one will realize the "sovereignty" (*îshvaratva*) associated with the great splendor of All-Selfhood, as well as unobstructed "lordship" (*aishvarya*) appearing eightfold [in the form of the great magical powers].[18] (10)

I bow to God Dakshinamûrti, the Lord, the teacher of the three worlds, who skillfully (*daksha*)[19] removes the suffering of birth and death and who, seated on the ground near the fig tree, swiftly bestows wisdom on a whole host of sages. (11)

Wonder! The disciples under the fig tree are old. The teacher is young. The teacher's silence is the instruction that destroyed the disciples' doubts. (12)

*Om.* Obeisance to the [hidden] purport of the *pranava*.[20] Obeisance to Dakshinamûrti, tranquil and undefiled, the sole embodiment of pure wisdom. (13)

Obeisance to Dakshinamûrti, the treasure house of all learning, the teacher of all the worlds, and the physician to those who are afflicted with [conditioned] existence. (14)

I worship the young Dakshinamûrti, Lord of preceptors, who imparts the truth of the Absolute through the instruction of silence, who is surrounded by a host of aged seers dedicated to [the realization of] the Absolute, whose hand is in the gesture of [bestowing] Consciousness,[21] who is of the form of Bliss, delighting in the Self, of joyous speech. (15)

## V. LEARNING BEYOND THE SELF —THE DISCIPLE

Traditionally, when a person—generally a male—had resolved to seriously take up spiritual life, he approached a master of Yoga "with fuel in hand," hoping that he would be accepted. The fuel sticks that he ceremoniously presented to his prospective teacher were an outward sign of his inner readiness to submit himself to the *guru*, to be consumed by the fire of spiritual practice. Yoga, or the spiritual process, has always been compared to a purificatory conflagration that consumes the ego-personality until the transcendental Self-Identity alone is left. Therefore, only foolhardy individuals would approach an adept unprepared—and were apt to be rejected, though perhaps not without having been taught some useful lessons about self-transcendence, love, obedience, nonattachment, and humility.

Once an aspirant presented himself to a master of Yoga, he was carefully scrutinized by the teacher for signs of emotional and spiritual maturity. The esoteric lore must never be passed on to an unqualified individual, lest it cause him or her harm or be abused by him or her to the detriment of others. Spiritual pupilage is always a demanding affair and, ultimately, a matter of life and death. As we can read in the *Mahâbhârata* (12.300.50):

> This great path of the wise priests is arduous. No one can tread it easily, O bull of Bharata! It is like a terrible jungle creeping with large snakes, filled with pits, devoid of water, full of thorns, and quite inaccessible.

What is at stake in the spiritual process is the conditional ego-personality itself, which fiercely struggles to survive but which must be surrendered in order for the transcendental Self to shine forth. Spiritual life demands a rebirth that is as dramatic as the transformation of a caterpillar into a butterfly. This transmutation does not happen without great inner sacrifices, and not all aspirants are able to complete the process. Some even become lost en route, succumbing to insanity or terminal disease.

Because the spiritual path is like a razor's edge, a responsible teacher will not accept an unprepared individual for discipleship. He or she will, rather, apply certain traditional and also common-sense criteria of competence (*adhikâra*). Nonetheless, a teacher may decide to take on an ill-prepared aspirant if he or she detects a certain spiritual potential. Such a student must not expect to receive more than exoteric teachings until he or she has been purified of personal weaknesses through much service and study.

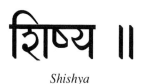

*Shishya*

Significantly, the Hindi word for "student" is *chela*, which also means "servant." The Sanskrit equivalent is *shishya*, which stems from the verbal root *shâs*, meaning "to instruct" but also "to chastise." The same root can be found in the words *shâsa* ("command"), *shâsaka* ("instructor"), *shâsana*

("instructing" or "chastising"), *shâstra* ("precept" or "textbook), *shâstrin* ("scholar"), *shishtatâ* ("learning"), and *shishyatâ* ("pupilage"). The double meaning of "instruction" and "chastisement" deserves comment. Modern education emphasizes reward rather than punishment as a goad to learning, which has been shown to lead to problems of its own. Children today expect to be rewarded and have little respect for authority. Ancient educators, however, were not immune to resorting to reprimand and, if necessary, physical chastisement, to correct a student's behavior. Authoritarianism of course always has the potential of abuse, but nonauthoritarian, democratized education also lends itself to abuse—on the part of students. While a punitive education system falls short of the nonviolent ethics promoted by Yoga, authority and respect for authority clearly have their place in teaching.

The *Shiva-Samhitâ* (5.17ff.) distinguishes four types of aspirants, classifying them according to the intensity of their commitment. The weak (*mridu*) practitioner is characterized as unenthusiastic, foolish, fickle, timid, ill, dependent, rude, ill-mannered, and unenergetic. This practitioner is fit only for Mantra-Yoga, consisting in the meditative repetition of a sacred syllable or phrase given and empowered by the teacher.

The mediocre (*madhya*) practitioner, who is said to be capable of practicing Laya-Yoga—the path of meditative absorption and subtle energy work—is said to be endowed with even-mindedness, patience, a desire for virtue, kind speech, and the tendency to take the middle path in all undertakings. The exceptional (*adhimâtra*) practitioner, who qualifies for the practice of Hatha-Yoga, is expected to demonstrate the following qualities: firm understanding, an aptitude for meditative absorption (*laya*), self-reliance, liberal-mindedness, bravery, vigor, faithfulness, the willingness to worship the teacher's lotus feet (both literally and figuratively), and delight in the practice of Yoga.

For the extraordinary (*adhimâtratama*) practitioner, who may practice all forms of Yoga, the *Shiva-Samhitâ* lists no fewer than thirty-one qualities: great energy, enthusiasm, charm, heroism, scriptural knowledge, the inclination to practice, freedom from delusion, orderliness, prime of youth, moderate eating habits, control over the senses, fearlessness, purity, skillfulness, liberality, the ability to be a refuge for all people, capability, stability, thoughtfulness, the willingness to do whatever is desired (by the teacher), patience, good manners, observance of the law (*dharma*), the ability to keep the struggle of practice to himself or herself, kind speech, faith in the scriptures, the willingness to venerate God and the *guru* (as the embodiment of the Divine), knowledge of the vows pertaining to his or her level of practice and, lastly, the practice of all types of Yoga.

After a person has been accepted by a teacher, he or she can expect to be tested again and again. There are even traditional prescriptions for such testing, although the teacher who is an advanced or even Self-realized adept is unlikely to need any guidelines for ascertaining a disciple's seriousness about spiritual life. At this point, a student may begin to live with or close to the teacher, serving and attending him or her constantly. Such a student is known as an *antevâsin*, that is, "one who abides near." In the company of a God-realized master, the practitioner is continuously exposed to the realizer's spiritualized body-mind, and by way of "contagion" his or her own physical and psychic being is gradually transformed. This can be understood in modern terms as a form of rhythm entrainment, where the *guru's* faster vibratory state gradually speeds up the disciple's vibration.

For this spontaneous process to be truly effective, the disciple must consciously cooperate with the *guru*, and this is accomplished by making the teacher the focus of attention. This is the great principle of *sat-sanga*. The word means literally "company of the True" or "relationship to the Real." *Sat-sanga* is the supreme means of liberation in *guru-yoga*. And since the *guru* has from ancient times been deemed essential to yogic practice, *sat-sanga* is at the core of all schools of Yoga. However, it would be inaccurate to say that all Yoga is *guru-yoga*, for not every school makes focusing on the teacher a central practice, though all call for proper respect for the teacher.

In practice, the aspirant must move from the stage of the student to that of the disciple and, in schools where *guru-yoga* is the norm, to that of the "devotee" (*bhakta*). At the student level, the aspirant still has an exoteric understanding of, and relationship to, the teacher. The student is inspired by listening to the teacher's discourses but has not yet seriously taken up spiritual life and wavers in his or her commitment to the yogic process; worldly life still exerts a strong pull. The disciple, by contrast, is more sensitive to the esoteric relationship between the *guru* and himself or herself, understanding that there is a continuous psychospiritual link to the teacher that must be honored and cultivated. The devotee, finally, *experiences* the *guru* as a spiritual reality rather than as a human personality and is therefore naturally inclined to assume a devotional attitude that acts as a powerful conduit between the *guru* and himself or herself. This is the essence of *guru-yoga*. Needless to say, not all schools calling for devotion to the teacher describe the mature disciple as a "devotee."

To enter into conscious relationship to the Real, in the form of the teacher, means more than to pay the *guru* attention in the conventional sense. What the scriptures call for is devotion to, or love for, the adept teacher. Thus, in the *Mandala-Brâhmana-Upanishad* (1.1.4), perhaps composed in the fourteenth century C.E., *guru-bhakti* or "devotion to the teacher" is listed as one of the constituents of the ninefold moral code (*niyama*) for *yogins*. And the *Yoga-Shikhâ-Upanishad* (5.53), which is of a similar age, declares:

> There is no one greater in the three worlds than the *guru*. It is he who grants "divine knowledge" (*divya-jnâna*) and should [therefore] be worshiped with supreme devotion.

Similarly, the *Tejo-Bindu-Upanishad* (6.109) regards devotion to the teacher as indispensable for the serious aspirant. And according to the *Brahma-Vidyâ-Upanishad* (30), devotion to the teacher should always be practiced, because the teacher is none other than the Divine. The equivalence of *guru* worship and worship of the Divine is emphasized in the *Shiva-Purâna* (1.18.95) and in numerous other Sanskrit texts—far too many to list here.

However, there are at least two scriptures exclusively dedicated to the theme of devotion to the spiritual master. The first stems from the tradition of Hinduism. This is the *Guru-Gîtâ*, which is widely circulated in India as an independent composition, but which belongs to the latter part of the vast *Skanda-Purâna*.[22] It consists of 352 stanzas that are delivered in the form of a didactic dialogue between God Shiva and his divine spouse Umâ (or Pârvatî). The second scripture is a favorite Buddhist text—namely Ashvaghosha's *Guru-Panca-Shikhâ*, which is extant only in a Tibetan

translation.[23] Ashvaghosha (c. 80 C.E.) was a celebrated poet and an eminent teacher of Mahâyâna Buddhism, who achieved fame through his artistic biography of Gautama the Buddha, called the *Buddha-Carita* ("Buddha's Conduct"), and a philosophical exposition entitled *Shraddhâ-Utpâda-Shâstra* ("Scripture on the Awakening of Faith"), of which the Sanskrit original appears to have been lost but which continues to be studied in Chinese.[24]

During the *antevâsin* period the devotee discovers the potency of the mutual love between himself or herself and the adept teacher, creating profound trust in the *guru* and faith in the spiritual process itself. The disciple's service (*sevâ, sevanâ*) becomes more demanding as his or her ability to take responsibility increases. According to the *Kula-Arnava-Tantra* (12.64) such service—the text actually uses the word *shûshrushâ*, meaning "obedience"—is fourfold: service through one's bodily self (*âtman*), through material means (*artha*), through respect (*mana*), and through a good disposition (*sadbhâva*). It is made clear that service is for the benefit of the devotee rather than the teacher.

In the meantime, the *guru* constantly monitors the disciple's progress, waiting for the right moment at which initiation (*dîkshâ*) can take place. As soon as the disciple is ready, the *guru* will begin to impart to him or her the secrets of the esoteric lineage. Only a fully qualified disciple, called *adhikârin*, is eligible for formal spiritual initiation. Only a fully enlightened adept is capable of empowering that initiation, so that the disciple's life is mysteriously guided toward the fulfillment of the "Atman project"— the impulse toward Self- or God-realization.

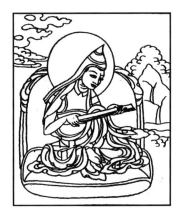

*Ashvaghosha*
*(from a woodblock)*

## VI. GIVING BIRTH TO A NEW IDENTITY—INITIATION

According to the *Kula-Arnava-Tantra* (10.1), it is impossible to attain enlightenment, or liberation, without initiation (*dîkshâ, abhisheka*), and there can be no real initiation without a qualified teacher.

# दीक्षा । अभिशेक ॥

*Dîkshâ, abhisheka*

In anthropological contexts, the term "initiation" stands for a person's transition to a new social grade or status, usually induction into a privileged group such as adult society or a secret brotherhood. Such initiation is frequently marked by special mandatory ceremonies involving tests and trials of courage for the initiate—from seclusion and mutilation to the observance of special vows. Often the initiatory process is symbolized as the initiate's death and subsequent rebirth. While these formal aspects of tribal initiation may also be associated with yogic initiation, the crux of *dîkshâ* is something more profound.

Rather than an induction into a new social status, the yogic *dîkshâ* is primarily a form of spiritual transmission (*sancâra*) by which the disciple's bodily, mental, and spiritual condition is changed through the adept's transference of spiritual "energy" or "consciousness." *Dîkshâ* means first and foremost "enhallowment." This is captured in the synonym *abhisheka*, meaning "sprinkling," which refers to the ceremonial act of sprinkling consecrated water on the devotee—a form of baptism. By means of initiation, which may occur informally or in a more ritual setting, the spiritual process is either awakened or magnified in the practitioner. It is always a direct empowerment, in which the teacher effects in the disciple a change of consciousness, a turnabout,

or *metanoia*. It is a moment of conversion from ordinary worldliness to a sacred life, which alters the being state of the new initiate. From then on the student's spiritual struggle has a new depth. The *Kriyâ-Samgraha-Panjikâ* ("Concise Compendium of Action"), a Buddhist Tantric scripture, quotes the following saying:

> The *yogin* who aspires to "yogihood" (*yogitva*) but has not been initiated is [like a person who] strikes out at the sky with fists and drinks the water of a mirage.[25]

Initiation creates a special link between the *guru* and the devotee—a spiritual connection that represents a unique responsibility on the teacher's part and a significant challenge for the practitioner. Through initiation, the aspirant becomes an integral part of his or her teacher's lineage (*paramparâ*), which is understood as a chain of empowerment that exceeds the world of space and time insofar as it continues after the death of both the teacher and the disciple. Admission to this chain must be earned through wholehearted dedication to the spiritual path, which is a form of self-surrender. This has been made clear by the well-known Tibetan teacher Chögyam Trungpa:

> Without abhisheka our attempts to achieve spirituality will result in no more than a huge spiritual collection rather than real surrender. We have been collecting different behavior patterns, different manners of speech, dress, thought, whole different ways of acting. And all of it is merely a collection we are attempting to impose upon ourselves. Abhisheka, true initiation, is born out of surrender. We open ourselves to the situation as it is, and then

we make real communication with the teacher. In any event, the guru is already there with us in a state of openness; and if we open ourselves, are willing to give up our collections, then initiation takes place.[26]

Thus, the disciple's emotional vulnerability, or openness, forms the basis for spiritual transmission. He or she must become like an empty vessel to be filled by the teacher's gift of transmission. According to the Tibetan tradition, an unsuitable vessel can be dirty (full of emotional and mental confusion), turned upside down (inaccessible to instruction), or leaking (incapable of retaining the transmitted wisdom). The teacher is admonished not to waste the precious teaching (*dharma*) on a student who is an unsuitable vessel.

What is it that is passed from teacher to disciple during initiation? The Tantric term *shakti-pâta*, which literally means "descent of the power," encapsulates the central occurrence during initiation. *Shakti-pâta* stands for the event and the experience of the descent of a powerful energy current into the body, usually starting from the crown of the head or the upper torso and moving down into the pelvic area (which is the location of an important psychospiritual center, the *mûlâ-dhâra-cakra*) and sometimes into the lower extremities.

By virtue of their enlightenment, or at least their advanced spiritual realization, the adept teachers have become a locus of concentrated psychospiritual energy. Whereas the ordinary body-mind represents a low-energy system, the adept's body-mind is like a powerful radio beacon. This is not a mere metaphor. Rather, it is an experiential fact that is recognized in many esoteric traditions. There is even a remarkable passage in Plato's works where a conversation is recorded between Socrates and his pupil

Aristeides. The latter confesses to Socrates that his philosophical understanding increases whenever he associates with the great philosopher, and that this effect is most pronounced when he sits close to him and touches him.

In Aristeide's case, it was intellectual insight that was deepened by sheer proximity to that great lover of wisdom, the saintly Socrates. In the case of the yogic initiate, a different transmission occurs. The initiate is inducted into the secret dimension of existence: He or she discovers that the apparent material cosmos, including his or her own body, is a vast sea of psychospiritual energy. In other words, the initiate begins to understand and experience the very actuality behind the mathematical models of modern quantum physics. The initiate's body-mind and the universe reveal themselves as indefinable patterns of light and energy, imbued with superconsciousness.

According to the *Kula-Arnava-Tantra* (14.39), there are seven kinds of initiation:

1. *Kriyâ-dîkshâ* — initiation through ritual, which is said to be eightfold, depending on the type of ceremonial implements used, such as the fire bowl or the water jar, etc.

2. *Varna-dîkshâ* — initiation through the alphabet, which has three versions, according to whether the alphabet used has 42, 50, or 62 letters. The teacher visualizes the Sanskrit letters in the aspirant's body and then gradually dissolves them again, until the disciple has gained the state of ecstatic unification with the Divine. Visualization is not ordinary mental picturing but a powerful tool that, on the level of energy, actually creates objects perceivable by yogic means.

3.  *Kalâ-dîkshâ* — initiation through the *kalâ*, which is a special emanation, a subtle form of energy, which the teacher projects into the aspirant's body-mind again by means of visualization. This energy is given different names, depending on its appearance in different areas of the body. Thus, it is called *nivritti* ("cessation") from the soles of the feet to the knees, *pratishthâ* ("foundation") from the knees to the navel, *vidyâ* ("knowledge") from the navel to the neck, *shânti* ("peace") from the neck to the forehead, and *shânti-atîta* ("peace-transcending," written *shântyatîta*) from the forehead to the crown of the head.[27] Next the teacher visualizes these energies as gradually dissolving together with the disciple's consciousness, until the mind reaches the zero-point of the manifest world itself, whereupon it flips over into the transcendental State.

4.  *Sparsha-dîkshâ* — initiation through touch (*sparsha*), which involves physical contact between the teacher and the disciple.

5.  *Vag-dîkshâ* — initiation through mantric utterance (*vâc*), which occurs when the teacher, with his or her attention firmly implanted in the Divine, utters a *mantra* or verse from the sacred scriptures.

6.  *Drig-dîkshâ* — initiation through gaze (*drik*), which the teacher performs by gazing into the very being of the disciple.

7.  *Mânasa-dîkshâ* — initiation through mere thought, which involves the projection of energy and consciousness through telepathic means.

Other classifications are also known, but they are all very similar.[28] What they have in common is the graceful transformative agency of the divine Power (*shakti*). Whether the initiate will realize the ultimate Reality at once or only gradually depends on his or her preparation and capacity.

When by the *guru's* mere glance, utterance, or touch the disciple instantly experiences the bliss of Reality, this is also known as *shambhavî-dîkshâ*.[29] The word *shâmbhavî* means "belonging to Shambhu," and Shambhu ("He who is benevolent") is a form of Shiva, the ultimate Being recognized in many schools of Tantra. Initiation by touch is compared to the slow nurturing by a bird that grants its fledglings the warmth of its wings. Initiation by glance is likened to the nurturing by a fish that protects its offspring through watchful eyes. Initiation by the mind alone is said to be similar to the nurturing by a tortoise that simply thinks of its young—a simile that means more to a Yoga practitioner than a biologist.

This type of instant initiation is generally contrasted with *shâktikâ-dîkshâ* on the one hand and *ânavî-dîkshâ* on the other. In the former type of initiation the teacher activates by esoteric means the disciple's innate capacity (*shakti*) for God-realization so that, after a period of time, enlightenment is spontaneously attained. The latter kind of *dîkshâ* involves spiritual instruction, including the imparting of a *mantra*, or sacred word or phrase, which the initiate then recites as directed. Thus, both *shâmbhavî-dîkshâ* and *shâktikâ-dîkshâ* are initiations that lead to realization spontaneously, but whereas the one is instant the other represents a delayed reaction, due to the gradual effect of the awakened *shakti*. Only *ânavî-dîkshâ* calls for a course of application on the disciple's part. He or she is given the teacher's empowerment, but has to cooperate with the

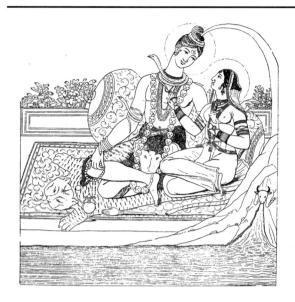

*Shiva and Pârvatî, with the River Gangâ (Ganges) issuing from Shiva's crown*

psychospiritual forces set in motion in him or her through the esoteric process of initiation. The word *ânavî* means "pertaining to *anu*," and *anu* ("atom") is a designation for the individual psyche in some schools of Tantra.

Many more intriguing facts about the ceremonial aspects of *dîkshâ* can be found in the *Mahânirvâna-Tantra* (chapter 10), a fairly recent scripture that is greatly valued by practitioners of Tantra-Yoga.[30]

Whether initiation occurs by yogic means or through the sheer presence of an enlightened adept, it always magnifies the disciple's native intuition of Reality, thus provoking a crisis in consciousness: Through the intensified sensitivity to the transcendental Condition, the initiate understands more deeply the mechanisms by which he or she perpetuates the state of unenlightenment. The disciple experiences the basic dilemma or suffering of ordinary existence, seeing how everything he or she does, thinks, and feels is governed by the principle of egoic separation.

Under the impact of the God-realized adept's spontaneous transmission, the practitioner undergoes spiritual crisis after crisis, awakening more and more to the sublime principle that he or she is presently free, enlightened, and blissful. As this recognition grows in the disciple, he or she finds that his or her egoic impulses, motivations, and obsessions are becoming increasingly obsolete. In this way the teacher's grace (*prasâda*) draws the initiate, step by step, into a radically different disposition—the disposition of enlightenment.[31] It is for this reason alone that initiation, or *dîkshâ*, is given such prominence in the esoteric schools of India.

> *Dîkshâ*, verily, releases [the aspirant] from the extensive bondage impeding [the realization of] the supreme Abode, and it leads [him] upward to Shiva's Domain.[32]

## VII. CRAZY WISDOM AND CRAZY ADEPTS

In Tibet there is a tradition known by the name "crazy wisdom." The phenomenon for which this term stands can be found in all the major religions of the world, though it is seldom acknowledged as a valid expression of spiritual life by the religious orthodoxy or the secular establishment. Crazy wisdom is a unique mode of teaching, which avails itself of seemingly irreligious or unspiritual means in order to awaken the conventional ego-personality from its spiritual slumber.

The unconventional means used by adepts who teach in this risky manner seem crazy or mad in the eyes of ordinary people, who seldom look beyond appearances. Crazy-wisdom methods are designed to shock, but their purpose is always benign: to reflect to the ordinary worldling (*samsârin*) the "madness" of his or her pedestrian existence, which, from the enlightened point of view, is an existence rooted in a profound illusion. That illusion is the ingrained presumption that the individual is an ego-identity bounded by the skin of the human body, rather than the all-pervasive Self-Identity, i.e., the *âtman* or Buddha-nature. Crazy wisdom is a logical extension of the deep insights of spiritual life in general, and it is at the core of the relationship between adept and disciple—a relationship that has the express function of undermining the disciple's ego-illusion.

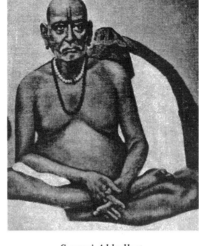

*Swami Akkulkot,
a contemporary avadhûta*

The crazy-wisdom message and approach are understandably offensive to both the secular and the conventionally religious establishments. Hence, crazy adepts have generally been suppressed. This was not the case in traditional Tibet and India, however, where the "holy fool" or "divine madman" has been recognized as a legitimate figure in the compass of spiritual aspiration and realization. Thus, the "saintly madman" (Tibetan: *lama myonpa*) has been venerated throughout the history of Tibet. The same is true of the Indian *avadhûta* who has, as the name suggests, "cast off" all concerns and conventional standards in his ecstatic intoxication.

The Christian equivalent of the saintly madman of Tibet and the Indian *avadhûta* is the "fool for Christ's sake." Yet the large conservative faction among both the clergy and the laity has long driven the unorthodox figure of the "fool" (Greek: *salos*) into oblivion. The modern Christian knows next to nothing about such remarkable "holy idiots" as St. Simeon, St. Isaac Zatvornik, St. Basil, or St. Isadora, the last being one of the few female examples. It was the apostle Paul who first used the phrase "fool for Christ's sake" in 1 Corinthians 4:10. He spoke of the wisdom of God that looks like folly to the world, whereas the world's wisdom is founded in pride. When Mark the Mad, a desert monk of the sixth century C.E., came to the city to atone for his sins, the townspeople considered him insane. But Abba Daniel of Skete instantly recognized his great sanctity, shouting to the crowd that they were all fools for not seeing that Mark was the only reasonable man in the entire city.

St. Simeon, another sixth-century fool for Christ's sake, was a skilled simulator of insanity. Once he found a dead dog on a dung heap. He tied his cord belt to the dog's leg and dragged the corpse behind him through town. The people were outraged, failing to understand that the mad monk's burden was a symbol of the excess baggage they themselves carried around with them—the ego, or conventional mind, lacking love and wisdom. The very next day, St. Simeon entered the local church and threw nuts at the congregation when the Sunday liturgy began. At the end of his life, the saint confessed to his most trusted friend that his eccentric behavior had been solely an expression of his utter indifference (Greek: *apatheia*, Sanskrit: *vairâgya*) to things of the world. Its purpose was to denounce hypocrisy and hubris.

The mad saint, who in his God-intoxication fearlessly steps beyond the mores of his era, made his appearance also in Islam among the masters of Sufism, and in Judaism among the Hasidic mystics. These holy fools represent a wide spectrum of spiritual attainment, ranging from the religious eccentric to the enlightened adept. The common denominator between them is that in their lifestyle, or at least in their occasional eccentric behavior, they invert or reverse the standards and conventions of society.

The most pristine manifestation of crazy wisdom is found in the Tibetan *lama myonpa* and Indic *avadhûta* traditions. The Tibetans distinguish different kinds of madness, including what one might call religious neurosis (Tibetan: *chos-myon*) with sociopathic and paranoid symptoms. These are carefully held apart from saintly madness. Some of the characteristics of saintly madness are not dissimilar to the symptoms of secular and religious madness. However, its nature and causes are quite distinct. The crazy adept's eccentric behavior is a direct expression not of any personal psychopathology, but of his or her spiritual attainment and profound desire to illumine fellow humans.

In Mahâyâna Buddhist terms, crazy wisdom is the articulation in life of the realization that the phenomenal world (*samsâra*) and the transcendental Reality (*nirvâna*) are coessential. Seen from the perspective of the unillumined mind, operating on the basis of a sharp separation between subject and object, perfect enlightenment is a paradoxical condition. The enlightened adept exists as the ultimate spaceless and timeless Being-Consciousness but appears to animate a particular body-mind in space-time. In the nondualist terms of Advaita Vedânta, enlightenment is the fulfillment of the two axioms that the innermost self (*adhyâtman*) is identical with the transcendental Self (*parama-âtman*), and that the ultimate Ground (*brahman*) is identical with the cosmos in all its levels of manifestation, including the self.

Thus the enlightened adept lives as the Totality of existence which, from the narrow perspective of the finite personality, is a veritable chaos. While this is the immediate "experience" of all enlightened masters who live consummately spontaneous (*sahaja*) lives, there are those whose appearance and behavior reflects more directly their divine madness. These are the crazy adepts who do not care to make sense and who, for the sake of instructing others, disregard conventional expectations, norms, and obligations.

They feel free to reject customary behavior and to be subversive, criticizing and poking fun at the worldly and religious establishment, dressing in bizarre ways or even going about naked, ignoring the niceties of social contact, ridiculing the narrow concerns of scholars and scholastics, cursing and using obscene language, employing song and dance, and using stimulants, intoxicants (like alcohol), and engaging in sexuality. They incarnate the esoteric principle of Tantra that liberation (*mukti*) is coessential with enjoyment (*bhukti*); that Reality transcends the categories of transcendence and immanence; that the spiritual is not inherently separate from the world.

In their wild and eccentric behavior, the crazy adepts constantly challenge the limitations that unenlightened individuals presume and thus confront them with the naked truth of existence: that life is mad and unpredictable, except for the inescapable fact that we are thrown into the chaos of manifestation for only a brief span of time. They are a perpetual reminder that our whole human civilization is an attempt to deny the inevitability of death, which makes nonsense out of even the noblest efforts to create a symbolic order out of the infinite plastic that is life.

Unlike conventional wisdom, which is meant to create a higher order or harmony, crazy wisdom has the primary function of disrupting humankind's model-making enthusiasm, its impulse to create order, structure, and meaning. Crazy wisdom is enlightened iconoclasm. What it smashes, in the last analysis, is the egocentric universe and its creator, the subjective sense of being a separate entity—the ego. Thus, as my book *Holy Madness* explains in more detail, crazy wisdom is spiritual shock therapy.[33]

The crazy adept's "naturalness" must be carefully distinguished from the mere impulsiveness of the child or the emotionally labile adult, just as it must be differentiated from the kind of learned spontaneity that is pursued in various humanistic therapies. Enlightened spontaneity (*sahaja*) implies more than enhanced awareness or integration of the body-mind as part of a comprehensive psychohygiene. The realized adepts are not just particularly successful egos. Their spontaneity is absolutely pure and coincides with the world process itself. They act out of the Whole, as the Whole.

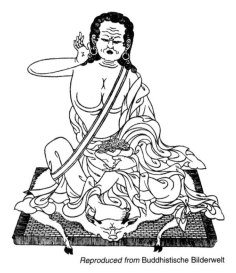

*Reproduced from Buddhistische Bilderwelt*

*Milarepa*

The best known crazy adept of the Tibetan tradition is undoubtedly Tibet's folk hero Milarepa (written Milaraspa, 1040–1123 C.E.), *yogin* and poet extraordinaire. His hard years of pupilage under Marpa "the translator" exemplify the ego-grinding tribulations of all authentic spiritual discipleship. Who would not be touched by the traditional Tibetan biography of Milarepa in which we see him rebuild the same tower again

and again, fighting physical pain, exhaustion, anger at the futility of it all, doubt about his *guru*, and spiritual despair? Already an accomplished magician and miracle worker by the time he met his teacher, Milarepa became an adept in his own right through Marpa's skillful guidance and grace.

Clad only in a white cotton robe, he traversed the borderland between Tibet and Nepal, teaching by way of his didactic poems and songs. Occasionally Milarepa would be found naked, and in one of his songs he observes that he knows no shame, since his genitals are natural enough. His disposition of crazy wisdom is indicated by the fact that, though living the life of a wandering renouncer, he is known to have initiated several of his female devotees into esoteric sexuality. To the common mind, sex and spirituality do not mix. Tantra, as we will see in Chapter 17, contradicts this popular assumption.

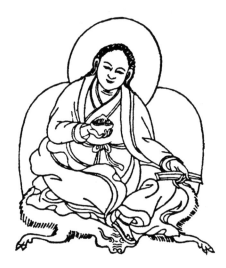

*Marpa (from a woodblock)*

Marpa (1012–1097 C.E.), the founder of the Kagyupa order of Vajrayâna Buddhism, was himself a crazy-wisdom master. A generous and humorous personage, he would often animate an angry disposition toward Milarepa to provoke in his beloved devotee the spiritual crisis that alone could lead to Milarepa's liberation. In addition to his chief wife, he also associated with eight Tantric consorts.

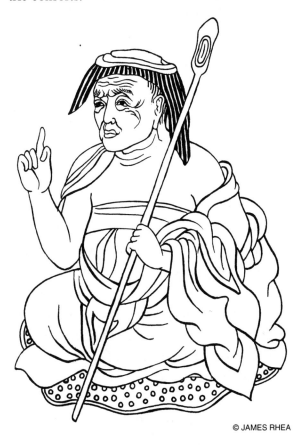

© JAMES RHEA

*Crazy adept Drukpa Kunleg*

The most exaggerated and outrageous crazy adept of Tibet was undoubtedly Drukpa Kunleg (1455–1570 C.E.), who, like many other saintly madmen, started out as a monk, but upon enlightenment adopted the life of a mendicant. His Tibetan biography, which contains much symbolic and legendary material, claims that he initiated no fewer than five thousand women into the sexual secrets of Tantra. His biographer portrays him as a fond consumer of *chung*, the Tibetan beer, and an accomplished raconteur who was a fearless and humorous critic of his monastic contemporaries and society at large.

The crazy-wisdom tradition of India revolves largely around the figure of the *avadhûta*. The Sanskrit word *avadhûta* means literally "cast off," referring to one who has abandoned all

the cares and concerns that burden the ordinary mortal. The *avadhûta* is an extreme type of renouncer (*samnyâsin*), a "supreme swan" (*parama-hamsa*) who, as the title indicates, drifts freely from place to place like a beautiful swan (*hamsa*), depending on nothing but the Divine. The designation *avadhûta* came into vogue during the Common Era, which saw the rise of Tantra in the form of such traditions as Sahajayâna Buddhism, Hindu Kaulism, and Nathism, followed by Hatha-Yoga.

Possibly one of the earliest references to the *avadhûta* can be found in the *Mahanirvâna-Tantra* (8.11). This work states that the "crazy" lifestyle of the *avadhûta* is to the *kali-yuga*—the present "dark age"—what the lifestyle of the *samnyâsin* was to the preceding epoch, where the moral fiber was still relatively strong. In the *kali-yuga*, more drastic means of awakening people are required because of their general insensitivity to the sacred dimension. The "shock therapy" of crazy wisdom is thus preferable to the quiet example of the world-renouncing ascetic, or *samnyâsin*.

The *Mahanirvâna-Tantra* distinctly associates the *avadhûta* with Shaivism, the religio-spiritual tradition that has God Shiva as its focus. This scripture (14.140ff.) speaks of four classes of *avadhûtas*. The *shaiva-avadhûta* has received full Tantric initiation, while the *brahma-avadhûta* employs the *brahma-mantra* "*Om*, the One Being-Consciousness, the Absolute" (*om saccid-ekam brahma*). Both categories are subdivided into those who are as yet imperfect—"wanderers" (*parivraj*)—and those who have attained perfection—the "supreme swans."

One of the earliest Hatha-Yoga scriptures, the *Siddha-Siddhânta-Paddhati*, contains many verses that describe the *avadhûta*. One stanza (6.20) in particular refers to his chameleon-like capacity to animate any character or role. Thus, he is said to behave at times like a worldling or even like a king, and at other times like an ascetic or naked renouncer. The appellation *avadhûta*, more than any other, came to be associated with the apparently crazy modes of behavior of some *parama-hamsas*, who dramatize the reversal of social norms, which is a behavior characteristic of their spontaneous lifestyle. In the *Avadhûta-Gîtâ*, a medieval work celebrating the crazy adept, the *avadhûta* is depicted as a spiritual hero who is beyond good and evil, beyond praise and blame, indeed beyond any of the categories that the mind can construct. One stanza (7.9) speaks of his transcendental status thus:

> As a *yogin* devoid of "union" (*yoga*) and "separation" (*viyoga*) and as an "enjoyer" (*bhogin*) devoid of enjoyment and nonenjoyment—thus he wanders about at leisure, filled with spontaneous Bliss [innate in his own] mind.

The same scripture (8.6–9) explains the designation *avadhûta* as follows:

> The significance of the letter *a* is that [the *avadhûta*] abides eternally in "Bliss" (*ânanda*), freed from the fetters of hope and pure in the beginning, middle, and end.

> The significance of the syllable *va* is that he dwells [always] in the present and that his speech is blameless, [and it applies to him] who has conquered desire (*vâsanâ*).

> The significance of the syllable *dhû* is that he is relieved of [the practice of] concentration

and meditation, that his limbs are gray with dust, that his mind is pure and he is free from disease.

> The significance of the syllable *ta* is that he is freed from [spiritual] darkness (*tamas*) and the I-sense (*ahamkâra*) and that he is devoid of thought and purpose, with his mind steadfast on Reality (*tattva*).[34]

The whole text, which belongs perhaps to the fifteenth or sixteenth century C.E., is written from a lofty nondualist point of view. It is similar to the *Ashtâvakra-Gîtâ* ("Ashtâvakra's Song") which, significantly, is also known as *Avadhûta-Anubhûti* ("Realization of the Crazy Adept") and which has been placed in the late fifteenth century C.E.[35] Both scriptures are ecstatic outpourings, and both celebrate the highest form of nondualist realization.

The *Avadhûta-Gîtâ* is ascribed to Dattâtreya, a semi-legendary spiritual master, who was elevated to the status of a deity.[36] Sage Dattâtreya's story is told in the *Mârkandeya-Purâna* (chapter

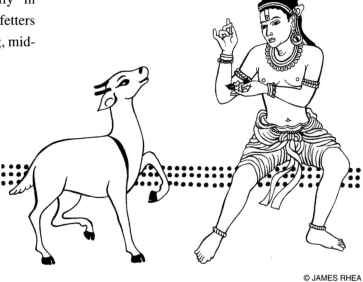

© JAMES RHEA

*Dattâtreya*

16), in a section that belongs perhaps to the fourth century C.E. It describes the miraculous birth of one of the great crazy-wisdom adepts of India.

According to this account, a certain brahmin named Kaushika lived a profligate life, losing both wealth and health as a result of his infatuation with a courtesan. His wife, Shândilî, however, was utterly faithful to him. One night she even carried her sick husband to the courtesan's house. On the way, with her husband riding on her shoulders, Shândilî accidentally stepped on Sage Mândavya, who was lying in the road barely alive. Mândavya, who was feared for his potent curses, promptly condemned the pair to die at sunrise. The chaste woman prayed with all her might, appealing to the sun not to rise at all so that her husband might live. Her pure-hearted prayer was answered. Now all the deities were in an uproar, and they enlisted the help of Anushuyâ, wife of the famous Sage Atri, to convince Shândilî to allow the universal order to be restored. Anushuyâ, herself a paragon of womanly virtue, won Shândilî over, on the condition that Kaushika's life would be spared when the sun rose.

In appreciation of her timely intercession, the gods granted Anushuyâ a boon. She asked for her husband's and her own liberation and then for the principal deities—Brahma, Vishnu, and Shiva—to be born as sons to her. After a period of time, while Anushuyâ was bowing to her husband, a light shone forth from Sage Atri's eyes and served as the seed for the three divine sons Soma, Durvâsa, and Datta—partial incarnations of Brahma, Shiva, and Vishnu respectively.

Other *Purânas* (popular encyclopedias) contain different narratives relating to Dattâtreya, but all involve the figure of Atri—hence the name Dattâtreya, "Datta, son of Atri." It is clear from some of the incidents in Dattâtreya's life that he was a rather unconventional figure. For instance,

he is said to have immersed himself in a lake, from which he emerged after many years in the company of a maiden. Knowing of Dattâtreya's perfect nonattachment, his disciples thought nothing of it. In order to test their faith in him, he began to consume wine with the maiden, but his devotees were not disturbed even by this.

Then again, various *Purânas*, including the *Mârkandeya-Purâna* (chapters 30–40), say that Dattâtreya taught the eight-limbed Yoga (*ashta-anga-yoga*) of Patanjali, which favors an ascetic lifestyle. Thus, Dattâtreya is associated with both ascetical motifs and with situations involving sexuality and alcohol—the two great ingredients of the Tantric ritual.[37]

Dattâtreya is the archetypal crazy adept. It is not clear how, from a quasi-Tantric sage, he was made into a full-blown deity. Nevertheless, both sage and deity are intimately connected with Avadhûtism. Even though mythology remembers Sage Dattâtreya as an incarnation of God Vishnu, his name is just as closely associated with the cultural sphere of Shiva, the Lord of *yogins* and ascetics. It would appear that this great spiritual hero served both the Vaishnava and the Shaiva tradition as a symbol of the God-realizer, whose state transcends all beliefs and customs.

Hence, it is not surprising that Dattâtreya should also be credited with the authorship of the *Jîvan-Mukta-Gîtâ* ("Song of Living Liberation"), a short tract of twenty-three stanzas that extols the *jîvan-mukta*, the adept who is liberated while still in the embodied condition. Likewise, the *Tripura-Rahasya* ("Tripura's Secret Teaching") is attributed to Dattâtreya. Considering this scripture's focus on the supreme mind-transcending disposition of enlightened spontaneity (*sahaja*), this attribution seems singularly appropriate.

Crazy wisdom is found to varying degrees in most schools of Yoga, because the *guru*'s prescribed task is to undermine the disciple's illusion of being an island unto himself or herself. Most teachers, especially if they are fully enlightened, will on occasion resort to unconventional behavior to penetrate the disciple's protective armor. Few teachers, however, tend to teach in the full-fledged mode of crazy wisdom as did, for instance, Marpa and Drukpa Kunleg. Today, individuals maintain more carefully defined ego-boundaries than in the past, and so crazy-wisdom methods tend to be experienced as interfering with the personal integrity of the disciple. Hence,

few teachers are willing to adopt a crazy-wisdom style of teaching. There also remains the broader question of whether this ancient way of teaching is still useful and morally justifiable today.[38]

This brief review of the crazy-wisdom dimension of Hindu and Buddhist spirituality completes Chapter 1, which explains the fundamental categories involved in the spiritual process of Yoga. The next chapter outlines the major approaches or schools within the yogic tradition.

---

**SOURCE READING 2**

# *Siddha-Siddhânta-Paddhati (Selection)*

The *Siddha-Siddhânta-Paddhati* ("Tracks of the Doctrine of the Adepts"), considered to be one of the oldest scriptures of Nâthism, is a composition comprising six chapters. The concluding chapter is dedicated to defining and eulogizing the *avadhûta*, who is distinguished from the spiritual types peculiar to traditions other than the Nâtha order. Of particular interest are the first twenty-one verses, translated here. Like most Hatha-Yoga scriptures, the text is deliberately written in defective Sanskrit, which makes it at times difficult to ascertain the precise meaning of a verse. The following verses are excerpted from the sixth chapter.

Now a description of the *avadhûta-yogin* is given. Tell me, then, who is this so-called *avadhûta-yogin*? The *avadhûta* is he who casts off all of Nature's modifications (*vikâra*). A *yogin* is one for whom there is "union" (*yoga*). *Dhûta* is [derived from] *dhû* [denoting "to shake"], as in trembling, that is, it has the meaning of "trembling." Trembling or shaking [occurs when] the mind is involved with the sense objects like bodies or bodily [states]. Having grasped [these sense objects] and then having withdrawn from them, the mind absorbed into the glory of its own "Domain" (*dhâman*) is devoid of phenomena and is free from the diverse "dwellings" (*nidhâna*) [i.e., the sense objects], which have a beginning, a middle, and an end. (1)

The sound *ya* is the seed syllable (*bîja*) of the wind [element]; the sound *ra* is the seed syllable of the fire [element]. Indistinct from both is the sound *om*, which is praised as the form of Consciousness. (2)

Thus he is clearly called: He who is shaven by cutting off the multitudinous[39] bonds of suffering (*klesha*), who is released from all states—he is styled an *avadhûta*. (3)

The *yogin* who, in his body, is adorned with the splendorous memory of the innate [Reality] and for whom [the serpent-power or *kundalinî-shakti*] has risen from the "support" [i.e., the *mûlâdhâra-cakra* at the base of the spine]—he is named an *avadhûta*. (4)

[That *yogin* who] is firmly stationed in the center of the world, devoid of all "trembling" [i.e., free from all attachment to the sense objects], who has freedom from dejection (*adainya*) as his loincloth and staff (*kharpara*)—he is named an *avadhûta*. (5)

[That *yogin*] by whom the doctrine (*siddhânta*) is preserved like the convergence of the sounds *sham* [designating] joy and *kham* [symbolizing] the supreme Absolute in the word *shamkha* [meaning "conch"]—he is named an *avadhûta*. (6)

Whose limit is [naught but] the supreme Consciousness, who has knowledge of the [ultimate] Object as his sandals, and the great vow as his antelope skin [upon which he is seated]—he is named an *avadhûta*. (7)

Who has perpetual abstention (*nivritti*) as his belt, who has the very Essence (*sva-svarûpa*) as his matted seat, [and who practices] abstention from the six modifications[40] [of Nature]—he is named an *avadhûta*. (8)

Who indeed has the Light of Consciousness and supreme Bliss as his pair of earrings and who has ceased recitation (*japa*) with a rosary (*mala*)—he is named an *avadhûta*. (9)

Who has steadiness as his walking stick, the supreme Space (*para-âkâsha*)[41] as his staff, and the innate power (*nija-shakti*) as his yogic armrest (*yoga-patta*)[42]—he is styled an *avadhûta*. (10)

Who is himself difference and identity [of world and Divine], who has alms as his delight in the taste of the six essences (*rasa*),[43] and who has the condition of being full of that [ultimate Reality] as his adultery—he is styled an *avadhûta*. (11)

Who moves with his inner being into the Unthinkable, the remote Region within, who has that very Place as his undergarment—he is named an *avadhûta*. (12)

Who [desires] to assimilate his own immortal body to the Infinite, the Immortal, who alone would drink this [draft of immortality]—he is named an *avadhûta*. (13)

Who devours the *vajrî*[44] abounding in defilements of desire and strong like a thunderbolt (*vajra*) [that is none other than] nescience (*avidyâ*)—he is named an *avadhûta*. (14)

Who always turns around fully into the very center of himself and who views the world with equanimity (*samatva*)—he is named an *avadhûta*. (15)

Who understands himself and who abides in his Self alone, who is fully established in effortlessness (*anutthâna*)—he is named an *avadhûta*. (16)

Who is conversant with [the art of] supreme repose and endowed with the foundation of effortlessness (*anutthâ*), and who knows the principle formed of Consciousness and contentment (*dhriti*)—he is styled an *avadhûta*. (17)

Who consumes the manifest (*vyakta*) and the unmanifest (*avyakta*) [realms of existence] and devours completely the entire manifestation (*vyakta*) [of Nature], while being [firmly established] in his inner being [and possessing] the Truth within—he is named an *avadhûta*. (18)

Who is firmly established in his own luminosity, who is [that] luster of the nature of [absolute] Radiance (*avabhâsa*), who delights in the world through play (*lîlâ*)—he is named an *avadhûta*. (19)

Who is sometimes an enjoyer, sometimes a renouncer, sometimes a nudist or like a demon, sometimes a king and sometimes a well-mannered [person]—he is named an *avadhûta*. (20)

Who is of the essence of the Innermost [Self] when thus performing different roles (*samketa*) in public, who fully pierces through to the Real in his essential vision of all doctrinal views—he is named an *avadhûta-yogin*. He is a true teacher (*sad-guru*). Because in his essential vision of all views he creates a [grand] synthesis (*samanvaya*)—he is an *avadhûta-yogin*. (21)

"In yoga . . . many may take one path as a key in order to experience self-realisation while others take another path, but I say that there is absolutely no difference between the various practices of yoga."

—B. K. S. Iyengar, *The Tree of Yoga*, p. 15

# Chapter 2
# THE WHEEL OF YOGA

## I. OVERVIEW

In its oldest known form, Yoga appears to have been the practice of disciplined introspection, or meditative focusing, in conjunction with sacrificial rituals. In this form we meet with Yoga in the four *Vedas*, the earliest and most treasured sacred scriptures of Hinduism. These four collections of hymns are thought to contain the revealed, or "superhuman" (*atimânusha*), knowledge of the archaic Sanskrit-speaking civilization of India, known as the Vedic civilization or, more recently, as the Indus-Sarasvatî civilization. The rites of the Vedic priests had to be performed with perfect exactitude, demanding the sacrificer's utmost concentration, and thus the custodians of the sacred lore had to undergo rigorous mental training. This is one of the taproots of later Yoga, which two or more thousand years later led to the consciousness technology of the *Upanishads*, the esoteric teachings of those who made meditation their principal approach to enlightenment.

Out of this Upanishadic Yoga evolved over many centuries an immense body of practices together with more or less elaborate explanations aimed at transcending the human condition. The heritage of Yoga was handed down from teacher to pupil by word of mouth. The Sanskrit term for this transmission of esoteric knowledge is *paramparâ*, which means literally "one after another" or "succession." As time progressed, much was added and much was left out or changed. Soon numerous

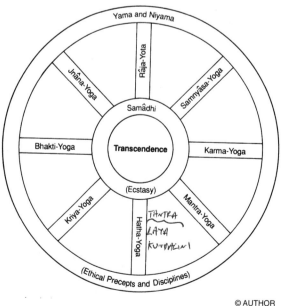

© AUTHOR

*The wheel of Yoga—various approaches to enlightenment*

35

schools had sprung up that represented distinct traditions, within which new splits and reformations took place.

Thus Yoga is by no means a homogeneous whole. Views and practices vary from school to school or teacher to teacher and sometimes cannot even be reconciled with each other. So, when we speak of Yoga we speak of a multitude of yogic paths and orientations with contrasting theoretical frameworks and occasionally even divergent goals, though all are means to liberation. For instance, the ideal of Râja-Yoga is to recover one's true Identity as the transcendental Self (*purusha*) standing eternally apart from the round of Nature, whereas the proclaimed ideal of Hatha-Yoga is to create an immortal body for oneself that permits total mastery of Nature. To give another example, some schools favor the cultivation of paranormal powers (*siddhi*), whereas others consider them obstacles on the path and exhort practitioners to shun them altogether.

Despite the colorful diversity within the Yoga tradition, all approaches are agreed on the need for self-transcendence for going beyond the ordinary personality with its predictable habit patterns. Yoga is indeed the technology of ecstatic transcendence. The differences relate more to the way in which this transcendence is accomplished and how it is conceptualized.

Historically speaking, the most significant of all schools of Yoga is the classical system of Patanjali, which is also known as *the* "view of Yoga" (*yoga-darshana*). This system, which came to be equated with Râja-Yoga, is the formalized résumé of many generations of yogic experimentation and culture. Besides this philosophical school there are numerous nonsystematic Yogas, which are often interwoven with popular beliefs and practices. There also are Yogas within the Jaina and Buddhist spheres of teaching, which are discussed in Chapters 6 and 7.

Within the realm of Hinduism, six major forms of Yoga have gained prominence. They are Râja-Yoga, Hatha-Yoga, Jnâna-Yoga, Bhakti-Yoga, Karma-Yoga, and Mantra-Yoga. To these must be added Laya-Yoga and Kundalinî-Yoga, which are closely associated with Hatha-Yoga but are often mentioned as independent approaches. These two are also subsumed under Tantra-Yoga.

The Yoga tradition has not ceased to change and grow, adapting to new sociocultural conditions. This is borne out by Sri Aurobindo's Integral Yoga, a unique modern approach that is based on traditional Yoga but goes beyond it by favoring an evolutionary synthesis.

Additionally, we find in the Sanskrit scriptures numerous compound words that end in -*yoga*. For the most part, these do not stand for independent schools. Rather the word *yoga* has here the more generic significance of "practice" or "disciplined application." For instance, the compound *buddhi-yoga* means the "practice of discriminative knowledge," and *samnyâsa-yoga* denotes "the practice of renunciation." Other instances are *dhyâna-yoga* ("practice of meditation"), *samâdhi-yoga* ("practice of ecstasy"), and *guru-yoga* ("practice that has the spiritual teacher as its focus"). Other compounds represent a more specific orientation, such as *nâda-yoga* ("Yoga of the inner sound"), *kriyâ-yoga* ("Yoga of ritual action"), the Vedântic *asparsha-yoga* ("intangible Yoga"), and so on. The last-mentioned Yoga, taught in the *Mândûkya-Kârikâ*, is so called because it consists in the direct contemplation of the intangible Absolute, which is the ever-present foundation of all existence.

If we liken Yoga to a many-spoked wheel, then the spokes represent the diverse schools and movements of Yoga, the rim symbolizes the moral requirements shared by all types of Yoga, while the hub stands for the ecstatic experience by virtue of which the Yoga practitioner transcends not only his or her own limited consciousness but cosmic existence itself. All authentic forms of Yoga are ways to a single center, the transcendental Reality, which may be defined differently by the various schools.

There also are *yogins* who aspire to the realization of states of consciousness that fall short of ultimate transcendence, or who seek to attain paranormal powers rather than enlightenment. Their orientation and teaching is magical rather than psychospiritual, as understood here. There is a strong magical component in the archaic tradition of asceticism (*tapas*) and also in Tantra, both of which are discussed later. The *yogin* has always been looked upon as a magus who is endowed with special faculties, notably the ability to bless and to curse effectively. Modern students are apt to dismiss the magical dimension of Yoga, but it is an integral aspect of yogic experience. Why else would Patanjali devote an entire chapter to paranormal powers (*siddhi*) in his *Yoga-Sûtra*? It is important, though, that we remain sensitive to the distinction between magical purposes and the great work of spiritual transformation, which goes beyond the attainment of paranormal experiences and abilities, just as it goes beyond mere mystical states of consciousness. The goal of authentic spirituality is Self- or God-realization, founded in self-transcendence.

## II. RÂJA-YOGA— THE RESPLENDENT YOGA OF SPIRITUAL KINGS

The designation *râja-yoga*, meaning "royal Yoga," is a comparatively late coinage that came in vogue in the sixteenth century C.E. It refers specifically to the Yoga system of Patanjali,

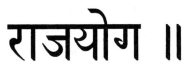

*Râja-yoga*

created in the second century C.E., and is most commonly used to distinguish Patanjali's eightfold path of meditative introversion from Hatha-Yoga. According to the *Yoga-Râja-Upanishad* (1–2),[1] a late work, there are four kinds of Yoga, namely Mantra-Yoga, Laya-Yoga, Hatha-Yoga, and Râja-Yoga. All are said to include the well-known practices of posture, breath control (here called *prâna-samrodha*), meditation, and ecstasy.

The idea behind the appellation *râja-yoga* is that this type of Yoga is superior to Hatha-Yoga. The latter is thought to be for those who cannot dedicate themselves exclusively to the sacred ordeal of meditative practice and renunciation. In other words, Râja-Yoga understands itself as the Yoga for the true heroes of mind training. However, we cannot fail to note that this qualification is not altogether true to fact. For Hatha-Yoga, too, has its intense meditative practices and can certainly be as much of an ordeal as Râja-Yoga. Unfortunately, both Indic and Western practitioners of Hatha-Yoga do not always respect the spiritual goals or even the ethical foundations of this approach and often tend to pursue Hatha-Yoga as a kind of calisthenics or body cosmetics.

Other explanations of the phrase *râja-yoga* are possible. It could refer to the fact that Patanjali's Yoga was practiced by kings, notably the tenth-century King Bhoja, who even wrote a well-known commentary on the *Yoga-Sûtra*. Switching over to a more esoteric level of explanation, we could also see in the word *râja* a hidden reference to the transcendental Self, which is the ultimate ruler, or king, of the body-mind. Moreover, the Self is traditionally described as "luminous" or "resplendent" (*râjate*)—an adjective that stems from the same verbal root as *râja*.

Or again, the term *raja* could refer to the "Lord" (*îshvara*), or God, who is recognized by Patanjali as a special Self among the countless transcendental Selves.

Finally, the *Yoga-Shikhâ-Upanishad* (1.136–138), composed perhaps in the fourteenth or fifteenth century C.E., gives a completely esoteric (Tantric) interpretation:

> In the middle of the perineum (*yoni*), the great place, dwells well-concealed *rajas*, the principle of the Goddess, resembling the [red] *japâ* and *bandhukâ* [flowers in color]. Râja-Yoga is so called owing to the union (*yoga*) of *rajas* and semen (*retas*). Having attained the [various paranormal powers] such as miniaturization through Râja-Yoga, [the *yogin*] becomes resplendent (*râjate*).

The red *rajas* principle mentioned in the above quote is sometimes identified as menstrual blood, sometimes as female hormonal secretions, and sometimes as ovum. The last interpretation makes the most sense symbolically, because the joining of semen and ovum leads to a new being—in this case, metaphorically, the condition of enlightenment. But hormonal secretions play a role in this Yoga as well, as they do in Taoism. Metaphysically speaking, *rajas* and *retas* are the feminine and masculine energetic principle respectively. Their perfect harmonization (*samarasa*) is thought to bring about the leap into unqualified ecstasy. But this esoteric explanation belongs to Tantric symbolism rather than Patanjali's philosophical school.

Râja-Yoga, or Classical Yoga, is treated at length in Chapters 9 and 10. Since its creation in the early centuries of the Common Era—some scholars, however, consider Patanjali to have lived in the pre-Christian period—Râja-Yoga has been one of the most influential schools of the Yoga tradition. It is the high road of meditation and contemplation. As Swami Vivekananda stated enthusiastically, "Râja-Yoga is the science of religion, the rationale of all worship, all prayers, forms, ceremonies, and miracles."[2] He added that the goal of Râja-Yoga is to teach "how to concentrate the mind, then how to discover the innermost recesses of our own minds, then how to generalize their contents and form our own conclusions from them."[3] In the end this meditative quest is intended to lead to the discovery of the transcendental Reality beyond thought and image, beyond worship and prayer, beyond ritual and magic.

## III. HATHA-YOGA—CULTIVATING AN ADAMANTINE BODY

The "forceful Yoga," or Hatha-Yoga, is a medieval development. Its fundamental objective is the same as that of any authentic form of Yoga: to transcend the egoic (or, to coin a phrase, egotropic) consciousness and to realize the Self, or divine Reality.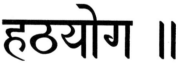

*Hatha-yoga*

However, the psychospiritual technology of Hatha-Yoga is particularly focused on developing the body's potential so that the body can withstand the onslaught of transcendental realization. We are prone to think of ecstatic states like *samâdhi* as purely mental events, which is not the case. Mystical states of consciousness can have a profound effect on the nervous system and the rest of the body. After all, the experience of ecstatic union occurs in the embodied state. The *hatha-yogin*, therefore, endeavors to steel the body—to "bake" it well, as the texts say.

Most importantly, enlightenment itself is a whole-body event. This has been made nowhere more clear than in the writings of the contemporary spiritual teacher Da Free John (Adi Da), who writes:

> The Enlightenment of Man is the Enlightenment of the whole and entire body-mind. It is literal, even bodily Enlightenment, or Translation of the whole and entire body-mind of the individual into the absolute Radiance, Intensity, Love, or Light that is prior and superior to all the speeds of manifest or invisible light and all the forms or beings that cycle in manifest light, whether subtle or gross.[4]

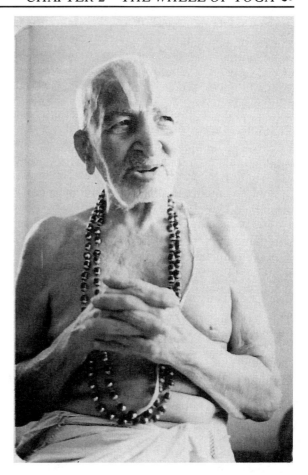

*T. S. Krishnamacharya, the greatest exponent of Hatha-Yoga in modern times*

Thus, the disciplines of Hatha-Yoga are designed to help manifest the ultimate Reality in the finite human body-mind. In this, Hatha-Yoga expresses the ideal of Tantra, which is to live in the world out of the fullness of Self-realization rather than to withdraw from life in order to gain enlightenment. Hatha-Yoga belongs on the side of integralism, as explained in the Introduction.

The Hatha-Yoga practitioner wants to construct a "divine body" (*divya-sharîra*) or "adamantine body" (*vajra-deha*) for himself or herself, which would guarantee immortality in the manifest realms. He or she is not interested in attaining enlightenment on the basis of prolonged neglect of the physical body. He or she wants it all: Self-realization *and* a transmuted body in which to enjoy the manifest universe in its diverse dimensions. Who would not sympathize with this desire? Yet, as can be imagined, the practitioners of Hatha-Yoga have sometimes sacrificed their highest spiritual aspirations and settled for lesser, perhaps magical, goals in service of the ego-personality. Magic, like exo-technology, is a way of manipulating the forces of Nature, whereas spirituality is about the transcendence of the manipulative ego-personality.

Narcissism, or body-oriented egocentrism, is as great a danger among *hatha-yogins* as it is among bodybuilders. A strong will is necessary in all spiritual traditions, but it can never be a substitute for discernment and renunciation, especially the renunciation of self-will. But *hatha-yogins*, like other practitioners of Yoga, occasionally end up with inflated rather than transcended egos. This has led some scholars to characterize Hatha-Yoga as a decadent teaching.

Thus, the German Sanskritist J. W. Hauer made this harsh judgment:

> A typical product of the period of decline of the Indian mind, which, in spite of all assurances to the contrary, is far from the ruthlessly honest urge toward full clarification, the liberation of the soul, and the experience of the ultimate Reality . . . Hathayoga has a strong touch of coarse suggestion and is intimately linked with magic and sexuality.[5]

This condemnation certainly applies to the vulgarized versions of Hatha-Yoga practiced in India, but it is unjustifiable in regard to the authentic teachings and teachers of this tradition.

Genuine Hatha-Yoga always demands that it should be understood as psychospiritual technology in service of transcendental realization. In the *Hatha-Yoga-Pradîpikâ* (4.102), the most popular manual of this school, this fact is expressed as follows:

> All means of Hatha[-Yoga] are for [reaching] perfection in Râja-Yoga. A person rooted in Râja-Yoga conquers death.

What this stanza suggests is that Hatha-Yoga and Râja-Yoga should be looked upon as complementary, and that the desire to conquer death is fulfilled in Self-realization alone. For, only the transcendental Self is deathless and immortal. Even a specially manufactured "divine" body, composed of subtle matter or energy, must sooner or later disintegrate, since all products of Nature are subject to the law of change, or entropy.

Hatha-Yoga reminds one of the many body-oriented therapies that have sprung up in recent years in Western countries. These have given us a new appreciation of the experiential or energetic dimension of bodily existence. However, the remarkable discoveries made by *yogins* centuries ago about esoteric or subtle anatomy still need to be fully appreciated. Especially the phenomenon of the serpent power (*kundalinî-shakti*), the psychospiritual force dormant in the unenlightened body-mind, is barely understood. Yet, as will be explained in Chapter 17 on Tantra-Yoga, it is central to the Hatha-Yoga practitioner's inner work and to his or her perceptions and insights into dimensions of existence that are just beginning to be of interest to modern science. The metaphysics and the practical path of Hatha-Yoga are dealt with in detail in Chapter 18.

## IV. JNÂNA-YOGA—SEEING WITH THE EYE OF WISDOM

The word *jnâna* means "knowledge," "insight," or "wisdom," and in spiritual contexts has the specific sense of what the ancient Greeks called *gnosis*, a special kind of liberating knowledge or intuition. In fact, the terms *jnâna* and *gnosis* are etymologically related through the Indo-European root *gno*, meaning "to know." Jnâna-Yoga is virtually identical with the spiritual path of Vedânta, the Hindu tradition

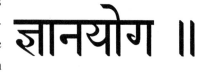

*Jnâna-yoga*

of nondualism. Jnâna-Yoga is the path of Self-realization through the exercise of gnostic understanding, or, to be more precise, the wisdom associated with discerning the Real from the unreal or illusory.

The term *jnâna-yoga* is first mentioned in the *Bhagavad-Gîtâ* (3.3), where Krishna declares:

Of yore I proclaimed a twofold way of life in this world, O guileless [Prince Arjuna]–Jnâna-Yoga for the *samkhyas* and Karma-Yoga for the *yogins*.

Karma-Yoga, as we will see shortly, is the Yoga of self-surrendered action, which is said here to be for the *yogins*. The *samkhyas* are the follower of the once-influential Sâmkhya tradition, which is the contemplative path of distinguishing between the products of Nature and the transcendental Self, until the Self (*purusha*) is realized in the moment of liberation. The Sâmkhya tradition, which has always been closely related to Yoga, is discussed in Chapter 3 in the section entitled "Yoga and Hindu Philosophy."

Vyâsa, the alleged author of the *Bhagavad-Gîtâ*, tried to bridge the gap between the two by having Lord Krishna reject the view that Yoga and Sâmkhya are completely separate approaches:

"Sâmkhya and Yoga are different" say the simpletons, not the learned. Resorting properly to one [or the other], one obtains the fruit of both. (5.4)

That state which is obtained by the *sâmkhyas* is also reached by the *yogins*. He who sees Sâmkhya and Yoga as one, sees indeed. (5.5)

It is clear from the context that Krishna, Arjuna's divine teacher, equates Jnâna-Yoga with Buddhi-Yoga. In my rendering of the *Bhaga-vad-Gîtâ*, I have translated the

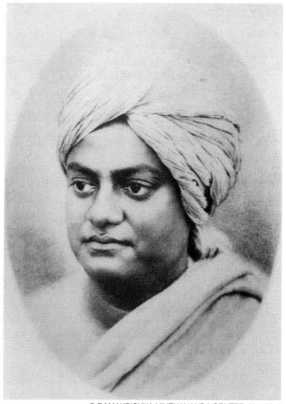

© RAMAKRISHNA-VIVEKANANDA CENTER, New York
*Swami Vivekananda, a great jnâna-yogin*

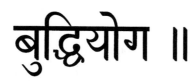
*Buddhi-yoga*

term *buddhi* as "wisdom faculty." It signifies illumined reason. Buddhi-Yoga is the path of Self-realization that applies discriminative wisdom, or higher intuitive knowledge, to all situations and conditions of life. For this reason, it goes hand in hand with Karma-Yoga. In the words of Lord Krishna:

Renouncing in thought all actions to Me, intent on Me, resorting to Buddhi-Yoga, be constantly "Me-minded" (*mac-citta*).[6] (18.57)

"Me-minded," you will transcend all obstacles by My grace. But if out of egotism (*ahamkâra*) you will not listen, you will perish! (18.58)

The "Me-mindedness" spoken of here is of course not a form of egotism but the practice of placing one's attention on the Divine. The "Me," in other words, is God Krishna himself, not the human personality.

In contrast to Râja-Yoga, which operates on the basis of a dualist (*dvaita*) metaphysics that distinguishes between the many transcendental Selves and Nature, the metaphysics of Jnâna-Yoga is strictly nondualist (*advaita*). As I have mentioned already, it is the path of the Vedânta tradition par excellence. It is the way taught in the *Upanishads* and is also known as the "road of wisdom" (*jnâna-mârga*). In the opinion of one scholar, Jnâna-Yoga

> is fundamentally different from all other forms and stands really unique in the history of the world. It is not the worship of God as an object different from the self and is not a discipline that leads to the attainment of anything distinct from one's own self. It may be described as *âtma-upâsana* (the worship of God as one's Self).[7]

The practitioner of Jnâna-Yoga, who is known as a *jnânin*, can be said to treat willpower (*icchâ*) and inspired reason (*buddhi*) as the two guiding principles by which enlightenment can be attained. In the words of Proverbs (4:7), "wisdom is the foundation." As this biblical book continues:

> Exalt her [i.e., Lady Wisdom], and she will exalt you; she will honor you if you embrace her. (4:8)

> She will place on your head a beautiful garland; she will bestow on you a crown of glory. (4:9)

> Keep hold of instruction; do not let go: Guard her, for she is your life. (4:13)

In the Near Eastern wisdom tradition, to which Proverbs belongs, wisdom allows a person to distinguish between right and wrong or wickedness and to walk the path of righteousness. The Hebrew *hokma* ("wisdom"), corresponding to the Greek *sophia*, is about the maintenance of order, balance, and harmony. So is *jnâna*, which upholds *dharma*—*dharma* being one of the most important concepts of Hinduism. According to the *Bhagavad-Gîtâ* (4.7), Lord Krishna takes ever new incarnations in order to restore *dharma* in the world whenever the cosmic order is threatened by human hubris and ignorance.

The *Tripura-Rahasya* (19.16ff.), a late but important Shâkta work on Jnâna-Yoga, distinguishes between three types of aspirant of Jnâna-Yoga, depending on the predominant psychic disposition (*vâsanâ*): The first type suffers from the fault of pride, which stands in the way of a proper understanding of the teachings of nonduality. The second type suffers from "activity" (*karma*), by which is meant the illusion of being an active subject, an ego-personality engaged in acts, which prevents equanimity and clarity as the basis of true wisdom. The third and most common type suffers from the "monster" of desire—that is, from motivations that run counter to the impulse toward liberation. Persons of this type, for instance, lose themselves in the hunger for power, the desire for fame, or in designs of sexual possession.

The prideful type of Jnâna-Yoga practitioner can overcome his or her fault by cultivating trust in the teaching and the teacher. The type who thinks of himself or herself as a doer of actions is simply in need of grace. The third, impulsive type must make a concerted effort to cultivate dispassion and discrimination through study, worship, and frequenting the illumined presence of the sages. Most practitioners of Jnâna-Yoga fall into the third group: those who are still confronting desires and motivations that conflict with the impulse toward emancipation. They are struggling to discern the real and the unreal and to uphold the former in everything they do, say, and think.

The *Tripura-Rahasya* (19.35) further states that the single most important factor of success is the actual urge toward emancipation. Philosophical study on its own is said to be like "dressing up a corpse." It comes alive only through the desire for liberation, and that desire must be deeply felt and not merely based on casual fascination or delusions of grandeur. Above all, the urge toward Self-realization must translate into consistent daily practice in order to bear fruit.

Depending on the practitioner's efforts and personality, Jnâna-Yoga can manifest differently in different individuals; although, as the unknown author of the *Tripura-Rahasya* (19.71) is quick to point out, these differences do not mean that wisdom itself is manifold. Rather, *jnâna* admits of no distinction. *Jnâna* is not different from the transcendental Reality itself.

This marvelous Sanskrit scripture next speaks of those *jnânins* who are liberated even while continuing to be present in the physical body. These great beings, called *jîvan-muktas* ("living liberated"), are quite unaffected by whatever dispositions or desires may arise in their conditional personalities. A second category comprises those advanced practitioners of Jnâna-Yoga who are so focused on the sacred work of self-transcendence that, in their single-mindedness, they appear to be mindless. These are the illustrious sages. Their "mindlessness" (*amanaskatâ*) manifests in a childlike quality that reflects their utter inner simplicity. They have no concerns or worries and no interest in acquiring knowledge or in displaying cleverness. The mind is useful to them only insofar as it allows them to handle the practicalities of their lives. Gradually it

is superseded by flawless spontaneity in all circumstances, without the intervening circuitry of the brain-mind.

The path of Jnâna-Yoga, which has been described as "a straight but steep course,"[8] is outlined with elegant conciseness by Sadânanda in his *Vedânta-Sâra* (15ff.), a fifteenth-century text.  Sadânanda lists four principal means (*sâdhana*) for attaining emancipation:

1. Discernment (*viveka*) between the permanent and the transient; that is, the constant practice of seeing the world for what it is—a finite and changeable realm that, even at its most enjoyable, must never be confused with the transcendental Bliss.

2. Renunciation (*virâga*) of the enjoyment of the fruit (*phala*) of one's actions; this is the high ideal of Karma-Yoga, which asks students to engage in appropriate actions without expecting any reward.

3. The "six accomplishments" (*shat-sampatti*), which are detailed below.

4. The urge toward liberation (*mumukshutva*); that is, the cultivation of the spiritual impulse. In Mahâyâna Buddhism the desire for liberation is kindled for the benefit of all other beings and is known as the "enlightenment mind" (*bodhi-citta*).

The six accomplishments are:

1. Tranquillity (*shama*), or the art of remaining calm even in the face of adversity.

2. Sense-restraint (*dama*), or the curbing of one's senses, which are habitually hankering after stimulation.

3. "Cessation" (*uparati*), or abstention from actions that are not relevant either to the maintenance of the body or to the pursuit of enlightenment.

4. Endurance (*titikshâ*), which is specifically understood as the stoic ability to be unruffled by the play of opposites (*dvandva*) in Nature, such as heat and cold, pleasure and pain, or praise and censure.

5. Mental collectedness (*samâdhâna*), or concentration, the discipline of single-mindedness in all situations but specifically during periods of formal education.

6. Faith (*shraddhâ*), a deeply inspired, heartfelt acceptance of the sacred and transcendental Reality. Faith, which is fundamental to all forms of spirituality, must not be confused with mere belief, which operates only on the level of the mind.

In some works a threefold path is expounded. A good example is Shankara's brilliant commentary on the *Brahma-Sûtra* (1.1.4). Together with the *Upanishads* and the *Bhagavad-Gîtâ*, the *Brahma-Sûtra* is considered the philosophical mainstay of the Vedânta tradition. This threefold path has the following means: listening (*shravana*), or reception of the sacred teachings, and considering (*manana*) their import, as well as contemplation (*nididhyâsana*) of the truth, which is the Self (*âtman*).[9]

Jnâna-Yoga, then, is the disciplined cultivation of the eye of wisdom (*jnâna-cakshus*), which alone can lead us, in the words of an ancient Sanskrit prayer, "from the unreal to the Real."[10]

**SOURCE READING 3**

# Amrita-Bindu-Upanishad

According to tradition, the *Amrita-Bindu-Upanishad* (written *Amritabindûpanishad*) is the twentieth in the classic list of 108 *Upanishads*. The title means "Secret Doctrine of the Seed of Immortality." The term *bindu* (lit. "dot" or "point"), here rendered as "seed," has all kinds of esoteric connotations. In the present context it probably stands for the mind (*manas*) itself, which is the seed or source of either liberation or bondage. This usage is also found in the *Yoga-Kundalî-Upanishad* (3.5). The underlying idea is expressed very well in the *Viveka-Cûdâmani* ("Crest Jewel of Discernment"), ascribed to Shankara, the great preceptor of Vedânta, as follows:

The mind continually creates all the objects that are experienced by oneself as coarse or very fine, [including] the differences of body, estate, stage of life or class, and the [various] qualities, actions, reasons, and fruits [of those actions]. (177)

The mind deludes the unattached form of [pure] Awareness [i.e., the Self] and binds it by means of the ropes of body, organs, and breath, thereby causing it to roam incessantly in the self-inflicted experience of the fruits [of one's actions] as "I" and "mine." (178)

Hence the learned who perceive the truth say that the mind is ignorance, by which alone the world is moved about, like cloud banks by the wind. (180)

[Therefore] the seeker of liberation should diligently effect the purification of the mind. When it is purified, liberation is as a fruit in one's hand. (181)

The position of the *Amrita-Bindu-Upanishad* is very similar. It too speaks of the mind as the source point of either bondage or spiritual liberation. The clouded mind is forever restless, agitated, unsatisfied, and deluded, obscuring the individual's true identity as the transcendental Self. Through diligent inner work, notably meditation, the mind can be cleansed of these impurities. When the aspirant finally achieves, in Lord Byron's words, "a mind at peace with all below," then consciousness acts like a highly polished mirror reflecting the splendor of the Self's pure Awareness. The fully controlled mind is said to be "nonexistent" or "destroyed," since it has lost its characteristic mode of creating unreality or illusion (*mâyâ*). However, the enlightened person is not mindless in the sense of being unconscious or unmindful. On the contrary, the mind is eclipsed by the superconsciousness of the transcendental Self.

The mind is said to be twofold; pure and impure. The impure [mind is driven by] desire and volition; the pure [mind] is devoid of desire. (1)

The mind alone is the cause of bondage and liberation (*moksha*) to humans. Attached to objects, [it leads] to bondage; freed from objects, it is deemed [to lead] to emancipation (*mukti*). (2)

The mind should always be made devoid of objects by the seeker of liberation, since the liberation of the mind devoid of objects is desirable. (3)

When the mind, freed from contact with objects and confined in the heart, reaches nonbeing (*abhâva*), then that is the supreme State. (4)

[The mind] should be checked until it meets with destruction in the heart. This is gnosis (*jnâna*); this is meditation (*dhyâna*). The rest is diffuse speculation. (5)

[The Absolute] is neither thinkable nor unthinkable; it is not thinkable and [yet] thinkable. [When one is] free from partial standpoints, then the Absolute (*brahman*) is attained. (6)

One should combine Yoga with the sound (*svara*). One should realize the Supreme as the Soundless (*asvara*). Through the realization of the Soundless, [there can be] no nonbeing (*abhâva*). Being is desirable. (7)

That verily is the impartite Absolute, [which is] formless and stainless. Knowing "I am the Absolute," the Absolute is surely attained. (8)

It is formless, infinite, devoid of cause or precedent, immeasurable and beginningless. Knowing this the sage is liberated. (9)

There is neither dissolution nor origination, neither the bonded nor the realizer (*sâdhaka*), neither the seeker of liberation nor the liberated. This is the supreme truth. (10)

The Self is to be thought of only as singular during waking, dreaming, and sleeping. For him who has transcended the three states [of waking, dreaming, and sleeping], there is no rebirth. (11)

The Elemental Self (*bhûta-âtman*)[11] residing in every being is but one. [It is] seen as unitary and manifold, like the moon's [reflection] in water. (12)

Just as the space (*âkâsha*) enclosed in a pot [is not transferred] when the pot is moved, or just as that space is not [affected] when the pot is destroyed—similarly, the psyche (*jîva*) resembles the space. (13)

Like the pot, [the individuated self] has diverse shapes, breaking apart again and again. Upon its disintegration, one does not know it and yet one knows it eternally [as the Self]. (14)

He who is surrounded by the illusion of verbalization, [blinded] by darkness, does not go to the Source of Plenty (*pushkara*).[12] When the darkness is dispelled, he verily beholds only Oneness (*ekatva*). (15)

The imperishable (*akshara*) sound [i.e., the sacred syllable *om*] is the supreme Absolute. When that has dwindled what [remains] is the Imperishable [itself]. Should the knower desire Self's peace, he should contemplate that Imperishable (*akshara*). (16)

The two [forms of] knowledge (*vidyâ*) to be known are the Sonic Absolute (*shabda-brahman*) and that which transcends it. He who is familiar with the Sonic Absolute reaches the supreme Absolute. (17)

The sage who, after studying the books, is intent on that [Absolute] through wisdom (*jnâna*) and knowledge (*vijnâna*) should discard all books, even as the husk [is discarded by a person] seeking the grain. (18)

There is but a single color for the milk of variously colored cows—thus he looks upon gnosis as on milk, and upon the [numerous] signs (*lingin*) as on cows. (19)

Knowledge (*vijnâna*) abides hidden in every being, as does butter in milk. By means of the mind as churning-stick, [every] being should constantly churn [this knowledge] within the mind. (20)

Employing the eye of wisdom (*jnâna-netra*), one should extract the Supreme, as fire [is extracted from wood by friction], remembering "I am that impartite, motionless, tranquil Absolute." (21)

That which, though dwelling in beings, is the dwelling-place of all beings, favoring all [beings]—that Vâsudeva[13] I am. (22)

## V. *BHAKTI-YOGA—THE SELF-TRANSCENDING POWER OF LOVE*

Râja-Yoga and Jnâna-Yoga approach Self-realization chiefly through the transcendence and transformation of the mind, whereas Hatha-Yoga aspires to the same goal through the transmutation of the body. In Bhakti-Yoga, the emotional force of the human being is purified and channeled toward the Divine. In

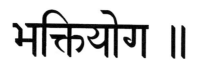

भक्तियोग ॥
*Bhakti-yoga*

their discipline of ecstatic self-transcendence, the *bhakti-yogins*—or *bhaktas* ("devotees")—tend to be more openly expressive than the typical *râja-yogin* or *jnânin*. The followers of Bhakti-Yoga do not, for instance, shy away from shedding tears of longing for the Divine. In this approach, the transcendental Reality is usually conceived as a supreme Person rather than as an impersonal Absolute. Many practitioners of this path even prefer to look upon the Divine as an Other. They speak of communion and partial merging with God rather than total identification, as in Jnâna-Yoga. This dualist orientation is beautifully expressed in one of Tukârâma's devotional songs:

> Can water drink itself?
> Can a tree taste its own fruit?
> The worshiper of God must
>     remain distinct from
>     Him.
> Only thus will he come to
>     know God's joyful love.
> But if he were to say that God
>     and he are one,
> that joy and love would
>     vanish instantly.

*Shândilya*

© AUTHOR

The seventeenth-century saint Tukârâma, about whom more will be said in Chapter 12, was one of the great representatives of the *bhakti-mârga*, or "way of love/devotion."

The term *bhakti*, derived from the root *bhaj* ("to share" or "to participate in"), is generally rendered as "devotion" or "love." Bhakti-Yoga is thus the Yoga of loving self-dedication to, and love-participation in, the divine Person. It is the way of the heart. Shândilya, the author of the *Bhakti-Sûtra* (1.2), defines *bhakti* as "supreme attachment to the Lord." It is the only kind of attachment that does not reinforce the egoic personality and its destiny. Attachment is a combination of placing one's attention on something and investing it with great emotional energy. When we confess that we are attached to various persons, we mean that we enjoy their company or even delight in simply thinking about them, so that when we contemplate their absence or loss, we become saddened. The loss of loved individuals, animals, or even inanimate objects seems to diminish our own being.

It is such energized love-attachment (*âsakti*) that *bhakti-yogins* consciously harness in their quest for communion or union with the Divine. At times when we are emotionally estranged from the Ground of existence, we similarly feel diminished in our being. In fact, the masters of Bhakti-Yoga would say that the confusion and unhappiness prevalent in the world are caused by our alienation from the Divine. St. Augustine undoubtedly intuited this when he exclaimed that "our heart is restless until it rests in Thee."[14]

In Bhakti-Yoga, the practitioner is always a devotee (*bhakta*), a lover, and the Divine is the

Beloved. There are different degrees of devotion, and the *Bhâgavata-Purâna*, composed in the ninth century C.E., delineates nine stages. These have been formalized by Jîva Gosvâmin, the great sixteenth-century preceptor of Gaudîya Vaishnavism, in his *Shat-Sandarbha* ("Six Compositions") as follows:[15]

1. Listening (*shravana*) to the names of the divine Person. Each of the hundreds of names highlights a distinct quality of God, and hearing them creates a devotional attitude in the receptive listener.

2. Chanting (*kîrtana*) praise songs in honor of the Lord. Such songs generally have a simple melody and are accompanied by musical instruments. Again, the singing is a form of meditative remembrance of the Divine and can lead to ecstatic breakthroughs.

3. Remembrance (*smarana*) of God, the loving meditative recalling of the attributes of the divine Person, often in his human incarnation—for instance, as the beautiful cowherd Krishna.

4. "Service at the feet" (*pâda-sevana*) of the Lord, which is a part of ceremonial worship. The feet are traditionally considered a terminal of magical and spiritual power (*shakti*) and grace. In the case of one's living teacher, self-surrender is frequently expressed by bowing at the *guru*'s feet. Here service at the Lord's feet is understood metaphorically, as one's inner embrace of the Divine in all one's activities.

5. Ritual (*arcanâ*), the performance of the prescribed religious rites, especially those involving the daily ceremony at the home altar on which the image of one's chosen deity (*ishta-devatâ*) is installed.

6. Prostration (*vandana*) before the image of the Divine.

7. "Slavish devotion" (*dâsya*)[16] to God, which is expressed in the devotee's intense yearning to be in the company of the Lord.

8. Feeling of friendship (*sâkhya*) for the Divine, which is a more intimate, mystical form of associating with God.

9. "Self-offering" (*âtma-nivedana*), or ecstatic self-transcendence, through which the worshiper enters into the immortal body of the divine Person.

These nine stages also are lucidly explained in Rûpa Gosvâmin's *Bhakti-Rasa-Amrita-Sindhu* ("Ocean of the Immortal Essence of Devotion").[17] They form part of a ladder of continuous ascent to ever more fervent devotion and thus to union with the Divine. Supporting this process is the disposition of faith (*shraddhâ*), which is true of all traditional forms of Yoga. In Vyâsa's *Yoga-Bhâshya* (1.20), faith is said to be like a good, protective mother. As noted before, faith is different from belief. Whereas belief is of the nature of an opinion, faith is the disposition of trust in the spiritual Reality and the yogic process leading to it. Faith is emphasized already in the ancient *Rig-Veda*:

With faith the [sacrificial] fire is kindled. With faith the oblation is offered.

With speech I glorify [the Goddess] Faith [who is seated] upon Bhaga's head. (10.151.1)

We invoke faith at dawn, faith at midday, faith at sunset. O Faith, establish faith within us! (10.151.5)

Remarkably, the *Bhâgavata-Purâna* (7.1.30) acknowledges the liberating power of emotions other than love—such as fear, sexual desire, and even hatred—so long as their object is the Divine. The secret behind this is simple enough: In order to fear God (as did Kamsa), feel hatred for the Divine (as did Shishupâla), or approach the Lord with burning sexual love (as did the cowgirls of Vrindavâna in the case of the God-man Krishna), a person must place his or her attention on the Divine. This focus creates a bridge across which the eternally given grace can enter and transform that person's life, even to the point of enlightenment, provided the emotion is intense enough. Thus the content of the emotion is less important than its object. The *Vishnu-Purâna* tells the story of King Shishupâla, who hated the Divine, in the form of Vishnu, so intensely that he thought about God constantly and in the process achieved enlightenment. This involuntary spiritual practice bears the name *dvesha-yoga*, meaning "Yoga of hatred."

In the path of Bhakti-Yoga, the devotee feels a growing passion (*rati*) for the Lord, and this helps him or her to break down one barrier after another between the human personality and the divine Person. This increasing love culminates in the vision of the cosmos penetrated, saturated, and sustained by the Lord. This is the kind of vision that overwhelmed and awed Prince Arjuna, as described in the famous eleventh chapter of the *Bhagavad-Gîtâ*. Witnessing the divine splendor of Lord Krishna, Arjuna exclaimed:

O God, in your Body I behold the deities and all the various kinds of beings, the Lord Brahma seated on the lotus throne, and all the seers and divine serpents! (11.15)

Everywhere I behold you [who are] of endless Form, with many arms, bellies, mouths, and eyes. I can see no end, middle, or beginning in you, O All-Lord, All-Form! (11.16)

I behold you with diadem, mace, and discus—a mass of brilliance, flaming all round. You are hard to see, for you are immeasurable, entirely a brilliant radiance of sun-fire. (11.17)

Beholding that great Form of yours, with its many mouths and eyes, its many arms, thighs, feet, bellies, and formidable fangs, O strong-armed [Krishna], the worlds shudder, and so do I. (11.23)

With flaming mouths, you lick up and devour all the worlds entirely. Filling the whole universe with your brilliance, your dread-inspiring rays blaze forth, O Vishnu. (11.30)

Tell me who you of dread-inspiring Form are. Salutations be to you! O foremost God, have mercy! I wish to know you [as you were] at first [in your human form], for I do not comprehend your Creativity (*pravritti*). (11.31)

The final moment of realization, when the devotee merges with the Divine, is described in the *Bhagavad-Gîtâ* as supreme love-participation (*para-bhakti*). Prior to that event, devotion requires that God be faced as an Other, who can be worshiped in song, ritual action, or meditation. After that moment, however, the Divine and the devotee are inseparably merged in love, though most schools of Bhakti-Yoga insist that this mystical merging is not one of total identification with God. The Divine is experienced as infinitely more comprehensive than the devotee, who is rather like a conscious cell within the incommensurable body of God.

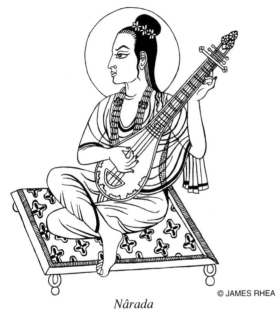

*Nârada*

© JAMES RHEA

In his *Bhakti-Sûtra*, Sage Nârada distinguishes between a primary and a secondary type of devotion. The latter is tinged by personal goals and ulterior motives, such as the desire to be protectively embraced by the Lord or to be aided by him in worldly affairs. It can express itself in many different ways. Depending on the predominance of one of the three qualities (*guna*) of Nature, the devotee's love for the Divine can be more or less self-centered and more or less active.[18] By contrast, primary devotion is total surrender to God, pure devotion free of selfish motivation. As Nârada puts it in the *Bhakti-Sûtra* (5), the true devotee "sees nothing but love, hears only about love, speaks only of love, and thinks

of love alone." The great scholar Surendranath Dasgupta characterized this advanced spiritual practitioner as follows:

> Such a person is so attached to God that there is nothing else for which he cares; without any effort on his part, other attachments and inclinations lose their hold over him. So great is his passion for God that it consumes all his earthly passion . . .
>
> The *bhakta* who is filled with such a passion does not experience it merely as an undercurrent of joy which waters the depths of his heart in his own privacy, but as a torrent that overflows the caverns of his heart into all his senses. Through all his senses he realizes it as if it were a sensuous delight; with his heart and soul he feels it as a spiritual intoxication of joy. Such a person is beside himself with this love of God. He sings, laughs, dances and weeps. He is no longer a person of this world.[19]

Bhakti-Yoga is often cited as an example of a typical dualist teaching, but dualism is not true of all schools of this branch of Yoga. Even though at the outset all devotees relate to the Divine as a Person who is a separate being, the final goal of some schools is to merge so completely with the Divine that there is utter forgetfulness of one's own being: The Lord is realized as the only Reality there is—a realization that annuls the illusion of the ego-personality and thus transcends the notion of being a separate entity, or devotee.

## The History of the Bhakti Ideal

The devotional approach in India has a fascinating history that we know only imperfectly. There are only a few hymns in the *Vedas* that suggest a passionate emotional relationship to the invoked deity. The imagery of the Vedic invocations is lofty but aloof, lacking the devotional pathos typical of the medieval *bhakti* literature. Yet devotionalism is by no means absent from the Vedic hymns.

Thus the opening hymn of the *Rig-Veda* is in praise of God Agni, who is said to be "worthy of praise by past and present seers" (1.2), and who is asked to make himself easily accessible "like a father is to a son" (1.9). Hymn 8.14.10 speaks of the praise of Indra rushing onward "like exhilarating waves of water." In hymn 1.171.1, Sage Agastya addresses Indra and the Maruts thus: "To you I come with this homage, and with a hymn I request the kindness of the mighty." The Vedic hymns are full of mythological allusions, poetic metaphors, and petitions, as well as demands. Above all, the seers were praying for immortality (*amrita*) in the company of the deities.

Let us recall here that the word *ric*, which for euphonic reasons is modified to *rig* in the compound name *Rig-Veda*, means "praise." This in itself reflects the basic devotional attitude of the ancient Vedic seers and priests. The Vedic hymns are invocations to various higher powers and reverential celebration, and in them we find the earliest historical roots of Bhakti-Yoga.

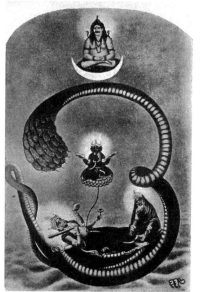

Reproduced from The Gods of India

*Nârâyana*

However, this Vedic devotionalism occurred in the context of an elaborate sacrificial religion that, over time, became ever more sophisticated and demanding. By the time of the *Brâhmanas*—texts explaining the Vedic rituals and mythological allusions—the exacting sacrificial ritualism seems to have stifled the devotional element. The proper performance of the various rituals and appeasement of the deities or their enlisting in the sacrificial tasks had become more important than personal devotion to the Divine. Perhaps the never-ending demands of ritualism caused many priests to be motivated more by a sense of duty than a heart overflowing with emotions of spiritual longing or gratitude.

Not surprisingly, the monotheistic Pancarâtra tradition early on attracted a growing number of people who found the Vedic pantheon of deities unconvincing or the impersonal Absolute (*brahman*) of the orthodox theologians too abstract, or who derived no emotional satisfaction from the brahmins' sacrificial ritualism. The Pancarâtra tradition catered to those who longed for personal intimacy with the Divine, and their worship revolved around God Vasudeva-Nârâyana-Vishnu. Already the *Shata-Patha-Brâhmana* (13.6.1) mentions a *pancarâtra* sacrifice in association with God Nârâyana, and the *Mahâbhârata* (12.335) speaks of Sage Nara as a devotee of Nârâyana and as hosting many sages well versed in the system of Pancarâtra.[20] Thus, this tradition originated long before the time of the Buddha, and it flourished at the margins of the ancient Indic society. Although it was certainly not looked upon favorably by the Vedic priesthood, it nevertheless made its mark within the orthodox fold.

It was largely because of the success of this religio-spiritual tradition—epitomized in the immense popularity of the *Bhagavad-Gîtâ* and the *Bhâgavata-Purâna*—that Hinduism came to be what it is today: a religious culture of temples, sacred imagery, and devotional worship. The Pancarâtra tradition, which is sometimes referred to as Bhâgavatism, also was instrumental in the post-Vedic development of Yoga. It introduced the concept and practice of *bhakti* into what was all too often a somewhat heady or dry approach to Self-realization.

Although the *bhakti* path was originally most intimately associated with the religious worship of God Vishnu, the word *bhakti* is used in the technical sense in an early scripture dedicated to God Shiva. This is the *Shvetâshvatara-Upanishad* (6.23), a powerfully monotheistic work usually assigned to the third or fourth century B.C.E., but probably belonging to the pre-Buddhist era. This text introduces the dual idea of love for God and love for the spiritual teacher, who should be loved in the same manner as the Divine, since he or she is its embodiment.

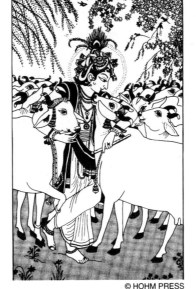

© HOHM PRESS

*Lord Krishna, lover of all creatures*

In order to appreciate the evolution of the *bhakti* path, we must understand that the monotheistic teachings were developed largely, though not exclusively, in two religious circles, namely Vaishnavism (largely carried by the Pancarâtra tradition) and Shaivism. The Vaishnavas celebrate God Vishnu—often in his Krishna incarnation—as the divine Person, and the Shaivas dedicate their lives to Lord Shiva. Both Vishnu and Shiva

are mentioned in the *Rig-Veda*, and we may assume that they have had worshipers since those early days. However, as full-fledged religious movements, Vaishnavism and Shaivism become fully visible only during the second half of the first millennium B.C.E. Early sects of the latter movement were the Pâshupatas, the Kâpâlikas, and the Kâlâmukhas, which are treated in Chapter 11.

A third significant strand of religious development, which also has its roots in the *Rig-Veda*, is known as Shaktism. It centers on the worship of the Divine in its feminine or power aspect—as Shakti. In this movement, too, *bhakti* plays an important role as part of the ritual worship of the Goddess, whether it be Mahâdevî, Kâlî, Durgâ, Pârvatî, Annapûrnâ, Cândî, Sâtî, or any of the other female deities of Hinduism. In the early centuries of the Common Era, Shaktism merged more and more with Tantra, though without losing its independent identity altogether.

The *Bhagavad-Gîtâ*, a Vaishnava scripture belonging possibly to the sixth century B.C.E., uses the word *bhakti* extensively. It stands for the proper relationship between the spiritual practitioner and the Divine (in the form of Lord Krishna). Significantly, however, in this work *bhakti* refers not only to the path of devotion but also to the goal of liberation. For Lord Krishna, *bhakti* is the alpha and omega of spiritual life. Vaishnavism became increasingly popular in the early centuries of the Common Era, attracting large numbers of adherents in both North and South India.

In medieval times, the Shaiva community created a counterpart to the ever more popular

*Bhagavad-Gîtâ*, namely the *Îshvara-Gîtâ*, which is embedded in the second part of the *Kûrma-Purâna* (chapter 11). This poetic composition, which is dated slightly later than the *Bhâgavata-Purâna* (c. 900 C.E.), belongs to an era in which the *bhakti* path was broadened into a cultural movement that swept across the entire Indian peninsula. A comparable event occurred in medieval Europe, in the thirteenth and fourteenth centuries, when thousands of Christian women discovered the power of the heart through Jesus mysticism.

The *bhakti* ideal found enthusiastic reception especially in South India, where the path of devotion was developed by both the Shaiva and the Vaishnava communities. Thousands of Tamil and Sanskrit works extolling the virtue of devotion in its various forms were created in the millennium between 200 B.C.E. and 800 C.E.

Among the Shiva devotees of Tamilnadu (South India), who created the theological system of Shaiva-Siddhânta, *bhakti* played an important role already in the centuries prior to the Common Era. Thus, in the wonderful *Tiru-Mantiram* ("Sacred Words") of Tirumûlar (often placed c. 200 B.C.E.–100 C.E., but probably 700 C.E.) the Tamil terms *patti* and *anpu* are explicitly mentioned; both these terms are synonyms of the Sanskrit word *bhakti*. Tirumûlar's work forms the tenth book of the *Tiru-Murai*, which has been called the Tamil Shaiva equivalent of the *Vedas* of North India. It was compiled fairly late (in the eleventh century C.E.) by Nambiyândâr Nambi. (The Vaishnavas of the South also claim a *"Veda"* of their own in the form of the *Tiru-Vâymoli*, which will be introduced shortly.) The *Tiru-Murukâr-Ruppatai* of Nakkîrar, a poetical composition found in the eleventh book of the *Tiru-Murai*, speaks of the *bhakta*'s quest for liberation at the feet of God Murukan (or Muruga).

Among the Vaishnava minority of South India, the *bhakti* ideal and the worship of God Vishnu were particularly promoted by the Âlvârs, a group of twelve saintly *bhaktas* (including only one woman). They sang their songs of praise in the seventh or eighth century C.E., though tradition places them as far back as the period 4203–2706 B.C.E. The northern branches of Vaishnavism and Shaivism likewise popularized the *bhakti* approach in their own distinct fashion.

The Âlvârs were followed by the so-called Âcâryas ("Preceptors"), who attempted to systematize the monotheistic theology of Vaishnavism. Foremost among them was Râmânuja (1017–1137 C.E.), a southern brahmin. He was the principal exponent of Vishishta-Advaita, or "Qualified Nondualism." His contribution to Hinduism equals that of Shankara, for what Râmânuja did was to make the idea of a suprapersonal divine Being logically consistent with the teaching of Vedântic nondualism. He succeeded in integrating the northern and southern traditions of Vaishnavism, thereby greatly strengthening the religious worship of Vishnu and paving the way for the medieval *bhakti-mârga*, or "way of devotion."

Râmânuja formulated a Yoga that is radically different from Patanjali's system in that the cultivation of *bhakti* is given prominence over meditation. For Râmânuja, devotion was not only the means to liberation but the goal of all spiritual endeavor. According to this school, there is no end to spiritual practice.

The history of the *bhakti* approach is vastly complex, and modern scholarship has only scratched the surface. In particular the traditions of South India have been badly neglected. What is clear, however, is that India has not only had its share of world-denying mystics but can also take pride in its many generations of thousands of love-intoxicated seekers and realizers.

The teachers of this movement hail *bhakti* as the easiest way to emancipation. Loving devotion to the Lord bears fruit readily when it is constant, unswerving, and purposeless. The *gopîs*, or cowgirls, of the Krishna legends symbolize that attitude perfectly. In their ardor for the God-man Krishna, they ignored everything—their husbands, children, family, friends, and daily duties. They were simply intoxicated with love, and it was their love that brought them closer to the divine essence of the beautiful young Krishna who was really God incarnate.

We will return to the Shaiva and Vaishnava communities and their devotional practices in Chapters 11 and 12.

---

**SOURCE READING 4**

## *Bhakti-Sûtra of Nârada*

The *Bhakti-Sûtra* of Sage Nârada is one of two *Sûtras* expounding the path of *bhakti*. This popular work was probably composed around 1000 C.E. It is thus slightly later than the *Bhakti-Sûtra* of Shândilya, which is more technical and abstruse. Nârada's scripture consists of eighty-four aphorisms (*sûtra*) distributed over five chapters. Unlike the *Bhagavad-Gîtâ*, it does not seek to integrate the distinct approaches of devotion, action, and knowledge. Instead it places *bhakti* above all other paths.

## Book I

Now then, we will expound love (*bhakti*). (1)

In this [book of aphorisms], this [love is understood to be of] the essence of supreme love (*para-prema*). (2)

And [it is of] the quintessence of immortality. (3)

Having obtained it, a man becomes perfect, becomes immortal, becomes content. (4)

Having reached it, he does not desire anything, does not grieve, not hate, not rejoice, and is not overactive. (5)

Having known it, he becomes intoxicated, he becomes immobilized [in ecstasy], he comes to delight in the Self. (6)

It is not of the nature of desire, because it is of the essence of restriction (*nirodha*).[21] (7)

Restriction, however, is the resignation of [all] secular and religious activities [to the Divine]. (8)

In that [resignation] is "non-otherness" and indifference toward [all things that are] antagonistic to that [love]. (9)

"Non-otherness" (*ananyatâ*) is the abandonment of [all] other refuges. (10)

Indifference (*udâsînatâ*) to secular and religious [things that are] antagonistic to that [love] is the performance [of actions that are] in consonance with that [love]. (11)

Let there be heedfulness about the teaching [even] after steadfastness of conviction [has been gained]. (12)

Otherwise [there is always] the possibility of falling [from grace]. (13)

Thus [there should be heedfulness] also about secular [activities] such as the activity of eating until the end of the maintenance of the body [due to natural death]. (14)

The characteristics of that [love] are described differently owing to differences of opinion. (15)

Pârâsharya [claims that love is] devotion to worship and so forth. (16)

Garga [states that love is devotion] to sacred stories (*kathâ*) and so forth. (17)

Shândilya [declares that love is that which is] not antagonistic to the Self's [innate] delight. (18)

Nârada, again, [insists that love is when] all conduct is consecrated to Him, [and that it also is the experience of] extreme agitation upon forgetting Him. (19)

There is [more than one example] of this. (20)

Like [the love] of the cowgirls of Vraja. (21)

Also, with regard to this, the imputation [that the cowgirls were] forgetful of the knowledge of [God's] glory [and merely loved the God-man Krishna for conventional reasons], is not [true]. (22)

Lacking that [knowledge of God's glory, they would have been] like adulterers. (23)

In such [adulterous passion], the happiness is not the happiness [innate to] this [glory]. (24)

# Book II

This [love] is even superior to ritual (*karma*), knowledge (*jnâna*), and the [conventional types of] Yoga. (25)

[This is so,] because [love is of] the essence of the fruit [of all these approaches]. (26)

Moreover, [love is superior to any other path,] because of the Lord's dislike for conceit and because of His fondness for [the devotee's mood of] humility (*dainya*). (27)

According to some, knowledge alone is the means for this [love]. (28)

According to others, there is interdependence of the various [means]. (29)

Brahmakumâra [i.e., Nârada, maintains that love is of] the essence of its own fruit. (30)

[This is so,] because there is the example of the king, the house, and the food, etc.[22] (31)

Not by that [recognition of his true parentage] is the king satisfied, nor [is there any satisfaction beyond] the appeasement of hunger. (32)

Therefore this [love] alone is to be followed by the seekers of liberation. (33)

# Book III

The teachers praise [the following] means for [realizing] it. (34)

That [love], however, [is realized] through the renunciation of objects and through the renunciation of clinging. (35)

[Love is realized] through constant dedication. (36)

[Love is further realized] through singing and hearing the Lord's attributes even [while engaged] in secular [activities]. (37)

[Love is realized] mainly through the grace of a great one or through a [mere] particle of the Lord's grace. (38)

But contact with a great one is difficult to obtain, [although his blessing] is incomprehensible and infallible. (39)

Even so, [love] is realized by the grace of these alone. (40)

[This is so,] because of the absence of difference in Him and in His creatures. (41)

That [love] alone is to be followed. That alone is to be followed. (42)

Bad company is to be avoided in every respect. (43)

[Bad company is to be avoided,] because it causes desire, anger, delusion, confusion of memory, and loss of wisdom. (44)

Even though these arise as [mere] waves, they become an ocean due to clinging (*sanga*). (45)

Who crosses, who indeed crosses [the ocean of] illusion (*mâyâ*)? He who abandons clinging, who frequents the great experience [of ecstatic love] free from [the sense of] "mine" . . . (46)

. . . who frequents solitary places, and who uproots the thralldom to the world becomes free of the triple qualities [of Nature] and abandons [all idea of] gain or hoarding . . . (47)

. . . who abandons the fruit of actions, [even] renounces actions, and thence becomes oppositeless (*nirdvandva*) . . . (48)

. . . who renounces even [the ritual actions enjoined] in the *Vedas*, and obtains undisturbed longing [for God] . . . (49)

—he crosses, he indeed crosses, he [even] saves the world. (50)

# Book IV

The essence of love is indescribable. (51)

Like the taste of a dumb [person]. (52)

[Love] is ever manifested in a [fit] recipient. (53)

[Love] is devoid of the qualities [of Nature], devoid of desire, continually growing, unbroken, extremely subtle, and of the essence of [transcendental] experience (*anubhava*). (54)

Having realized that [love], he sees only that, he hears only that, [he speaks only that], he ponders only that. (55)

Secondary [love] is threefold due to the distinctions in the qualities [of Nature] or due to the distinctions of being distressed, and so forth. (56)

Each preceding [quality of Nature: *sattva*, *rajas*, *tamas*] is [more conducive] to the good than each subsequent [quality].[23] (57)

In [comparison with this secondary] love, the other [i.e., the supreme love] is more easily realizable. (58)

[The supreme love is more easily realizable,] because it is independent from other evidence and owing to its self-evident [character]. (59)

[This is also true] because [the supreme love is of] the essence of peace and of the essence of supreme bliss (*parama-ânanda*). (60)

In the event of worldly lack, worry is not to be entertained, because the self is to be surrendered in [all] secular and religious [activities]. (61)

Upon attaining that [supreme love], secular activity is not to be abandoned, but the renunciation of the fruit [of one's actions should be practiced], and the means for it [are to be diligently cultivated]. (62)

The conduct of women, wealthy folk, and atheists should not be listened to.[24] (63)

Conceit, hypocrisy, and so forth should be abandoned. (64)

The consecration of one's conduct to Him, [including] desire, anger, conceit, and so on, are to be directed toward Him alone. (65)

Love consisting of constant devotion as of a servant or constant [devotion] as of a wife, preceded by the dispersion of the three types [of reactivity, as mentioned in the preceding aphorism], should be practiced; love alone should be practiced. (66)

# Book V

The radical (*ekântin*) devotees are foremost. (67)

Conversing with each other with choking throat and tears of ecstasy, they purify their families and the earth. (68)

They render sacred places (*tîrtha*) sacred; they render actions right; they endow scriptures with true meaning. (69)

They are filled with Him. (70)

The ancestors rejoice, the Gods dance, and this earth obtains a protector [in a true devotee]. (71)

In them there is no distinction of birth, knowledge, beauty, family, wealth, profession, and so forth. (72)

Because they are His. (73)

Controversy is not to be engaged. (74)

[This is demanded] because there is room for diversity and owing to the translogical nature (*aniyatatva*) [of God]. (75)

The scriptures on love are to be pondered; actions awakening it are to be taken. (76)

When "marking" time—having given up pleasure, sorrow, desire, gain, and so forth—not even half an instant should be spent uselessly. (77)

Practices like nonharming, truthfulness, purity, liberality, faith (*âstikya*), and so on should be cultivated. (78)

The Lord should ever be worshipped with one's entire being by a carefree [devotee]. (79)

He, being praised, swiftly manifests to the devotees and makes them realize [His true nature beyond space and time]. (80)

Only love for the triple truth is greater; only love is greater. (81)

[Love], though singular, is elevenfold: [It takes] the forms of attachment (*âsakti*) through the glorification of [God's] attributes; attachment to His beauty; attachment through worship; attachment through remembrance [of His names]; attachment through service; attachment through friendship [with Him]; attachment through affection [for Him]; attachment of a lover; attachment of self-surrender; attachment of uniformity [with His ultimate nature]; attachment in one's separation from the Supreme. (82)

Thus declare the preceptors of love unanimously and fearless of people's prattle: Kumâra, Vyâsa, Shuka, Shândilya, Garga, Vishnu, Kaundinya, Shesha, Uddhava, Âruni, Bali, Hanumat, Vibhîshana, and so forth. (83)

He who trusts and believes this auspicious exposition declared by Nârada, he becomes loving; he reaches the Beloved; he reaches the Beloved. (84)

## VI. *KARMA-YOGA—FREEDOM IN ACTION*

To exist is to act. Even an inanimate object such as a rock has movement. And the building blocks of matter, the atomic particles, are in fact no building blocks at all but incredibly complex

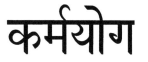
*Karma-yoga*

patterns of energy in constant motion. Thus, the universe is a vast vibratory expanse. In the words of philosopher Alfred North Whitehead, the world is *process*. It is on this insight, commonplace as it may seem, that Karma-Yoga is founded.

The word *karma* (or *karman*), derived from the root *kri* ("to make" or "to do"), has many meanings. It can signify "action," "work," "product," "effect," and so on. Thus Karma-Yoga is literally the Yoga of Action. But here the term *karma* stands for a particular kind of action. Specifically, it denotes an inner attitude toward action, which is itself a form of action. What this attitude consists in is spelled out in the *Bhagavad-Gîtâ*, which is the earliest scripture to teach Karma-Yoga.

Not by abstention from actions does a man enjoy action-transcendence, nor by renunciation alone does he approach perfection. (3.4)

For, not even for a moment can anyone ever remain without performing action. Everyone is unwittingly made to act by the qualities (*guna*) issuing from Nature. (3.5)

He who restrains his organs of action but sits remembering in his mind the objects of the senses is called a self-bewildered hypocrite. (3.6)

So, O Arjuna, more excellent is he who, controlling the senses with his mind, embarks unattached on Karma-Yoga with his organs of action. (3.7)

You must do the allotted action, for action is superior to inaction; not even your body's processes (*yâtrâ*) can be accomplished by inaction. (3.8)

This world is action-bound, save when this action is [intended] as sacrifice. With that purpose, O son of Kuntî, engage in action devoid of attachment. (3.9)

Therefore always perform unattached the proper (*kârya*) deed, for the man who performs action without attachment attains the Supreme. (3.19)

Then God Krishna, who communicates this teaching to his pupil Arjuna, points to himself as the archetypal model of the active person:

For Me, O son of Pritha, there is nothing to be done in the three worlds, nothing ungained to be gained—and yet I engage in action. (3.22)

For, if I were not untiringly ever to abide in action, O son of Pritha, everywhere people would follow My "track" [that is, My example]. (3.23)

If I were not to perform action, these worlds would perish, and I would be the author of chaos, destroying [all] creatures. (3.24)

Just as the unwise act attached to action, O son of Bharata, the wise should act unattached, desiring the world's welfare. (3.25)

By the qualities (*guna*) of Nature, actions are everywhere performed. [Yet, he whose] self is deluded by the ego (*ahamkâra*) thinks: "I am the doer." (3.27)

But, O strong-armed one, the knower of Reality [who understands] the relationship between the qualities and action is unattached and thinks: "Qualities dwell upon qualities." (3.28)

Always performing all [allotted] actions and taking refuge in Me, he attains through My grace the eternal, immutable State. (18.56)

Renouncing in thought all actions to Me, intent on Me, resorting to Buddhi-Yoga, be constantly "Me-minded." (18.57)

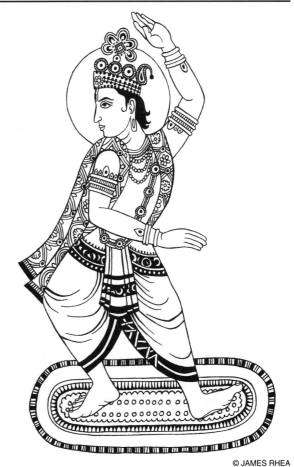

© JAMES RHEA

*Krishna*

What Krishna, the divine Lord in human form, is saying here is that all activity arises spontaneously as part of the program of Nature (*prakriti*). The idea that "I do this or that" is delusional, a fatal presumption that we habitually superimpose on what is actually occurring. Thus, even our thoughts are not really generated by us. Thoughts, like all processes of Nature, are simply arising. We decide to type into a computer, play the piano, ride a bicycle, or speak to a friend—but these activities, according to Krishna (and the spiritual authorities of Hinduism in general), are not effects of the ego-personality in relation to which they seem to be occurring. In fact, the ego-sense itself arises as one of the spontaneous activities of Nature, presuming itself to be the actor of certain deeds and then presuming itself to suffer their consequences.

The objective of Karma-Yoga is stated to be "action freedom." The actual Sanskrit term is *naishkarmya*, which literally means "nonaction." But this literal meaning is misleading, because it is not inactivity that is meant to be expressed here. Rather, *naishkarmya-karman* corresponds to the Taoist notion of *wu-wei*, or inaction in action. That is to say, Karma-Yoga is about freedom *in* action, or the transcendence of egoic motivations. When the illusion of the ego as acting subject is transcended, then actions are recognized to occur spontaneously. Without the interference of the ego, their spontaneity appears as a smooth flow. Hence, truly enlightened beings have an economy and elegance of movement about them that is generally absent in unenlightened individuals. Behind the action of the enlightened being there is no author; or we could say that Nature itself is the author.

Since, by definition, life is action, even any apparent inaction must be understood as a form of action. The principle of Karma-Yoga applies universally. This means that even the renouncers in the tradition of *samnyâsa*, who formally abstain from secular activity, are still bound *to* action and bound *by* their actions, unless their withdrawal from the world is done in the spirit of Karma-Yoga.

Through Karma-Yoga, whether one lives the life of a householder or of a renouncer, every action is turned into a sacrifice. What is sacrificed is, in the last analysis, the self or ego. So long as the ego (*ahamkâra*) is the author behind actions or inactions, these actions or inactions have a binding power. They reinforce the ego and thereby obstruct the event of enlightenment. Egoic action or inaction generates karma.

The word *karma* has become part of the English language, and *Webster's* explains it as "the force generated by a person's actions held in Hinduism and Buddhism to perpetuate transmigration and in its ethical consequences to determine his destiny in his next existence." This definition is essentially correct. Karma is not only action but also its invisible result that shapes a person's destiny.

The underlying idea is that we are what we are because of what we do or, rather, *how* we do it. In our actions, we express who or what we are (or presume ourselves to be). In other words, we externalize our inner being, so that our actions are a reflection of ourselves. But they are not only reflections. There is a "feedback loop" between our actions and our being. Every action acts upon our self and contributes to the entire structure of the person we tend to be.

Thus, put simply, if someone tends to be a good-hearted, benign individual, his or her actions are apt to be what would be judged good or benign, and they in turn reinforce that person's native good-heartedness and benignity. On the other hand, if someone tends to be mean and destructive, his or her actions are likely to be of the kind that would be judged mean and destructive, and they in turn reinforce that individual's native meanness and destructiveness.

Actions and inactions have their immediate, visible results, which may or may not have been intended. But just as important is their invisible aftereffect on the quality of our being, about which we in the West are mostly ignorant. We may send in our monthly donation to our favorite charity and thereby obtain various advantages such as a tax break—the visible results of our action—but we also set in motion invisible forces that shape and transform our being and thus our future destiny: We reap what we sow. That India's religious geniuses have understood this very clearly is evident from the karma doctrine.

The link between action and its feedback effects is thought to be an iron law—or what has been called the law of moral causation. It appears that the karmic law is the only immutable aspect of our world of constant change, the *samsâra*. It governs the cosmos on all its countless levels, and only the transcendental Reality itself is free of this peculiar arrangement.

This teaching is closely associated with another widespread belief, shared by all Hindu, Buddhist, and Jaina schools. This is the notion that the human being is a multidimensional structure or process, which does not come to an abrupt end with the death of the physical body. Diverse traditions have offered varying explanations for this postmortem continuity, and the interpretations range from naive to rather sophisticated. According to some, the surviving consciousness is clothed in a nonmaterial body awaiting its renewed incarnation on the material plane in another physical body, or on one of the supramaterial (or "subtle") planes in a supraphysical body. According to others, the ego-consciousness does not survive the death of the body, so that there is, strictly speaking, no stable transmigrating entity but only a continuity of different "karmic" forces.

All schools are agreed that the mechanics of destiny on the physical plane and on any other level of existence are controlled by the quality of a person's action or, more accurately, his or her *intention*. Karma-Yoga is the art and science of "karmically" aware and responsible action and intention. Its immediate purpose is to prevent the accumulation of unfavorable karmic effects and to reverse the effects of existing karma.

Karma-Yoga implies a complete reversal of human nature, for it demands that every action is performed out of a disposition that is radically distinct from our everyday mood. Not only are we asked to assume responsibility for appropriate (*kârya*) action but also to offer up our work and its fruit (*phala*) to the divine Person. Such offering (*arpana*), however, necessarily entails a self-offering, or the surrender of the ego. Karma-Yoga thus involves considerably more than doing one's duty. It goes beyond conventional morality and involves a profound spiritual attitude. The "easy" discipline of Karma-Yoga, when adopted conscientiously, becomes a fiery practice of self-transcendence.

Action performed in the spirit of self-surrender has benign invisible effects. It improves the quality of our being and makes us a source of spiritual uplift for others. Lord Krishna, in the *Bhagavad-Gîtâ*, speaks of the *karma-yogin*'s working for the welfare of the world. The Sanskrit phrase he uses is *loka-samgraha*, which literally means "world gathering" or "pulling people together." What it refers to is this: Our own personal wholeness, founded in self-surrender, actively transforms our social environment, contributing to its wholeness. But this is not the ultimate goal of the *karma-yogin*, only an intermediate effect of the practice of inaction in action.

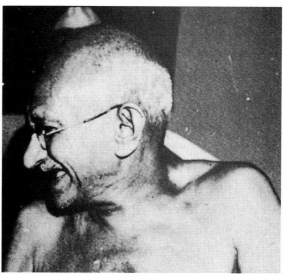

*Reproduced from* Traveler's India

*"Mahatma" Gandhi, a consummate karma-yogin*

"Mahatma" Gandhi was modern India's most superb example of a *karma-yogin* in action. He worked tirelessly on himself and for the welfare of the Indian nation. In pursuing the lofty ideal of Karma-Yoga, Gandhi had to give up his life. He did so without rancor, with the name of God—"Ram"—on his lips. He embraced his destiny, trusting that none of his spiritual efforts could ever be lost, as is indeed the solemn promise of Lord Krishna in the *Bhagavad-Gîtâ*, which Gandhi read daily. Gandhi believed in the inevitability of karma, but he also believed in the freedom of the human will.

It should be noted here that the law of karma does not intrinsically encourage fatalism, even though some individuals and schools of thought have taken this stance. On the contrary, it is a call to assume responsibility for one's destiny. This call is made in all the psychospiritual traditions of India, which, as liberation teachings, insist on the freedom of will: We are free to turn toward the transcendental Reality or toward conditional existence under the thrall of karma.

The fulcrum of Karma-Yoga is that we can transcend all karmic necessity *in our consciousness*. We still have to endure certain karmic results (such as illness, misfortune, and of course death), but these need not determine our being: In our essence we are free, and the *yogin* who has realized the Self is abundantly aware of this truth. Action can improve the quality of our being and destiny, and this is the intent behind conventional religiosity: A person does good deeds because he or she wants to be spared the terrible blows of bad karma and instead enter one of the delightful celestial realms after dropping the physical body.

Karma-Yoga, however, aims at the transcendence of all possible destinies in the conditional realms of the multilevel cosmos. The *karma-yogin* aspires to the Unconditional beyond good and evil, pain and pleasure, beyond karmic necessity and embodiment. For when the Self is realized there is only bliss, and from this position the machine of Nature cannot touch our true being. A Self-realized *yogin* may still suffer all kinds of adversities—Sri Ramana Maharshi, one of modern India's greatest sages, died of cancer—but he knows himself to be infinitely above the arising qualities of conditional existence. The enlightened adept is the eternal Essence behind all possible qualities—whether desirable or undesirable—that impinge upon the physical body or the personality associated with it. Herein lies his triumph over the body, the mind, and all other finite aspects of human nature.

Historically, Karma-Yoga can be regarded as the countering response of the conservative forces in ancient India to the growing social movement of world renunciation. Spiritually, however, it is much more than a compromise solution between conventional life (whether religious or secular) and the life of a forest-dwelling ascetic or wandering mendicant. It is an integral teaching that transcends both worldliness and otherworldliness.

Therefore, the *Bhagavad-Gîtâ* with its integrated Karma-Yoga, Bhakti-Yoga, and Jnâna-Yoga represents a genuine innovation.[25] Its teachings have had a lasting influence on many other Hindu traditions. This wonderful scripture is dealt with in more detail in Chapter 8.

Another work that must be mentioned in the present context is the *Yoga-Vâsishtha*, composed well over a thousand years after the dialogue between Krishna and Arjuna. Although it espouses a form of nondualism that is so radical as to regard the world to be entirely illusory, it nevertheless favors an outlook that affirms mundane existence. For in this scripture, the *yogin* is encouraged to fully participate in the activities of his family and society. Wisdom (*jnâna*) and action (*karma*) are compared to the two wings of a bird; it needs both to fly. Emancipation is said to be achieved by the harmonious development of both means. More will be said about this in Chapter 14.

A similar teaching can be found in the *Tri-Shikhi-Brâhmana-Upanishad*, a late medieval work:

> Yoga is deemed twofold: Jnâna-Yoga and Karma-Yoga. Now then, O best of brahmins, listen to the Yoga of action (*kriyâ-yoga*). The binding of the undistracted consciousness (*citta*) to an object, O best among the twice-born [i.e., brahmins], is union (*samyoga*). It is attained in two ways: The constant binding of the mind (*manas*) to prescribed action—since action is to be performed—is called Karma-Yoga. The continual binding of consciousness to the supreme Object [i.e., the Self] should be known as Jnâna-Yoga, which is auspicious and yields all accomplishments. He whose mind is immutable,

even though the twofold Yoga characterized here [is followed], goes to the supreme Good, which is of the nature of liberation. (2.23–28)

Karma-Yoga is the most grounded of all yogic approaches. Its great ideal of inaction in action (*naishkarmya-karma*) applies to all other spiritual disciplines and is as relevant today as it was when India's sages first formulated it well over two thousand years ago.

## VII. MANTRA-YOGA—SOUND AS A VEHICLE OF TRANSCENDENCE

Sound is a form of vibration, and it was known as such to the yogis of both ancient and medieval India. According to the dominant theory of the science of sacred sound—known as *mantra-vidyâ* or *mantra-shâstra*—the universe is in a state of vibration (*spanda* or *spandana*). The

## मन्त्रयोग । मन्त्रविद्या । मन्त्रशास्त्र ॥

*Mantra-yoga, mantra-vidyâ, mantra-shâstra*

discovery that sound, particularly repetitive sound, affects consciousness was made a very long time ago, perhaps in the Stone Age. We may safely assume that some form of simple chanting and drumming, possibly with animal bones as drumsticks, was associated with paleolithic rituals. It is not surprising, therefore, that by the time the Vedic civilization was flowering in India, sound (both as ritual speech or chanting and as music) had become a rather sophisticated means of religious expression and spiritual transformation.

The hymns of the *Vedas* are traditionally referred to as *mantras*. There is no adequate

English equivalent for the word *mantra*. It is derived from the root *man* ("to think" or "be intent"), which also is found in the terms *manman* ("to ponder intently"), *manas* ("mind"), *manisha* ("understanding"), *manu* ("wise" or "man"), *mana* ("zeal"), *manyu* ("mood" or "mind"), *mantu* ("ruler"), and *manus* ("human being"). The suffix *tra* in *mantra* suggests instrumentality. However, according to an esoteric explanation it stands for the word *trâna*, meaning "saving." Thus a *mantra* is that which saves the mind from itself, or which leads to salvation through the concentration of the mind.

A *mantra* is sacred utterance, numinous sound, or sound that is charged with psychospiritual power. A *mantra* is sound that empowers the mind, or that is empowered by the mind. It is a vehicle of meditative transformation of the human body-mind and is thought to have magical potency. Ernest Wood (alias Swami Sattwikagraganya), an early Western exponent of Yoga, wrote:

It may be said that there is in all material forms—those that appeal to the ear as well as those that affect the eye—the presence and power of the divine. Everything affects us, according to its form. For example, if you go into a room largely decorated with forms composed of straight lines, you will find that it stimulates your mentality; but if you enter one full of curved and flower-like forms, it will be found to stir the emotions. When, through any of those forms we catch a glimpse of the divine, we call it beauty. Beauty is the power of God touching us direct in material things . . . Mantras, then, are forms of sound prescribed for repetition, calculated to link man with the divine by assisting him in his emotional and mental aspirations. All good poetry is something of a mantra, because it conveys more than the common meaning of its words. All beauty affects us mantrically, but the power of its impressions is often lost by the presence of too much variety and confusion and rapid change.[26]

In his *Tantra-Âloka* (7.3–5), the tenth-century adept and scholar Abhinava Gupta explains the function of *mantras* with the aid of the following simile: A single waterwheel, turning endlessly under the power of the flowing river, can move a series of mechanical contraptions coupled to it. Similarly, a single *mantra*, repeated over and over again, can activate the deities (*devatâ*) associated with it, which then—without further effort on his or her part—become an auspicious force in the transformation of the practitioner's consciousness.

This seems to have been fully understood in Vedic times already. The Sanskrit hymns of the *Vedas*, "visualized" by highly gifted seers, were composed in fifteen different meters that called for punctilious recitation in ritual contexts and required carefully regulated breathing to ensure the necessary accuracy. It is here that we may look for the origins of the later yogic technique of breath control (*prânâyâma*) and Mantra-Yoga. One of the four Vedic hymnodies, the *Sâma-Veda*, contains a large number of hymns that were sung by special priests during the great sacrificial rites; the songs, which are still sung today, sound somewhat like medieval plainchants.

It is a well-known fact that prolonged and concentrated chanting leads to alterations in consciousness. When this effect is combined with the "intoxicating" *soma* draft used in the daily rituals, it is easy to understand why the Vedic seers were experts on altered states of consciousness. It is not known from which plant the *soma* juice was pressed. Some authorities think it was *Asclepias acida*, while others identify it with the fly agaric mushroom,[27] but the latter hypothesis does not seem to be borne out by the Vedic descriptions of the plant and the method of pressing it. That the *soma* draft had a consciousness-altering effect is clear from the hymns themselves, although, at the same time, the "real" *soma* was not the plant pressed and poured during the ritual, but the heavenly nectar of immortality. This hidden *soma*, declares the *Rig-Veda* (10.85.3), "no one tastes." That higher *soma* is said to be brought forth by "skillful visionary thought." The physical *soma* draft merely acts as a trigger for the vision of the divine *soma*.

The most remarkable speculation about sound is found in the Rig-Vedic hymn 1.164, which speaks of Vâc (Latin *vox*, "speech"), a feminine deity, as the "mother" of the *Vedas*. She is said to have four "feet" (*pâda*), or aspects. Three of these are beyond the ken of mortals, and only one is known, belonging to human speech. Only the seers (*rishi*) know how to track down Vâc in her secret dimension. A second hymn (10.71.4) expresses regret at those who see and hear without seeing and hearing Vâc.

In other hymns, Vâc is related to the sacred cows (*vâcas*) who are called "auspiciously voiced." Some experts think that the mooing of cows was associated with the sacred syllable *om*, which is the primal sound of the cosmos. Such an association may well have existed, but to suggest that the sound of an animal, however much it may have been appreciated by the Vedic people, somehow gave rise to the metaphysical speculations surrounding the sacred syllable seems farfetched. At any rate, in these archaic hymns we clearly have the foundations of the later Mantra-Yoga.

The single most important sound in Vedic ritual chanting was *om*, and it is to this day the most widely recognized and venerated sacred phoneme of Hinduism. It is even found in Buddhist Tantrism (e.g., in the Tibetan mantric formula *om mani padme hûm*, "*Om*, jewel in the lotus, *hûm*"). The syllable *om*, which contains "a whole philosophy which many volumes would not suffice to state,"[28] is held to be or to ex-

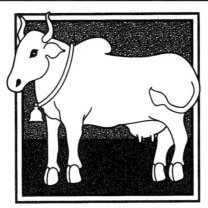

© HINDUISM TODAY
*Sacred cow*

press the pulse of the cosmos itself. It was through meditative practice rather than intellectual speculation that the seers and sages of Vedic times arrived at the idea of a universal sound, eternally resounding in the universe, which they saw as the very origin of the created world. The Vedic seers inwardly heard that sound in their moments of deepest meditation when they had successfully blocked out all external sounds.

The late Agehananda Bharati, a Western Swami and professor of anthropology, made the important observation that a *mantra* is a *mantra* only when it has been imparted by a teacher to a disciple during an initiatory ritual.[29] Thus, the sacred syllable *om* is not a *mantra* to the uninitiated. It acquires its mantric power only through initiation. The *Mantra-Yoga-Samhitâ* (1.5), a work possibly of the eighteenth century C.E, acknowledges this fact when it states:

> Initiation (*dîkshâ*) is the root of all recitation (*japa*);[30] initiation is likewise the root of asceticism; initiation by a true teacher accomplishes all things.

*Mantras*, which may consist of single sounds or a whole string of sounds, can be employed for many different purposes. Originally, *mantras* were undoubtedly used to ward off undesirable powers or events and to attract those that were deemed

desirable, and this is still their predominant application. In other words, *mantras* are used as magical tools. But they are also employed in spiritual contexts as instruments of empowerment, where they aid the aspirant's search for identification with the transcendental Reality. Thus, a Vedântic *mantra* like *aham brahma-asmi*,[31] "I am the Absolute," is a potent affirmation of our fundamental identity as the Self (*âtman*), which also is the Ground of the objective world.

The beginnings of Mantra-Yoga, as we have seen, lie far back in the era of the *Vedas*. But Mantra-Yoga proper is a product of the same philosophical and cultural forces that also gave rise to Tantra in medieval India. In fact, Mantra-Yoga is a principal aspect of the Tantric approach and is treated in numerous works belonging to that spiritual heritage. For this reason its metaphysical or esoteric basis will be discussed in Chapter 17.

There also are a number of scriptures that specifically expound Mantra-Yoga, notably the encyclopedic *Mantra-Mahodadhi* ("Ocean of *Mantras*"), which was composed by Mahîdhara in the late nineteenth century. This text comes complete with an autocommentary entitled *Naukâ* ("Boat"). Other popular and relatively recent works are the *Mantra-Mahârnava* ("Great Ocean of *Mantras*"), the *Mantra-Mukta-Âvalî* ("Independent Tract on *Mantras*"), the *Mantra-Kaumudî* ("Moonlight on *Mantras*"), the *Tattva-Ânanda-Taranginî* ("River of the Bliss of Reality") of the sixteenth-century adept Pûrnânanda, and the *Mantra-Yoga-Samhitâ* ("Compendium of Mantra-Yoga"), authored in the seventeenth or eighteenth century. To these must be added several dictionaries that endeavor to explain the esoteric meaning of *mantras*—a rather dubious enterprise, as is borne out by the fact that these reference works frequently contradict one another. Of these scriptures, only the *Mantra-Mahodadhi* and the *Mantra-Yoga-Samhitâ* are available in English.

According to the last-mentioned text, Mantra-Yoga has sixteen limbs:

1. Devotion (*bhakti*), which is threefold: (a) prescribed devotion (*vaidhi-bhakti*), (b) devotion involving attachment (*râga-âtmika-bhakti*)—that is, which is tainted by egoic motives, and (c) supreme devotion (*para-bhakti*), which yields superlative bliss.

2. Purification (*shuddhi*), which is distinguishable by the following four factors: body, mind, direction, and location. This practice entails (a) cleansing the body, (b) purifying the mind (through faith, study, and the cultivation of various virtues), (c) facing in the right direction during recitation, and (d) using an especially consecrated location for one's practice.

3. Posture (*âsana*), which is meant to stabilize the body during meditative recitation; it is said to comprise two principal forms, namely *svastika-âsana* and the lotus posture (*padma-âsana*),[32] which are both depicted in Chapter 18.

4. "Serving the five limbs" (*panca-anga-sevana*), the daily ritual of reading the *Bhagavad-Gîtâ* ("Lord's Song") and the *Sahasra-Nâma* ("Thousand Names") and reciting songs of praise (*stava*), protection (*kavaca*), and heart-opening (*hridaya*). These five are

thought of as the "limbs" of the Divine; their practice is understood as a powerful means of granting attention and energy to the Divine and thereby becoming assimilated into it.

5. Conduct (*âcâra*), which is of three kinds: divine (*divya*), or that which is beyond worldly activity and renunciation; "left-hand" (*vâma*), which involves worldly activity; and "right-hand" (*dakshina*), which involves renunciation.

6. Concentration (*dhâranâ*), which may have an external or an internal object.

7. "Serving the divine space" (*divya-desha-sevana*), which has sixteen constituent practices that convert a given place into consecrated space.

8. "Breath ritual" (*prâna-kriyâ*), which is said to be singular but accompanied by a variety of practices, such as the various types of placing (*nyâsa*) the life force into different parts of the body.

9. Gesture or "seal" (*mudrâ*), which has numerous forms. These hand gestures are used to focus the mind. They are described in more detail in Chapter 17.

10. "Satisfaction" (*tarpana*), which is the practice of offering libations of water to the deities, thereby delighting them and making them favorably disposed toward the *yogin*.

11. Invocation (*havana*), or calling upon the deity by means of *mantras*.

12. Offering (*bali*), which consists in making gifts of fruit, etc., to the deity. The best offering is deemed to be the gift of oneself.

13. Sacrifice (*yâga*),[33] which can be either external or internal. The inner sacrifice is praised as superior.

14. Recitation (*japa*), which is of three kinds: mental (*mânasa*), quiet (*upâmshu*), and voiced (*vâcika*).

15. Meditation (*dhyâna*), which is manifold, because of the great variety of possible objects of contemplation.

16. Ecstasy (*samâdhi*), which is also known as the "great state" (*mahâ-bhâva*) in which the mind dissolves into the Divine or the chosen deity as a manifestation of the absolute Being.

As is evident from this outline of the sixteenfold path of Mantra-Yoga, this school has a pronounced ritualistic orientation. This reflects well the overall bias of Tantra. Today, when *mantras* are widely sold and published, it is perhaps good to remember that they originated in a sacred setting. Mantra-Yoga has through the ages been presented as the easiest of all approaches to Self-realization. What could possibly be easier than to recite a *mantra*? Yet, it is obvious that this Yoga, in the final analysis, is as demanding as any other. The mindless repetition of *mantras*, especially by the uninitiated, can hardly lead to enlightenment or bliss. Paradoxically, we must be intensely attentive in order to transcend the game of attention and realize the ultimate Being-Consciousness-Bliss. Mantra-Yoga demands the same self-sacrifice as all other forms of Yoga.

## VIII. LAYA-YOGA—DISSOLVING THE UNIVERSE

Laya-Yoga makes meditative "absorption" or "dissolution" (*laya*) its focus. The word *laya* is derived from the root *lî*, meaning "to become dissolved" or "vanish" but also "to cling" and "to remain sticking."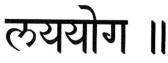

*Laya-yoga*

This dual connotation of the verbal root *lî* is preserved in the word *laya*. The *laya-yogins* seek to meditatively *dissolve* themselves by *clinging* solely to the transcendental Self. They endeavor to transcend all memory traces and sensory experiences by dissolving the microcosm, the mind, into the transcendental Being-Consciousness-Bliss. Their goal is to progressively dismantle their inner universe by way of intense contemplation, until only the singular transcendental Reality, the Self, remains.

The spiritual process has long been understood as one of gradual resorption of "later" aspects of the psychocosmologic evolution into "earlier" ones—that is, the involution of the Many into the One through a progressive simplification of the psyche, or mind. The *Katha-Upanishad* (1.3.13), for instance, speaks of controlling "speech" in the mind (*manas*), the mind in the knowledge identity (*jnâna-âtman*), the knowledge identity (i.e., the sense-derived knowledge) in the "great one" (*mahân*), and the great one (i.e., the higher mind, or *buddhi*) in the supreme Self. Similarly, the *Prashna-Upanishad* (4.8) states that all the various principles of existence, such as the material elements, the subtle elements, the senses, the mind, the higher mind, the ego-sense, awareness (*citta*), and the life force, must be realized as residing in the supreme Self.

Laya-Yoga is a frontal attack on the illusion of individuality. As Shyam Sundar Goswami, who has written the most authoritative book on the subject, explained:

> Layayoga is that form of yoga in which yoga, that is *samâdhi*, is attained through *laya*. *Laya* is deep concentration causing the absorption of the cosmic principles, stage by stage, into the spiritual aspect of the Supreme Power-Consciousness. It is the process of absorption of the cosmic principles in deep concentration, thus freeing consciousness from all that is not spiritual, and in which is held the divine luminous coiled power, termed *kundalinî*.[34]

The spiritual work of the *laya-yogin* appears to have been misunderstood already in medieval times. This is evident from the following stanza found in the *Hatha-Yoga-Pradîpikâ* (4.34), one of the standard manuals of Hatha-Yoga:

> They exclaim "absorption, absorption," but what is the character of absorption? Absorption is the nonremembering of objects as a result of the nonemergence of previously [acquired] impressions (*vâsanâ*).

The "nonremembering of objects" is not a temporary lapse of memory but the condition of objectless or transconceptual ecstasy, or what in Vedânta is called *nirvikalpa-samâdhi*. This state roughly corresponds to *asamprajnâta-samâdhi* in Classical Yoga. In yogic circles, memory is explained as a network of subliminal impressions (*vâsanâ*). These are rather like the scent lingering in the nose after one has smelled a fragrant flower, though they are far less benign, as they

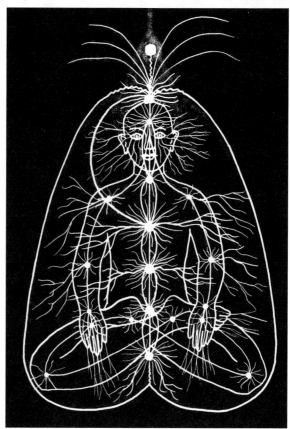

© AUTHOR

*The luminous conduits or currents of the subtle body*

keep us imprisoned in the world of change. Because they are highly dynamic forces, which continually give rise to mental activity, they also are known as "activators" (*samskâra*). In the highest ecstatic state, these subliminal forces are neutralized, preparing the mind for its own dissolution (i.e., transcendence) in the state of enlightenment.

The *laya-yogins* are concerned with transcending these karmic patterns within their own mind to the point at which their inner cosmos becomes dissolved. In this endeavor they utilize many practices and concepts from Tantra-Yoga, which also can be found in Hatha-Yoga, especially the model of the subtle body (*sûkshma-sharîra*) with its psychoenergetic centers (*cakra*) and currents (*nâdî*).

Central to Laya-Yoga, moreover, is the important notion of the *kundalinî-shakti*, the serpent power, which represents the universal life force as manifested in the human body. The arousal and manipulation of this tremendous force also is the principal objective of the *hatha-yogin*. In fact, Laya-Yoga can be understood as the higher, meditative phase of Hatha-Yoga.

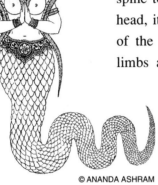

As the awakened *kundalinî* force ascends from the psychoenergetic center at the base of the spine to the crown of the head, it absorbs a portion of the life energy in the limbs and trunk. This is esoterically explained as the reabsorption of the five material elements (*bhûta*) into their subtle counterparts.

© ANANDA ASHRAM

*A pictorial representation of the serpent power*

The body temperature drops measurably in those parts, whereas the crown feels as if on fire and is very warm to the touch. The physiology of this process is not yet understood. Subjectively, however, *yogins* experience a progressive dissolution of their ordinary state of being, until they recover the ever-present Self-Identity (*âtman*) that knows no bodily or mental limits. Also, at the climax of microcosmic dissolution, breathing automatically stops or becomes imperceptible. This is known as "absolute retention" (*kevala-kumbhaka*).

The process of absorption is common to all forms of meditative Yoga, which consists in a progressive withdrawal from the external world and the increasing unification of one's inner environment. However, in Laya-Yoga special attention is paid to the psychoenergetic aspect of

this process. The significance of this will become clearer after reading Chapters 17 and 18.

## IX. INTEGRAL YOGA—A MODERN SYNTHESIS

All the schools of Yoga described so far were creations of premodern India. With Sri Aurobindo's Integral Yoga we enter the modern era. His Yoga is a vivid demonstration that the Yoga tradition, which has always been highly

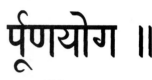

*Pûrna-yoga*

adaptive, is continuing to develop in response to the changing cultural conditions. Integral Yoga is the single most impressive attempt to reformulate Yoga for our modern needs and abilities.

While intent on preserving the continuity of the Yoga tradition, Sri Aurobindo was eager to adapt Yoga to the unique context of the Westernized world of our age. He did this on the basis not only of his own European education but also his profound personal experimentation and experience with spiritual life. He combined in himself the rare qualities of an original philosopher and those of a mystic and sage.

Aurobindo saw in all past forms of Yoga an attempt to transcend the ordinary person's enmeshment in the external world by means of renunciation, asceticism, meditation, breath control, and a whole battery of other yogic means. As I have explained in the Introduction, many traditional schools of Yoga favor an approach that can conveniently be described as "verticalism": They are pathways to the transcendental Reality, Spirit, Self, or the Godhead, which is conceived as being

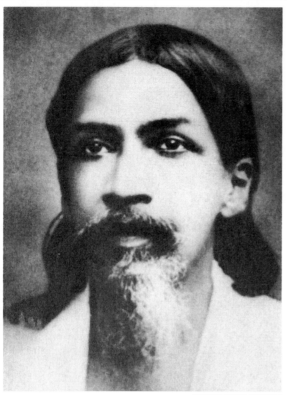

© AUROBINDO ASHRAM

*Sri Aurobindo, father of Integral Yoga,
in his younger years*

in some sense apart from the material world. The verticalist Yogas all seek to rise beyond conventional life by an ascent of attention.

In his magnificent work *The Life Divine*, Aurobindo speaks of the earlier Yogas as being characterized by "the refusal of the ascetic."[35] This refusal consists in the ascetics' downgrading the material world as a result of their overpowering experience of the supramundane dimensions of existence, especially the splendorous domain of the Spirit itself. This negative attitude toward the world is encapsulated in the Vedântic teaching of illusionism, known as *mâyâ-vâda*.

The term *mâyâ* refers to the unreality of the manifest universe—a notion that has typically been understood to mean that the cosmos itself is illusory. This metaphysical axiom has generally been coupled with the idea that worldly existence is shot through with suffering, pain, distress, or sorrow, and therefore is utterly worthless. As a

consequence, the verticalist philosophers and sages have recommended various paths that involve one or another form of external renunciation.

By contrast, Integral Yoga—which is called *pûrna-yoga* in Sanskrit—has the explicit purpose of bringing the "divine consciousness" down into the human body-mind and into ordinary life. It seeks to overcome the traditional paradigm that pits the Spirit against matter, which, according to Aurobindo, commenced with Buddhism some 2,500 years ago. He acknowledged that the Indian philosophers and sages made periodic efforts to overcome this influential paradigm, but, as he noted, "all have lived in the shadow of the great Refusal and the final end of life for all is the garb of the ascetic."[36] To quote Aurobindo's insightful and eloquent remarks more fully:

The general conception of existence has been permeated with the Buddhistic theory of the chain of Karma and with the consequent antinomy of bondage and liberation, bondage by birth, liberation by cessation from birth. Therefore all voices are joined in one great consensus that not in this world of the dualities can there be our kingdom of heaven, but beyond, whether in the joys of the eternal Vrindavan or the high beatitude of Brahmaloka, beyond all manifestations in some ineffable Nirvana or where all separate experience is lost in the featureless unity of the indefinable Existence. And through many centuries a great army of shining witnesses, saints and teachers, names sacred to Indian memory and dominant in Indian imagination, have borne always the same witness and swelled always the same lofty and distant appeal,—renunciation the sole path of knowledge, acceptation of physical life the act of the ignorant, cessation from birth the right use of human birth, the call of the Spirit, the recoil from Matter.[37]

While Aurobindo certainly did not deny the value of asceticism, he sought to assign to it its proper place within the context of an integral spirituality. He argued that the ancient Hindu thinkers and sages took very seriously the Vedântic axiom that there is only a single Reality but failed to do proper justice to the correlated axiom that "all this is Brahman." In other words, they typically ignored the presence of the nondual Divine in and as the world in which we live.

Aurobindo's critique of traditional Hindu metaphysics and Yoga is essentially correct, although he chose to ignore those sporadic efforts, such as the Sahajayâna ("Vehicle of Spontaneity"), which clearly aims at a more integral worldview and ethics. Thus the ideal of sahaja ("spontaneity") could be said to be an attempt at overcoming the limitations of the traditional verticalism. It is true, however, that even some Sahajayâna schools contain a strong ascetical element, and they definitely cannot be said to subscribe to an evolution-based ethics of world affirmation, as is the case with Integral Yoga.

Aurobindo's "supramental Yoga" revolves around the transformation of terrestrial life. He wanted to see paradise on Earth—a thoroughly transmuted existence in the world. As he wrote:

The fundamental difference is in the teaching that there is a dynamic divine Truth and that into the present world of Ignorance that Truth can descend, create a new Truth-consciousness and divinise Life. The old Yogas go straight from mind to the absolute Divine,

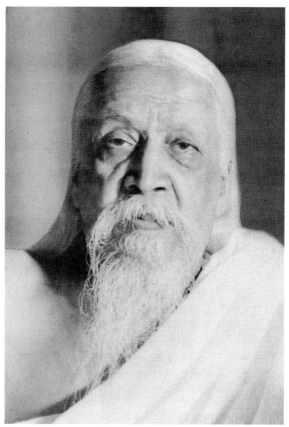

© AUROBINDO ASHRAM

*Sri Aurobindo*

regard all dynamic existence as Ignorance, Illusion or Lila; when you enter the static and immutable Divine Truth, they say, you pass out of cosmic existence . . . My aim is to realise and also to manifest the Divine in the world, bringing down for the purpose a yet unmanifested Power,—such as the Supermind.[38]

What is the Supermind? It is what Aurobindo calls the Truth-Consciousness—*rita-cit* in Sanskrit—behind the ordinary mind. It is "the real creative agency of the universal Existence."[39] It is the dynamic conduit between the eternal Being-Consciousness-Bliss and the conditional cosmos. The Supermind is the creator of the world, for it is the absolute principle of will and knowledge, organizing itself into the structures of the subtle and the coarse (or manifest) dimensions of existence.

According to Aurobindo, it is the Supermind that powers evolution, which he understands as a steady progression toward ever higher forms of consciousness. As such it also is responsible for the manifestation of the human brain-mind. The mind has the innate tendency to go beyond itself and to grasp the larger Whole. Yet it is destined to fail in this program, as is powerfully driven home by the history of philosophy and science. The most the human mind can do is to recognize its inherent limitations and open up to the higher reality of the Supermind. But this act of opening up is always experienced as the death of the mind-bound ego-personality—a terrifying experience for the spiritually immature individual. In his works, Aurobindo describes his own inner experience of the mind-shattering event of the Supermind's descent:

> . . . to reach Nirvana was the first radical result of my own Yoga. It threw me suddenly into a condition above and without thought, unstained by any mental or vital movement; there was no ego, no real world—only when one looked through the immobile senses, something perceived or bore upon its sheer silence a world of empty forms, materialized shadows without true substance. There was no One or many even, only just absolutely That, featureless, relationless, sheer, indescribable, unthinkable, absolute, yet supremely real and solely real. . . . I lived in that Nirvana day and night before it began to admit other things into itself or modify itself at all, and the inner heart of experience, a constant memory of it and its power to return remain until in the end it began to disappear into a greater Superconsciousness from above. But meanwhile realization added itself to realization and fused itself with this original experience. At an early stage the aspect of an illusory world gave place to one in which illusion is only a small surface phenomenon with an immense Divine Reality behind it and a supreme Divine Reality above it and an intense Divine Reality in the heart of everything that had seemed at first only a cinematic shape or shadow.[40]

Aurobindo regarded the person transformed by the Supermind as the pinnacle of evolution. Nature, which is a form of the Divine, struggles to produce the truly spiritual being, who exceeds the "vital man" and the "mental man." This yogic evolutionism is not widely understood in India, and Aurobindo's work also is not as widely known among Western spiritual seekers as it deserves to be. But Integral Yoga is a living spiritual force that, in the words of philosopher Haridas Chaudhuri, "goes on fertilizing the spiritual soil of the world."[41]

On the practical level, Integral Yoga is a matter of the synchronized action of personal aspiration "from below" and divine grace "from above." The essence of aspiration, however, is self-surrender, which must be complete for grace to do its transformative work. Aurobindo contrasted this with the arduous self-effort made on the path of asceticism (*tapasya*).

Integral Yoga has no prescribed techniques, since the inward transformation is accomplished by the divine Power itself. There are no obligatory rituals, mantras, postures, or breathing exercises to be performed. The aspirant must simply open himself or herself to that higher Power, which Sri Aurobindo identified with The Mother. This self-opening and calling upon the presence of The Mother is understood as a form of meditation or prayer. Aurobindo advised that practitioners should focus their attention at the heart, which has anciently been the secret gateway to the Divine. Faith, or inner certitude, is deemed a key to spiritual growth. Other important aspects of Integral Yoga practice are chastity (*brahma-carya*), truthfulness (*satya*), and a pervasive disposition of calm (*prashânti*).

The Mother was for Aurobindo not some abstract principle or otherworldly deity, but the force of grace embodied in his own lifelong partner. He understood himself as Consciousness and her as divine Power or Shakti manifesting in physical form.

> "Yoga is a spirituality rather than a religion. As a spirituality it has influenced the entire range of Indian religious and spiritual development."
>
> —Thomas Berry, *Religions of India*, p. 75

# Chapter 3

# YOGA AND OTHER HINDU TRADITIONS

## I. A BIRD'S-EYE VIEW OF THE CULTURAL HISTORY OF INDIA

The Indian subcontinent is the home of thousands of local cults that have been described as "animistic" and "polytheistic," paralleling the richness of the shamanic cultures of the African continent. But India also has spawned four major spiritual traditions that rank among the world religions—Hinduism, Buddhism, Jainism, and Sikhism. Thus, India's contribution to world spirituality is second to none. More than any other people, the Indians have demonstrated an incredible versatility in spiritual matters, which has inspired many other nations and which in our century has led to a much-needed enrichment of our spiritually ailing Western civilization.

The dominant tradition of the Indian subcontinent has for centuries been Hinduism, which today has more than 780 million adherents around the world. In India, which

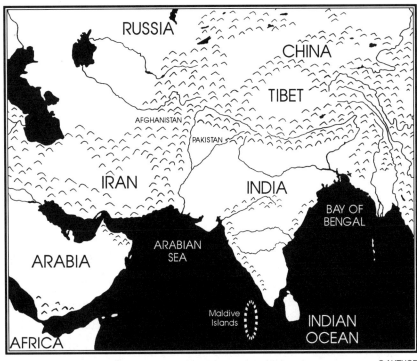

*Map of India (Bharatavarsha) and surrounding countries* © AUTHOR

79

now has a population of around 900 million, there are estimated to be roughly 750 million Hindus. The second largest religious group are the Muslims, who number around 100 million, followed by around 25 million Christians, and 20 million Sikhs. The Buddhists are a small minority in India but are strongly represented in Sri Lanka (former Ceylon), Tibet, and South East Asia.

The term "Hinduism" is ambiguous. Sometimes it is used to refer to the total culture of all the inhabitants of the peninsula apart from those who belong to such clearly defined religions as Buddhism and Christianity. More specifically, the name applies to the numerous traditions that are historically and ideologically connected with the ancient Vedic culture of six thousand and more years ago and that assumed their characteristic form at the beginning of the first millennium C.E. In this volume, the designation "Hinduism" is understood in the broader sense.

Hinduism is more than a religion. Like the other world religions, it is an entire culture with its distinct lifestyle, characterized by a unique social structure: the caste system. For thousands of years, Hindu society has been organized into four estates (*varna*), which are often wrongly referred to as castes: the priestly or *brâhmana* estate or class; the warrior or *kshatriya* class; the "common people" or *vaishya* class (made up of agriculturalists, traders, and artisans), and the servile or *shûdra* class. This arrangement is explained as having its precedent in the divine order itself. Thus in the "Hymn of Man" (*purusha-sûkta*) of the *Rig-Veda* (10.90.12), the primordial being or macranthropos is described as giving birth to the four estates as follows:

> The brahmin is His mouth; the warrior
> was fashioned from His arms; he who
> is merchant is His thighs, and from His
> feet the servant was born.

The members of the servile estate were systematically excluded from learning the sacred lore and eventually came to be considered outcasts. The feet are symbolically "dirty," and the assignment of the *shûdras* to the lower limbs of the Cosmic Man bespeaks their low social status. However, the feet are an integral part of a fully functional human being, and so the servile estate is likewise important to the well-being of society. Yet, from the Vedic point of view, the *shûdras* are karmically preordained for menial labor rather than intellectual work, leadership, or creative work, because their consciousness is of a darker hue (*varna*). It has often been wrongly assumed that the term *varna* ("color") refers to skin color and that the four estates were separated from each other by ethnic boundaries. But all four estates belong to the social body of the Vedic Aryans, who, judging from the *Rig-Veda*, paid more attention to the soul's color than to racial characteristics.

Only the top three estates are considered "twice-born" (*dvija*), that is, "born again" through proper initiation into the Vedic tradition. This occurred traditionally at the ages of eight, eleven, and twelve for boys *and* girls of the priestly, military, and agricultural/mercantile estates respectively. It was then that they underwent the ritual of investiture (*upanayana*) in which they were given a sacred thread (*yajna-upavîta*, written *yajno-pavîta*)[1] to be worn permanently over the left shoulder, hanging diagonally across the chest.

Permitted intermarriage between members of different estates led to the creation of social subdivisions, which are properly called castes (*jâti*). These, in turn, spawned an increasing number of subcastes. This social hierarchy is governed by elaborate conventions that carefully regulate the behavior and activities between members of different castes. Inevitably this stratification gave rise to marginal groups, which are deemed outcastes or "untouchables."

This vast social edifice has frequently been challenged by visionaries and reformers. Gautama, the founder of Buddhism, was among the first to reject it. Yet it continued to persist over the centuries and to exert a compelling influence on all other traditions of the subcontinent. Social innovators who rejected the caste system generally also had to reject the Vedic revelation that sanctioned it. For the pious Hindu, the caste system with its social inequality is as natural as democracy is to us. Just as we justify democratic principles by pointing to the worth of the individual, the caste system is justified by invoking the law of karma: Each person has his or her station in life because of former volitions and actions. Brahmins are brahmins because of their virtuous and spiritual pursuits in previous lifetimes. Outcastes are outcastes perhaps because of their past lack of motivation toward a higher life or because of serious misdeeds.

The caste system may offend our modern Western sensibilities, but not too long ago our forebears held opinions and values similar to those of the traditional Hindus. It was only with the emergence of a pronounced individualism during the Renaissance that the ancient social order, which was pointedly hierarchical, came to be questioned, challenged, and finally abolished. Of course, even our modern so-called egalitarian societies are not free from social stratification, with a super-wealthy elite at one end and a great number of underprivileged people at the other.

The rigidity of the caste system has been balanced by a strong tendency toward ideological flexibility. Thus Hinduism has demonstrated an amazing capacity for assimilating even the most extreme opposites within itself. For instance, at one end of the spectrum we find the radical nondualist school of Shankara and at the other end the strict dualist school of Classical Sâmkhya, which despite its atheism is still counted as one of Hinduism's six major philosophical systems (*darshana*). Another example of such widely contrasting philosophical positions is the "cool" contemplative approach of nondualist Jnâna-Yoga of the *Upanishads* on one side and the fervent emotionalism of some schools of monotheistic Bhakti-Yoga on the other. The medieval path of devotionalism (*bhakti-mârga*) is strongly syncretistic and has incorporated, among other things, elements from Islamic Sufism. Typical of this all-inclusive spirit of Hinduism is the *Allah-Upanishad*, a late work composed under Muslim influence.

The spongelike absorptive power of Hinduism is such that even a well-defined religious tradition like Christianity fell under its spell and, in the sixteenth and seventeenth centuries, had to be rescued by Jesuit missionaries from complete Hinduization. Sometimes the Hindu tendency of inclusiveness is misinterpreted as a universal kind of tolerance, which is not the case. Throughout India's history there have been numerous instances of intolerance between various schools or factions of Hinduism, and one might mention the long-standing tension between the Vaishnavas and the Shaivas as an example.

Hinduism is best understood as a complex sociocultural process that has unfolded in the dynamics between continuity and discontinuity, or the persistence of ancient forms and the assimilation of new expressions of cultural and religious life. Thus, from one point of view, Hinduism can be said to have commenced with the Vedic civilization (possibly as early as the fifth millennium B.C.E.). From another point of view, there are real and important differences between the Vedic sacred culture and Hinduism as we know it today. Yet, overall, the continuity has been astonishing and more significant than the changes introduced in the course of history.

Until recently, most Western and Indian scholars tended to emphasize the element of discontinuity in India's cultural evolution. In particular, they saw a clash between the civilization of the Indus valley and the Vedic "Aryan" culture, which they thought originated outside India. However, this long-standing theory of the Aryan invasion is now being vigorously challenged. A growing number of scholars, both in India and the West, regard this historical model as a scientific myth, which was constructed in the absence of adequate evidence and which has adversely influenced our understanding of ancient India's history and culture. This important change in scholarly opinion is documented in the book *In Search of the Cradle of Civilization.*[2]

All the evidence points to the fact that the Sanskrit-speaking Aryans, who composed the *Vedas*, were not primitive nomads who came from outside India, bringing death and destruction to the indigenous population. Rather, the available evidence points to their having been true natives of India. Moreover, there are good reasons for assuming that the Vedic civilization, as reflected in the *Rig-Veda* and the other three Vedic *Samhitâs*, was largely or even completely identical with the so-called Indus civilization. More will be said about this in Chapter 4.

In light of this new understanding, the historical development of Hindu India can conveniently be organized into nine periods, expressing distinguishable cultural styles. The following chronology is very tentative, and to some degree the periodization is arbitrary, since history is largely continuous. The dating of the first four historical periods is admittedly speculative, but so is the standard chronology found in college textbooks. The *Vedas* clearly must be assigned to an era well before the benchmark date of 1900 B.C.E., which will be explained shortly. How much earlier is not yet known with any degree of certainty, though astronomical references in the *Vedas* themselves, together with

the dynastic genealogies (from the *Purânas*) and the list of sages in the *Brâhmanas* and *Upanishads*, justify a date at least two thousand or more years prior to 1200 B.C.E., which is the commonly accepted but patently wrong date for the composition of the *Rig-Veda*. Just as the *Vedas* must be assigned to an earlier period, the composition of the original *Brâhmanas* for very similar reasons must be pushed back in time before 1900 B.C.E. Likewise the oldest *Upanishads*, generally thought to have been created shortly before the time of the Buddha, ought to be placed much earlier in light of all this.

## 1. Pre-Vedic Age (6500–4500 B.C.E.)

Recent archaeological work in eastern Baluchistan (Pakistan) has brought to light a city the size of Stanford in California, which has been

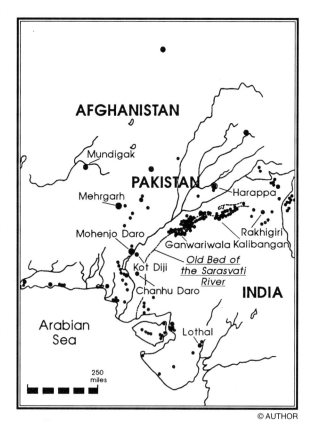

© AUTHOR

*Archaeological sites of the Indus-Sarasvatî civilization*

dated to the middle of the seventh millennium B.C.E. This early Neolithic town, labeled Mehrgarh by archaeologists, in many ways foreshadowed the later urban civilization along the two great rivers of northwestern India: the Indus and the now dried-up Sarasvatî east of it.

Mehrgarh's population is estimated to have been around 20,000 individuals, which was huge for that period. Apart from having been a thriving marketplace for imported and exported goods, the town also appears to have been a center of technological creativity and innovation. The industrious people of Mehrgarh cultivated cotton as early as the fifth millennium B.C.E. and mass-produced good-quality pottery by the fourth millennium B.C.E. Terra-cotta figurines dated to c. 2600 B.C.E. clearly evince a marvelous stylistic continuity with the art of the Indus-Sarasvatî civilization and also with later Hinduism.

## 2. *Vedic Age (4500–2500 B.C.E.)*

This period is defined by the creation and cultural prominence of the wisdom tradition embodied in the hymns of the four *Vedas*. Certain astronomical references in the *Rig-Veda* suggest that the bulk of the hymns were composed in the fourth, with some hymns possibly dating back to the fifth, millennium B.C.E. The absolute lower limit of the Vedic period is fixed by a great natural disaster: the drying up of the mighty Sarasvatî River, apparently as a result of tectonic and climatic changes over a period of several hundred years. Around 3100 B.C.E., the Yamunâ River apparently changed its course and ceased to pour its waters into the Sarasvatî; instead it became a tributary of the Ganges. Around 2300 B.C.E., the Sutlej, the biggest tributary of the Sarasvatî, also started to flow into the Ganges. By 1900 B.C.E., the Sarasvatî, once the greatest stream of Northern

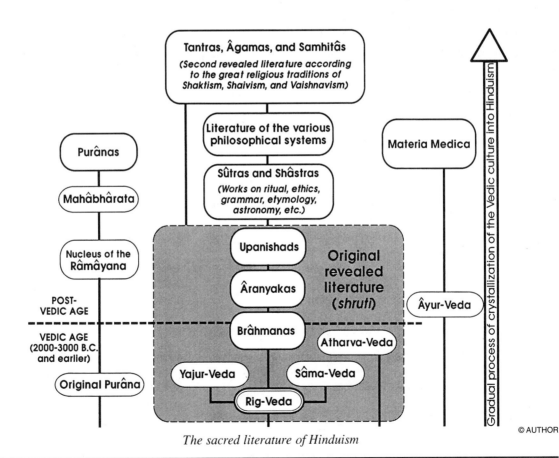

*The sacred literature of Hinduism*

India, had dried up. Soon the numerous settlements along its banks were abandoned and finally covered with the sands of the vast Thar Desert.

Given the antiquity of the Vedic hymns and the fact that the Sanskrit-speaking Aryans, as noted above, were not foreign invaders, we can reach only one conclusion: The Vedic people were present in India simultaneously with the so-called Indus civilization. More than that, the archaeological remains of that civilization in no way contradict the cultural world as it is mirrored in the Vedic hymns. Hence we must conclude that the citizens of Harappa and Mohenjo-Daro, as well as the hundreds of other towns of the Indus and Sarasvatî rivers, and the Vedic Aryans were one and the same people.

Also, as has been shown, Vedic mathematics influenced the mathematics of Babylonia, which means that the nucleus of the *Shulba-Sûtras* containing Vedic mathematical theory must have existed around 1800 B.C.E. Since the *Sûtras* are deemed later than the *Brâhmanas*, the date of the *Vedas* can be pushed back to the third millennium B.C.E. to allow sufficient time for these developments. According to some scholars, the *end* of the Vedic Age (including the *Brahmanas* and the *Upanishads*) is marked by the famous war remembered in the *Mahâbhârata*, which is traditionally dated to 3102 B.C.E.).[3] This coincides with the beginning of the *kali-yuga*, the dark age spoken of in the later *Purânas*, *Tantras*, and other scriptures. This date, however, is likely too early, and a date of c. 1500 B.C.E. for the war and the final redaction of the four Vedic hymnodies is more probable.

## 3. The Brahmanical Age (2500–1500 B.C.E.)

With the collapse of the settlements along the Sarasvatî and the Indus, the center of the Vedic civilization shifted further east to the fertile banks of the Ganges (Gangâ) River and its tributaries. The environmental conditions in the new settlement areas not surprisingly caused changes in the social system, which became increasingly complex. In this period, the priestly class developed into a highly specialized professional elite that soon dominated the Vedic culture and religion. The theological-mythological speculations and ritual preoccupations of the priesthood are captured in the *Brâhmana* literature, after which this period is generally named. The concluding centuries of this era also saw the creation of the *Âranyakas* (ritual texts for forest-dwelling ascetics) and the extensive *Sûtra* literature dealing with legal and ethical issues and also the arts.

## 4. The Post-Vedic/Upanishadic Age (1500–1000 B.C.E.)

With the appearance of the earliest *Upanishads* we enter a new period with its own distinct metaphysical and cultural flavor. They introduced the ideal of internalized ritualism—"inner sacrifice" (*antar-yajna*)—combined with renunciation of the world. In these anonymously authored sacred scriptures—forming the third stage of the Vedic revelation (*shruti*)—we can see the beginnings of India's psychospiritual technology proper. Yet, the *Upanishads* do not, as is sometimes maintained, represent a radical departure from Vedic thought, but rather merely explicate what is hinted at or present in a rudimentary way in the *Vedas*. The conclusion of the Post-Vedic Age coincides with the emergence of the non-Vedic traditions of Jainism and Buddhism.

## 5. *The Pre-Classical or Epic Age (1000–100 B.C.E.)*

During the fifth period in the present chronological scheme, India's metaphysical and ethical thought was in considerable ferment. It had reached a degree of sophistication that led to a fertile confrontation between the various religio-philosophical schools. At the same time, we can witness a healthy tendency toward integrating the many psychospiritual paths, notably the two great orientations of world renunciation (*samnyâsa*) on one side and the acceptance of social obligations (*dharma*) on the other. This is the area of the pre-classical developments of Yoga and Sâmkhya. The integrative, syncretistic spirit is best exemplified in the teachings found in the *Mahâbhârata* epic, in which the earliest complete Yoga work, the *Bhagavad-Gîtâ*, is embedded. During this period, the massive *Mahâbhârata* as we know it was created, though its nucleus, which commemorates the great war of the Pândavas and Kauravas, belongs to a much earlier era. Because of the significance of the epic for this period, it may also be referred to as the Epic Age.

The *Râmâyana* epic is later than the *Mahâbhârata*, although its historical core belongs to an age antedating that of the *Mahâbhârata* by nearly thirty generations.

## 6. *The Classical Age (100 B.C.E.–500 C.E.)*

During this era the six classical schools of Hindu philosophy intensified their long-drawn struggle for intellectual supremacy. Halfway through this period the *Yoga-Sûtra* of Patanjali and the *Brahma-Sûtra* of Bâdarâyana were composed, and its end is marked by the composition of the *Sâmkhya-Kârikâ* of Îshvara Krishna. This is also the period in which Mahâyâna Buddhism crystallized, leading to a very active dialogue between Buddhists and Hindus. The end of the Classical Age coincides with the decline of the Gupta dynasty, whose last great ruler, Skandagupta, died around 455 C.E. Under the Gupta kings, whose rule began in 320 C.E., the arts and sciences flourished extraordinarily. Even though the kings were devout adherents of Vaishnavism, they practiced tolerance toward other religions, which allowed especially Buddhism to thrive and leave its mark on India's culture. The Chinese pilgrim Fa-hien was greatly impressed with the country and its people. He writes of prosperous towns and numerous charitable institutions, as well as rest houses for travelers on the highways.

## 7. *The Tantric/Puranic Age (500–1300 C.E.)*

Around the middle of the first millennium C.E., or slightly earlier, we can witness the beginnings of the great cultural revolution of Tantra, or Tantrism. This tradition, whose extraordinary psychotechnology is discussed in Chapter 17, represents the impressive outcome of many centuries of effort to create a grand philosophical and spiritual synthesis out of the numerous divergent approaches in existence at the time. In particular, Tantra can be seen as integrating the highest metaphysical ideas and ideals with popular (rural) beliefs and practices. Tantra understood itself as the gospel of the dark age (*kali-yuga*). By the turn of the first millennium C.E., Tantric teachings had swept across the entire Indian subcontinent, influencing and transforming the spiritual life of Hindus, Buddhists, and Jainas alike.

On one hand, Tantra simply continued the millennia-long process of amalgamation and synthesis; on the other hand, it was genuinely innovative. Although it added little to India's philosophical repertoire, Tantra was of the utmost significance on the level of spiritual practice. It promoted a spiritual lifestyle that was in contrast to most of what had hitherto been considered legitimate within the fold of Hinduism, Buddhism, and Jainism. In particular, Tantra lent philosophical respectability to the feminine psychocosmic principle (known as *shakti*), which had long been acknowledged in more local cults of Goddess worship.

This era could also be referred to as the Puranic Age, because during this time the great encyclopedic compilations known as the *Purânas* were created on the basis of much older Puranic traditions (dating back to the Vedic era). At their core the *Purânas* are sacred histories around which a web of philosophical, mythological, and ritual knowledge has been woven. Many of these works show the influence of Tantra, and many contain valuable information about Yoga.

## 8. *The Sectarian Age (1300–1700 C.E.)*

The Tantric rediscovery of the feminine principle for philosophy and yogic practice set the stage for the next phase in India's cultural history: the *bhakti* movement. This movement of religious devotionalism was the culmination of the monotheistic aspirations of the great sectarian communities, notably the Vaishnavas and Shaivas; hence the title Sectarian Age. By including the emotional dimension in the psychospiritual process, the devotional movement—or *bhakti-mârga*—completed the pan-Indian synthesis that had been initiated during the Pre-Classical/Epic Age.

## 9. *Modern Age (1700–Present)*

The ferment created by the syncretistic *bhakti* movement was followed by the collapse of the Mughal empire in the first quarter of the eighteenth century and by the growing political presence of European nations in India, culminating in Queen Victoria assuming the title Empress of India in 1880. The Queen was fascinated with Hindu spirituality and welcomed visits from *yogins* and other spiritual figures. Ever since the founding of the East India Company in London in 1600 and the Dutch East India Company two years later, there has been a growing impact of Western secular imperialism upon the age-old religious traditions of India. This has led to a progressive undermining of the native Indic value system through the introduction of a Western-style (science-oriented and essentially materialistic) education combined with new technologies. On this point the following remark by Carl Gustav Jung springs to mind:

> The European invasion of the East was an act of violence on a grand scale, and it has left us with the duty—*noblesse oblige*—of understanding the mind of the East. This is perhaps more necessary than we realize at present.[4]

India's creative genius, however, has not suffered these developments passively. There has been a promising spiritual renaissance, which, among other things, has created for the first time in history a missionary sense among Hindus: Ever since the appearance of the imposing figure of Swami Vivekananda at the Parliament of Religions in Chicago in 1893, there has been a steady flow of Hindu wisdom, especially Yoga and Vedânta, to the Euro-American countries. As Jung, with characteristic perceptiveness, observed:

We have never yet hit upon the thought that while we are overpowering the Orient from without, it may be fastening its hold upon us from within.[5]

Much more could be said about the modern revival of the Hindu tradition and its impact in the West, but this subject lies beyond the scope of the present book.

The above attempt at periodization is only an approximation, and the dates given are flexible. India's chronology is notoriously conjectural until we come to the nineteenth century. The Hindu historiographers have seldom been concerned with recording actual dates and tended to freely mingle historical fact with mythology, symbolism, and ideology. Western scholars have often remarked on the "timelessness" of Hindu consciousness and culture. Yet, this notion has proven a veritable blind spot, because it has blocked the serious study of the chronological information contained in the Hindu scriptures, especially the *Purânas*.[6]

In addition to the division into religio-spiritual traditions and chronological periods, a useful distinction can also be made between the fundamental orientations of asceticism (*tapas*), renunciation (*samnyâsa*), and mysticism (*yoga*) in the broadest sense of the term. These cut across all the religious and philosophical schools of India. The differences and similarities between these major approaches will be made clear in the sections immediately following.

## II. THE GLOW OF PSYCHIC POWER—YOGA AND ASCETICISM

Long before the word *yoga* acquired its customary meaning of "spirituality" or "spiritual discipline," the sages of India had developed a body of knowledge and techniques that aimed at the transformation and transcendence of ordinary consciousness. This stock of ideas and practices formed the matrix out of which grew the complex historical phenomenon that later came to be called Yoga. In a certain sense, Yoga may be looked upon

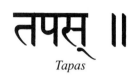
*Tapas*

as internalized asceticism. Where the earlier ascetic stood stock-still under the burning sun in order to win the favor of a deity, the *yogin* or *yoginî*'s work occurs primarily in the laboratory of his or her own consciousness.

A typical example of the ascetic is the royal sage Bhagîratha, whose exploits are told in the *Mahâbhârata*. In ancient times, during a long spell of drought, he took it upon himself to stand on one foot for a thousand years and, for another

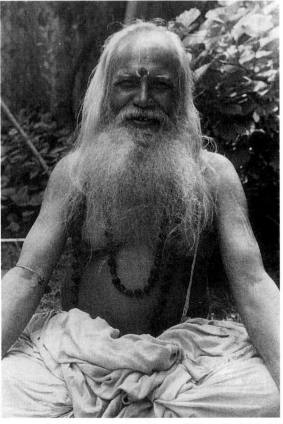

© MATTHEW GREENBLATT
*Contemporary Hindu ascetic*

thousand, hold his arms up high. In this manner he compelled the Gods to grant his request that the heavenly river Ganges (Gangâ) release its waters to flood and regenerate the parched earth. The downpour from the celestial river was so great that God Shiva had to slow its speed by catching the water on his head. The water ran through his tangled hair, forming the riverine basin of the Ganges (Gangâ) River of northern India.

The earliest term for Yoga-like endeavors in India is *tapas*. Literally, this ancient Sanskrit word means "heat." It is derived from the verbal root *tap* meaning "to burn" or "to glow." The term is often used in the *Rig-Veda* to describe the quality and work of the solar orb (or its corresponding deity, God Sûrya), or of the sacrificial fire (or its corresponding deity, God Agni). In these contexts it is frequently implied that the heat of sun and fire is painful and distressing in its burning intensity. We can see in this the root of the subsequent metaphoric usage of *tapas* as psychic heat in the form of anger and aggression, but also as fervor, zeal, or painstaking self-application.

Thus, the word *tapas* came to be applied to the religious or spiritual struggle of voluntary self-discipline through the practice of austerities. The term *tapas* is therefore frequently rendered as "asceticism," or "austerities." The earlier hymns of the *Rig-Veda* still refer to *tapas* in its naturalistic or psychological connotations. But the tenth book, which is thought to belong to the concluding phase of the Vedic Age, contains many references to its spiritual significance.

In one of the most exquisite hymns of the *Rig-Veda* (10.129), which is an early philosophical treatment of the theme of creation, the manifest worlds are said to have been produced by virtue of the excessive self-heating (*tapas*) of the primordial Being.[7] This self-exertion and self-sacrifice by the incommensurate Being that abides prior to space and time is the great archetype for spiritual practice in general. That the Vedic seers and sages were aware of this is borne out by the above-mentioned "Hymn of Creation" and many other hymns.

The *Rig-Veda* documents the emergence of *tapas* as a religious means of creating inner heat or the kind of creative tension that yields ecstatic states, visions of the deities, perhaps even transcendence of object-dependent consciousness itself. The Vedic sacrificial ritual (*yajna*) involved tremendous concentration, for success depended on the correct pronunciation and intonation of the prayers and on the accurate performance of the ceremony. It is easy to see how the Vedic ritual should have given rise not only to a whole sacrificial mysticism but also to ascetic practices designed to prepare the sacrificer for the actual ritual. The *Rig-Vidhâna* (1.8) of Shaunaka, an old text on mantric magic belonging to the Epic Era, recommends that all twice-born persons should be intent on *tapas* and study of the *Vedas*, as well as cultivate compassion toward all beings.[8]

However, the typical ascetic (*tapasvin*) in the Vedic era is not the dutiful householder-sacrificer or even the exalted seer (*rishi*), but the ecstatic *muni*. The *muni* belongs to what one might call the Vedic counterculture, composed of religious individuals and groups (like the Vrâtyas) who pursued their sacred aspirations at the margins of Vedic society. The *muni* has frequently been regarded as the prototype of the later *yogin*. In his ecstatic oblivion he resembles a madman. Many elements in his lifestyle anticipate the unconventional behavior of the later *avadhûta*, as celebrated in the *Avadhûta-Gîtâ* and other medieval Sanskrit works.

*Tapas* continued as an independent tradition alongside Yoga. This parallel development is documented, for instance, in the *Mahâbhârata* epic. It relates many stories of such renowned *tapasvins* as Vyâsa, Vishvâmitra, Vashishtha, Cyavana,

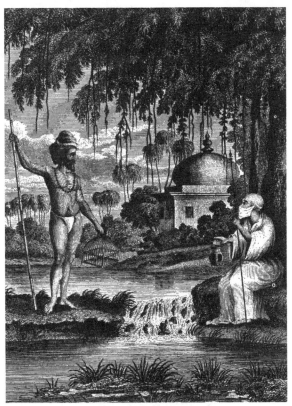

*Reproduced from* Hindu Religion, Customs and Manners

*Hindu and Jaina ascetics*

Bharadvâja, Bhrigu, and Uttanka. Indeed, in many parts of the epic, the tradition of *tapas* is given preeminence over Yoga, which can be taken as an indication of the early age of these passages.

*Tapas* is generally pursued through the observance of chastity (*brahmacarya*) and the subjugation of the senses (*indriya-jaya*). The frustration of the body-mind's natural inclinations is held to generate psychophysical effulgence (*tejas*), radiance (*jyotis*), great strength (*bala*), and vitality (*vîrya*). Another term closely associated with asceticism since Vedic times is *ojas* (apparently related to the Latin *augustus*, "majestic"). It stands for a particular kind of numinous energy that charges the entire body-mind. *Ojas* is generated especially through the practice of chastity, as a result of the sublimation of sexual energy. It is held to be so potent that the ascetic can influence and change his or her destiny and the destiny of others. According to the

*Atharva-Veda* (11.5–19), the deities themselves acquired their state of immortality through the practice of chastity and austerities.

*Tapas* is typically associated with the acquisition of psychic powers (*siddhi*), which often proved the downfall of unwise ascetics who abused their extraordinary capabilities. The tradition of *tapas*, both in the Vedic Age and the Epic Age, unfolded against the backdrop of a magical worldview according to which the cosmos is filled with personalized sources of psychic power. Thus the *tapasvins*, or *tâpasas*, are frequently depicted as combating evil spirits or as pitting themselves against various deities to win a boon from them. More often than not, the ascetics emerge as victors, and only pride or sexual profligacy are held to diminish their formidable puissance. To this day, the practitioners of *tapas* are thought of by the villagers of India as magicians able to accomplish any feat—from reading people's minds, to predicting the future, to stopping the sun in its course.

Yoga spiritualized the orientation of the earlier tradition of *tapas* by emphasizing self-transcendence over the acquisition of magical powers. At the same time, the *yogins* adopted and adapted many of the techniques and practices of the older tradition of *tapas*. Chastity remained central to its practice, as is clear from the eight-limbed path outlined in the *Yoga-Sûtra*. In this work, Patanjali states (2.38) that the *yogin* who is grounded in chastity gains vigor (*vîrya*). He also mentions (2.32) *tapas* as one of the five observances or restraints (*niyama*) and declares (2.43) that through asceticism the body and its senses are perfected. Manifestly, *tapas* is here relegated to the status of a preparatory practice. The real concern of Yoga is meditation and its intensified form, ecstatic transcendence (*samâdhi*).

The tradition of *tapas* flourished alongside the schools of Yoga for centuries, and this is no different today. The remarkable story of a modern *tapasvin* and saint, who reputedly lived for 185 years, is told in the hagiography *Maharaj.*[9] The hero of the story, known as Tapasviji Maharaj, was born around 1820 into a princely family but left everything behind in his late fifties and girded himself with a loincloth. During his lifetime he was widely hailed as a mighty ascetic and miracle worker. He performed startling feats of endurance, conquering both pain and boredom. For three years he stood on one leg, with one arm stretched upward; for another twenty-four years he never lay down, while also walking many miles every day. In the 1960s, this saint attracted much attention in the United States because of his extreme longevity, which he claimed was the result of undergoing on three different occasions the *kâya-kalpa* or rejuvenating treatment known to native Indian medicine. The success of this treatment depends largely on the disposition of the individual, who must be able to endure long periods of almost complete isolation. Only a skilled meditator of the stature of Tapasviji Maharaj could possibly cope with the ordeal of self-denial involved. Clearly, Western medicine has much to learn from the *tapasvins* of ancient and modern India.

## III. DELIGHT IN NOTHING—YOGA AND THE WAY OF RENUNCIATION

*Tapas*, as we have seen, represents a more magical-shamanic type of spirituality. Unlike Yoga, which is primarily concerned with the achievement of contemplative states and self-transcendence, the technology of *tapas* focuses on the attainment of inner strength, visionary experiences, and magical powers. The cultivation of willpower is crucial to this approach. By contrast, Yoga embodies a more

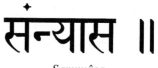

*Samnyâsa*

refined orientation to psychospiritual growth. It recognizes, for instance, the need for the transcendence of the will, which is a manifestation of the egoic personality.

Nevertheless, many facets of *tapas* have found their way into the yogic tradition, and the popular image of the *yogin* or *yoginî* is that of a thaumaturgist, or miracle-working ascetic. Yet Yoga is closer in spirit to another tradition, that of renunciation (*samnyâsa*) of worldly life, which first appeared as an ideal worthy of pursuit in the Post-Vedic Age. Suddenly, or so it appears, a growing number of householders left the villages and cities to live out the rest of their days in the wilderness, often on their own but occasionally also with their spouses.

These renouncers are known as *samnyâsins*, practitioners of *samnyâsa*. The word *samnyâsa* is composed of the prefixes *sam* (expressing the idea of "union," similar to the Greek *syn-* or the Latin *com-*) and *ni* (denoting "down"), as well as the verbal root *as* (meaning "to cast" or "to throw"). Thus, it signifies one's "casting down" or "laying aside" of all worldly concerns and attachments.

Although renunciation can be identified as a lifestyle, it cannot be performed as one might perform austerities or meditation. It is primarily a fundamental *attitude* to life. Hence the tradition of renunciation can be said to be counter-technological: It aims at leaving everything behind, including, if it is pursued rigorously enough, all methods of seeking. The German indologist Joachim Friedrich Sprockhoff rightly described renunciation as "a phenomenon at the margin of life,"[10] and compared it to other borderline experiences, such as fatal illness or old age.

Renunciation is a response to the insight that human existence, and cosmic existence in general, is either morally inferior or altogether illusory.

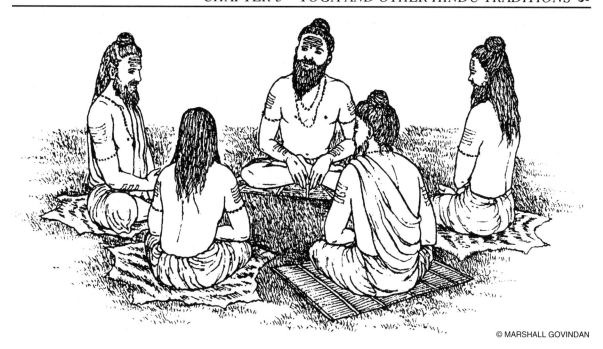

*Hindu renouncers*

In either case, the renouncer seeks to realize a higher state of being, which is equated with Reality itself. Depending on whether the world is regarded as illusory or merely morally unworthy (but still rooted in the Divine), renunciation can be expressed in at least two principal ways. On one side is what can be called literal renunciation; on the other is symbolic renunciation. The former position understands renunciation, pure and simple, as the abandonment of ordinary life: The renouncer leaves everything behind—wife, children, property, work, social respectability, worldly ambitions, and any concern for the future. The latter position perceives renunciation in metaphorical terms as primarily an inner act: the voluntary letting go of all attachments and, in the final analysis, of the ego itself.

Both approaches have had their advocates throughout the long history of Indian spirituality. In the *Bhagavad-Gîtâ* (3.3ff.) we find the earliest record of an attempt to reconcile the two routes. Thus, the God-man Krishna taught Prince Arjuna the distinction between mere abandonment and inner renunciation, clearly favoring the latter. In response to Arjuna, who was confused about the difference between renunciation of actions and renunciation in action, Krishna explained that anciently he taught both paths. One is the path of *samnyâsa*, which Krishna identifies with the Yoga of Wisdom (*jnâna-yoga*); the other is the Yoga of Action (*karma-yoga*). Both, he emphasized, lead to the highest goal, but of the two he deemed the Yoga of Action more excellent. He said:

> He who does not hate or desire is forever to be known as a renouncer. (5.3a)

> But renunciation, O strong-armed [Arjuna], is difficult to attain without Yoga. The sage (*muni*) yoked in Yoga approaches the Absolute without delay. (5.6)

> Yoked in Yoga, with the self purified, with the self subdued, and the senses conquered—he whose self has become

the Self of all beings, even though he is active, is not defiled. (5.7)

"I do nothing whatsoever"—thus reflects the yoked one, the knower of Reality, [even as he is] seeing, hearing, touching, smelling, eating, walking, sleeping, breathing, talking, excreting, grasping, opening and closing [his eyes], and thinking "the senses abide in the sense objects." (5.8–9)

He who acts, assigning [all] actions to the Absolute, and having abandoned attachment (*sanga*), is not defiled by sin (*pâpa*), just as a lotus leaf [is not stained] by the water. (5.10)

The symbolic interpretation of renunciation was, understandably, favored by the orthodox Hindu authority, which was greatly concerned about the growing mood of world resignation. If it had only been the older generation that found the eremitic existence in forests or caves attractive, the priestly establishment would have had little cause to worry. But the ideal of flight from the world also appealed strongly to the middle-aged population and even to young men (and, more rarely, women). Their renunciation of worldly life led to abandoned families and fields, as well as kingdoms, we are told. The sociocultural reasons for this trend are ill understood; some scholars have blamed the hot, dry climate of many parts of the peninsula, but this seems reductionistic.

In psychohistorical terms, the ideal of literal relinquishment reflects what I have elsewhere called the "mythical" (verticalist) variant of Yoga.[11] In contradistinction, the ideal of life-positive *samnyâsa* suggests a more integral attitude. Mythic Yoga is founded in a radical and abrupt break with the conventional universe: One either abstains from

all mundane activities and thoughts and dedicates one's life to the contemplation of the supramundane Reality, or one engages ordinary life and reaps the doubtful rewards of an earth-bound existence. For the practitioner of Mythic Yoga, there can be no in-between state. He or she must choose either the transcendental Self or the conditional self, God or the world, abiding happiness or daily sorrow. The contrasting idea that the finite cosmos is a manifestation of the Divine and therefore not merely sorrowful but also an abode of joy belongs to the more integral world perception of Tantrism, Sahajayâna, and especially Sri Aurobindo's Integral Yoga.

In the *Maitrâyanîya-Upanishad* (1.2ff.), a work in the tradition of mythic Yoga belonging to the centuries just before the beginning of the Common Era, King Brihadratha is portrayed as suffering from excessive existential ennui. He articulated a sentiment that, at one time or another, must have overwhelmed thousands of other ascetics when he said:

In this ill-smelling, pithless body, which is a conglomerate of bone, skin, muscle, marrow, flesh, semen, blood, mucus, tears, rheum, feces, urine, wind, bile, and phlegm—what good is the enjoyment of desires? In this body, which is afflicted with lust, anger, greed, delusion, fear, despondency, jealousy, separation from what is loved, union with what is unloved, hunger, thirst, senility, death, illness, grief, and the like—what good is the enjoyment of desires?

We see that all this is perishable, like these gnats, mosquitoes, and so on, like the grass and the trees that grow and decay. Indeed, what of these? There are the great ones, mighty warriors, some of them rulers of empires like Sudyumna,

Bhuridyumna . . . and kings like Marutta, Bharata, and others, who, before the eyes of their whole family, surrendered their great wealth and passed on from this world to the next.

Radical relinquishment of conventional existence at times clearly threatened the social fabric and established order. Consequently, the Hindu lawgivers discouraged what they considered premature renunciation and instead proposed the alternative social ideal of the stages of life (*âshrama*)—studentship (*brahmacarya*), householder stage (*gârhastya*), forest-dweller existence (*vâna-prasthya*), and finally total renunciation. In this new hierarchical framework, renunciation was fully sanctioned, but only after a person had fulfilled his or her obligations as a householder (*grihastha*, from *griha* "house" and *sthâ* "to abide").

Two levels of renunciation came to be distinguished. The first, known as *vâna-prasthya* ("forest-dwelling"), is the stage of the hermit who practices a kind of esoteric ritualism in the seclusion of the forest. He or she is called a "forest-dweller" (*vâna-prastha*). The second stage, known as *samnyâsa*, consists in leaving behind even the forest-dweller's sedentary existence and sacrificial ritualism, taking up a life of constant wandering. These two lifestyles anticipated the modern custom of retirement, though by turning the evening of an individual's life into a sacred opportunity, the Hindu orthodoxy granted older people—at least in theory—a dignity that they are denied by our own Western society.

The tradition of renunciation has been as persistent a feature of Indian spirituality as has been the tradition of asceticism. Often the two overlapped. Although the word *samnyâsa* is first mentioned in the *Mundaka-Upanishad* (3.2.6), which is commonly thought to belong to the third or second century B.C.E. but may be earlier, the idea and

ideal is much older. Thus, the *Brihad-Âranyaka-Upanishad* (4.4.22), which is reckoned as the oldest work of the Upanishadic genre, speaks of the *pravrâjin*, the person who has "gone forth" (*pra + vraj* "to wander"), that is, who has left house and home and is wholly intent on Self-realization. In a memorable passage, Yâjnavalkya, the grand old man of Upanishadic wisdom, instructs a disciple as follows:

> That which is beyond hunger and thirst, sorrow and delusion, old age and death [is the transcendental Reality]: The brahmins who know That as the very Self overcome the desire for sons, the desire for wealth, the desire for the worlds, and they lead a mendicant's life. The desire for sons is the desire for wealth, and the desire for wealth is the desire for the worlds; thus both these are merely desires. Therefore let a brahmin despair of scholarship and desire to live [in innocence] as a child. When he has despaired both of scholarship and childlikeness, then he becomes a sage (*muni*). When he despairs both of sagehood (*mauna*)[12] and nonsagehood (*a-mauna*), then he becomes a [true] brahmin. (3.5.1)

Thus, Yâjnavalkya characterized renunciation as the transcendence of attachment to every conceivable desire, including the desire for renunciation itself. Elsewhere in the same scripture (3.8.10) he is remembered as expressing his doubts about the usefulness of asceticism (*tapas*). According to him, even a millennium of austerities will be of no avail unless the Absolute is intuited first. This statement enunciates a perennial paradox of the spiritual path: We only seek that which we have, in some sense, found already. To put it differently: To realize the Self, our innermost reality, we must simply stand perfectly still and remember.

Even though the Hindu orthodoxy made provisions for those who felt an irresistible urge to "drop out," renunciation was always at best condoned, never actively encouraged. And in some quarters renunciation was viewed as unlawful. In the *Mahâbhârata* (12.10.17ff.), for instance, there is the story of Yudhishthira, who, fatigued from the brutalities of the great Bharata war, felt moved to embrace the life of a forest eremite. His teacher Bhîshma reminded him, as Krishna had reminded Arjuna, that renunciation was inappropriate for a warrior. Bhîshma also aired the cynical opinion (no doubt based in part on reality) that only those assailed by misfortune adopt such a lifestyle.

That renouncers were not all of the same sort becomes readily apparent when one delves into the various Sanskrit scriptures dealing with renunciation, notably the so-called *Samnyâsa-Upanishads*. The *Jâbala-Upanishad*, dated c. 300 B.C.E. and thus being one of the oldest works of this genre, differentiates between renouncers who maintain the sacred fire and those who do not—that is, between those who in their retirement continue to engage the Vedic sacrificial ritualism and those God-seekers who simply leave it all behind. This work celebrates the *parama-hamsa* ("great swan"), who drifts through life unconcerned by any of its problems, as the foremost of all renouncers. Some six hundred years later, the *Vaikhânasa-Smârta-Sûtra* (chapter 8) furnishes a more detailed picture. It mentions four types of forest

> "Fasting is better than eating only at night. Unrequested food is better than fasting. Begged food is better than unrequested food. Therefore [the renouncer] should subsist on begged food."
>
> —*Brihat-Samnyâsa-Upanishad* 265

anchorites and four types of wandering renouncers. The forest-dwelling ascetics can be married, whereas the wandering renouncers must live on their own, seeking nothing but Self-realization.

An almost identical list is found in the *Âshrama-Upanishad* (c. 300 C.E.). This scripture mentions four types of forest eremite:

1. Vaikhânasas, who perform the traditional fire ritual (*agnihotra*) and live on wild grain and vegetables available in their forest environment. The appellation *vaikhânasa* is derived from the prefix *vi* ("dis-") and the word *khâna* ("food"). It hints at the dietary discipline adopted by these renouncers.

2. Audumbaras, who sustain themselves by eating wild grain and fruit, especially figs (*udumbara*).

3. Vâlakhilyas, who get their name from wearing their hair (*vâla*) in a tuft (*khilya*). Their diet is as meager as that of the other renouncers, but they gather food for only eight months of the year and basically fast during the remaining months. This ascetical practice is known as *catur-mâsya* ("the four months").

4. Phenapas, whose name means literally "froth-drinkers." Perhaps this curious designation stems from their practice of drinking the morning dew from leaves. Their diet is stark, consisting

chiefly of certain kinds of fruit. Unlike the other eremites, the Phenapas have no fixed abode.

The wandering renouncers (*parivrajaka*) comprise the following categories:

1. Kuticakas: The name refers to their wearing of a tuft but has other connotations as well. Thus the word *kuti* can mean both "house" or "home" and "sexual intercourse," whereas the stem *caka* means "to tremble." Hence the *kuticaka* is one who trembles when he ponders the householder existence, especially the lure of sexual attachment, that is, he practices chastity. He wanders from place to place, wearing a loincloth and carrying a renouncer's staff and water vessel. He practices meditation by means of sacred syllables or chants (*mantra*).

2. Bahûdakas: Their lifestyle is as simple as that of the Kuticakas. They subsist on eight morsels a day, which they gather from different places "like a bee." The appellation means literally "abundant water" (*bahu* "much," *udaka* "water") and refers to the fact that renouncers of this type tend to frequent sacred places along rivers.

3. Hamsas: These itinerant ascetics are so named because they live like "swans." (Strictly speaking, the word *hamsa* refers to the male of India's species of wild geese.) They do not even beg their food but live from the products of cows, including urine and dung.

4. Paramahamsas: The way of life of these "supreme swans" is still more Spartan. They are described as smearing their entire body with ashes as a sign of their total renunciation of conventional existence. Various scriptures prescribe different rituals for them, such as wearing a single loin cloth or carrying a bamboo staff. But the important fact about the *parama-hamsas* is that they are considered to be fully Self-realized beings. According to some texts, such as the *Vaikhânasa-Smârta-Sûtra*, the *parama-hamsas* wander about in the nude and frequent graveyards. This strange custom foreshadowed the later left-hand rituals of Tantra, which will be introduced in Chapter 17.

The *Nârada-Parivrâjaka-Upanishad* (c. 1200 C.E.) adds two more classes to the above schema—the *turîyâtitas* and the *avadhûtas*. Both are Self-realized adepts. The former, whose name means "transcending the Fourth," live on the little food that is placed directly in their mouths—a practice that is called "cow-face" (*go-mukha*). The latter depend equally on the charity of others. The most telling distinction between the two is that the *avadhûtas* walk about naked, thus demonstrating their ecstatic obliviousness to all differences: There is only the One Reality, which is sexless. All else has, as the name *avadhûta* suggests, been "cast off."

As can be seen, the term "renunciation" covers a wide range of possible lifestyles—from the householder who simply performs an inner or symbolic renunciation to the forest-dweller who continues to observe certain ritual obligations, to the naked wanderer whose way of life can be described as a form of sacred anarchy. Some of these renouncers practiced one or the other form of Yoga, while others simply contemplated the mystery of the Self, without any external aids. All these different types have, over the millennia, contributed to the rich tapestry of Indian spirituality.

## IV. YOGA AND HINDU PHILOSOPHY

In Hinduism the distinction between philosophy and religion is not as clear-cut as it is in our contemporary Western civilization. Sanskrit, the sacred language of Hinduism, does not have straightforward equivalents for either the term "philosophy" or "religion." The closest synonym for "philosophy" is *ânvîkshikî-vidyâ* ("science of examination"). The related term *tarka-shâstra* ("discipline of reasoning") is generally applied only to the Nyâya school of thought, which deals with logic and dialectics. Modern pundits use the term *tattva-vidyâ-shâstra* ("discipline of knowing reality") to express what we mean by "philosophical inquiry."

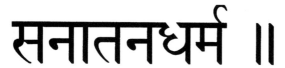

*Sanâtana-dharma*

The concept of "religion" is captured in the Sanskrit term *dharma*, which means "law" or "norm" (with many other connotations). Hindu religion is referred to as *sanâtana-dharma* ("eternal law"), which corresponds to the Western notion of *philosophia perennis*.

For the Hindu, philosophy is not a matter of purely abstract knowledge but metaphysics that has moral implications. In other words, whatever one's theoretical conclusions about reality may be, they must be applied in daily life. Thus philosophy is always regarded as a way of life and is never pursued as merely an inconsequential exercise in rational thinking. More than that, Hindu philosophy (and Indian philosophy as a whole) has a spiritual thrust. With the exception of the materialist school, which is known as Lokâyata or Cârvâka, all philosophical schools acknowledge the existence of a transcendental Reality and agree that a person's spiritual well-being is dependent on how he or she relates to that Reality. Hindu philosophy is therefore closer to the spirit of the ancient Greek *philosophia* ("love of wisdom") than to the contemporary academic discipline of conceptual analysis, which goes by the name of philosophy but is not particularly concerned with life-enhancing wisdom.

Hindu philosophy comprises the same areas of rational inquiry that also have preoccupied the philosophers of the West since the time of Socrates, Plato, and Aristotle—namely, ontology (which deals with the categories of existence), epistemology (which is concerned with the knowledge processes by which we come to know what there is "in reality"), logic (which defines the rules of rational thought), ethics (which critically examines the philosophical basis of action), and aesthetics (which seeks to understand beauty). However, as is true for instance of Christian philosophy, Hindu philosophy is greatly concerned with the ultimate spiritual destiny of humankind. Hence it often describes itself as *âtma-vidyâ* ("science of the Self") or *âdhyâtmika-vidyâ* ("spiritual science").

The earliest philosophical speculations or intuitions of Hinduism are found in the ancient *Rig-Veda*, though mature self-critical systems appear to be the product of the time after the emergence of Buddhism in the sixth century B.C.E. Traditionally, six systems are distinguished, which are referred to as "viewpoints" or "visions" (*darshana*, from the verbal root *drish* "to see"). This phrase hints at two significant things about Hindu philosophy: Each system is not merely the product of rational thinking but also of visionary-intuitive processes, and each system is a particular perspective from which the same truth is viewed, which suggests a position of tolerance (at least in theory, if not in practice). And that identical Truth is what has been handed down by word of mouth (and by esoteric initiation) as the ultimate or transcendental Reality, whether it is called God (*îsh, îsha, îshvara*, all meaning "ruler"), the Self (*âtman, purusha*), or the Absolute (*brahman*).

Tradition is a key element in Hindu philosophy, and tradition means the Vedic revelation (*shruti*), particularly the *Rig-Veda*. In order to establish their respective schools within the orthodox fold, the Hindu philosophers had to defer, or at least pay lip service, to the ancient Vedic heritage. The six principal schools recognized by the Hindu orthodoxy as representing valid points of view within the context of the Vedic revelation are the following: Pûrva-Mîmâmsâ (which puts forward a philosophy of sacrificial ritualism), Uttara-Mîmâmsâ or Vedânta (which is the nondualist metaphysics espoused especially in the *Upanishads*), Sâmkhya (whose principal contribution concerns the categories of existence, or *tattvas*), Yoga (which here refers specifically to the philosophical school of Patanjali, the author of the *Yoga-Sûtra*), Vaisheshika (which, similar to the Sâmkhya school, is an attempt to grasp the categories of existence, though from a different angle), and Nyâya (which is primarily a theory of logic and argument). I will briefly describe each school and highlight its relationship to the Yoga tradition.

## Pûrva-Mîmâmsâ

The school of Pûrva-Mîmâmsâ ("Earlier Inquiry") is so called because it interprets the "earlier" two portions of the Vedic revelation: the ancient Vedic hymnodies themselves and the *Brâhmana* texts that explain and develop their sacrificial rituals. It is contrasted to the Uttara-Mîmâmsâ ("Later Inquiry"), represented by the nondualist teachings of the *Upanishads*. The Pûrva-Mîmâmsâ school was given its distinct form by the *Mîmâmsâ-Sûtra* of Jaimini (c. 200–300 B.C.E.). It expounds the art and science of moral action in keeping with Vedic ritualism. Its focal point is the concept of *dharma*, or virtue, insofar as it affects the religious or spiritual destiny of the individual. The secular applications of *dharma* are left to the authorities of ethics (*dharma-shâstra*) to define and explain. There have been several renowned Jaiminis, and the author of the *Sûtra* must be distinguished especially from the sage who was a disciple of Vyâsa at the time of the Bhârata war.

The Mîmâmsâ thinkers, or *mîmâmsâkas*, regard ethical action as an invisible, extraordinary force that determines the appearance of the world: The human being is intrinsically active, and action determines the quality of human existence both in the present incarnation and in future incarnations. Good actions (actions in keeping with the Vedic moral code, which is thought to mirror the universal order itself) bring about positive life circumstances, whereas bad actions (actions contradicting the Vedic moral code) lead to negative life circumstances.

The purpose of living a morally sound life is to improve the qualities of one's existence in the present, in the hereafter, and in subsequent embodiments. Because the individual has free will, he or she can accumulate positive results, and even annul existing negative results, through good actions. Free will is guaranteed by the fact that the essential Self is transcendental and eternal. In contrast to Vedânta, the Mîmâmsâ school postulates many such essential Selves (*âtman*). These are deemed intrinsically unconscious and come to consciousness only in conjunction with a body-mind. Consciousness is, therefore, always I-consciousness (*aham-dhî*) for the Mîmâmsâ thinkers. There is no God over and above those many eternal and omnipresent Selves, although from the fifteenth century on, some representatives of this school started to believe in a Creator God.

Since the Self is held to possess neither consciousness nor bliss, the earlier *mîmâmsâkas* naturally found the ideal of liberation pursued by other schools quite undesirable. This orientation was rejected by the eighth-century philosopher Kumârila Bhatta and his pupil Prabhâkara. They both taught that abstention from the prohibited and merely optional actions and the dutiful performance of the prescribed actions automatically lead to the dissociation of the Self from the body-mind—that is, liberation. They looked upon the Self as consciousness, though failed to fully develop the metaphysical implications of their position.

The practice of yogic techniques has no place in Mîmâmsâ, which extols the ideal of duty for duty's sake. Sarvepalli Radhakrishnan, a former president of India and a great scholar, remarked about this school of thought that "as a philosophical view of the universe it is strikingly incomplete . . . There is little in such a religion to touch the heart and make it glow."[13] However, Pûrva-Mîmâmsâ was one of the cultural forces encountered by the Yoga tradition, and therefore it needs to be taken into account here.

By Western standards, this system of thought would hardly be called philosophical, though Pûrva-Mîmâmsâ was instrumental in developing logic and dialectics. Apart from Jaimini, Kumârila, and Prabhâkara, the most outstanding thinker of this school, which has a rather comprehensive literature, is Mandana Mishra (ninth century C.E.), who later became converted to Shankara's school of Advaita Vedânta and assumed the name Sureshvara.

The story of the electrifying encounter between Shankara and Mandana Mishra is told in the fourteenth-century *Shankara-Dig-Vijaya*, a spurious biography of Shankara. According to this legend, the young Shankara, who had adopted the life of a renouncer, visited Mandana Mishra's stately mansion just as the great scholar of Vedic ritualism was about to embark on one of his ceremonies. He was annoyed with Shankara, who wore neither the traditional hair tuft nor the sacred thread across his chest. After a barrage of insulting remarks, which Shankara took calmly and not without amusement, Mandana Mishra, rather proud of his learning, challenged the visitor to a debate. They agreed, as was customary in those days, that whoever lost the debate was to assume the lifestyle of the winner.

Their combat of knowledge and wit lasted over several days and drew large crowds of scholars. Mandana Mishra's wife, Ubhayâ Bhâratî (who was none other than Sarasvatî, the Goddess of Learning, in disguise), was appointed umpire. Before long, she announced the defeat of her husband but then promptly argued that Shankara had defeated only one half; for his victory to be real, he would also have to defeat her. Slyly, she challenged the young renouncer to a discussion about sexuality.

Without losing his composure, Shankara asked for an adjournment so that he could acquaint himself with this area of knowledge. It so happened that the ruler of a neighboring kingdom had just died, and Shankara, wasting no time, used his yogic powers to enter the corpse and reanimate it. Under the joyous exclamations of the king's relatives, he returned to the palace. In the spirit of Tantra, Shankara enjoyed and explored for a period of time the delights of sexual love among the dead king's wives and courtesans. As the legend goes, he got so absorbed in this new life that his disciples had to steal into the palace and remind him of his former life as a renouncer.

Restored to his true identity, Shankara deftly dropped the king's body and resumed the debate with Mandana Mishra's wife. Of course, he won. Mandana Mishra declared himself a pupil of Shankara, whereupon his wife Ubhayâ Bhâratî revealed her true identity. Shankara's victory is generally seen as a victory of his superior nondualist metaphysics over the less sophisticated philosophy of Pûrva-Mîmâmsâ. This may be so, but it was primarily a triumph of yogic experientialism over intellectualism.

## Uttara-Mîmâmsâ

The many-branched school of Uttara-Mîmâmsâ ("Later Inquiry"), also known as Vedânta ("Veda's End"), gets its name from the fact that it evolved around the consideration of the "later" two portions of the Vedic revelation: the *Âranyakas* (forest treatises composed by hermits) and the *Upanishads* (esoteric gnostic scriptures composed by sages). Both the *Âranyakas* and the *Upanishads* represent a metaphoric reinterpretation of the ancient Vedic heritage: They preached the internalization of the archaic rituals in the form of meditation. Especially the Upanishadic teachings gave rise to the whole consciousness technology associated with the Vedânta tradition.

The literature of the Uttara-Mîmâmsâ school, or Vedânta, comprises the *Upanishads* (of which there are over two hundred texts), the *Bhagavad-Gîtâ* (which is given the sacred status of an *Upanishad* and may belong to c. 500–600 B.C.E.), and the *Vedânta-* or *Brahma-Sûtra* of Bâdarâyana (c. 200 C.E.), which systematizes the often contradictory teachings of the *Upanishads* and the *Bhagavad-Gîtâ*.

Vedânta is metaphysics par excellence. Its various subschools all teach one or another form of nondualism, according to which Reality is a single, homogeneous whole. The fundamental idea of Vedântic nondualism is articulated in the following stanzas from the *Naishkarmya-Siddhi* ("Perfection of Action-Transcendence"), composed by Sureshvara (the former Mandana Mishra):

Nonrecognition of the singular Self-hood [of all things] is [spiritual] ignorance (*avidyâ*). The mainstay of [that ignorance] is the experience of one's own self. It is the seed of the world-of-change. The destruction of that [spiritual ignorance] is the liberation (*mukti*) of the self. (1.7)

The fire of right knowledge (*jnâna*) arising from the brilliant Vedic utterances burns up the delusion of [there being an independent] self. Action does not [remove ignorance], because it is not incompatible [with ignorance]. (1.80)

Because action arises from ignorance, it does not do away with delusion. Right knowledge [alone can remove ignorance], since it is its opposite, rather like the sun is [the opposite of] darkness. (1.35)

Upon mistaking a tree stump for a thief, one becomes frightened and runs away. Similarly, one who is deluded superimposes the Self upon the *buddhi* [i.e., the higher mind] and the other [aspects of the human personality], and then acts [on the basis of that mistaken view]. (1.60)

Advaita Vedânta stood the earlier Vedic ritualism on its head. It is a gospel of gnosis: not intellectual or factual knowledge but the liberating intuition of the transcendental Reality.

The two greatest exponents of Vedânta were Shankara (c. 788–820 C.E.)[14] and Râmânuja (1017–1127 C.E.). The former succeeded in constructing a coherent philosophical system out of the Upanishadic teachings and has largely been responsible for the survival of Hinduism and the displacement of Buddhism from India. Râmânuja, on the other hand, came to the rescue of the Advaita Vedânta tradition when it was threatened with losing itself in dry scholasticism. His notion of the Divine as entailing rather than transcending all qualities encouraged the popular thrust toward a more devotional expression within Hindu spirituality. Both Shankara and Râmânuja, as well as many other Vedânta teachers, have had strong links with the Yoga tradition. This is explored in Chapter 12.

## Sâmkhya

The tradition of Sâmkhya ("Enumeration"), which comprises many different schools, is primarily concerned with enumerating and describing the principal categories of existence. This approach would be called "ontology," or the "science of being," in Western philosophy. In their metaphysical ideas, Sâmkhya and Yoga are closely akin and in fact once formed a single pre-classical tradition. But whereas the followers of Sâmkhya use discrimination (*viveka*) and renunciation as their chief means of salvation, the *yogins* proceed mainly through the combined practice of meditation and renunciation. Sâmkhya is often characterized as the theoretical aspect of Yoga practice, but this is incorrect. Both traditions have their own distinct theories and practical

approaches. Because of its emphasis on discriminative knowledge rather than meditation, Sâmkhya in later times has tended toward intellectualism, whereas Yoga has always been exposed to the danger of deviating into mere magical psychotechnology.

Next to Vedânta, the Sâmkhya philosophy has been the single most influential system of thought within the fold of Hinduism, and Shankara regarded it as his main opponent. Sâmkhya is said to have been founded by the Sage Kapila, who is credited with the authorship of the *Sâmkhya-Sûtra*. Although a teacher by that name is likely to have lived during the Vedic Era, the *Sâmkhya-Sûtra* appears to have been composed according to some

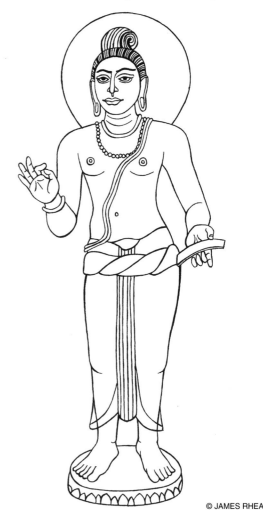

*Kapila, originator of the Sâmkhya tradition*

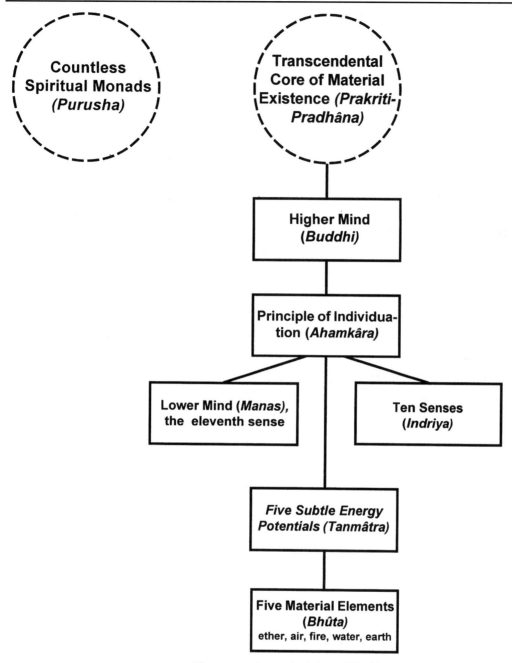

*The twenty-four principles of Sâmkhya*

scholars as late as the fourteenth or fifteenth century C.E.

In the framework of the six *darshanas*, the Sâmkhya referred to is the school of Îshvara Krishna (c. 350 C.E.), author of the *Sâmkhya-Kârikâ*. In striking contrast to Vedânta and the earlier Sâmkhya schools mentioned in the *Mahâbharâta* epic, Îshvara Krishna taught that Reality is not singular but plural. On one side are the countless mutable and unconscious forms of Nature (*prakriti*), and on the other side are the innumerable transcendental Selves (*purusha*), which are pure Consciousness, omnipresent and eternal. Looked at more closely, this pluralism is illogical. If countless Selves are all omnipresent, they must also be infinitely intersecting each other, so that logically they should be considered identical. This problem has been tackled again and again by various philosophers, and while Shankara's nondualism is intellectually the most elegant, Râmânuja's qualified nondualism perhaps best satisfies both reason and intuition.

Îshvara Krishna further taught that Nature (*prakriti*) is a vast composite or multidimensional structure created by the interplay of three primary forces, the dynamic qualities (*guna*). The word *guna* means literally "strand" but has a wide range of connotations. In the context of Yoga and Sâmkhya metaphysics, the term denotes the irreducible ultimate "reals" of the cosmos. The *gunas*, which are of three types, can be said to resemble the energy quanta of modern physics. The three *gunas* are called *sattva*, *rajas*, and *tamas*. They underlie all material as well as psychomental phenomena. In the *Sâmkhya-Kârikâ*, their respective characters are delineated as follows:

> The [three types of] *gunas* are of the nature of joy, joylessness, and dejection and [respectively] have the purpose of illuminating, activating, and restricting. They overpower each other, are interdependent, productive, and cooperative in their activities. (12)

> *Sattva* is regarded as buoyant and illuminating. *Rajas* is stimulating and mobile. *Tamas* is inert and concealing. The activity [of the *gunas*] is purposive like a lamp [made up of various parts that together produce the single phenomenon of light]. (13)

The *gunas are* Nature, just as the atoms *are* matter-energy. Together they are responsible for the immense variety of natural forms on all levels of existence other than that of the transcendental Selves, which are unqualified Consciousness. The

German Sanskritist Max Müller observed about the *gunas*:

> We can best explain them by the general idea of two opposites and the middle term between them, or as Hegel's thesis, antithesis and synthesis, these being manifested in nature by light, darkness, and mist; in morals by good, bad, and indifferent, with many applications and modifications.[15]

According to the *Sâmkhya-Kârikâ*, the *gunas* are in a state of balance in the transcendental dimension of Nature, known as *prakriti-pradhâna* ("Nature's foundation"). The first product or evolute to appear in the process of evolution from this transcendental matrix to the multiplicity of space-time forms is *mahat*, meaning literally "great one," or great principle. It has the appearance of luminosity and intelligence, and is therefore also known as *buddhi* ("intuition" or "cognition"), standing for higher wisdom. But, in reality, *mahat* is in itself quite unconscious (as are all aspects of Nature), and it represents only a particularly refined form of matter-energy. It depends on the transcendental Self-Consciousness for its "light" of intelligence.

Out of the *mahat*, or *buddhi*, emerges *ahamkâra* ("I-maker"), the principle of individuation, which ushers in the distinction between subject and object. This existential category, in turn, causes the appearance of the lower mind (*manas*), the five cognitive senses (sight, smell, taste, touch, and hearing), and the five conative senses (speech, prehension, movement, excretion, and reproduction). The *ahamkâra* principle further gives rise to the five subtle essences (*tanmâtra*) underlying the sensory capacities. They, in turn, produce the five gross material elements (*bhûta*), namely earth, water, fire, air, and ether.

Thus, Classical Sâmkhya recognizes twenty-four categories of material existence in all. Beyond the *guna* triad and its products are the countless transcendental Self-monads, which are untouched by the ramifications of Nature.

The entire evolutionary process is triggered by the proximity of the transcendental Selves (*purusha*) to the transcendental matrix of Nature. Moreover, the process is for the sake of the liberation of those Selves that, mysteriously and wrongly, identify themselves with a particular body-mind rather than their intrinsic condition of pure Consciousness.

The psychocosmological evolutionism of the Sâmkhya tradition is not meant so much to explain the world as to help transcend it. It is a practical framework for those who desire Self-realization and who encounter the diverse levels or categories of existence in the course of their meditation practice.

## Yoga

In the context of the six schools of Hindu philosophy, Yoga signifies specifically the school of Patanjali, the author of the *Yoga-Sûtra*. This school, frequently referred to as Classical Yoga, is considered a cousin of the Sâmkhya school of Îshvara Krishna. Both are dualist philosophies, which teach that the transcendental Selves (*purusha*) are radically separate from Nature (*prakriti*) and that the former are eternally unchanging, whereas the latter is forever undergoing transformation and is therefore not conducive to lasting happiness. We need not go into further detail here, because Patanjali's school is presented at length in Part Three.

## Vaisheshika

The school of Vaisheshika ("Distinctionism") is concerned with the distinctions (*vishesha*) between things. It teaches that liberation is attained through a thorough understanding of the six primary categories of existence:

1. Substance (*dravya*), which is ninefold: earth, water, fire, air, ether, time, space, mind (*manas*), and Self (*âtman*)

2. quality (*guna*), of which there are twenty-three types, such as color, sensory perceptions, magnitude, and so on

3. action (*karma*)

4. the universal (*sâmânya* or *jâti*)

5. the particular (*vishesha*)

6. inherence (*samâvaya*), which refers to the necessary logical relationship between wholes and parts, or substances and their qualities, and so on.

The Vaisheshika school was founded by Kanâda, the author of the *Vaisheshika-Sûtra*, who lived perhaps around 500 or 600 B.C.E. The name Kanâda appears to be a nickname, meaning literally "particle eater." Presumably it refers to the kind of philosophy elaborated by him, though some Sanskrit authorities suggest that the name immortalizes the fact that this mighty ascetic lived on particles (*kana*) of grain. Perhaps both interpretations are correct.

The origins of Kanâda's school of thought are quite obscure. Some scholars regard it as an offshoot of the older Mîmâmsâ school, others see in it a development of the materialist tradition, and yet others have proposed that it has its earliest roots in a schismatic branch of Jainism. In its general orientation as well as its metaphysics, the Vaisheshika school is close to the Nyâya system, with which it is traditionally grouped. Both these schools come closest to what we in the West understand by philosophy. They made a lasting contribution to Indian thought, but neither school has retained a prominent position. The Vaisheshika school is virtually extinct, and the Nyâya school has only a few representatives, mostly in Bengal.

## Nyâya

The Nyâya ("Rule") school of thought was founded by Akshapâda Gautama (c. 500 B.C.E.), who lived in an age of great controversy between Vedic ritualism and such heterodox developments as Buddhism and Jainism—an era in which critical thinking and debating were, as in Greece, at an all-time peak. His was one of the earliest attempts to formulate valid rules for logic and the art of rhetoric.

Akshapâda is a nickname suggesting perhaps that Gautama was in the habit of looking down at his feet (perhaps while being immersed in thought or in order to purify the ground while walking). He is attributed with the authorship of the *Nyâya-Sûtra*, which had many commentaries written on it. The oldest extant commentary is that of Vâtsyâyana Pakshilasvâmin (c. 400 C.E.), written at a time when Buddhism was still strong in India. Another valuable commentary is Bharadvâja's or Uddyotakara's *Nyâya-Vârttika*, which has a fine subcommentary by Vâcaspati Mishra, who also wrote on Yoga. Nyâya entered its period of flowering around 1200 C.E., which is the beginning of the so-called Nava-Nyâya (or "New Nyâya").

Akshapâda Gautama proceeded from the insight that in order to live rightly and to pursue meaningful goals, we must first determine what constitutes right knowledge. True to the Indic flair for classification, he elaborated sixteen categories deemed important for anyone desiring to know the truth. These range from the means by which valid knowledge (*pramâna*) can be acquired, to the nature of doubt, to the difference between debate and mere wrangling. This is not the place to examine these categories more closely. What is of interest is the metaphysics of the Nyâya school.

According to the followers of Nyâya, there are numerous transcendental Subjects, or Selves (*âtman*). Each infinite Self is the ultimate agent behind the human mind, and each Self enjoys and suffers the fruits of its actions in the finite world. God is considered a special *âtman*, as in Classical Yoga, and he alone is conscious. Despite the fact that the human Selves are all considered unconscious, as in the Mîmâmsâ school, the Nyâya philosophers proposed the pursuit of liberation (*apavarga*) as the noblest goal in life. Of course, their opponents did not fail to point out the undesirability of a liberation that would lead to a rocklike, insentient existence. How little the adherents of Nyâya were convinced by their own metaphysics is evident from the fact that they looked for spiritual refuge in the religious teachings of Shaivism.

There are several points of contact between Nyâya and Yoga. Yoga is mentioned in the *Nyâya-Sûtra* (chapter 4) as that condition in which the mind is in contact with the Self alone, as a result of which there is mental equilibrium and insensitivity to bodily pain. In discussing various forms of perception, Vâtsyâyana Pakshilasvâmin noted that the *yogins* are able to perceive remote and even future events, a skill that can be cultivated by the regular practice of meditative concentration. Liberation is called *apavarga*, and this term is also found in the *Yoga-Sûtra* (2.18) where it is contrasted with the idea of world experience (*bhoga*).

A further curious parallel is that both Nyâya and Classical Yoga subscribe to the doctrine of *sphota*. This term refers to the eternal relationship between a word and its sound. The idea here is that, for instance, the letters *y*, *o*, *g*, and *a*, or even the entire word *yoga*, cannot explain the knowledge we have of the thing called "Yoga." Over and above these letters or sounds, there is an eternal concept, the essence of a thing. Upon hearing a sequence of sounds, this eternal essence "bursts forth" (*sphuta*) or reveals itself spontaneously in our mind, leading to comprehension of the thing thus denoted.

A final connecting point is that an adherent of Nyâya is also known as *yauga*, that is, "one who has to do with Yoga." It is not clear what is hidden in this designation.

The division of Hindu philosophy into six schools is somewhat artificial. There are many other schools—notably those associated with certain sectarian movements—that at one time or another played an important role in the evolution of Indian thought. We will encounter some of them in later chapters. What should be borne in mind is that Yoga influenced most of these approaches and traditions, though it did so more as a loose body of ideas, beliefs, and practices than as the philosophical system (*darshana*) articulated by Patanjali.

## V. YOGA, ÂYUR-VEDA, AND SIDDHA MEDICINE

Âyur-Veda ("Science of Life")—usually written as one word in English, *Âyurveda*—is the name given to the native Indian system of medicine. Âyur-Veda is essentially naturopathic medi-

cine, emphasizing prevention but also having an extensive curative repertoire. It is practiced in India alongside modern medicine and is put forward as a way of life for those wishing to enjoy good health and longevity. Although Âyur-Veda cannot be regarded as a philosophical tradition, it is founded in Hindu metaphysics. Âyur-Veda is traditionally considered to be supplementary knowledge to the ancient *Atharva-Veda*. In this sacred scripture we find the earliest recorded speculations on anatomy and on curative and preventive medicine. Because of its cultural importance, Âyur-Veda has sometimes been regarded as a fifth branch, or "collection," of the Vedic heritage.

The Âyur-Vedic body of knowledge is said to have originally amounted to 100,000 stanzas, gathered in a book of over one thousand chapters. While medicine was undoubtedly practiced in the early Vedic era, no work of such comprehensiveness has survived into our time. The earliest extant medical works of encyclopedic scope are the *Sushruta-Samhitâ* and the *Caraka-Samhitâ*. In its oldest portions the former work dates back to pre-Buddhist times, but it was completed in its present form only in the early centuries of the Common Era. Sushruta is remembered in the *Mahâbhârata* (1.4.55) as the grandson of King Gâdhi and son of the sage Vishvâmitra, which in the revised chronology adopted in this volume would place him roughly sixty-two generations before the Bharata war, that is, c. 3000 B.C.E. Sushruta's name means literally "well heard," suggesting that he was particularly capable of receiving and understanding the transmitted knowledge. How much of the original medical knowledge can be found in the extant *Sushruta-Samhitâ* is anyone's guess. We know, however, from hymns in the *Rig-Veda* and *Atharva-Veda* that there were skilled physicians during the Vedic Era.

The latter medical collection, which also was frequently revised, was probably given its present shape around 800 C.E. However, its reputed author, Caraka, probably lived many centuries earlier, since he is said to have been the court-physician of King Kanishka (78–120 C.E.). Caraka's name reminds us that the ancient physicians—though perhaps not the renowned Caraka himself—used to travel (*cara*) from place to place offering their medical services.

Like Classical Yoga, which is comprised of eight "limbs," the Âyur-Vedic system of medicine is—according to the *Sushruta-Samhitâ* (1.1.5–9)—divided into eight branches: (1) surgery; (2) treatment of diseases of the neck and head; (3) treatment of physical diseases of the torso, arms, and legs; (4) treatment of childhood diseases; (5) processes for counteracting baneful occult influences; (6) toxicology; (7) processes for rejuvenating the body, known as *rasâyana*; and (8) techniques for sexual revitalization (*vâjikarana*).

The formal similarity between Âyur-Veda and Patanjali's eightfold Yoga, remarked on by the Hindu authorities, is purely coincidental, though some traditional authorities have paid attention to this parallel. There are, however, a number of important concepts and techniques that Âyur-Veda and Yoga have in common. Most significantly, the authors and editors of the above-mentioned medical reference works availed themselves of the philosophy of the Yoga-Sâmkhya tradition. Thus, at one point the *Sushruta-Samhitâ* appears to have been revised in light of Îshvara Krishna's dualist system of thought, as propounded in his *Sâmkhya-Kârikâ*. The *Caraka-Samhitâ*, on the other hand, contains echoes of epic Sâmkhya-Yoga metaphysics. Here it should also be mentioned that some of the ancient Sanskrit commentators believed that the same Patanjali who composed the *Yoga-Sûtra* also wrote a famous treatise on grammar and one on medicine.

Both Âyur-Veda and Yoga insist on the interactive unity of body and mind. Physical diseases can affect the mind adversely, and mental imbalance can lead to illnesses of all kinds. Âyur-Veda's notion of a healthy life includes that it must be both happy (*sukha*) and morally good (*hita*). A happy life, by Âyur-Vedic definition, is one that is physically and mentally hale and vigorous as well as moral and even wise. The intimate relationship between ethical conduct and happiness is emphasized in the Yoga literature as well.

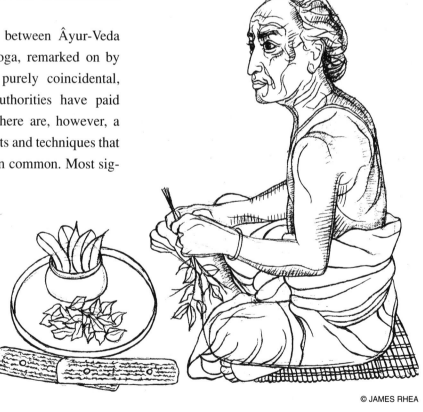

© JAMES RHEA

*Caraka*

The authorities of Âyur-Veda recommend the cultivation of tranquillity, self-knowledge, and prudence. Today we might say that the Hindu physicians incorporated self-actualization (in Abraham Maslow's sense[16]) into their medical theory and practice. We can readily appreciate that such a life would form a sound basis for the pursuit of the spiritual value of Self-realization (*âtma-jnâna*). In his book *Ayurveda and the Mind*, David Frawley goes so far as to say:

> Ayurveda is the healing branch of yogic science. Yoga is the spiritual aspect of Ayurveda. Ayurveda is the therapeutic branch of Yoga.[17]

A strong connecting point between Âyur-Veda and Yoga is the theory of the various life currents (*vâyu*) in the body, which originated at the time of the *Atharva-Veda*. The medical authorities generally list thirteen conduits (*nâdî*) along or in which the different types of life force (*prâna*) are thought to travel, whereas the Hatha-Yoga scriptures usually mention fourteen such principal pathways. Often a distinction is made between these conduits and larger ducts (called *dhamanî*) carrying fluids such as blood, etc. The Âyur-Vedic model of this network of channels is quite different from the Tantric model, which is more specific to the subtle body.

In Hatha-Yoga, the importance of commencing the practice of breath control in the right season is recognized. The medical basis for this custom is furnished by Âyur-Veda, according to which the bodily humors (*dosha*) undergo changes in the different seasons. The concept of the *doshas* also is referred to in a number of Yoga works, such as the fifth-century *Yoga-Bhâshya* (1.30), where illness is defined as an "imbalance of the constituents (*dhâtu*) or the activity of the secretions (*rasa*)." In his ninth-century gloss on

this text, Vâcaspati Mishra explains that the constituents are air (*vâta*), bile (*pitta*), and phlegm (*kapha*), in other words the *doshas*. This is medical language.

The *doshas* are also often referred to in the literature of Hatha-Yoga, which is concerned with the optimal functioning of the body. Health is deemed a matter of the proper balance between the bodily constituents.[18] These exist throughout the body but are present in different concentrations at various places. Thus, *vâta* is preeminent in the nervous system, heart, large intestines, lungs, bladder, and pelvis; *pitta* predominates in the liver, spleen, small intestines, endocrine glands, blood, and perspiration; *kapha* in the joints, mouth, head and neck, stomach, lymph, and adipose tissue. *Vâta* tends to accumulate below the navel, *kapha* above the diaphragm, and *pitta* between the diaphragm and navel.

In addition to the three *doshas*, Âyur-Veda also recognizes seven types of tissue (*dhâtu*) and three impure substances (*mala*). The *dhâtus* are blood plasma (*rasa*), blood (*rakta*), flesh (*mâmsa*), fat (*meda*), bone (*asthi*), bone marrow (*majjan*), and semen (*shukra*). The *malas*, or waste materials, are feces (*purîsha*), urine (*mûtra*), and perspiration (*sveda*, lit. "sweat"). These bodily components are occasionally mentioned in the Yoga literature as well.

This is also true of the vulnerable or sensitive zones (*marman*), which are already mentioned in the *Rig-Veda* (6.75.18). According to Âyur-Veda, there are 107 *marmans*, which are vital connections between flesh and muscle, bones, joints, and sinews, or between veins. A hard blow to some of these *marmans* can cause death, as is part of the secret knowledge of the Chinese and Japanese martial arts. The South Indian martial arts practice of *kalarippayattu* recognizes 160 to 220 such sensitive points in the body. This system regards the body as being constituted of three layers, namely the fluid body (including tissue and waste products); the solid body of muscles, bones, and the *marmans*; and the subtle body consisting of the channels and gathering points of vital energy. Injury to a *marman* interrupts the flow of the wind element, thus causing severe physical problems that may result in death. Sometimes a vigorous slap to the injured area, administered promptly, can restore the flow of the life force and thus prevent the worst. The *marmans* depend on the flow of *prâna*, and without *prâna* there are no *marmans*. The flow of the life force through these sensitive spots is controlled by the moon. A similar teaching is present in ancient Hindu sexology, which recommends stimulating certain sensitive areas on the woman's body only on particular lunar days.[19]

Some Yoga scriptures, such as the *Shândilya-Upanishad* (1.8.1f.), speak of eighteen *marmans*, and according to the *Kshurikâ-Upanishad* (14), the *yogin* should cut through these vital spots by means of the "mind's sharp blade." In other words, here the *marmans* appear to be understood as blockages in the flow of the life force, which are removed through concentration and breath control.

An important concept shared by Âyur-Veda and Yoga is that of *ojas*, or the energy of vitality, which is mentioned already in the *Atharva-Veda* (2.17.1). Both systems seek to increase *ojas* (that is, the "lower" variety) by various means. In Yoga, the most frequently recommended method for enhancing one's vital power is sexual abstinence. *Ojas* decreases with age and is reduced through hunger, poor diet, overwork, anger, and worry—all the physical and mental circumstances that sap one's zest for living. Their opposite conditions generate *ojas* and thus ensure good health. When *ojas* is low for longer periods, it gives rise to degenerative diseases and premature aging.

*Ojas* is present in the entire body but is especially stored in the heart, which is also the physical anchorage of consciousness. Cakrapâni, in his commentary on the *Caraka-Samhitâ*, mentions that while there is half a handful of "lower *ojas*" in the body, there are only eight drops of the "higher *ojas*" in the heart. The slightest waste of this precious vital energy is thought to cause death, and it cannot be replenished.

Furthermore, Hatha-Yoga and Âyur-Veda share certain purificatory techniques, notably the practice of self-induced vomiting (*vamana*) and physical cleansing (*dhauti*). These techniques have, among other things, a salutary effect on the body's metabolism. Âyur-Veda, moreover, knows of thirteen kinds of internal heat (*agni*), of which the digestive heat (*jâthara-agni*) is often mentioned by the authorities of Hatha-Yoga.

Physical well-being (*ârogya*) is definitely one of the prerequisites and intermediate goals of Hatha-Yoga. Even Patanjali, in his *Yoga-Sûtra* (3.46), mentions "adamantine robustness" of the body as one of the aspects of bodily perfection (*kâya-sampad*). In another aphorism (2.43), Patanjali speaks of the perfection of the body and the senses as a result of the dwindling of impurities by virtue of asceticism. Moreover, he states (2.38) that vitality (*vîrya*) is gained through chastity. In aphorism 1.30, again, Patanjali lists sickness (*vyâdhi*) as one of the distractions (*vikshepa*) of the mind that prevent progress in Yoga.

The *Shiva-Svarodaya*, a yogic work that is several hundred years old, promotes breath control as the foremost means of achieving or maintaining well-being and for gaining occult knowledge and powers, as well as wisdom and even liberation. In one verse (314), the technique of *svarodaya*—from *svara* ("sound [of the breath]") and *udaya* ("rising")—is stated to be a science promulgated by the *siddha-yogins*.

In the *Sat-Karma-Samgraha* ("Compendium of Right Acts"), a Yoga text authored by Cidghanânanda, a disciple of Gaganânanda of the Nâtha sect, a whole range of purificatory practices is outlined. These are intended to either stave off or cure all kinds of illnesses resulting from sheer misfortune or from carelessness in observing the prescribed dietary and other rules, such as those relative to the proper location and time. Cidghanânanda advises the *yogin* first to use postures (*âsana*) and occult medications to heal himself. When these fail, he should proceed with the techniques disclosed in the text.

The link between Yoga and Âyur-Veda is clearly acknowledged in the sixteenth-century work by Yogânanda Nâtha, entitled *Âyur-Veda-Sûtra*, in which the author specifically makes use of Patanjali's *Yoga-Sûtra* and also explores diet and fasting as efficient means to health. Food is examined in light of the relative predominance of the three *gunas* in it. The *gunas*—*sattva*, *rajas*, and *tamas*—are also part of the medical theory of Âyur-Veda. Imbalance in the bodily constituents or the humors suggest an imbalance in the *gunas*, and vice versa. All finite existence, in a way, is the result of a disequilibrium of the *gunas*; only at the transcendental level of Nature (*prakriti-pradhâna*) are they in a perfect balance. Sometimes the three humors (*dosha*) are regarded as somatic defects and the three *gunas* as mental flaws. They are correlated as follows: wind — *sattva*; bile — *rajas*; phlegm — *tamas*.

# सत्त्व । रजस् । तमस् ॥

*Sattva, rajas, tamas*

One of the practices of Âyur-Veda that meshes closely with Hatha-Yoga's ideal of creating a long-lived, if not immortal, body is *kâya-kalpa*. This is a difficult ritual of rejuvenation requiring prolonged isolation in darkness, rigorous dietary constraints, and secret potions. The modern saint Tapasviji Maharaj reportedly underwent this treatment on several occasions, each time emerging from his solitary confinement in a dark hut looking and feeling thoroughly rejuvenated.

The close connection between Âyur-Veda, Yoga, and alchemy (*rasâyana*, from *rasa* "essence" or "mercury" and *ayana* "course") is particularly apparent in the medieval Siddha tradition of northern India. The adherents of this important tradition sought after bodily immortality through a sophisticated psychophysiological technology known as *kâya-sâdhana*, or "body cultivation." Out of this grew the various schools of Hatha-Yoga, which, on one level, can almost be looked upon as the preventative branch of Hindu medicine. Interestingly, one book on medicine—by a certain Vrinda—has the title *Siddha-Yoga*. Another medical treatise, ascribed to Nâgârjuna, bears the title *Yoga-Shataka* ("Century [of Verses] on Yoga").

South India has produced a second independent medical system that is the equivalent of Âyur-Veda. This system is associated with the Siddha tradition as it has developed in the Tamil-speaking countries. Even more than Âyur-Veda, it has a strong connection with alchemy and employs a large number of remedies derived from vegetables and chemicals. Its three principal diagnostic and therapeutic tools are astrology, mantras, and drugs, known in the Tamil language respectively as *mani*, *mantiram*, and *maruntu*. It also makes use of postures (*âsana*) and breath control.

This rival system of medicine, which has scarcely been researched, was founded by the legendary Sage Akattiyar (Sanskrit: Agastya), to whom over two hundred works are attributed. He is the first of the eighteen *siddhas*, or fully accomplished adepts, venerated in the south of the Indian peninsula. There was an ancient seer

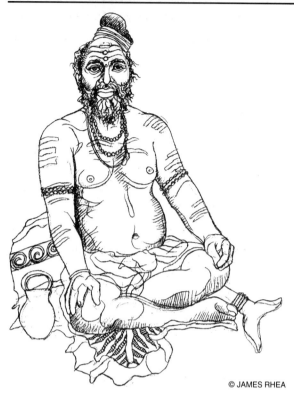

© JAMES RHEA

*Agastya, the dwarfish sage*

called Agastya, who composed several hymns of the *Rig-Veda*, and this archaic scripture (1.179) has even preserved a conversation between him and his wife Lohâmudrâ. He is remembered as having been of small stature and in iconography is typically depicted as a dwarf. His name has anciently been associated with South India, where he is held in the same high esteem that Matsyendra Nâtha enjoys in the North.

Teraiyar, who is traditionally considered one of Agastya's disciples but probably lived as late as the fifteenth century C.E., was an adept and a renowned healer. Of his many works only two are still available: the *Cikamanivenpa* and the *Natikkottu* (on pulse diagnosis). A fragment of the *Noyanukaviti* (on hygiene) also has survived. The last-mentioned work contains the following stanzas:

> We will eat only twice, not three times
> a day;

we will sleep only at night, not during
   the day;
we will have sexual intercourse only
   once a month;
we will drink water only at meals,
   though we may feel thirsty;
we will not eat the bulbous root of any
   plant except that of karanai;
we will not eat any unripe fruit except
   the tender plantain;
we shall take a short walk after a
   friendly meal;
what has death then to do with us?

Once in six months we shall take an
   emetic;
we shall take a purgative once in four
   months;
once in a month and a half, we shall
   take naciyam;[20]
we shall have the head shaved twice in
   a fortnight;
once every fourth day we shall anoint
   ourselves with oil and bathe;
we shall apply collyrium to the eyes
   every third day;
we shall never smell perfumes or flowers in the middle of the night;
what has death then to do with us?[21]

It is clear from the above lines that the *siddhas* of South India, like their northern counterparts, were greatly interested in longevity, and were even aspiring to immortality in a transubstantiated body. More will be said about their teachings in Chapters 17 and 18.

## VI. YOGA AND HINDU RELIGION

Yoga is not religion in the conventional sense but rather spirituality, esotericism, or mysticism.

Yet, whether we look at Hinduism, Buddhism, Jainism, or Sikhism, Yoga is as a rule intimately connected with the cosmologies as well as the religious beliefs and practices of these distinct traditions. This has proven a stumbling block for many Western Yoga practitioners, who neither are informed about these traditions nor, perhaps, are on good terms with their own religious heritage, be it Christianity or Judaism. In particular, they are startled by the numerous deities of the Hindu, Buddhist, and Jaina pantheons and are wondering how they relate to actual Yoga practice and to the teaching of nondualism (*advaita*) characteristic of most forms of Yoga. Those students who have monotheistic leanings may even be concerned about succumbing to polytheism, which is considered a sin in the Judeo-Christian tradition. Since the focus of this book is on Hindu Yoga, I propose to introduce the major Gods and Goddesses of Hinduism, which make their appearance here and there in the Sanskrit and vernacular literature of Yoga. The Jainas by and large have retained the same deities, and many Hindu deities also form part of the expansive Buddhist pantheon.

The various deities are invoked and worshiped as manifestations or personifications of the ultimate Reality, and in the eyes of their worshipers *are* each the supreme Godhead. Worshipers of God Shiva, for instance, regard Shiva as transcendental, formless, and qualityless (*nirguna*), but for the purpose of worship bestow upon this featureless Being certain anthropomorphic features or qualities (*guna*)—such as goodness, beauty, power, and grace. In relation to Shiva, all other deities are looked upon as high beings occupying various heavenly realms (*loka*). In Christian terminology, they are archangels or angels. For the community of Vishnu devotees, the situation is reversed. For them, Vishnu is the supreme Godhead, while all other deities— including Shiva—are merely *devas*, "shining ones," who have a status equivalent to that of angelic beings in the Judeo-Christian and Islamic traditions.

Early on, the deities were interpreted from three perspectives: their material (*âdhibhautika*), psychological (*adhyâtmika*), and spiritual (*âdhidaivika*) significance. For instance, the Vedic God Agni signifies the actual sacrificial fire, the sacrificer's inner fire (related to the serpent power or *kundalinî-shakti*), and the divine fire or transcendental Light. Whenever we consider a deity, we must bear all three aspects in mind. Thus far, most scholars have focused only on the first aspect, which has caused them to view (and sometimes dismiss) the Vedic spirituality as merely "naturalistic." Upon closer study, however, we realize that the Vedic seers and sages were steeped in symbolism and were greatly skilled in the use of metaphoric language. It is our understanding, not their symbolic communication, that is inadequate.

Since Vedic times, India's "theologians" have spoken of thirty-three deities, though in actual practice there have long been many more mentioned in the scriptures. The following brief discussion focuses on only a few deities who are especially associated with Yoga.

To begin with Shiva ("Benign one"), who is mentioned already in the *Rig-Veda* (1.114; 2.33): He is the focal point of Shaivism, that is, the Shaiva tradition of worship and theology. He is the deity of *yogins par excellence* and is often depicted as a *yogin*, with long, matted hair, a body besmeared with ashes, and a garland of skulls—all signs of his utter renunciation. In his hair is the crescent moon symbolizing mystical vision and knowledge. His three eyes symbolize sun, moon, and fire, and they reveal to him everything in the past, present, and future. The central or "third" eye, located at the forehead, is

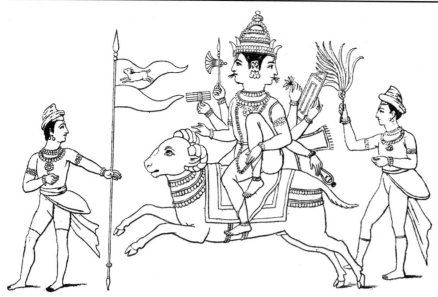

*Agni*

connected with the cosmic fire, and a single glance from this eye can incinerate the entire universe. The serpent coiled around his neck symbolizes the mysterious spiritual energy of *kundalinî.*

The Gangâ (Ganges) River that cascades from the crown of Shiva's head is a symbol of perpetual purification, which is the mechanism underlying his gift of spiritual liberation bestowed upon devotees. The tiger skin on which he is seated represents power (*shakti*), and his four arms are a sign of his perfect control over the four cardinal directions. His trident represents the three primary qualities (*guna*) of Nature, namely *tamas*, *rajas*, and *sattva*. The animal commonly associated with him is the bull called Nandin ("Delightful"), a symbol of sexual energy, which Shiva has mastered perfectly. The lion often shown in images of Shiva symbolizes greed for food, which he also has conquered.

Shiva has from the beginning been closely associated with Rudra ("Howler"), a deity especially connected with the air element and its diverse manifestations (i.e., wind, storm, thunder, and lightning but also life energy and the

breath, etc.). Rudra, however, is also understood to be a great healer, and the same function is hinted at in Shiva's name. In later Hinduism, Shiva became the destructive aspect of the famous trinity (*tri-mûrti*), the other two being Vishnu (representing the principle of preservation) and Brahma (standing for the principle of creation). As such, Shiva is often called Hara ("Remover"). He is typically pictured as dwelling on Mount Kailâsa with his divine spouse Pârvatî ("She who dwells on the mountain"). In many *Tantras*, he figures as the first teacher of esoteric knowledge. As the

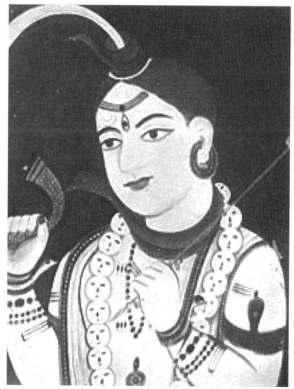

*Shiva*

ultimate Reality, the Shaivas invoke him as Maheshvara ("Great Lord," from *mahâ* "great" and *îshvara* "lord"). As the giver of joy or serenity he is called Shankara, and as the abode of delight he is given the name Shambhu. Other names are Pashupati ("Lord of the beasts"), Îshana ("Ruler") and, not least, Mahâdeva ("Great God").

Another symbol typically connected with Shiva and having many associations is the *linga*. This word is often translated as "phallus," but it literally means "sign" and stands for the principle of creativity per se. The *linga* (sometimes rendered as "lingam" in English) is the creative core of cosmic existence (*prakriti*), which is undivided and causal. Its counterpole is the feminine principle of *yoni* ("womb," "source"). Together, both these principles weave the tapestry of space-time. Some Shaivas—notably the Lingâyatas—wear the *shiva-linga* as an amulet, and in Tantric contexts, stone or metal representations of the *linga* set in *yoni* bowls remind practitioners of the bipolar nature of all manifest existence: The world is a play of Shiva and Pârvatî (Shakti), or Consciousness and Energy.

Vishnu ("Pervader") is the object of worship among the Vaishnavas. Vaishnavism has its roots in Vedic times, as Vishnu is mentioned already in the *Rig-Veda* (e.g., 1.23; 154; 8.12; 29). His most important other names are Hari ("Remover"), Nârâyâna ("Abode of humans"), and Vâsudeva ("God of [all] things"). Between the successive periods of world creation, mythology pictures Vishnu as resting in a formless state on the cosmic serpent Shesha (or Ananta) floating in the infinite ocean of unmanifest existence.

Vishnu, like Shiva, is often represented

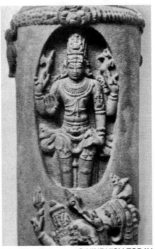

© HINDUISM TODAY

*Shiva-linga*

with four arms signifying his omnipresence and omnipotence. His attributes include the conch (symbol of creation), the discus (standing for the universal mind), the lotus (representing the universe), the bow and arrows (symbolizing the ego sense and the senses), the mace (standing for the life force), the lock of golden hair on the left side of his chest (representing the core of Nature), the chariot (symbolizing the mind as the principle of action), and his black or dark blue color (suggesting the infinite expanse of ether/space, the first of five elements).

In order to restore the moral order (*dharma*) on Earth, Vishnu is said to have incarnated several times. His ten incarnations (*avatâra*, "descent") are:

1. Matsya ("Fish") incarnated with the specific purpose of saving Manu Satyavrata, the progenitor of the human race during the deluge at the beginning of the present world age.

2. Kûrma ("Tortoise") took form out of Vishnu's infinitude in order to recover various treasures lost during the deluge, notably the elixir of life. Both the deities (*deva* or *sura*) and the counter-deities (*asura*) collaborated in churning the world ocean by using the cosmic serpent (Ananta) as a rope and the cosmic mountain Mandara as a churning rod. Kûrma served as the pivot for the rod. Through their churning, all the lost treasures were recovered, thus restoring the universal order and balance.

3. Varâha ("Boar") was born with the mission to destroy the demon Hiranyâksha ("Golden-Eyed") who had flooded the entire earth.

4. Nara-Simha ("Man-Lion") manifested in order to destroy the evil emperor Hiranyakashipu ("Golden Vestment") who had tried unsuccessfully to kill his son Prahlâda, a great devotee of Vishnu. As a result of a boon granted by God Brahma, Hiranyakashipu could not be killed by day or by night, by a deity, human being, or beast, and neither inside nor outside the walls of his palace. Thus, Nara-Simha appeared at twilight, as a lion-headed human, and within a pillar. With his claws he tore open the king's body, destroying him.

5. Vamâna ("Dwarf") incarnated specifically in order to destroy the demonic Bali, who had ousted the deities and gained dominion over the universe. He requested from Bali as much land as he could cover with three steps. Amused by such a request, the demon emperor granted his wish. Vamâna took two steps and encompassed all of creation, and with his third step placed his foot on Bali's head, pushing him into the hell realms. Because Bali was not entirely devoid of virtues, Vamâna granted him rulership of the nether regions. Vishnu's three steps are referred to already in the *Rig-Veda* (e.g., 1.23.17–18, 20).

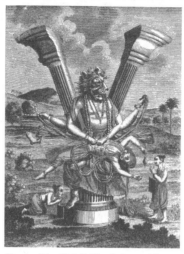

*Reproduced from* Hindu Religion, Customs and Manners

*Vishnu as Nara-Simha*

6. Parashu-Râma ("Râma with the Ax") was a warlike incarnation. He destroyed the warrior estate twenty-one times, which suggests a great struggle between the *kshatriyas* and the brahmins in early Vedic times.

7. Râma ("Dark one" or "Pleasing one"), also called Râmacandra, was a wise and just ruler of Ayodhyâ and a younger contemporary of Parashu-Râma. His life story is told in the *Râmâyana* epic. His wife was Sîtâ ("Furrow"), who is often identified with the Goddess Lakshmî ("Good Sign") and who symbolizes the principle of marital fidelity, love, and devotion. She was kidnapped by the demon-king Râvana, whose kingdom may have been located in Sri Lanka (formerly Ceylon), and rescued by the monkey-headed demigod Hanumat, who represents the principle of faithful service.

8. Krishna ("Puller") was the God-man whose teaching is featured in the *Bhagavad-Gîtâ* and many other sections of the *Mahâbhârata* epic. Krishna's death inaugurated the *kali-yuga*, which is still in full swing and will last many thousands of years.

9. Buddha ("Awakened one") was born in order to mislead evil-doers and demons. Some authorities question whether this refers to Gautama the Buddha, but there can be little doubt

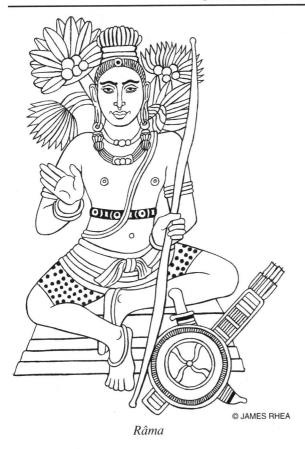

© JAMES RHEA

*Râma*

Shaivism or Vaishnavism, are often described as Smârtas, or adherents of the *Smritis* (nonrevelatory literature).

Closely associated with God Shiva is Ganesha ("Lord of the hosts"), the elephant-headed God, who is called by many other names, including Ganapati (having the same meaning) and Vinâyaka ("Leader").[22] In 1995, Ganesha made the headlines of the *New York Times* and other prominent newspapers around the world for what has been dubbed the "milk miracle" (*kshîra-camatkâra*). On September 21 that year, an otherwise ordinary Hindu in New Delhi dreamed that Ganesha was craving some milk. When the man got up in the morning, he went straight to the nearest temple and, with the priest's permission, offered a spoonful of milk to this deity's statue. To his and the priest's astonishment, the milk vanished. Within hours, news had traveled around the country, and tens of millions of devout Hindus flocked to the temples. Apparently, countless others—including shocked skeptics—

that this was the intent of the brahmins who created the doctrine of ten incarnations.

10. Kalki ("Base one") is the *avatâra* yet to come. He is described in various *Purânas* as riding a white horse and brandishing a blazing sword. His task will be to bring about the destruction of the present world (*yuga*) and the birthing of the next Golden Age, or Age of Truth (*satya-yuga*).

Of the Hindu trinity, God Brahma is the most abstract and consequently has not captured the imagination of the brahmins. He simply is the Creator of the world. He must be carefully distinguished from *brahman*, which is the nondual transcendental Reality. Those who do not belong to the great religious communities, such as

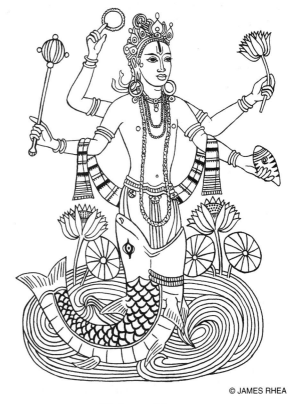

© JAMES RHEA

*Vishnu as Matsya*

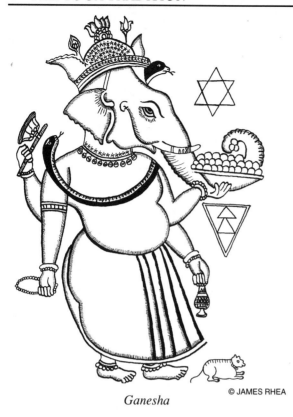

*Ganesha*
© JAMES RHEA

saw the miracle repeated in many sacred spots and even not-so-sacred locations (such as Ganesha figurines on automobile dashboards). Within twenty-four hours the miracle ceased as suddenly as it had begun.

Whatever view we may take of this event, it affords us the opportunity to ponder the symbolism of the milk offering. In ancient Vedic times, milk was often mixed into the fabled *soma* draft before it was offered into the sacred fire for the deities' enjoyment, or was imbibed by the sacrificial priest to facilitate his communion with the deities. In subsequent times, *soma* sacrifices were understood and practiced merely metaphorically. *Soma* became the nectar of immortality generated within the human body itself through intense concentration. Milk, as a product of the sacred cow, is full of symbolic associations. Ganesha is particularly connected with the symbolism of the life force (*prâna*) and the serpent energy (*kundalinî*), which, when it has fully risen to the psychospiritual center at the crown of the

head, causes the ambrosial liquid to irrigate the *yogin*'s body.

Of the various female deities, we must single out Durgâ ("She who is difficult to cross"), who represents the cosmic energy of destruction, particularly the removal of the ego (*ahamkâra*), which stands in the way of spiritual growth and ultimate liberation. She is a nurturing mother only for those who walk the path of self-transcendence; all others experience her wrathful side.

Kâlî ("Dark One"), a personification of Durgâ's wrath, is one of a group of ten major Goddesses known as the "Great Wisdoms" (*mahâ-vidyâ*). The others are Târâ, Tripurâ-Sundarî, Bhuvaneshvarî, Chinnamastâ, Bhairavî, Dhûmâvatî, Bagalâmukhî, Mâtangî, and Kamalâ. Of these, Chinnamastâ ("She whose head is cut off") holds special significance for Yoga. This fierce Goddess is typically depicted in the nude and with a garland of skulls around the stump of her neck from which spout two fountains of

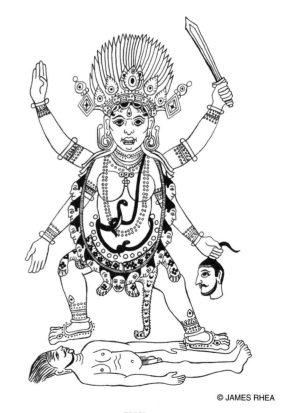

© JAMES RHEA

*Kâlî*

blood. She holds her severed head in her left hand. Various myths seek to explain her unusual condition, but they all are agreed that the Goddess cut off her own head in order to feed her two attendants, called Dâkinî and Varninî, or Jayâ and Vijayâ. Yogically interpreted, this primal sacrifice of the divine Mother stands for the left and right current—*idâ* and *pingalâ*—which must be sacrificed in order to induce the free flow of the psychospiritual energy through the central channel (*sushumnâ-nâdî*). The head—symbol of the mind—must be severed, that is, transcended, in order for enlightenment to occur. This yogic symbolism is suggested in this Goddess's alternative name, Sushumnâsvara-Bhâsinî, meaning "She who shines with the sound of the central channel."

The benign aspect of the Ultimate in its feminine form is emphasized in the Goddess Lakshmî, whose name is derived from *lakshman* ("sign") and means "Good Sign" or "Fortune." The South Indian Goddess Lalitâ Tripurâ-Sundarî ("Lovely Beauty of the Triple City") expresses the same aspect of the Divine. She is described as benevolent (*saumya*) and beautiful (*saundarya*), rather than terrifying (*ugra*) and horrifying (*ghora*). Yet, since Lakshmî and Lalitâ are conceived as the ultimate Reality, they also necessarily include the destructive aspect. From

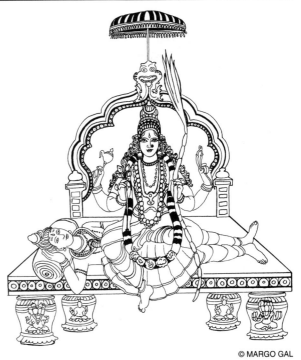

© MARGO GAL

*Tripurâ*

our limited human point of view, the Divine is neither merely positive nor exclusively negative, but it transcends all such categories. The most important Hindu work extolling the Divine in its feminine aspect is the voluminous *Devî-Bhâgavata*, a Shâkta counterpart of the Vaishnava *Bhâgavata-Purâna*, which has been dated between the seventh to twelfth centuries.[23] Here the great Goddess is introduced as the eternal essence of the universe.

## Part Two
# PRE-CLASSICAL YOGA

"Yoga is present everywhere—no less in the oral tradition
of India than in the Sanskrit and vernacular literatures . . .
To such a degree is this true that Yoga has ended by becoming a characteristic dimension of Indian spirituality."

—Mircea Eliade, *Yoga: Immortality and Freedom*, p. 101

"This immutable Yoga I proclaimed to Vivasvat. Vivasvat imparted it to Manu, and Manu declared it to Ikshvâku. Thus handed down from one to another, the royal seers learned it."

—*Bhagavad-Gîtâ* (4.1–2)

# Chapter 4

# YOGA IN ANCIENT TIMES

## I. HISTORY FOR SELF-UNDERSTANDING

Yoga has been called a living fossil. It belongs to the earliest manifestations of India's cultural heritage. Thanks to the missionary efforts of Hindu swamis, it has entered a new phase of flowering in our century, both in India and in other parts of the world. Today, hundreds of thousands of Westerners are actively practicing some form of Yoga, though they do not always have a clear understanding of its traditional goals and purposes. To a large extent this is because they are generally uninformed about Yoga's richly textured history. Therefore, Part Two of this volume is dedicated to outlining the essential developments in the long and complex evolution of Yoga.

History provides a vital context for understanding the world, especially human culture. More than that, history tells us about ourselves, because our beliefs and attitudes are largely shaped by the culture to which we belong. We are what we are, not only because of our own personal history but also because of the collective history of human civilization. As the German philosopher and psychiatrist Karl Jaspers commented:

> No reality is more essential to our self-awareness than history. It shows us the broadest horizon of mankind, brings us the contents of tradition upon which our life is built, shows us standards by which to measure the present, frees us from unconscious bondage to our own age, teaches us to see man in his highest potentials and his imperishable creations . . . We can have a better understanding of our present experience if we see it in the mirror of history.[1]

Without adequate understanding of the historical unfoldment of Yoga, it is hard to imagine that we could arrive at a genuine appreciation of its spiritual treasures, or could practice it meaningfully and with ultimate effectiveness. A study of the history of Yoga gives us a broader picture than we can glean from most of the popular literature on the subject.

To learn about the historical evolution of Yoga is more than an academic exercise; it actually furthers our self-understanding and hence our efforts to swim free of the boundaries of the ego-personality. The following chapters will reveal some of the glory of the Yoga tradition, which has generated an immense wealth of insight into the human condition. It is, of course, impossible to capture even on a few hundred pages everything that scholarship has brought to light. Indeed, no one has so far attempted to integrate all the available data, which would require mastery of several languages (especially Sanskrit and Tamil) and a truly encyclopedic knowledge. Therefore, what I will attempt in this book is the more modest goal of erecting a preliminary framework for our understanding of Yoga.

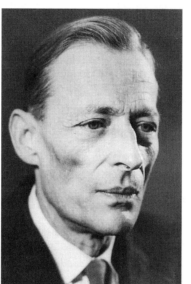

In the previous chapter we have seen how the history of Hinduism can conveniently be arranged into nine periods, extending from the Pre-Vedic Age to our Modern Age—a span of over 8,000 years. In reading the following chapters it will be helpful to bear that schema in mind. Since yogic ideas and

© RUDOLF HÄMMERLI

*Jean Gebser*

practices are not unique to Hinduism but also are found, for instance, in Buddhism and Jainism, it would be possible to write quite different histories. However, given the superlative position of Hinduism in the historical development of India's civilization, this would only add needless complication. In the following, therefore, the development of Yoga is presented from the point of view of Hinduism, though I have included short chapters on Buddhism and Jainism. These two traditions are treated in their relative chronological sequence: Jainism appears after the earliest *Upanishads* and is followed by Buddhism.

Before beginning the panoramic treatment of the history of Yoga, I would like to briefly introduce a useful evolutionary perspective: the Gebserian model of structures of consciousness.

## *History and Consciousness*

In its fully developed form, the psychospiritual technology of Yoga belongs to what Karl Jaspers called the "axial age," the crucial period around the middle of the first millennium B.C.E.— the age of Lao Tzu and Confucius in China, Mahâvîra and Gautama the Buddha in India, and Pythagoras, Socrates, Plato, and Aristotle in Greece.[2] These geniuses and a host of other pathmakers of that time ushered in a new paradigm or style of thought.

What this new orientation means in the overall history of human civilization has been brilliantly articulated by the Swiss cultural philosopher Jean Gebser.[3] According to him, humanity has traversed a series of four structures of consciousness, or cognitive styles, which he characterized as follows:

1. *Archaic consciousness:* This is the simplest and earliest identifiable cognitive style, which has the least degree of self-awareness and is still almost completely instinctual. Historically, it takes us back to the time of *Australopithecus* and *Homo habilis*. Today, this consciousness manifests in us, for instance, as the impulse toward self-transcen-

dence. Also, it is activated in some types of ecstatic experience (*samâdhi*) or even certain drug-induced altered states of awareness, where the barrier between subject and object is temporarily lifted.

2. *Magical consciousness:* Emerging from the archaic consciousness, the magical consciousness is still pre-egoic, with a diffuse awareness. It operates on the principle of identity, as it is expressed in analogical thinking, which is a gut-level (archetypal) response that relates apparently disjointed elements into a whole. This type of consciousness may have characterized *Homo erectus*, over one-and-a-half million years ago. It is still effective in us today whenever we are spellbound or in sympathy with someone or something. It manifests negatively in such diverse situations as blindly falling in love or temporarily losing one's judgment (and sometimes one's humanity) under the hypnotic influence of a large crowd. The magical consciousness also is strongly present in those aspects of Yoga that involve extreme inward concentration, leading to loss of body awareness. Of course, it also is the cognitive basis for all forms of sympathetic magic, which is an ingredient of some yogic paths, notably those schools of Tantrism that emphasize the cultivation of paranormal powers, or *siddhis*.

3. *Mythical consciousness:* This represents a more pronounced degree of self-awareness, corresponding to, though not identical with, that of a child. Thinking operates on the principle of polarity rather than magical identity or mental duality. It unfolds through symbol rather than calculus, myth rather than hypothesis, feeling or intuition rather than abstraction. The Neanderthals and Cro-Magnons may largely have embodied the mythical consciousness. Like the other structures of consciousness, it continues to be effective to this day and was a principal factor in the creation of the immense variety of sacred traditions, including Yoga. We activate the mythical consciousness whenever we close our eyes and immerse ourselves into the imagery of the mind, or when we give poetic expression to our deep-felt thoughts. The mythic component is strong in most traditional approaches of Yoga, and they can usefully be grouped together under the label of Mythic Yoga, as opposed to a more integrative orientation, such as Sri Aurobindo's Integral Yoga. Mythic Yoga follows the verticalist motto of "in, up, and out." I have explored all this more fully in *Wholeness or Transcendence?*[4]

4. *Mental consciousness:* As the name suggests, this cognitive style is the domain of the thinking, rational mind, operating on the principle of duality ("either/or"). Here self-consciousness is acute, and the world is experienced as split up into subject and object. Since the European renaissance, this cognitive style has dominated our lives and has in fact become a destructive force. Today, the mental consciousness,

which is inherently balanced, has degenerated into what Gebser calls the rational mode.

The mental consciousness at its best was still at work when Patanjali wrote his *Yoga-Sûtra* or when Vyâsa composed his commentary on it. Thus, Yoga by no means excludes this particular cognitive style, but all traditional schools of Yoga call for the transcendence of the mind, both in its lower form as *manas* and in its higher form as *buddhi*. The truth is always considered to lie beyond the mind and the senses. In what I have dubbed Mythic Yoga, the mind is frequently portrayed as the arch enemy of the spiritual process. This notion, however, is a limitation that is not present in more integrative forms of Yoga. Intellectual work is not necessarily detrimental to spiritual growth, although, in order to realize the Self, the mechanism of the mind must indeed be transcended and freed from its egoic anchorage.

In his magnificent work *The Ever-Present Origin* and in several of his other books, Gebser argued that today we are witnessing the emergence of a fifth structure of consciousness, which he called the integral consciousness. This is not the place to furnish a detailed description of this emerging modality of the human mind. I merely wish to mention that, in Gebser's view, this new consciousness is an antidote to the one-sidedness of the exaggerated rational mentality that is a degradation of the original mental consciousness. The rational consciousness, in Gebser's sense of the term, is excessively egoic and is at odds with the spiritual Reality. The integral consciousness, by contrast, is inherently ego-transcending and open to what Gebser called the "Origin," that is, the Ground of Being. There are obvious parallels here to Sri Aurobindo's philosophy, and Gebser admitted to standing in the spiritual gravity field of that great sage.

The task before us—individually and collectively—is to help this emerging integral consciousness to take effect in us and in our human civilization as a whole. Only in this way can we hope to restore the balance between the various structures of consciousness, allowing each to express itself according to its inherent values. It is my belief that the Yoga tradition—as well as other spiritual traditions—contains many elements that, applied judiciously to our contemporary situation, can assist greatly in this challenging work of integration.

## II. FROM SHAMANISM TO YOGA

Cultural heroes like Gautama the Buddha or the Upanishadic sages stood at the threshold of the mental structure of consciousness, which they helped usher in. Thus, the psychospiritual technology of Yoga is the product of the early mental structure of consciousness. Prior to that we find the Proto-Yoga of the *Vedas*, couched in heavily symbolic terms. Before that we have the ecstatic technology of Shamanism extending back to the Stone Age. Although Shamanism has been dated to around 25,000 B.C.E., it is probably very much older. As we know from other contexts, the absence of artifacts does not necessarily imply the absence of the belief system with which they are associated.

Shamanism is the sacred art of changing one's awareness in order to enter nonordinary realms of reality, which are experienced to be populated by spirits. The word *shaman* is of Siberian (Tungusic) origin and describes a seasoned traveler in the spirit realms. Mostly by listening to the monotonous sound of a drum, click stick, or other percussion instrument, or by means of psychotropic substances (such as the fly agaric mushroom), shamans achieve a radical shift in their perceptual field. They do this in order to communicate with the spirit world. Their purpose is not idle curiosity; rather, they hope to retrieve power and information that are vital to the psychological and bodily welfare of their community.

According to some authorities, notably Mircea Eliade, Shamanism is of Siberian origin. Others regard Shamanism as a worldwide tradition that has arisen independently in diverse cultures. I favor the former view, which associates Shamanism especially with the cultural backdrop of Siberia and Central Asia. In a similar vein, Yoga is essentially an Indic phenomenon, and the spiritual traditions of other cultures should be given their own distinct name. Thus, strictly speaking, we should not speak of African Shamanism, unless it can be demonstrated that it is a descendant of Siberian Shamanism, which is true of the shamanic tradition of the Eskimos and Hopi Indians. Similarly, we should not speak of a Christian Yoga, unless it is indeed a hybrid between Christianity and Hinduism. Terms like "sorcery," "witchcraft," or "magic" may be applied in contexts other than Siberian or Siberian-derived spirituality, and "mysticism" or "spiritual esotericism" may be used in connection with Yoga-like traditions other than those traceable to India.

Some scholars have suggested that Yoga grew directly out of Shamanism, but this is difficult to prove. While Yoga contains shamanic elements, it absorbed many other teachings as well. According to Michael Harner, the transition from Shamanism to Yoga occurred at the time of the early city states in the East, when shamans were

> "Shamans are usually aroused during their journey and may dance or become highly agitated . . . In yogic samadhi, calm may become so profound that many mental processes cease temporarily."
>
> —Roger Walsh, *The Spirit of Shamanism,* p. 229

suppressed by the representatives of the official religion.[5] In order to avoid detection, they had to cease drumming loudly and instead elaborated quiet methods of altering consciousness. Out of this, in Harner's reconstruction of ancient history, evolved the tradition of Yoga.

While Harner's hypothesis is intriguing, the waning of the shamanic tradition was probably more connected with the fact that the rise of the city states coincided with the collapse of the tribal communities that were served by the shamans. This collapse, in turn, is best understood as a shift in consciousness toward a more individuated self-awareness, associated with the emerging mental structure of consciousness.[6]

The shaman is a privileged sacred technician who acts on behalf of his (or more rarely her) community. This aspect is shared by the brahmin (*brâhmana*), who performs his sacrifices and other rituals for the sake of others, whether it be the ancestral spirits, his own living family, or the community at large. However, the *yogin* is a sacred technician who first and foremost seeks his own salvation. He does not, as a rule, endeavor to make any direct social contribution. If anything, he has dropped out of the social game. Yet, indirectly by their exemplary behavior and benevolent aura, the *yogins* of India have contributed significantly not only toward their own society but also to human civilization as a whole.[7] Even in Karma-Yoga, the ideal of benefiting the world (*loka-samgraha*), as mentioned earlier, is primarily in the interest of the *yogin*'s own spiritual growth. Only the *bodhisattva* ideal of Mahâyâna Buddhism embodies the intention to improve our collective human destiny. But, unlike the shaman, the *bodhisattva* is chiefly concerned with the *spiritual* welfare of people, not merely their bodily or emotional well-being or their material prosperity. Even those practitioners of the *bodhisattva* path who are healers understand their healing ministry as a spiritual service to others: By helping people re-establish physical health or emotional balance, these healers hope to create in them the proper conditions for spiritual practice.

While the hypothesis that derives Yoga from (officially suppressed) Shamanism is problematical, clearly many aspects and motifs of Shamanism have survived in Yoga. Eliade, who pioneered research on both Yoga and Shamanism, furnished the following characteristics for the shamanic tradition:

Among the elements that constitute and are peculiar to shamanism, we must count as of primary importance: (1) an initiation comprising the candidate's symbolical dismemberment, death, and resurrection, which, among other things, implies his descent into hell and ascent to heaven; (2) the shaman's ability to make ecstatic journeys in his role of healer and psychopompos (he goes in search of the sick man's soul, stolen by demons, captures it, and restores it to the body; he conducts the dead man's soul to hell, etc.); (3) "mastery of fire" (the shaman touches red-hot iron, walks over burning coals, etc., without being hurt); (4) the shaman's ability to assume animal forms (he flies like the birds, etc.) and to make himself invisible.[8]

Yoga, as we have seen in Chapter 1, is an initiatory tradition. Its entire course is governed by the idea of the progressive transcendence

("dismemberment") of the human ego-personality. Later we will encounter the *Kshurikâ-Upanishad* ("Secret Doctrine of the Dagger"), a work that explains the yogic process in terms of a step-by-step dismantling of ordinary consciousness. This corresponds to the dismemberment associated with the shamanic rope trick, which has been described as a form of mass hypnosis. This involves the shaman, a sharp blade in his mouth, climbing up the vertically extended rope in hot pursuit of a young boy until both are out of sight. After a while, the boy's severed limbs rain down from high above. The drama ends with the boy's resurrection by the shaman. Cameras will only capture the shaman sitting on the ground, alone and perhaps with a knowing smile.

The *yogin*'s ecstatic introversion and mystical ascent is the equivalent of the shaman's ecstatic flight, and the *yogin*'s teaching function corresponds to the shaman's role as a guide of souls. Furthermore, many of the shamanic powers also are recognized in Yoga, where they are known as *siddhis* ("accomplishments"), including the ability to become invisible, with which shamans are also credited. Finally, the shaman's mastery of fire—an external feat—is paralleled by the yogic mastery of the "inner fire," especially the psychophysiological heat generated during the arousal of the life force in Kundalinî-Yoga. This is the basis for the Tibetan practice of *tumo*, which allows practitioners of this yogic discipline to sit naked for many hours in the frozen snow blanketing the mountain peaks of the Himalayas.

One of the best known techniques of Yoga—sitting cross-legged in one of the many yogic postures (*âsana*)—has its shamanic precursor. In her book *Where the Spirits Ride the Wind*, the American anthropologist Felicitas Goodman examined a number of shamanic postures that have been used to induce ecstatic states or out-of-body experiences.[9] Apparently, each posture has its own distinct effect on the mind, and she and her students are capable of entering various states of consciousness by using specific shamanic postures.

The previous chapter introduced the tradition of asceticism (*tapas*), the precursor of Yoga, which has many striking parallels to Shamanism: Where shamans demonstrate their mastery of fire by touching burning coals, *tapasvins* excel in the act of "self-heating"—that is, in disciplining themselves to the point where sweat pours from all pores. One ancient ascetic practice (called *panca-agni*, written *pancâgni*) is to sit surrounded by four lit fires, in the middle of summer, while the sun is burning down from above. In recent years, Swami Satyananda Saraswati of the Bihar School of Yoga practiced this age-old technique over a long period. Whether through prolonged retention of the breath or through transmutation of the sexual drive into vital energy (*ojas*), *yogins* similarly seek to frustrate the natural tendencies of the body-mind and thereby create an inner pressure that translates into physiological heat. They feel as if they are burning up. Then, at the peak of this experience, a radical breakthrough occurs whereby their whole being is illumined. They discover that they *are* that light, which has no apparent source but is the Source of everything.

The condition of illumination, or enlightenment, is to the *yogin* what the magical journey into other realms is to the shaman. Both experiences represent a radical departure from conventional reality and consciousness. Both have a profoundly transformative effect. Yet only the *yogin*, who travels inward, discovers the ultimate futility of all journeying, because he realizes that he is never traveling outside the very Reality that is the goal of his spiritual odyssey.

The environment of the shaman is composed of the subtle realms of existence, which he strives to master. "The distinctive feature of the shamanic ecstasy," writes the American psychiatrist Roger Walsh, "is the experience of 'soul flight' or 'journeying' or 'out-of-body experience.' That is, in their ecstatic state shamans experience themselves, or their soul or spirit, flying through space and traveling either to other worlds or to distant parts of this world."[10] The shamanic journeys are for the sake of obtaining knowledge or power, or to effect changes in the material realm by altering the conditions in the subtle realms. The *yogin*'s ultimate purpose, however, is to go beyond the subtle levels of existence explored by the shaman, and to realize the transcendental Being, which is transdimensional and unqualified, and which the *yogin* knows to be his innermost identity. Thus, whereas the shaman is a healer or miracle-worker, the *yogin* is primarily a transcender. But in the spiritual ascent to the transcendental Reality, the *yogin* is likely to gather a great deal of knowledge about the subtle realms (*sûkshma-loka*). This explains why many *yogins* have demonstrated extraordinary abilities and have long been looked upon by the Indian people as miracle workers and magicians. From the yogic point of view, however, the paranormal abilities possessed by many adepts are insignificant by comparison with the ultimate attainment of Self-realization, or enlightenment.

## III. YOGA AND THE ENIGMATIC INDUS-SARASVATÎ CIVILIZATION

### The Vedic Aryans: A Revolutionary New View

Yoga as we know it today is the product of several millennia. The earliest beginnings are lost in the obscurity of ancient Indian prehistory. Rightly, the *Bhagavad-Gîtâ* (4.3), essentially composed in its present form perhaps around 500–600 B.C.E., calls Yoga "archaic" (*purâtana*).[11] Western scholars have generally underestimated the antiquity of Yoga, and until recently the consensus has been to connect it with the esotericism of the *Upanishads*, which have been placed as late as the sixth or seventh century B.C.E., but which are much older.

Recent studies have clearly shown the presence of Yoga, as a loose structure of ideas and practices (which we might conveniently call "Proto-Yoga"), at the time of the *Rig-Veda*. More importantly, the age of the Vedic canon itself has been pushed back considerably. The bulk of the *Rig-Veda*, the most important of the four Vedic hymnodies, was composed long prior to 1900 B.C.E. I will discuss the significance of this date shortly.

Several generations of Western scholars have subscribed to the so-called Aryan invasion model, which has now been refuted by the new evidence. According to this outdated model, the Sanskrit-speaking Vedic tribes invaded India between 1500 and 1200 B.C.E., causing death and destruction among the native (supposedly Dravidian) population. This hypothesis, favored especially by the influential scholar Max Müller, quickly acquired the status of a popular dogma that has proven extremely resilient even in the face of abundant contradictory evidence.

The first challenge to the Aryan invasion theory came when, in 1921, archaeologists discovered the ancient cities of Harappa and Mohenjo-Daro at the banks of the Indus River in Pakistan. However, instead of questioning their assumptions about the origin of the Vedic Aryans, most researchers simply adjusted the date for the alleged invasion by several hundred years to take into account the archaeological record. Under the influence of the invasion model, they overinterpreted certain archaeological findings, notably

the apparent signs of violence in some strata of Mohenjo-Daro. In the meantime, most archaeologists have abandoned this particular explanation, but many Indologists continue to rely on the outdated interpretations.

The reason for this is that the alternative, which is strongly suggested by the facts themselves, requires a total revision of our understanding of India's early civilized history: That is, the invasion of India by the Vedic Aryans never occurred! Rather, they have long been established in India. The overwhelming evidence refuting the Aryan invasion model has been presented and discussed in some detail in the book *In Search of the Cradle of Civilization.*[12] Therefore it will not be necessary to review all the facts again, and a broadly painted picture should suffice.

The Vedic Aryans belonged to the Indo-European language family, whose numerous members undoubtedly also shared many ethnic features. The Vedic Aryans are related to the Celts, the Persians, the Goths, and several other linguistic-cultural groups that no longer exist. They also are distant cousins of those of us whose native tongue is English, French, German, Spanish, Russian, and a host of other languages that originated in Eurasia.

The Indo-European speakers all are thought to be descendants of the Proto-Indo-Europeans, who are now placed as early as the seventh millennium B.C.E. Scholars are not agreed about their homeland, but it is generally located somewhere in Central Asia or Eastern Europe. According to one influential linguist, Colin Renfrew, the Proto-Indo-Europeans originally had their home in Anatolia (modern Turkey) and from there spread to the north, the west, and the east.[13] At any rate, it is now considered probable that the Proto-Indo-European communities were well established in Eurasia by 4500 B.C.E. or earlier still. Thereafter, the various dialects crystallized into separate languages,

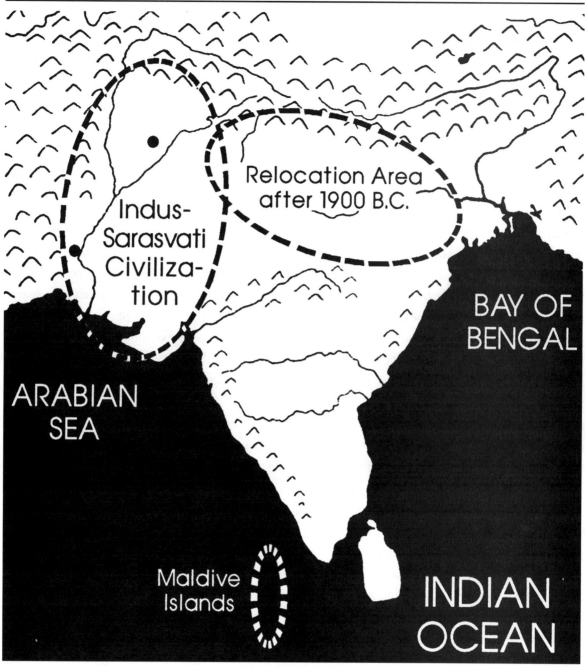

*Map of Vedic India*                                                    © AUTHOR

including Vedic Sanskrit. According to Renfrew and others, by at least 3000 B.C.E. Indo-European languages and their various dialects were spoken throughout Europe, and a strong Indo-European presence continued to exist in Anatolia, as is evident from the Hittite empire of 2200 B.C.E.

In light of this and other evidence, we can safely jettison the idea that the Vedic Aryans arrived in India as late as 1500 B.C.E. They could easily have been resident there several millennia earlier, growing out of an existing branch of the Proto-Indo-European community present on the subcontinent. This is exactly what is suggested by the archaeological evidence and also by the internal evidence of the *Rig-Veda*.

Very significantly, as aerial photographs have revealed, the most celebrated river of the *Rig-Veda*—the Sarasvatî, which was situated to the east of the Indus river—ceased to exist around 1900 B.C.E. The catastrophic drying up of this huge river, which may have been caused by a major tectonic upheaval followed by climatic and environmental changes, occurred over many centuries. It led to the abandonment of numerous towns and villages, and the relocation of the heart of the Vedic civilization to the Ganges (Gangâ) River. In other words, the *Rig-Veda* must have been composed prior to the disappearance of the Sarasvatî. In fact, astronomical references in this archaic hymnody point to the third, fourth, and even fifth millennium B.C.E., but these have typically been ignored or dismissed as later inventions. However, astronomical back calculations are notoriously difficult, and there is no reason to brand the references to solstices in the *Rig-Veda* and other early scriptures as subsequent interpolations, especially considering that virtually all scholars marvel about the high degree of fidelity with which the Vedic hymnodies have been transmitted through the millennia.

Another very important finding is that Babylonian mathematics (c. 1700 B.C.E) was profoundly influenced by India's mathematical geniuses. This conclusion was arrived at by A. Seidenberg, a historian of mathematics who had no particular fealty to India.[14] Indic mathematics appears to have grown out of the brahmins' ritual culture, particularly the construction of complex altars that were symbolically related to the structure of the macrocosm. Mathematical ideas made their first appearance in the *Brâhmanas*, and subsequently were elaborated and codified in the *Shulba-Sûtras*.[15] The first *Brâhmanas* cannot be dated much later than 2000 B.C.E. Some researchers assign them to 3000 B.C.E. and the *Vedas* to 4000–5000 B.C.E. and earlier still. In this book I have opted for a tentative date of 2500 B.C.E. for the earliest *Brâhmanas*.

These facts raise anew the important question of the relationship between the Sanskrit-speaking Aryan tribes and the so-called Indus civilization, which flourished from around 2800 B.C.E. to 1900 B.C.E. It must also be noted here that the date of 2800 B.C.E. is purely provisional since the earliest strata of Mohenjo-Daro have not yet been excavated because of permanent flooding. The foundations of that city, which lie under twenty-four feet of mud, could be many centuries older. Nor have the more than two thousand other sites along the Indus and the Sarasvatî been excavated. It is possible that some of these towns, most of which are situated at the banks of the former Sarasvatî (rather than the Indus), could be older still. The city of Mehrgarh in the extreme northwest of India has been dated back to 6500 B.C.E., thus providing the earliest step in an astonishing continuity of cultural expression.

More and more investigators are inclined to regard that great civilization as a creation of the Vedic Aryans themselves. Indeed, there is nothing in the *Vedas* themselves to contradict such an identification. Those passages that previous generations of scholars have always taken as proof for the violent invasion of India can easily and more sensibly be interpreted in other ways. The battles mentioned in some of the Rig-Vedic hymns are either mythological or, if historical, clearly recollect intertribal Aryan conflicts and not the supposed conquest of the native population by the Vedic Aryans as foreign aggressors.

Scholars have frequently commented on the remarkable continuity in the symbolism and cultural motifs between the Indus-Sarasvatî civilization and later Hinduism. When we identify the Vedic Aryans with the people who inhabited the towns and villages of the Indus and the Sarasvatî, this continuity becomes perfectly intelligible. When the bias of the Aryan invasion

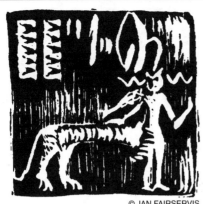
© JAN FAIRSERVIS
*Seal from the Indus-Sarasvatî civilization*

model is removed, we can readily see that the Vedic oral/scriptural tradition matches the archaeological evidence. No longer do we have to deal with the mystery of great cities without a literature, and a great literary heritage without a material base. These new findings also revolutionize our understanding of the history of Yoga.

Most contemporary scholars agree that there are traces of an early Yoga in the Indus cities. In the past, this has always been taken as confirmation for the non-Vedic origin of the Yoga tradition, but this assumption was made possible only because of a complete misunderstanding of the spirituality of the Vedic Aryans. We find as many proto-yogic notions in the *Vedas* as we find in the Indus-Sarasvatî artifacts. The nature of this Proto-Yoga will be discussed shortly.

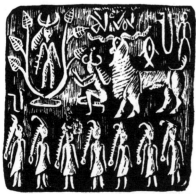
© JAN FAIRSERVIS
*Seal from the Indus-Sarasvatî civilization*

The archaeological findings and the literary evidence of the *Vedas*, particularly the *Rig-Veda*, are, as far as we can tell, perfectly complementary. Together they provide us with a substantial glimpse into what appears to be the oldest *continuous* civilization on Earth—starting with the early Neolithic culture represented by the town of Mehrgarh in the seventh millenium B.C.E. and extending to modern Hinduism.

But the Vedic/Indus/Sarasvatî civilization is not only the oldest on Earth, it also was the largest civilization of early antiquity, much larger than Sumer, Assyria, and Egypt combined. From what we know (and archaeology has mere-

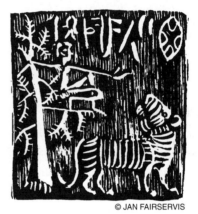
© JAN FAIRSERVIS
*Seal from the Indus-Sarasvatî civilization*

ly scraped the surface thus far), by the end of the third millennium B.C.E. this enormous civilization covered an estimated area of some 300,000 square miles—an area larger than Texas, the second-largest of the United States of America.

## The Splendor of the Indus Settlements

The gigantic Indus-Sarasvatî civilization (as the Indus civilization should properly be called) was chanced upon in the early 1920s, just after the savant world had settled down to the

131

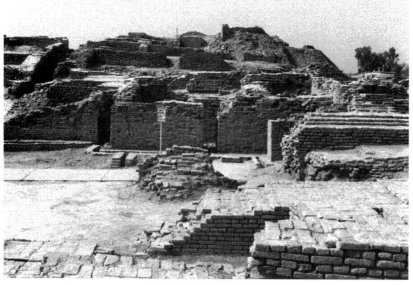

*The ruins of Mahenjo-Daro*

© S. P. GUPTA

*Indus-Sarasvatî glyphs*

striking cities are Mohenjo-Daro in the south and Harappa, 350 miles farther north. The Indus River once served as their main artery of communication. Mohenjo-Daro, the bigger of the two metropolises excavated in the Indus valley, covered an area of about a square mile, which is enough living space to accommodate at least 35,000 people. Both cities show meticulous planning and a high degree of standardization, suggesting a sophisticated sociopolitical organization.

The excavations have brought to light an elaborate drainage system, complete with rubbish shoots, which is unique for pre-Roman times. They also revealed an abundance of bathrooms, and this suggests the kind of ritual ablution that is typical of modern Hinduism. The mostly windowless buildings, including three-story houses, were made from kiln-fired bricks, one of the finest known building materials. In both big cities the nucleus consists of a huge citadel, some 400 by 200 yards in extent, built on an artificial mound. In the case of Mohenjo-Daro, it includes a large bath (230 by 78 feet), halls of assembly, a large structure that was presumably a college for priests, and a great granary (grain storage was a governmental function). The urban layout, as well as the standardized brick sizes and weights, point to a centralized authority, undoubtedly of a priestly nature.

Although no temples have so far been definitely identified, we must assume that religion played a very important role in the lives of these early people. This is mainly borne out by finds—not least motifs on soapstone seals—that show a

comforting belief that, with the surprise discovery of the Hittite empire, they had found the last of the great civilizations of the ancient world. The Indus-Sarasvatî civilization outstripped the keenest imagination of modern scholarship.

So far, only some 60 of a total of more than 2,500 known sites have been excavated. The largest sites are Mohenjo-Daro, Harappa, Ganweriwala, Rakhigarhi, Kaliban-gan, Dholavira, and the harbor city of Lothal (located on the Kathiawar peninsula near the city of Ahmadabad in Gujarat). The most remarkable resemblance to the religious motifs of later Hinduism and also agree with early Vedic symbolism. Apart from this, the *Vedas* mention no temples, as the Vedic people practiced their religion at home and only came together in public for great official events affecting their particular tribe or clan.

The reticence of archaeologists in pronouncing certain sites as having been intended for ritual or sacred usage is difficult to understand, given the central role of religion in other comparable cultures of that period. Significantly, recent excavations at Lothal and Kalibangan have unearthed fire altars whose structure agrees in principle with the information we have about Vedic fire altars—a finding that must not be underestimated.

Not surprisingly, the seven great rivers fertilizing the Indus-Sarasvatî civilization were a stimulus not only to ship building, but also to maritime trade with Middle Eastern empires like Sumer, and probably more distant countries. Active seafaring, as can be expected, also is reflected in the *Rig-Veda*, which has often been wrongly viewed as the product of an unlettered seminomadic people who lived as herders and enriched themselves by periodic raids on the wealthy cities of the Indus.

The two great cosmopolitan environments of Mohenjo-Daro and Harappa, which incidentally have a common ground plan, flourished for around 800 years, during which span there was astonishingly little change in technology, written language, or artistic creativity. This feature prompted the British archaeologist Stuart Piggott to remark:

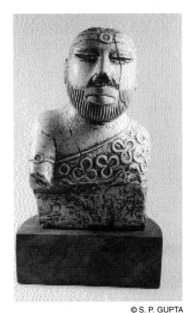

© S. P. GUPTA

*Soapstone sculpture of a chief priest or nobleman*

There is a terrible efficiency about the Harappa civilization which recalls all the worst of Rome, but with this elaborately contrived system goes an isolation and a stagnation hard to parallel in any known civilization of the Old World.[16]

But continuity need not necessarily be a sign of stagnation. It could also be its opposite—a sign of strength. Perhaps the Indus-Sarasvatî people were grounded in a spiritual tradition so profound that it required no major change to provide generation after generation with meaning and succor. Such a spiritual tradition is indeed present in the *Rig-Veda*, the literary counterpart to the archaeological artifacts found in the Indus-Sarasvatî cities. When we interpret, in light of the *Vedas*, the cultural artifacts unearthed by archaeologists, we can make better sense of both the material and the literary evidence.

Of special interest are the numerous steatite seals—used by merchants—that depict animals, plants, and mythological figures reminiscent of later Hinduism. A number of the over two thousand terra-cotta seals that have been found show horned deities seated in the manner of the later *yogins*. One seal in particular, the so-called *pashupati* seal, has attracted attention and excited the imagination of archaeologists and historians. It portrays a divinity enthroned on a low seat and surrounded by four animals: an elephant, a tiger, a rhinoceros, and a buffalo. Beneath the seat is a pair of antelope-like creatures. This figure has been widely identified as God Shiva, the arch-*yogin* and lord (*pati*) of the beasts

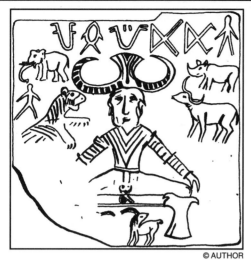

*The so-called pashupati seal*

(*pashu*). While some of the interpretations proffered do not hold up under closer scrutiny, there is little doubt that the figure (whether male or female) represents a sacred being in a ritualized posture that has not been conclusively identified, but that resembles *bhadra-* or *goraksha-âsana.*[17]

There also is good evidence for the existence of a Goddess cult at that time. One seal depicts a female from whose womb a plant grows, which suggests fertility beliefs and rituals, as one would expect of an early agricultural society. Associated with this are objects reminiscent of the later Tantric male generative symbol (*linga*) and the female generative symbol (*yoni*). Seals depicting the fig tree, which to this day is held sacred in India, and trees with a humanoid figure standing in its branches, readily allow one to make connections to the hymns of the *Vedas.* Most importantly, all this is continuous with the religious world of rural India today.

## IV. SACRIFICE AND MEDITATION—THE RITUAL YOGA OF THE RIG-VEDA

As interesting as the artifactual evidence of the Indus-Sarasvatî civilization is, it is not sufficient in itself to conclusively prove the existence of some form of Yoga in that early period. However, the situation changes considerably when we read the artifacts in conjunction with the evidence found in the hymns of the *Rig-Veda.* The picture that emerges is that of a highly ritualistic culture containing many proto-yogic ideas and practices.

The renowned Indian scholar Surendranath Dasgupta rightly categorized the Vedic religion as "sacrificial mysticism."[18] For sacrifice (*yajna*) is at the heart of the religious beliefs and practices of the Indus-Sarasvatî civilization. Two types of sacrifical rites were distinguished: *griha* or domestic sacrifices and *shrauta* or public sacrifices. The former were private ceremonies involving a single household and only one fire. The latter required numerous priests, three fires, and large crowds of

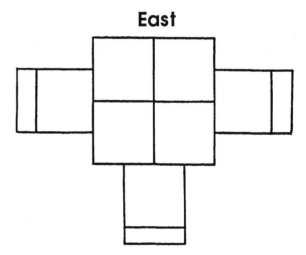

*Vedic fire altar in the shape of a bird*

silent participants. They extended over several days and sometimes weeks and months. On special sacrificial occasions, the entire village or tribe would congregate to participate in large-scale sacrifices, such as the famous *agni-shtoma* (fire sacrifice) and the *ashva-medha* (horse sacrifice), which was performed only rarely and in order to ensure the continued reign of a great king and the tribe's or country's prosperity.

Every "twice-born" (*dvija*) household—a family belonging to the brahmin, warrior, or agricultural/trading class—was obliged to perform the fire sacrifice (*homa*) every day at sunrise and at sunset. This relatively simple sacrifice was performed by husband and wife together and was attended by the immediate family and any resident disciples. The main offering consisted of milk mixed with water, which was then poured into the fire. The ceremony was accompanied by recitations.

The inner purpose of the various sacrifices was always to recreate the universal order (*rita*) within the body of the sacrificing priest, the patron of the sacrifice, and the spectators. Outwardly, the sacrifice was intended to win the favor of a particular deity. The deities were mostly male Gods, such as Indra, Agni, Soma, Rudra, and Savitri, but a few of the Vedic hymns were addressed to Goddesses, notably Vâc (Speech), Ushâ or Ushas (Dawn), Sarasvatî (the river of that name and its cosmic counterpart), and Prithivî (Earth).

As noted before, the Vedic people did not appear to have had temples, and the public sacrifices were performed outdoors. Their religiosity bore the stamp of a great immediacy and vitality, and in their prayers they were petitioning for a long, healthy, and prosperous life in harmony with the cosmic order. As is clear from the Vedic hymns, however, there were also those who had a more mystical bent, aspiring to communion with their favorite God or Goddess, or even to merging with the ultimate Being (*sat*) that has no name and was also described, because it is not limited

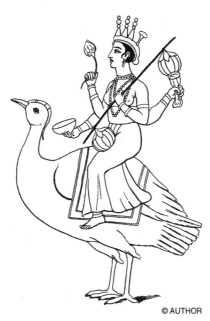

*The Vedic Goddess Sarasvatî*

by any finite form, as Non-being (*asat*), corresponding to the later concept of the Void (*shûnya*).

The spiritual heroes of the Vedic people were not the priests, though they were held in high esteem, but the sages or seers (*rishi*) who "saw" the truth, who perceived with the inner eye the hidden reality behind the smoke screen of manifest existence. Many of them belonged to the priestly class, but some were members of the three other social classes. They were the illumined sages, whose wisdom burst forth in rhythmic poetry and highly symbolic language: the astounding hymns of the *Vedas*. These seers, who were also called poets (*kavi*), revealed to the ordinary, unenlightened individual the luminous Reality beyond all spiritual darkness. They also showed the pathway to that eternal Being, which is singular (*eka*) and unborn (*aja*) but is given many names. The Vedic seers won their sacred visions by their own hard inner work—their austerities and their deep impulse toward spiritual enlightenment. They regarded themselves as "children of light" (*Rig-Veda* 9.38.5) and had their hearts set on reaching the "heavenly light," or ultimate Light-Being (*Rig-Veda* 10.36.3).

Those who were free of sin or guilt could look forward to a happy existence in the hereafter. Sinners, however, were thought to be hurled into the dark pit of hell, though the Rig-Vedic hymns do not overly dwell on this unfortunate fate. As the British scholar Jeanine Miller observed, the Vedic seers preferred an optimistic viewpoint. She also remarked:

Two trends of thought are perceptible: The wish for life on earth with its corollary avoidance of death—even though physical life and immortality are generally not equivalent. The quest of the latter was ultimately the quest of every mortal. In the meanwhile the ordinary man was content with a full life of a hundred years of vitality, a boon for which one finds many a prayer, hence, one step at a time sums up the attitude: enjoyment of this earthly life first, then the heavenly reward.[19]

The 1,028 hymns of the *Rig-Veda*, totaling 10,600 verses, contain numerous passages that are of special relevance to the study of the Vedic Proto-Yoga.[20] In particular, the following hymns deserve close attention by Yoga researchers:

**1.164:** (=*Atharva-Veda* 9.9–10): This hymn, consisting of fifty-two verses, is a collection of profound mystical riddles. The sixth verse, for instance, asks about the nature of the One that is unborn and is yet the cause of the manifested universe. Verses 20–22 speak of the two birds that occupy the same tree. The one is said to eat of its fruit, whilst the other merely looks on. The tree can be read as a symbol of the world. The unenlightened being devours the tree's fruit, impelled by egoic desires. The enlightened being, or the sage, however, abstains and merely looks on dispassionately. The tree could also be seen as a symbol of the tree of knowledge, of whose fruit the sage partakes but not the uninitiated. A more strictly Vedântic interpretation is the following: The onlooking bird is the uninvolved Self beyond the realm of nature; the other is the embodied being enmeshed in conditioned existence. In verse 46, we find the astonishing and oft-quoted utterance that the nameless one Being is called differently by the sages.

The author, or "seer," of this particular Rig-Vedic hymn is known by the name Dîrghatamas ("Long Darkness"). He was undoubtedly one of the deepest thinkers, or envisioners, of that early period. The Indian scholar Vasudeva A. Agrawala, who has written a detailed study of this so-called *asya-vamiya-sûkta*, remarked:

> Dîrghatamas is the type of all men of philosophy and science who have cast their eyes of comprehension on the visible world. Their vision is focused on the invisible source, the First Cause which was Mystery of yore and a Mystery now. Dîrghatamas stands at the apex of them all asking: "Where is the Teacher, knowing the solution? Where is the pupil, coming to the Teacher for revelation?" . . . He takes quick snaps of the Cosmos itself, pointing to many symbols that carry the tale of its secret. The Seer seems to take the confident view that the imprisoned divine splendour, although a veritable Mystery, is present in every manifest form and is open to understanding.[21]

**3.31:** This invocation to God Indra, translated below, contains many key elements of Vedic metaphysics.

**3.38:** This hymn, rendered below, gives us insight into the sacred task of crafting vision-based hymns of praise, which was integral to the Vedic Yoga of the *rishis*.

**3.57:** This hymn, rendered below, is in praise of the "Single Cow," which provides ample spiritual sustenance for deities and humans alike.

**4.58:** This hymn reveals the esoteric symbolism of the ghee (*ghrita*) used in the fire sacrifice. Ghee is said (verse 5) to flow from the ocean of the heart. Its secret name is given as "tongue of the Gods" or "navel of immortality." *Soma* is called (verse 2) a "four-horned buffalo," who has three feet, two heads, and seven arms. "The whole world," declares verse 11, "is stationed in your splendor (*dhâman*) within the ocean, within the heart, in the life-span."

**5.81:** This hymn, translated below, introduces the Solar Yoga that is central to the spirituality of the Vedic civilization.

**6.1:** Vedic spirituality is unthinkable without God Agni, who is the sublime essence behind the sacrificial fire that carries oblations to the divine realms. This hymn brings out some of the profound symbolism revolving around Agni and the fire ritual.

**6.9:** This beautiful invocation to God Agni as Vaishvânara speaks of him as the "immortal Light among mortals," "swifter than the mind," and "stationed in the heart."

**8.48:** Dedicated to Soma, the God of the ambrosia of immortality, this hymn offers many insights into Vedic spirituality. A translation is found in the following Source Reading.

**10.61:** Consisting of twenty-seven verses, this relatively long hymn is replete with Vedic symbolism relating to the mystery of the sun. It was composed by Nâbhânedishtha, whose name means "he who is nearest to the navel," the navel being an esoteric designation of the sun, as is made clear in verse 18. According to a legend told in the *Aitareya-Brâhmana* (5.14), this and hymn 10.62 (also composed by Nâbhânedishtha) helped the Angirases to attain Heaven. In verse 19, the great seer affirms his identity with the sun, exclaiming ecstatically, "I am all this, the twice-born, the first-born of the [cosmic] Order."

**10.72:** This is another cosmogonic hymn, addressing the riddle of the universe's origin. In the third and fourth verse the term *uttânapâd*, "one whose feet are turned upward," is mentioned, which is a name of the Goddess Aditi ("Boundless") who gave birth to the world. This peculiar expression is reminiscent of the *uttâna-carana* posture referred to in Yâjnavalkya's *Smriti* (3.198), a text on ethics and jurisprudence that is generally dated to the early centuries C.E. but undoubtedly contains materials that are very much older. This posture is executed by raising the legs above the ground, as in the shoulderstand.

**10.90:** Of the various cosmogonic hymns that are important for a study of archaic Yoga inasmuch as they describe not only the evolution of the cosmos but also the genesis of the human psyche, the *purusha-sûkta,* or "Hymn of Man," is one of the most striking. In the first verse the primeval male (*purusha*) is said to have covered the entire creation and extended ten digits beyond it. This is meant to suggest that the Creator transcends his creation, that the manifest world emanates from the transcendental Reality but does not define it. A more elaborate version of this hymn is found in the *Atharva-Veda* (15.6).

**10.121:** The seer of this hymn envisions the universe as arising out of the Golden Germ (*hiranya-garbha*). The great singular Being, whose "shadow is immortality," is declared to be the ruler of the world who has firmly fixed both Heaven and Earth. Nine of the ten verses of this hymn end in the refrain "Which God shall we worship with oblations?"

**10.129:** Known as the *nâsadîya-sûkta,* or the "Hymn of Creation," this cosmogonic hymn foreshadows the later metaphysical speculations of the Sâmkhya school of thought that was so closely allied with Yoga. A translation is given below.

**10.136:** This is known as the *keshî-sûkta,* or "Hymn of the Long-hair," which is also rendered into English below. The *keshin* is a special type of non-Vedic ascetic in whom some scholars have seen a forerunner of the later *yogin.* According to the later Sanskrit commentators, each verse of this hymn was composed by a different sage: Jûti, Vâtajûti, Viprajûti, Vrishânaka, Karikrata, Etasha, and Rishyashringa.

**10.177:** This short hymn, rendered below, proffers a valuable glimpse into the Vedic spiritual practice of visionary, ecstatic intuition (*manishâ*).

As we begin to understand the enigmatic poetry of the *rishis* better, we also learn to appreciate more the complexity of their spiritual culture. The small selection of Rig-Vedic hymns given in Source Reading 5 provides only a rudimentary picture of Vedic spirituality and its Proto-Yoga. Further information can be found in some of the books by Sri Aurobindo and more recently David Frawley.[22]

Miller has examined the *Rig-Veda* from the point of view of spiritual practice, and she concludes that the discipline of meditation (*dhyâna*), as the fulcrum of Yoga, goes back to the Rig-Vedic period. She observes:

> The Vedic bards were *seers* who *saw* the *Veda* and sang what they saw. With them vision and sound, seership and singing are intimately connected and this linking of the two sense functions forms the basis of Vedic prayer.[23]

Vedic Sanskrit has two words for prayerful meditation—*brahman* and *dhî.* The former is derived from the verbal root *brih* meaning "to grow," or "to expand," whereas the latter stands for intensive thought, inspired reflection, or meditative vision. Miller describes the brahmic meditation as follows:

> This is the essence of the Vedic *brahman*—the Vedic magic: an invocation and an evocation, an active participation, by means of mental energy and spiritual insight, in the divine process, rather than a mere passive reception of external influences; a deliberate drawing forth out of a probing deep within the *psyche*, and the appropriate formulation thereof; the words themselves into which the orison [prayer], now mentally conceived, is finally couched, being but the form in which is clothed the *inspiration—vision—action.*[24]

According to Miller, the meditative practice in Vedic times displays three distinct but overlapping aspects, which she calls "mantric meditation," "visual meditation," and "absorption in mind and heart" respectively. By "mantric meditation," she means mental absorption via the vehicle of sound, or sacred utterance (*mantra*). Visual meditation, again, is epitomized in the concept of *dhî* (the later *dhyâna*), in which a particular deity is envisioned. Finally, absorption in mind and heart is the highest meditative stage in which the seer, on the basis of what Miller calls a "seed-thought," explores the great psychic and cosmic mysteries that led to the composition of the remarkable cosmogonic hymns, such as the "Hymn of Creation" (*Rig-Veda* 10.129).

Meditation, when successful, leads to illumination, the discovery of the "fearless Light" (*Rig-Veda* 6.47.8). Thus, Sage Atri in one Rig-Vedic hymn (5.40.6) is said to have "found the sun

hidden by darkness" in the course of the fourth stage of prayer, which can be equated with ecstasy (*samâdhi*). Miller sees in this the "culmination of the Vedic quest for truth."[25] She concedes that the full meaning of this fourth stage is not given in the *Rig-Veda* itself, and she relates it to a later key teaching of Vedânta, as embodied especially in the *Mândûkya-Upanishad*, which speaks of the Absolute as the Fourth (*turîya*).

Miller's exacting and sensitive studies have revealed hitherto mostly unsuspected depths of spiritual practice among the Vedic settlers, and a spectacular world of symbols and ideas that bespeak a people who were as fond of introspection and contemplation as they were of earthly delights. The recent work of David Frawley in a way complements Miller's and is equally helpful in bringing out the profound spiritual dimension of the *Vedas*.[26]

The hymns are expressions of the deep spirituality of the Vedic Aryans. To compose a hymn meant to envision it in a state of contemplation. The envisioner was known as a *rishi*, or seer, by virtue of his sacred vision. By performing the prescribed sacrifices, the "mind-yoked" (*mano-yuja*) seer "sent forth" his vision (*dhî*) to the Divine. Frawley says of the Vedic seers that they "were the incarnation of the love of truth, of a free and open creativity, of a great ardor of life and awareness."[27] He continues enthusiastically:

> In stature they were like great mountains; in movement like great streams. Their powers of perception extended through all the realms of cosmic existence. Their creative force manifested in many worlds. Yet they were as humble and serviceable as a cow, as impartially beneficent as the sun . . . They were our spiritual fathers, the makers of civilisation, and as long as

civilisation upheld their inner sand spiritual values, there was true harmony on earth.[28]

The Proto-Yoga of the *rishis* contains many of the elements characteristic of later Yoga: concentration, watchfulness, austerities, regulation of the breath in connection with the recitation of the sacred hymns during rituals, painstakingly accurate recitation (foreshadowing the later Mantra-Yoga), devotional invocation (finding full flowering in the medieval Bhakti-Yoga), visionary experience, the idea of self-sacrifice (or surrender of the ego), the encounter with a Reality larger than the ego-personality, and the continuous enrichment of ordinary life by that encounter (heralding the later Sahaja-Yoga).

Because the *Vedas* were created by seers of extraordinary spiritual aptitude, they are more than poetry and more than a depository of history. They are sacred utterances, testimonies to the spiritual potential of our species, and therefore we must read them accordingly. Miller, Frawley, and also Sri Aurobindo, who was himself modern India's finest seer-poet, consequently have championed a spiritual interpretation of the Vedic hymns. Aurobindo wrote:

> The Veda possesses the high spiritual substance of the Upanishads, but lacks their phraseology; it is an inspired knowledge as yet insufficiently equipped with intellectual and philosophical terms. We find a language of poets and illuminates to whom all experience is real, vivid, sensible, even concrete, not yet of thinkers and systematisers to whom the realities of the mind and soul have become abstractions . . . Here we have the ancient psychological science and the art of spiritual living of which the Upanishads are the philosophical outcome.[29]

---

"Awesome are the seers.
Obeisance be to them!
What vision is theirs
and what truth is in their
mind!"

—*Atharva-Veda* 2.35.4

---

Aurobindo pushed the symbolic interpretation of the *Vedas* as far as possible, and any unbiased reading of these scriptures will bear him out. Thus he insisted that the this-worldly tone of many of the Vedic hymns, which petition the deities for a long life, health, and wealth, must not be understood as mere materialistic requests. Rather, we should read them in metaphoric terms. Aurobindo's approach to Vedic interpretation is far sounder than the literalist reading favored by many scholars, who see in the *Vedas* little more than primitive poetry. However, we can easily appreciate the Vedic *rishis'* spiritual wisdom, lofty idealism, and overall metaphysical orientation without denying that they also prayed for things in this world. Not everything in the *Vedas* is necessarily written in code, though a good deal appears to be. In relation to the latter, Subhash Kak has shown that the hymns of the *Rig-Veda* are organized according to an astronomical code, which demonstrates the superlative significance of astronomy in the ritual life of the Vedic Aryans.[30] This code also informed the construction of the five-layered fire altars. Thus we can begin to appreciate that the Vedic worldview was a consistent whole based on extensive microcosmic-macrocosmic correspondences.

## Of Seers and Ecstatics

The ancient brahmins, like their modern Hindu counterparts, represented the conservative arm of the Vedic religion. By contrast, the *rishis* were the creative force that constantly infused into the Vedic ritualism the lifeblood of their concrete visions of the deities and their realization of the ultimate Being. Later, with the waning influence of the visionary culture of the *rishis*, who tested their visions in verbal combat with each other, the brahmanical ritualism quickly rigidified under the heavy hand of priestly conservatism.[31] The sacrifices became more important than the visions and higher spiritual realizations. The meaning of the Vedic hymns was lost sight of, to the point that Kautsa, an ancient ritualist, was able to declare, "*Mantras* are meaningless." By *mantras* he meant the sacred hymns, which, in his opinion, contained many nonsensical utterances. By this attitude he anticipated the stance of not a few modern scholars who fail to perceive the spiritual import behind the dictionary definitions of Vedic Sanskrit words.

Be that as it may, as is evident from the *Upanishads*, mystical esotericism continued to break forth here and there outside the fold of the priestly orthodoxy. Even at the time of the *rishis* there were those who, like the *munis*, pursued the spiritual quest at the margins of Vedic society. The *munis* were ecstatics who remained close to the shamanic heritage. In the "Hymn of the Long-hair" (*Rig-Veda* 10.136), translated below, the *muni* is said to ride the winds and to benefit his fellow beings, both of which are typical shamanic motifs. At the time of the *Upanishads*, the wisdom tradition, with its emphasis on ecstatic self-transcendence and Self-realization, was often transmitted not by brahmins but by members of the warrior estate—rulers like Ajâtashatru, Uddâlaka, and the latter's son Shvetaketu. Let us not forget here that the *Bhagavad-Gîtâ*, which is called an esoteric teaching (*upanishad*) in the colophons to its eighteen chapters, was communicated by Lord Krishna to Prince Arjuna, son of King Pându. Of course, there were also great brahmins at the dawn of the Upanishadic Age—foremost among them the great sage Yâjnavalkya—who also taught the secrets of the inner sacrifice.

**SOURCE READING 5**

# *Rig-Veda (Selection)*

The language of the *Rig-Veda* is mantric, poetic, and often allegorical and esoteric. Unless this is appreciated, we cannot hope to grasp the message of the Vedic hymns. The following renderings of just a handful of the 1,028 hymns found in the *Rig-Veda* are based in the recognition that the seer-bards were not mere "primitives" but master wordsmiths who, moreover, were profoundly skilled in the art of ecstatic self-transcendence through ritual, prayer, and sound.

These readings from the most ancient part of the Vedic corpus have been selected because they are particularly relevant to a discussion of Vedic Proto-Yoga. They give us a basic idea of the Vedic approach to the sacred. They also show that the *rishis* had developed an elevated spiritual metaphysics anticipating the teachings of the *Upanishads*, the *Bhagavad-Gîtâ*, and other Sanskrit scriptures fundamental to Vedânta and Vedântic Yoga.

The Vedic hymns are pregnant with symbolism and mythology, which were the vehicles for the *rishis'* expression of deeper spiritual truths, although we do not know enough about the Vedic worldview to completely "unpack" the hymns' dense symbolism and metaphoric language. Ultimately, even with an arsenal of scholarly elucidations to draw from, the modern student of the *Vedas* must rely on his or her personal intuition in trying to comprehend the hymns.

## 3.31

God Indra, who is at the center of Vedic spirituality, is frequently invoked in the *Rig-Veda*. Commonly interpreted as a thunderstorm deity, Indra is a truly Protean God who is associated with a variety of phenomena—from thunder, lightning, and rain to sky, fire, and sun, as well as the year. In this hymn, Indra is revealed as the divine agent who slays Vritra, the demon of darkness, and releases the imprisoned cows. For the Vedic people, the word *go* meant a great many things apart from "cow," including "life-giving water," "light rays," and "sacred speech." The present hymn can be read in many ways, and the various meanings may all have been present in the mind of the *rishi* who composed it. There is obviously an intentional play on the experience of the dawning light at daybreak and at the

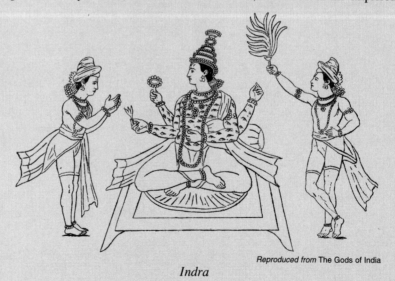

Reproduced from The Gods of India

*Indra*

moment of spiritual illumination. Both occurrences are aided by the sacrificial ritual honoring Indra, destroyer of darkness. Again we have here an indirect reference to Solar Yoga, the Yoga of tuning into the radiance of the great heavenly being the ancients knew as Sûrya.

Sri Aurobindo understood Indra as a symbol for the purified and thus empowered human mind that can release us from bondage (i.e., ignorance) and shower us with the blissful divine Light. When we are thus freed from egoic constraints, we can experience great spiritual intuitions, which become translated into inspired speech.

The driver [i.e., God Agni who carries the oblation to the divine realms] wise in the law came, speaking devoutly as he chastened his daughter's daughter. When the father strove to pour into his daughter [i.e., the sacrificial ladle], his heart eagerly consented. (1)

The son of the body did not leave the inheritance [i.e., the sacrificial butter] to the sister; he made her womb [i.e., the bowl of the sacrificial ladle] a treasure house for the winner. When the mothers [i.e., the kindling sticks] give birth to the driver, one of the two who do good deeds is the maker [i.e., the priest], and the other [i.e., the sacrificer] derives the gain. (2)

With his tongue quivering, Agni was born to honor the sons [i.e., the priests of the Angiras family] of the great rosy one [i.e., the sky at dawn]. Great was the embryo, great was their birth, and great the growth, through sacrifice, of the Lord [Indra] of bay horses. (3)

The conquerors surrounded the challenger; they brought forth great light out of darkness. The Dawn Goddesses recognized him and came to meet him; Indra became the only Lord of cows. (4)

The wise ones [i.e., the priestly sages] struck a path for those who were in the cave; the seven priests drove them on with thoughts pressing forward. They found all the paths of the right way; the knowing one entered [the cave], bowing low. (5)

If Saramâ [i.e., Indra's horse] finds the breach in the mountain, she will complete her earlier great pathfinding. The swift-footed one led out the head of the undying syllables [i.e., the cows]; knowing the way, she was the first to go toward the cry. (6)

The most inspired one [i.e., Indra?] came, behaving like a friend. The mountain made ripe the fruit [i.e., the cows] of its womb for the one who performed great deeds. The young hero, proving his generosity, won success with the youths; then [Sage] Angiras at once became a singer of praise. (7)

The image of this creature and that creature, he knows all who are born. Standing in the forefront, he killed Shushna [i.e., the Demon of Drought]. Knowing the path of the sky, longing for cows, he went before us, singing. The friend freed his friends from dishonor. (8)

With a heart longing for cows, they sat down while with their songs they made the road to immortality. This is their very seat, still often used now, the lawful way by which they wished to win the months. (9)

Glancing about, they rejoiced in their own possessions as they milked out the milk of the ancient seed. Their shout heated the two worlds. They arranged the offspring, dividing the cows among the men. (10)

With songs, he himself, Indra the killer of Vritra, released the rosy cows together with the offspring and the oblations. Stretching far, the cow was milked of the sweet honey-like butter that she had held for him. (11)

They made a seat for him as for a father, for these great deeds revealed a great, shining seat. They propped their two parents [i.e., sky and earth] apart with a pillar; sitting down, they raised the wild one high up. (12)

When Dhishanâ [i.e., the bowl of the sky?] determined to crush down the one who had grown great in a single day and had pervaded the two world halves, all irresistible powers came to Indra, in whom flawless praises come together. (13)

I long for your great friendship, for your powerful help. Many gifts go to the killer of Vritra. Great is praise; we have come to the kindness of the lord. Generous Indra, be good to us as our shepherd. (14)

He won great land and much wealth, and he sent the booty to his friends. Radiant with his men, Indra gave birth to the sun, the dawn, motion [i.e., the passage of the sun?], and fire. (15)

This house-friend has loosed into a single channel even the wide dispersed waters that shine with many colors, the honeyed waters made clear by the inspired filters. Rushing along by day and night, they drive forward. (16)

The two dark bearers of treasure [i.e., day and night], worthy of sacrifice, follow Sûrya with his consent when Your beloved, impetuous friends embrace Your splendor to draw it to them. (17)

Killer of Vritra, be the lord of lovely gifts, the bull who gives life to songs of praise for a whole life span. Come to us with kind and friendly favors, with great help, quickly, O Great One! (18)

Like Angiras I honor him and bow to him, making new for the ancient one a song that was born long ago. Thwart the many godless lies, and let us win the sun, generous Indra. (19)

The mists that were spread about [by Vritra] have become transparent; guide us safely across them. You, our charioteer, must protect us from injury. Soon, Indra, soon, make us winners of cows. (20)

The Killer of Vritra, Lord of cows, has shown us cows. He went among the dark ones [i.e., the dark forces] with His rosy forms. Revealing lovely gifts in the right way, He has opened up all his own gates. (21)

For success in this [psychocosmic] battle in which there are prizes to be won, we will invoke the generous Indra, most manly and brawny, who listens and gives help in combat, who kills enemies [i.e., evil forces] and wins riches [i.e., spiritual treasures]. (22)

### 3.38

Like a carpenter, craft an intuition (*manishâ*), proceeding like a well-yoked steed. Intent on what is desirable and most worthy,[32] I desire to behold the well-inspired (*sumedha*) seer-poets (*kavi*) [who are in the celestial realms]. (1)

Ask of the glorious race of seer-poets, [who] firm-minded and acting well, have created Heaven. May these praises, swelling and fast as the mind, duly reach You. (2)

Understanding what is hidden here [in this world], they have anointed both worlds [i.e., Heaven and Earth] for [their] dominion—limited them by measure, connected them together, widespread and vast, and fixed the intermediate realm for support (*dhur*). (3)

All adorned Him [i.e., God Indra] ascending [in his celestial chariot]. He moves self-radiant and clothed in splendor. Great is the name of that Asura, showerer (*vrisha*) [of countless blessings]. Multiform, He resides among the immortals. (4)

The Primal one, elder, and showerer [of blessings] has generated [the Waters]. These are the abundant healing draughts. O grandsons in Heaven, by your visions (*dhî*) you have acquired dominion over the splendid sacrifices. (5)

O rulers, attend and fill the three splendid sacrifices. I saw in my mind that the *gandharvas*, with hair blowing [in the wind], have gone to the rite. (6)

For the showerer [of countless blessings] they milk the agreeable [milk] of the cow of [many] names. Invested with various kinds of power (*asurya*), the builders (*mâyin*) put a form (*rûpa*) upon Him.[33] (7)

No one holds apart my golden luster from Savitri's in which he has taken refuge. Through praise He manifests both all-pervading worlds [i.e., Heaven and Earth] as a woman cherishes her offspring. (8)

Of the ancient ones, you two [i.e., Maruts] promote the power that spreads all around us as divine well-being. All the builders behold the many deeds of Him who stands still and whose tongue is protected. (9)

For success in this [psychocosmic] battle where there are prizes to be won, we will invoke the generous Indra, most manly and brawny, who listens and gives help in combat, who kills enemies [i.e., evil forces] and wins riches [i.e., spiritual treasures]. (10)

### 3.57

This hymn speaks of the *rishi's* discovery of the Single Cow, the cosmic Female, who is the wielder of power similar to the Shakti of later Hinduism. Like a mother, this great force in the universe provides sustenance for the spiritual pilgrim. She nurtures even the Gods, the sons of immortality, to whose abode the *rishi* aspires. Through Agni, the God of the sacrificial fire, the seer-bard's spiritual impulse is carried on high to yield the desired celestial vision or communion.

My finely discerning intuition (*manishâ*) has discovered the Cow (*dhenu*) roaming singly without herdsman, who instantly yields abundant milk for sustenance; hence Indra and Agni praise Her. (1)

Indra and Pûshan, vigorous and deft-handed, have indeed joyously milked the Ever-Flowing [Cow] of heaven. When all the Gods have delighted in Her, there, may I find grace (*sumnam*). (2)

The sisters who desire the Power (*shakti*) of the Seeder-Bull (*vrisha*), go [to Him] with reverence and recognize the seed (*garbha*) in Him. The cows come eagerly to the son [i.e., Soma?], who bears many forms (*vapûmshi*). (3)

I glorify the well-made Heaven and Earth, as I prepare the stones during the sacrifice [by means of] intuition (*manishâ*). These flames of Yours—visible and adorable—rise upward with abundant boons for humankind. (4)

O Agni, Your honeyed tongue, exceedingly wise, is said to be the Broad [i.e., the earth] among the Gods. By Her make all the adorable ones sit down here to drink the honey-brew. (5)

God Agni, Knower of [all] birth, bestow upon us She who is to You like a variegated, inexhaustible stream of a mountain—[She who is] knowledge (*pramati*), wisdom (*sumati*), [belonging to] all people. (6)

### 5.81

The sun, as the visible manifestation of the transcendental Light, is a central image of Vedic Proto-Yoga. This hymn reveals some of the elements of the Solar Yoga of the *rishis*. Spiritual realization is literal enlightenment, or the illumination of the inner world of consciousness by the unmanifest Light, which is the supreme Being.

The sages (*vipra*) of the greatly inspired Sage [i.e., Savitri] harness the mind; they harness their visions (*dhî*). He alone who is versed in the rules [of sacrifice] assigns the priesthood. Great indeed is the praise of God Savitri. (1)

The seer-poet (*kavi*) releases all forms and provides auspiciousness for the two-legged and the four-legged [creatures]. Most adorable Savitri has illumined the Heaven and governs brightly (*rajati*) with vitality (*ojas*) after Dawn's passage. (2)

After the passage of that God, the other Gods follow [in order to obtain] majesty with vigor (*ojas*). He who measured the earthly [regions] by his greatness is the resplendent God Savitri. (3)

You traverse the three luminous spheres; or You mix with Sûrya's rays; or You encompass Night on both sides; or You, O God, are Mitra because of Your [benign] qualities (*dharma*). (4)

You alone rule over creation (*prasava*). You, O God, are Pûshan because of Your movements. You govern brightly (*rajasi*) over this whole world. [Sage] Shyâvâshva has offered praise to You, O Savitri. (5)

### 8.48

Vedic sacrificial ritualism is unthinkable without the mysterious *soma* draft, celebrated in this hymn. The pressed and filtered *soma* juice, mixed with milk and water, is the single most important oblation in special public (*shrauta*) sacrifices. This ambrosial draft is here invoked as King Soma, the guardian of the body, who bestows immortality upon his worshipers in the company of the Gods. He is also addressed as the Drop (*indu*), which reminds one of the "seed-point" (*bindu*) of later Tantra-Yoga.

I have consumed the delicious drink of life, knowing that it inspires good thoughts and joyous expansiveness and which all the deities and mortals seek together, calling it honey. (1)

And going within, You become boundless (*aditi*), and You will avert the wrath of deities. Rejoicing in Indra's friendship, O Drop, create riches [for us] like an obedient racer [i.e., a horse] carrying a burden. (2)

We have drunk the Soma. We have become immortal. We have gone to the Light. We have found the Gods. What can enmity do to do us now, and what injury by a mortal, O Immortal one? (3)

When we have drunk You, O Drop, pacify our heart. O famous Soma, be kind like a father toward his son, thoughtful like a friend toward a friend. O praiseworthy Soma, extend our life so that we may live long. (4)

I have drunk these glorious [drops of *soma*] that widen me. [Yet] my limbs are tied together like bullocks yoked to a cart. Let them protect my foot from stumbling and may they ward off lameness because of [imbibing] the Drop. (5)

Inflame me like a fire kindled by friction. Make us farseeing. Make us richer, better. For when I am intoxicated with You, O Soma, I consider myself rich. Draw near and make us thrive! (6)

Impelled by a powerful mind, may we enjoy You like wealth [inherited] from a father. O King Soma, extend our life as the sun [expands] the days of spring. (7)

King Soma, have mercy on us for our welfare. Know that we are devoted to Your laws (*vratya*). O Drop, passion and enthusiasm are stirred up. Do not deliver us to the whim of the enemy. (8)

For You, O Soma, are the guardian of our body. Watching over men, You have settled down in every limb. If we break Your laws, O God, have mercy on us like a good friend, [making us] better. (9)

Let me join closely with my compassionate friend so that He will not injure me when I have drunk [the Drop]. O Lord of bay horses, for the Soma that is stationed in us I approach Indra to prolong our life span. (10)

Weaknesses and diseases have gone. The forces of darkness have fled in terror. Soma has climbed up in us, expanding. We have arrived where our life span is prolonged. (11)

The Drop that we have drunk has entered our hearts, an immortal within mortals. O forefathers, let us serve that Soma with the oblations and abide in His mercy and kindness. (12)

Uniting in agreement with the forefathers, O Soma, You have extended Yourself through Heaven and Earth. O Drop, let us serve with an oblation. Let us be masters of riches. (13)

You protecting Gods, speak out for us. Do not let sleep or harmful speech seize us. Let us, always dear to Soma, speak as men of power in the sacrificial gathering. (14)

O Soma, You give us the force of life on every side. You who have found Heaven and watch over men, enter into us. O Drop, summon Your helpers and protect us front and back. (15)

## 10.129

The "Hymn of Creation" is often hailed as one of the few truly philosophical hymns of the *Rig-Veda*, but, although it reflects a particularly poignant cosmogonic inquiry, it does not stand alone. Rather, once we have jettisoned the bias that the Vedic hymns represent basically "primitive poetry," we can see profound philosophizing throughout the Vedic corpus. We need, however, to appreciate that Vedic philosophy is multifaceted and integrally interwoven with Vedic spirituality. Thus, even the present hymn must be read as proffering probing questions not only about the origin of the external universe but also our inner world. Vedic cosmogony is psychocosmogony—a characteristic that has been preserved in the subsequent philosophical traditions of Yoga, Sâmkhya, and Vedânta, which (in their own unique ways) postulate a transcendental Ground from which arise both the multiplicity of objective realities and the multistructured minds apperceiving them.

Existence or nonexistence was not then. The bright region was not, nor the space (*vyoman*) that is beyond. What encompassed? Where? Under whose protection? What water was there—deep, unfathomable? (1)

Death or immortality was not then. There was no distinction between night and day. That One breathed, windless, by itself. Other than That there was nothing more. (2)

In the beginning there was darkness concealed by darkness. All this was [cosmic] water without distinction. The One that was covered by voidness emerged through the might of the heat-of-austerity (*tapas*). (3)

In the beginning, desire—the first seed of mind—arose in That. Seer-poets, searching in their heart with wisdom, found the bond of existence in nonexistence. (4)

Their [visions'] ray stretched across [existence and nonexistence]. Perhaps there was a below; perhaps there was an above. There were givers of seed; there were powers: effort below, self-giving above. (5)

Who knows the truth? Who here will pronounce it whence this birth, whence this creation? The Gods appeared afterward, with the creation of this [world]. Who then knows whence it arose? (6)

Whence arose this creation, whether it created itself or whether it did not? He who looks upon it from the highest space, He surely knows. Or maybe He knows not. (7)

## 10.136

The "Hymn of the Long-hair" (*keshî-sûkta*) gives us a glimpse of the shamanic ecstatic in Vedic times. The *keshin*, who, as the name indicates, wears long hair, is said to exult in his seeing of, and participation in, truths that are concealed from the ordinary mortal. He is as compassionate as he is mindlessly God-intoxicated or "God-impelled" (*deva-ishita*, written *deveshita*).

The word *keshin* is also applied to the sun whose long "hair" is its luminous rays reaching across space to the earth. The long-haired human sage is sunlike in nature, and perhaps his radiant aura was blinding to those sensitive enough to see it.

There are several obscure phrases and statements in this hymn. In interpreting them, I have largely followed Jeanine Miller's lead, though in a few instances I am putting forward my own divergent views and intuitions. The "tawny dirt" with which the *keshin* clothes himself could refer to the Hindu practice of smearing sandal paste on certain parts of the body, especially the forehead. This is held to have more than symbolic or ritual significance.

The phrase "wind-girt" has generally been interpreted to mean "nude." But this could also have deeper symbolic significance. As is clear from other verses of this hymn, the *keshin* is closely associated with Vâyu, God of the wind, or the life force. If we read this hymn from a yogic point of view, we could easily wrest from this phrase a different meaning: that the *keshin* armed himself with the breath, that is, he practiced breath control. This would explain the first-person exclamation "upon the winds we have ascended." In that case, it is through the regulation of the breath that the *keshin* enters a different state of consciousness (and its corresponding reality).

It is not clear what is meant by the "unbendable" (*kunamnamâ*) in the concluding stanza (the only place where this word appears). Miller speculates that it may be the "gross aspect" of the human body-mind, that is, the material vehicle that resists psychospiritual transformation. God Vâyu, the master of the life force (*prâna*), is said to have "churned" and "pounded" the "badly bent one" (*kunamnamâ*) for the *keshin*. Perhaps we can even see in this an early reference to the dormant psychospiritual power of the human body, which later came to be known as the *kundalinî-shakti*.

We must remember here that some three thousand years later the Goddess Kubjikâ was worshipped in some schools of Tantrism. She is said to reside with her divine spouse Shiva on the peak of the sacred Mount Kailâsa in the Himalayas. According to this Tantric tradition, Kubjikâ is closely associated with the *kundalinî*, which is said to be her body. The syllable *ku* in Kubjikâ's name is taken to represent the earth element, which is traditionally placed in the lowest psychoenergetic center, the *mûlâdhâra-cakra*, at the base of the spine. This is also the place of the coiled serpent power, or *kundalinî-shakti*.

The Sanskrit word *kubjâ* means literally "crooked one." This appears to be the meaning also of the Vedic word *kunamnamâ*. The Goddess Kubjikâ, who is also known as Vakreshvarî ("Crooked Princess"), is sometimes depicted as an old woman, in addition to her two other forms—that of a girl and that of a young woman.[34] Is it possible that we have here an esoteric tradition about the hidden spiritual power coiled within the human body that goes back to Vedic times?

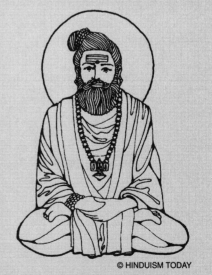

© HINDUISM TODAY

*Long-haired ascetic*

The long-hair [endures] fire; the long-hair [endures] poison; the long-hair endures Heaven-and-Earth (*rodasî*) [both physical and psychic]; the long-hair gazes fully on Heaven (*svar*); the long-hair is said to be that [transcendental] Light. (1)

The wind-girt sages (*muni*) have donned the tawny dirt (*mala*). Along the wind's course they glide when the Gods have penetrated [them]. (2)

Exulted by our silence (*mauna*), upon the winds we have ascended. Behold, you mortals, our bodies [only]. (3)

Through the mid-region (*antariksha*) flies the sage illuminating all forms; for his goodness, he is deemed the friend of every God. (4)

The wind's steed, Vâyu's friend, is the God-intoxicated sage; within both oceans he dwells, the upper and the lower. (5)

In the paths of *apsarases* [female spirits], *gandharvas* [male spirits], and beasts wanders the long-hair, knower of [the most hidden] thoughts, a gentle friend, most exhilarating. (6)

For him has Vâyu churned and pounded the badly bent one (*kunamnamâ*), when the long-hair drank with Rudra from the poison cup. (7)


### 10.177

With their heart (*hrid*), with their mind (*manas*), the wise see the Winged-one (*patanga*) endowed with Asura's magic (*mâyâ*). The seer-poets (*kavi*) recognize [Him] inside the ocean. The sages desire the footprint of [His] rays. (1)

With the heart, the Winged-one carries the Word (*vâc*) that the *gandharva* pronounced inside the womb. The seer-poets protect this thunderous (*svarya*) flashing intuition (*manishâ*) in the abode (*pada*) of the [cosmic] order (*rita*). (2)

I have seen the protector who untiringly approaches and withdraws along the paths. Clothed with convergent and divergent [forces], He revolves within the worlds.[35] (3)

## V. SPELLS OF TRANSCENDENCE— THE MAGICAL YOGA OF THE ATHARVA-VEDA

The *Atharva-Veda* contains sacred knowledge (*veda*) collected by the magus and fire-priest Atharvan, who may have been a native of what is now Bihar. As a collection, the *Atharva-Veda* is at least several centuries younger than the *Rig-Veda*, but much of its contents is probably as old as the oldest hymns of the *Rig-Veda*. Even though the *Atharva-Veda* was undoubtedly widely resorted to, for a long time it was not counted as part of the sacred Vedic canon, and even after its incorporation it was never granted by the orthodox priesthood the same status as the *Rig-Veda*, *Yajur-Veda*, and *Sâma-Veda*.

The *Atharva-Veda* consists of around six thousand verses and one thousand lines in prose, most of which deal with magical spells and charms designed to either promote peace, health, love, and material and spiritual prosperity, or to call down disaster on an enemy. Here are three excerpts that epitomize the magical side of this hymnody:

As the creeper has completely embraced the tree, so may you embrace me. May you love me. May you not withdraw from me.

As the eagle, flying forth, beats its wings toward the earth, so I beat down your mind. May you love me. May you not withdraw from me.

As the sun travels swiftly in [the space between] sky and earth here, so do I go about your mind. May you love me. May you not withdraw from me. (6.8.1–3)

* * *

Having harnessed the chariot [of my mind], here has come forth the thousand-eyed curse, seeking after my curser, as a wolf [seeks out] the dwelling of a shepherd.

O curse, avoid us like a burning fire [avoids] a pool. Strike our curser here, as the [lightning] bolt from the sky [strikes] a tree.

Whoever shall curse us not cursing, and whoever shall curse us cursing, him [who is] whithered I cast unto death, as a bone [is cast to] a dog. (6.37.1–3)

* * *

Night after night, we bring to You, O Agni, [our offerings] without mixture, as fodder to a standing horse. Let us, Your neighbors, not experience harm, [but] enjoy abundance of wealth and food.

Whatever arrow [of destiny] of You who are good is in the air, that is Yours. With it, be gracious to us. Let us, Your neighbors, not experience harm, [but] enjoy abundance of wealth and food.

Evening after evening, Agni is our household's lord. Morning after morning, He is the giver of good intentions. May You be for us the giver of good of every kind. May we adorn ourselves by kindling You.

Morning after morning, Agni is our household's lord. Evening after evening, He is the giver of good intentions. May You be for us the giver of good of every kind. May we thrive a hundred winters by kindling You.

May I not fall short of food. To the food-eating Lord of Food, to Agni [who is Rudra] be homage. (19.55.1–5)

The first of the above hymns is a love charm, the second is a spell against curses, and the third is an incantation addressed to Agni for prosperity. These prayers and spells give some indication of the range of concerns expressed in the "fourth" *Veda*.

Of the many mystical passages in the *Atharva-Veda*, most of which defy full comprehension, the following selection of hymns appear to imply some esoteric knowledge that could feasibly be linked to Proto-Yoga and the related Proto-Sâmkhya tradition.

**2.1:** This hymn speaks of the seer Vena of whom it is said that he saw that which is the highest secret, "where everything becomes of one form."

**4.1:** This is another enigmatic hymn, which tells of Vena's mystic Realization. Vena is said to have uncovered the womb (*yoni*) of being and nonbeing.

**5.1:** This hymn is purposely obscure and probably grammatically corrupt in many parts. However, judging from the sophisticated concepts expressed, its composer was evidently aware of a deep mystical tradition.

**7.5:** This *sûkta* teaches of the inner sacrifice, which became the main theme of the early *Upanishads*. It starts with the line, "By the sacrifice the Gods sacrificed to the sacrifice." That is, the deities themselves performed sacrifices, and their sacrifices had no other purpose than the action of sacrifice, which is the giving of oneself. The sacrifice is described as being the overlord of the Gods who extended, or taught, the sacrifice to human beings.

**8.9:** This cosmogonic hymn, which extols Virâj, poses a number of esoteric riddles. Virâj is the female (in other hymns also male) creative principle, which the anonymous author declares can be seen by some and not by others. "Breathless, She goes by the breath of breathing ones."

**8.10:** The subject of this hymn is again Virâj, who is said to ascend and descend into the householder's fire. The householder who knows this secret is said to be "house-sacrificing" (*griha-medhin*).

**9.1:** This cosmogonic hymn intimates the secret of the "honey whip" (*madhu-kashâ*). This mysterious substance is said to have sprung from the elements that were generated by the Gods and upon which the sages contemplate. From what we can gather from the difficult passages, the honeyed whip corresponds to the later idea, found in Tantra and Hatha-Yoga, of the internal ambrosia, the nectar of immortality held to drip from a secret place near the palate. The Vedic seers aspired to win the honey, to experience the transcendental splendor within their own body-mind. The honey doctrine (*madhu-vidyâ*) can be met with in the ancient *Brihad-Âranyaka-Upanishad* (2.5.14), where we find this passage:

> The Self (*âtman*) is honey for all things, and all things are honey for this Self. This shining, immortal Person who is in this Self, and, with reference to oneself, this shining, immortal Person who exists as the Self—he is just this Self, this Immortal, this Absolute, this All.

**10.7:** This is a mystical hymn, which consists of a series of probing questions, and which discloses the secret doctrine of the World Pillar (*skambha*) that sustains all of creation: In what part of Him resides austerity (*tapas*)? Where in Him abides the [cosmic] Order? Where vows? Where faith? In what part of Him is truth stationed? How far has the Divine penetrated its own creation? How much of the Divine has entered the past? How much the future?

According to verse 17, the Divine, or World Pillar, is known by those who know the transcendental Reality (*brah-*

*man*) within their own heart. Verse 23 mentions that thirty-three deities protect the secret treasure, that is, the Divine. "Only the knowers of *brahman*," declares verse 27, "know these thirty-three deities." This is pure Vedânta. The Divine, at the center of the world, is attainable through the practice of austerities (*tapas*) states verse 38. Verse 40 tells us that in the seer who has reached this spiritual zenith are all the lights. In verse 15, the *nâdîs* (the currents or "rivers" of the life force) are mentioned, which shows the age of such notions about the subtle or energetic body.

**10.8:** This is a hymn hinting at the author's occult understanding about the origin of the cosmos and expressing wonder at the complexity of creation. A translation is given in Source Reading 6.

**11.4:** This *sûkta* extols the life force (*prâna*), which is said to clothe man, as a father could clothe his dear son (verse 11).

**11.5:** Here the Vedic novice (*brahmacarin*) is spoken of, and the symbolism of his initiation and subsequent spiritual practice are briefly discussed.

**15.1–18:** This is the famous *Vrâtya-Khânda* ("Book of the Vrâtyas"), which will be discussed in the next section.

**SOURCE READING 6**

## *Atharva-Veda (Selection)*

From a spiritual point of view, the following hymn (10.8) is one of the most significant of the *Atharva-Veda* and appears to be intimately connected with hymn 10.7, divulging the secret lore about the World Pillar (*skambha*). In its deep symbolism, which we can only barely grasp, the present hymn reminds one of Dîrghatamas's riddles in the *Rig-Veda* (1.164).

Obeisance to the foremost *brahman* to whom alone belongs Heaven, who presides over past, future, and all [things]. (1)

Established by the Pillar (*skambha*), Heaven and Earth are propped apart. This entire [universe], whatever breathes or closes down (*nimesha*), is embodied (*âtmanvat*) in the Pillar. (2)

Three [kinds of] creatures have gone forth [into transmigration], while others have entered completely into the sun (*arka*).[36] The Great one remains, measuring out the sky. The Golden one [i.e., the sun] has entered the golden [regions].[37] (3)

Twelve rims, one wheel (*cakra*), three naves: Who has understood this? Three hundred and sixty spokes and [the same number of] pins, which are firmly set. (4)

Consider this well, O Savitri: six twins [and] one born singly. They desire relationship with the one who is born singly.[38] (5)

It is manifest and yet is established in the hidden (*guhâ*). Its name is "Aged," "Great Place." In That this entire [universe] is fixed. What moves and breathes is established [in That]. (6)

The one wheel turns with a single rim, with one thousand imperishables (*akshara*),[39] rising in front [i.e., the east] and setting in the back [i.e., the west]. With one half it has engendered the entire world, but what has become of its [other] half? (7)

A carriage of five [horses] conducts the First[-born],[40] with harnessed side-horses pulling along [as well]. What has not been traversed is invisible; not so what has been traversed. What is above [the horizon] is closer; what is below [the horizon] is more remote. (8)

The opening of the vessel is on the side, and its bottom is above. Therein dwells the all-formed glory. There the seven seers,[41] who are the protectors of this Great one, are seated together. (9)

I ask you about the praise (*ric*) that is yoked (*yujyate*) front and back, that is yoked everywhere all round, and by which the sacrifice (*yajna*) is spread out to the east.[42] (10)

That which stirs, flies, stands still, breathes, or breathes not, closes [the eyes] but exists, sustains the earth and, being all-formed, is singular only. (11)

That which is endless is extended in every direction: the endless and the ending come together. These the Guardian [i.e., the sun] of the firmament (*nâka*), who knows past and future, continues to hold apart. (12)

Prajâpati [i.e., the Lord of Creatures] stirs in the [cosmic] womb (*garbha*). Invisible, He is born manifold. With one half He has engendered the whole universe, but what bright indication is there of His other half?[43] (13)

That Water Bearer who carries up the water in a pot,[44] all see Him with the eye, but not all know [Him] with the mind.[45] (14)

The great Spirit (*yaksha*) at the center of the universe dwells afar in wholeness, and afar He vanishes through lack—to Him the rulers [of the world] bear oblations. (15)

Whence the sun rises and where it goes to set, that verily I deem the Foremost (*jyeshtha*). Nothing exceeds That! (16)

Those who presently, formerly,[46] and anciently speak knowingly everywhere of the *Veda*, they all speak only of Âditya [i.e., the sun], the second Agni and threefold swan (*hamsa*).[47] (17)

A thousand days' journey stretches out His wings, the golden swan flying across the sky. He, placing all the Gods in His chest, moves about, overseeing all the worlds. (18)

In whom the Foremost rests, He glows up above through truth, He looks down through prayer (*brahman*), and He breathes crosswise [in the form of the wind] through the life force (*prâna*). (19)

He who indeed knows the churning sticks by which the [precious] thing (*vasu*) [i.e., the fire] is kindled, he may deem to know the Foremost; he should know the great *brâhmana*. (20)

Footless He was born in the beginning. In the beginning, He brought forth Heaven (*svar*).[48] Having become four-footed[49] and capable of eating, He took to Himself all food.[50] (21)

He who worships the eternal supreme God (*deva*) shall become capable of eating and shall eat many [kinds of] food. (22)

They call Him eternal; indeed, He may even now be renewed: Day and night are regenerated out of each other's forms. (23)

A hundred, a thousand, a myriad, a hundred million, countless [numbers of] His own dwell in Him. That of Him they consume[51] while He only looks on. Therefore this God is radiant thus. (24)

The One is finer than a hair;[52] the One is not even visible. Hence the deity (*devatâ*) who is more embracing [than this universe] is dear to me. (25)

This beautiful unaging [deity] is in the house [i.e., in the body] of a mortal. He for whom [this deity] was made lies [still]; he who has made [this deity] has become old.[53] (26)

You are woman. You are man. You are boy or a girl. You who are aged totter with a staff. When born, You face everywhere.[54] (27)

You are their father and also their son. You are their superior (*jyeshtha*) and their inferior. The one God, who has entered the mind, is born first and [yet] He is within the [cosmic] womb. (28)

From the Whole (*pûrna*) He turns up the Whole. The Whole pours forth as the Whole. Now may we also know That from which it is poured out. (29)

She, the eternal one, was born from eternity. She, the ancient one, encompassed all. The great Goddess (*devî*), radiant at dawn,[55] gazes at everyone in the twinkling [of an eye]. (30)

The deity named Avi[56] abides, enveloped by the [cosmic] order (*rita*). These golden[57] trees are turned golden because of Her form. (31)

[Because one is] close, one cannot abandon [that deity]; [although] being close, one does not see [that deity easily].[58] Behold the wisdom (*kâvya*) of the God. He did not [ever] die, nor does He grow old. (32)

The words impelled by the unpreceded [deity] speak [the truth] as it is.[59] Wherever they go speaking that, they declare the great *brâhmana*. (33)

That in which Gods and humans are fastened like spokes in a nave—that in which [the world?] is placed by [divine] magical powers (*mâyâ*), I ask of you, Flower of the Waters.[60] (34)

They who impel the wind to blow, who yield the five directions together, the Gods who deemed themselves above the [sacrificial] offering, the leaders of the waters—who were they? (35)

One of them dwells in this earth. One has become the mid-region (*antariksha*) all round. He who is the dispenser among them gives the sky (*diva*). Some protect all regions. (36)

He who may know the stretched-out thread (*sûtra*) into which these creatures are woven, who may know the thread of the thread, he may [indeed] know the great *brâhmana*. (37)

I know the stretched-out thread into which these creatures are woven. Likewise I know the thread of the thread, which is the great *brâhmana*. (38)

When Agni went burning across Heaven and Earth, consuming all, when the wives [i.e., the flames] of a single [husband, i.e., fire] stood higher than [everything], where then was Mâtarîshvan?[61] (39)

Mâtarîshvan had entered into the [cosmic] waters [while] the Gods were in the oceans. Great indeed was the measurer (*vimâna*) of the sky. The purifier (*pavamâna*) entered the golden ones.[62] (40)

Higher, as it were, than the *gâyatrî*, He went to immortality (*amrita*). Those who know well chant (*sâma*) by chant, where did they see the Unborn (*aja*)[63] ? (41)

Sheltering and assembling [all] things (*vasu*), God Savitri as it were [possesses] the quality of truth (*satya*). As Indra He stands [firm] in the battle for [spiritual] riches. (42)

The lotus of nine doors [i.e., the body and its nine orifices] covered with the three strands (*guna*) [i.e., skin, nails, and hair?]—whatever embodied (*âtmanvat*) Spirit (*yaksha*) is within it, that verily the knowers of *brahman* know. (43)

Desireless, wise, immortal, self-abiding (*svayambhu*), content with the essence (*rasa*), lacking nothing—knowing that wise, unaging, youthful Self (*âtman*), one is not afraid of death.[64] (44)

## VI. THE MYSTERIOUS VRÂTYA BROTHERHOODS

Ancient India holds many riddles for the modern historian. The spiritual brotherhood of the Vrâtyas is perhaps the most intriguing enigma. The statements about the Vrâtyas in Indian literature are confusing and often contradictory, and their intellectual legacy appears to have been suppressed and to an unknown degree distorted by the post-Vedic orthodoxy. Little wonder that most scholars have shied away from a frontal attack on their problematic nature. The only really comprehensive study is that by the German Yoga researcher Jakob Wilhelm Hauer (1927), who never completed the announced second volume. The importance of the Vrâtyas for the present survey lies in the fact that they were connected with the early evolution of Yoga and were in fact instrumental in the transmission of Yoga-like knowledge.

The single most important text containing perhaps largely authentic Vrâtya wisdom is the *Vrâtya-Khânda* (book 15) of the *Atharva-Veda*. Unfortunately, most of its hymns are scarcely intelligible. Nevertheless, there are a number of well-established points that, when viewed together, result in at least a rough picture of these people. The Vrâtyas were one of the many communities that did not belong to the orthodox kernel of Vedic society but had their own set of customs and values.[65] They roamed the country, mostly the northeast of India, in groups (*vrâta*) united by a vow (also *vrâta*). Some of them apparently traveled on their own and were known as *eka-vrâtyas*, the word *eka* meaning "singular" or "solitary."

In the eyes of their orthodox cousins, who upheld the Vedic sacrificial religion, the Vrâtyas were despicable outcasts who spoke the same tongue by accident and who were fit to become victims in human sacrifice (*purusha-medha*), which may have been enacted literally in the early Vedic period. This is the pervasive attitude in the early *Sûtra* literature, such as the *Grihya-Sûtras* and also the *Dharma-Sûtras* of Âpastamba, Baudhâyana, and Yâjnavalkya. Nevertheless, the Vrâtyas must have been numerous and influential, for later on the orthodox priesthood, the *brâhmanas* (brahmins in English), introduced special rites by which a Vrâtya could be purified and accepted into the mainstream of Vedic society. After their conversion most seem to have settled down and taken up a trade.

The Vrâtyas frequented especially the country of Mâgadha (modern Bihar) in northeastern India—the country of the two great heresies of Buddhism and Jainism, and later also of Tantra. They also appear to have had a vital relationship with the *kshatriya*, or warrior, class that played a substantial role in the formation of early Upanishadic thought. Thus, according to one hymn of the *Atharva-Veda* (15.8), the (deified) solitary Vrâtya was the originator of the warrior (*râjanya*) class. Indeed, kings like Ajâtashatru and the fabulously wealthy Janaka were among the first to promote the teaching of nondualism that is associated with the Vedânta of the *Upanishads*, and it would not be too farfetched to surmise that in many cases they might have been inspired directly by the Vrâtyas. Noteworthy is the case of the mighty King Prithu, who,

> "He stood erect for a year. The Gods said to him: 'Vrâtya, why do you stand?' He said: 'Let them bring me a seat.' They brought a seat for that Vrâtya. Summer and spring were two of its legs, autumn and the rains were [the other] two."
>
> —*Atharva-Veda* 15.3.1-4

according to the *Jaiminîya-Upanishad-Brâhmana*, received instruction about the sacred syllable *om* from the seer Vena, who is called the "divine Vrâtya."

The Vrâtyas apparently traveled in groups of thirty-three, and each group had its own leader. Members were distinguished on the principle of seniority. Some are said to have "quietened the penis"—that is, mastered their sexual drive. The ancient Sanskrit phrase for this accomplishment is *shamanica medhra*, which reminds one of the yogic state of *ûrdhva-retas*; that is, the upward conduction of semen in those who are adepts in celibacy. Interestingly enough, the phrase *ûrdhva-retas* is also employed in conjunction with God Rudra, whom the Vrâtyas worshiped together with Vâyu, the God of Wind and ecstatic flight.

The Vrâtyas wore simple garments, with red or black borders, tied to their loins, and a red turbanlike headdress. They used silver ornaments for neck or breast, wore sandals, and carried a whip and a small bow but no arrows. This and other evidence point to the fact that the Vrâtyas were organized into sacred brotherhoods, perhaps of a military origin. They traveled in primitive carts drawn by a horse and a mule; during their religious ceremonies the carts served as sacrificial altars. Each group was accompanied by a professional bard, known as *mâgadha* or *suta*, and a female called *pumshcalî* ("man-mover"). The bard and the sacred prostitute performed the sexual rite in the great midsummer ceremony, the so-called *mahâ-vrata* ("great vow"), which also involved railing and obscene dialogues. Without question, the bard and the sacred prostitute enacted the creative play between God and Goddess. Anticipating the bipolar metaphysics of later Tantra, the Vrâtyas pictured God Rudra ("Howler" or "Roarer") as being accompanied by a drum-beating female deity reminiscent of the Goddess Kâlî of Hinduism.

This important fertility (agricultural) ritual also included the use of a swing, which was regarded as a "ship bound for heaven." The leader swung on this apparatus while muttering prayers, which included references to the three types of life force that were thought to animate the body—*prâna*, *apâna*, and *vyâna*.

The Vrâtyas were experts in magical matters, and some of their magical lore has survived in the hymns of the *Atharva-Veda*. In view of the unorthodox nature of the Vrâtya beliefs and practices, the Vedic priests did everything to obscure or obliterate as much of the sacred lore of the Vrâtyas as possible, and it is something of a miracle that the *Vrâtya-Khânda* has survived at all.[66]

From the yogic point of view, the most interesting feature of Vrâtya lore is the Vrâtyas' apparent practice of *prânâyâma* and other similar austerities. It is in such practices that we can detect one of the taproots of later Yoga and Tantra. Thus, the *Atharva-Veda* (15.15.2) mentions the Vrâtyas' knowledge of seven *prânas*, seven *apânas*, and seven *vyânas*. These are the various functions of the life force circulating in the body and are related to the breath as it is inhaled, exhaled, and retained. The three sets of seven are analogically linked with a variety of different things as follows:

The seven *prânas* are (1) *agni* or fire, (2) *âditya* or sun, (3) *candramâ* or moon, (4) *pavamâna* or wind, (5) *âp* or "the waters," (6) *pashava* or cattle, and (7) *prajâ* or creatures. The seven *apânas* are (1) *paurnamâsî* or full moon, (2) *ashtakâ* or the day of the moon's quarter, (3) *amâvâsyâ* or the day of the new moon,

(4) *shraddhâ* or faith, (5) *dîkshâ* or consecration, (6) *yajna* or sacrifice, and (7) *dakshinâ* or sacrificial gift. The seven *vyânas* are (1) *bhûmi* or earth, (2) *antariksha* or "mid-region," (3) *dyau* or sky, (4) *nakshatra* or stellar constellations, (5) *ritu* or the seasons, (6) *ârtava* or "that which pertains to the seasons," and (7) *samvatsara* or the year.

Such magical psychocosmic associations are characteristic of the archaic mentality preserved in the *Vedas*.[67] The following extract from the *Atharva-Veda* (15.1) is another typical example of this style of analogical thinking:

[Once] there was a Vrâtya roaming about. He stirred up Prajâpati [Lord of Creatures]. (1)

He, Prajâpati, beheld gold within Himself. He brought it forth. (2)

That [gold] became the One; that became the Forehead-sign-bearer (*lalâma*); that became the Great (*mahat*); that became the Foremost (*jyeshtha*); that became the *brahman*; that became the creative power (*tapas*); that became Truth (*satya*); by this He brought [Himself] forth. (3)

He grew; He became the Great (*mahân*); He became the Great God (*mahâ-deva*). (4)

He surrounded [? *pari* + *ait*] the supremacy of the Gods; He became [their] ruler. (5)

He became the One Vrâtya; He took a bow; that was Indra's bow. (6)

Its belly was blue; red the back. (7)

With the blue [side of the bow] He encompasses hostile clans; with the red [side] He pierces the hateful [enemy]. Thus say the teachers of *brahman*. (8)

It is impossible to make strict rational sense of the above hymn. Its composer moved in a different frame of reality, that of mythopoeic thought rather than linear reasoning. He delighted in mystical equations and analogies, and he was obviously aware of esoteric meanings that we can only dimly intuit.

To summarize, the Vrâtyas were prominent representatives of the countercultural stream in Vedic and early post-Vedic times. A portion of their spiritual heritage was assimilated into the *Atharva-Veda*, perhaps because this hymnody itself has from the beginning had a marginal status within the Vedic revelation. But it is here that we find many formative ideas and practices that much later went into the making of Tantra, carried for centuries by those living at the edge or even completely outside orthodox Hinduism, as upheld by the brahmins. In some respects, the Vrâtyas can be seen as the forerunners of such marginal but significant religio-spiritual groups as the Pâshupatas, which arose in the Epic Age. It is even possible that the Vrâtyas were primarily responsible for the further development of Proto-Yoga in the early Post-Vedic Era

"Verily, this entire [world] is the Absolute (*brahman*). Tranquil, one should worship It [through contemplation], for one comes forth from It."

—*Chândogya-Upanishad* (3.14.1)

# Chapter 5

# THE WHISPERED WISDOM OF THE EARLY UPANISHADS

## I. OVERVIEW

Some historians regard the period from the collapse of the Indus cities (around 1500 B.C.E.) to the time of the Buddha a whole millennium later as the Dark Ages of India. But this designation is as inappropriate here as it is in the European context, for those days were far from decadent or sinister. Rather, they were a time of great cultural adventure in which the Vedic civilization reconfigured itself after what must have been centuries of hardship that necessitated a major relocation from the dried-up Sarasvatî River to the fertile Gangetic planes. More than anything, the expression "Dark Ages" betrays our lack of detailed and accurate historical knowledge for that period. Fortunately, our ignorance about that seminal period is less today than it was even a few years ago.

The bulk of the Vedic hymns was probably completed by the time of King Bharata, after whom India is named. He lived during the *tretâ-yuga*, around fifty generations prior to the five Pândava princes who fought for their patrimony in the great war chronicled in the *Mahâbhârata*. This war occurred perhaps around 1500 B.C.E. This was also the era of Vyâsa, who is traditionally said to have "arranged" not only the *Mahâbhârata* and the *Purânas* but also the four Vedic hymnodies.

By this time much of the inner knowledge of the Vedic *Samhitâs* seems to have been lost, and also the rituals accompanying them had been modified. A period of active interpretation and reinterpretation of the Vedic heritage followed, leading to the creation of the *Brâhmanas*, the *Âranyakas*, and the *Upanishads*—all regarded as an integral part of the sacred revelation—as well as the voluminous *Kalpa-Sûtra* literature to which belong the various *Shrauta-Sûtras*, *Grihya-Sûtras*, *Dharma-Sûtras*, and *Shulba-Sûtras*. The conclusion of this post-Vedic phase roughly coincided with the final drying up of the Sarasvatî River between 2100 and 1900 B.C.E. and the displacement of the center of the Vedic civilization from the Sarasvatî and Indus to the Ganges and its many tributaries.

165

We have seen in the previous chapter that proto-yogic ideas and practices were present both in the sacrificial ritualism of the Vedic priesthood and in the religious world of the nonbrahmanical circles at the fringe of the Vedic society, particularly in the mysterious Vrâtya brotherhoods. As the ritualism of the orthodox priesthood became more sophisticated and exclusive, the lay people increasingly hungered for their own inner relationship to the sacred reality. In ever larger numbers they turned to teachers who offered an emotionally and spiritually more satisfying approach to the Divine. Many of those teachers stood outside the fold of the sacerdotal orthodoxy, as they still do in India today. People continued to consult brahmins for the major sacramental ceremonies, such as birth, marriage, and death, but they also opened their minds and hearts to religious cults in which the Divine was worshiped in personal rather than impersonal terms, and to esoteric schools, such as those of the *Upanishads*, that promised mystical union with the Divine. The post-Vedic Yoga tradition appears to have taken shape largely among these marginal and even "heretical" groups.

## The Brâhmanas

The *Brâhmanas* (c. 2500-1500 B.C.E.) are prose works expounding and systematizing the Vedic sacrificial rituals and their accompanying mythology. They are the creations of the Vedic sacerdotal elite and are thoroughly orthodox in their orientation. Of the numerous *Brâhmanas* that once existed, only a few have survived. The *Rig-Veda* has attached to it the *Aitareya-* and the *Kaushîtaki-* (or *Shânkhâyana*)-*Brâhmana*; the *Sâma-Veda* has the *Panca-Vimsha-* (or *Tândya-*

*Mahâ*)-, the *Shadvimsha-*, the *Chândogya-*, and the *Jaiminîya-* (or *Talavakâra*)-*Brâhmana*; the *Yajur-Veda* has the *Kâthaka-*, the *Taittirîya-*, and the *Shata-Patha-Brâhmana*; and the *Atharva-Veda* has the *Go-Patha-Brâhmana*. In the case of the White (*Shukla*) *Yajur-Veda*, these explanatory works form independent texts, whereas in the case of the Black (*Krishna*) *Yajur-Veda*, they are interwoven with the actual Vedic hymnody. The oldest *Brâhmana* appears to be the *Aitareya-Brâhmana*, which consists of forty chapters and is traditionally attributed to Mahidâsa Aitareya. It deals mainly with the *soma* sacrifice and secondarily with the fire sacrifice (*agni-hotra*) and the royal consecration (*râja-sûya*). In many ways the most fascinating of these texts is the voluminous *Shata-Patha-Brâhmana*, which consists of one hundred chapters and is extant in two recensions—that of the Kânvas and that of the Mâdhyandinas.

In the latter recension of this comparatively late exegetical scripture (c. 1500 B.C.E.), the sages Yâjnavalkya (sections 1-5) and Shândilya (sections 6-14) figure as the principal teachers. Shândilya is particularly associated with the *agni-rahasya* ("fire mystery"), discussed at length in Section 10 (comprising c. 120 pages in English). The mystery is about the construction of the fire altar and its psychocosmic significance. Shândilya affirms a magical correlation between Prajâpati (the Creator), God Agni, the sun, the fire altar, and the year.

The fire altar consists of six layers of bricks and six layers of mortar, which together represent the twelve months. The first layer of bricks is associated with inhalation (*prâna*), the second with exhalation (*apâna*), the third with the diffusive breath (*vyâna*), the fourth with the upward breath (*udâna*), and the fifth with the mid-breath (*samâna*), while the sixth layer is connected with speech (*vâc*). As the fire is lit and the golden flames shoot upward toward the firmament (symbolizing Heaven), the sacrificer, through a process of mystical identification, simultaneously obtains a "golden" body. He becomes the Golden Creator (*hiranmaya-prajâpati*).

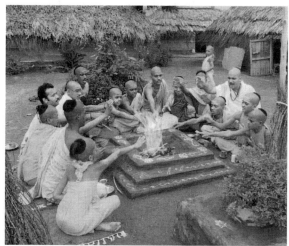

*The Vedic fire altar symbolizes the macrocosm*

The 101 bricks out of which the altar is constructed symbolize the 101 elements or aspects that comprise the sun. Since the fire altar is not only the cosmic body but also the body of the sacrificer, we may look for a somatic correlation of this number. Indeed, the *Brihad-Âranyaka-Upanishad* (4.2.3) provides an answer when it speaks of 101 conduits (*nâdî*) found in the human body, of which only one leads to immortality. That special channel is none other than the central pathway (the so-called *sushumnâ-nâdî*) through which flows, according to later Tantra, the *kundalinî-shakti* from the lowest psychoenergetic center at the base of the spine to the center at the crown of the head. Interestingly, the *Shata-Patha-Brâhmana* (10.2.4.4) speaks in this connection also of the seven celestial realms, which afford a comparison to the seven centers (*cakras*) of some schools of Tantra and Hatha-Yoga.

The *Shata-Patha-Brâhmana* in a way bridges the gap between the strictly ritualistic worldview of the *Brâhmanas* and the symbolic, internalized ritualism of the *Upanishads*. It contains speculations about the world ground, life force (*prâna*), and rebirth—all woven into the general fabric of Vedic sacrificial mysticism. Although Yoga is not mentioned in the *Brâhmana* scriptures, we can see in their ritualism one of the contributing sources of the later Yoga tradition. Thus, the *Shata-Patha-Brâhmana* (9.4.4.1ff.) reveals the details of the mystical process of *agni-yojana* or "yoking the fire [-altar]." Here the sacrificer "controls" the forces connected with the fire altar, that is, utilizes it in a disciplined manner involving great concentration and breath control. The goal is for the sacrificer to rise with the birdlike flames and smoke heavenward. As he pours the *soma* into the flames, the sacrificer "anoints" the fire and, by sipping the *soma* draught, at the same time consecrates himself, thereby becoming immortal. This is definitely a proto-yogic practice.

Similarly, the treatment of the ceremony of *prâna-agni-hotra* (written *prânâgni-hotra*), the "fire sacrifice of the breaths," which consists in the offering of food to the various kinds of breath, shows lines of thought that prepare the ground for the yogic theory and practice of breath control (*prânâyâma*). The *prâna-agni-hotra* is a symbolic substitute for the earlier Vedic fire ritual (*agni-hotra*), the most popular of all rites. In the *prâna-agni-hotra*,[1] the life force takes the place of the ritual fire and is identified with the transcendental Self, the *âtman*. However, this is not yet a full-fledged mental sacrifice, as are yogic meditation or lifelong celibacy, since the *prâna-agni-hotra* was enacted bodily. This important sacrifice was a decisive stepping-stone toward what historians of religion have called the interiorization of sacrifice—the conversion of external rites to inner or mental rites.

## The Âranyakas

The *Âranyakas,* or "forest teachings," which are of a very similar nature to the *Brâhmanas,* were meant as ritual "books" for the orthodox brahmin who retired to the forest (*aranya*) to live in solitude, dedicated to a life of quiet contemplation and mystical rituals. These forest-dwellers—*vâna-prasthas,* as they were later called—are the first step in the increasingly powerful trend in ancient India toward world renunciation (*samnyâsa*). Most of the *Âranyakas* have been lost, but the following are still extant: the *Aitareya-* and the *Kaushîtaki-Âranyaka* (both belonging to the *Rig-Veda*); the *Taittirîya-Âranyaka* (belonging to the Black *Yajur-Veda*); the *Brihad-Âranyaka* (belonging to the White *Yajur-Veda*). No *Âranyakas* for the *Sâma-Veda* and the *Atharva-Veda* are extant. These forest "books," which were deemed too sublime or sacred to be imparted in the villages or towns, prepared the ground for the still more esoteric teachings of the *Upanishads* and also the subsequent Yoga tradition in its more ascetical mode.

## The Dawn of the Upanishadic Age

The nuclei of the oldest *Upanishads*—*Brihad-Âranyaka-*, *Chândogya-*, *Kaushîtaki-*, *Aitareya-*, and *Kena-Upanishad*—appear to date back over three thousand years ago.[2] The Upanishadic sages initiated what was to become an ideological revolution. They internalized the Vedic ritual in the form of intense contemplation, or meditation. This is best illustrated in the following passage from the *Kaushîtaki-Brâhmana-Upanishad* (2.5):

Now next [follows the practice of] self-restraint according to Prâtardana, or the inner fire sacrifice, as they call it. Verily, as long as a person (*purusha*) is speaking, he is unable to breathe. Then he is sacrificing the breath to speech. Verily, as long as a person is breathing, he is unable to speak. Then he is sacrificing the speech to the breath. These are the two unending, immortal oblations. In sleeping and in waking, he sacrifices them continuously. Whatever other oblations there are, they are limited, for they consist in [ritual] actions. Understanding this, the ancestors did not offer the fire sacrifice [literally].

The last line suggests that this symbolic fire sacrifice was practiced already by the predecessors of the composer of this passage, that is, the sages behind the composition of the *Brâhmanas,* and very probably even earlier by the seers of the Vedic *Samhitâs.* But with the *Upanishads,* the symbolic aspect of sacrifice acquired paramount significance. Henceforth the Divine could be worshiped purely with the mind or heart, without external paraphernalia.

Who were these innovative sages? They were a diverse group: Some were prominent brahmins, like the famous Yâjnavalkya, who instructed the nobility; others were less well-known brahmins living in isolation as forest-dwellers; yet others were powerful kings, like Janaka and Ajâtashatru (the ruler of Kashi, modern Benares or Varanasi). What they had in common was a penchant for esoteric wisdom, or what in classical Greece was called *gnosis,* transcendental knowledge that could lift them beyond mundane life, even beyond Vedic ritualism and its promised heavens, to the realization of the unconditional Reality. That Reality they preferred to name *brahman,* the Absolute. The word *brahman* is derived from the verbal root *brih*, meaning "to grow." It denotes the inexhaustible vastness of the supreme Being.

Most significantly, the Upanishadic sages turned unanimously to meditative practice, or inner worship (*upâsana*), as the chief means of obtaining transcendental knowledge. In contrast to this, the meditation practiced by orthodox brahmins continued to be intimately bound up with sacrificial rituals, which, as we have seen, were given supreme status in the ancient Vedic religion. Even the forest-dwelling ascetics continued to adhere to the sacrificial cult of mainstream Vedic society; they merely retired from the hustle and bustle of ordinary life.

The idea that behind the reality of multiple forms—our ever-changing

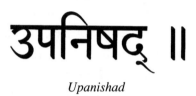

*Upanishad*

universe—there abides an eternally unchanging single Being was communicated already in Rig-Vedic times. What was new was that this grand discovery transcended the legacy of sacrificial ritualism. Understandably, the Upanishadic sages were careful to communicate this insight judiciously—in an esoteric setting requiring proper initiation. This is suggested by the word *upanishad* itself, which means "sitting down near" (*upa* "near," *ni* "down," *shad* "to sit") one's teacher. The Upanishadic teachings were not public knowledge, and those desiring to hear them were expected to approach the sages with proper respect and humility. Unless they came well prepared, they had to submit to years of discipleship before any hidden knowledge was imparted to them. The esoteric wisdom of the *Upanishads* was whispered rather than proclaimed aloud. Today these most precious teachings are made available in paperback books, and we tend to read the *Upanishads* as entertaining

or, at best, inspired and inspiring literature, seldom approaching these ancient teachings with the reverence and integrity they once commanded.

The Upanishadic teachings revolve around four interconnected conceptual pivots: *First*, the ultimate Reality of the universe is absolutely identical with our innermost nature; that is to say, *brahman* equals *âtman*, the Self. *Second*, only the realization of *brahman/âtman* liberates one from suffering and the necessity of birth, life, and death. *Third*, one's thoughts and actions determine one's destiny—the law of karma: You become what you identify with. *Fourth*, unless one is liberated and achieves the formless existence of *brahman/âtman* as a result of higher wisdom (*jnâna*), one is perforce reborn into the godly realms, the human world, or lower (demonic) realms, depending on one's karma.

Many scholars maintain that the doctrine of reincarnation (*punar-janman*, lit. "rebirth") and its corollary doctrine of moral causation (karma) were unknown in early Vedic times and were adopted from the Dravidians. Some researchers alternatively have proposed that the Upanishadic sages themselves discovered the cycle of births and deaths governed by the iron law of karma, rather than borrowed the idea from supposedly native tribes. However, both these views ignore the Vedic evidence, which suggests that already the Rig-Vedic *rishis* believed in reincarnation and karma.

Be that as it may, both esoteric teachings became a prominent feature of Hinduism, Buddhism, Jainism, and Sikhism. Each tradition of course has its own interpretations of how reembodiment works, and how the self-perpetuating mechanism of karma can be outwitted through spiritual practice. Early on, the escape from the round of successive births became a principal motive behind India's spirituality, and we will therefore meet this idea again and again in the remaining chapters of this book.

In the *Vedas*, the doctrine of the transcendental Self is nowhere clearly enunciated, though it is implied in many mystical passages. In the *Brâhmanas* and *Âranyakas*, however, we find amidst much theological speculation about the ritual and its cosmological correspondences the first scattered references to the Self, which is omnipresent. But only in the *Upanishads* is this precious teaching fully articulated.

What is the Self? Sage Yâjnavalkya put it thus in the *Brihad-Âranyaka-Upanishad* (3.4.1):

He who breathes with your inhalation (*prâna*) is your Self (*âtman*), which is in everything. He who breathes with your exhalation (*apâna*) is your Self, which is in everything. He who breathes with your diffusive breath (*vyâna*) is your Self, which is in everything. He who breathes with your up-breath (*udâna*) is your Self, which is in everything. He is your Self, which is in everything.

When asked how that Self is to be conceived, Yâjnavalkya continued:

You cannot see the Seer of seeing. You cannot hear the Hearer of hearing. You cannot think the Thinker of thinking. You cannot understand the Understander of understanding. He is your Self, which is in everything. Everything other than Him is irrelevant. (3.4.2)

---

"This immeasurable constant [Self] must be seen as singular. The Self is taintless, unborn, great, constant, beyond space [and time]."

—*Brihad-Âranyaka-Upanishad* 4.4.20

---

This passage epitomizes the essence of the Upanishadic mystery teachings, which were passed from Self-realized teacher to disciple by word of mouth: The transcendental ground of the world is identical with the ultimate core of the human being. That supreme Reality, which is pure, formless Consciousness, cannot be adequately described or defined. It must simply be *realized*. Upon realization, the Self will be found to be infinite, eternal, utterly real, and free, as well as unqualifiedly blissful (*ânanda*).

How *can* the Self be realized? The Upanishadic sages emphasized the need for world renunciation and intensive contemplation. They dismissed the idea that action (*karman*) can lead to liberation, insisting that only wisdom (*jnâna*) has the power to free us from bondage, because it is of the same nature as the transcendental Self. Yet, surprisingly, the earliest *Upanishads* contain few practical instructions about the art of introspective meditation. This was apparently a matter to be settled between the teachers and their disciples. We know, however, that the spiritual path included extensive service to the teacher and constant discrimination between the Real and the unreal—all sustained by a burning desire for Self-realization and a willingness to transcend the ego.

Despite their radical orientation, the *Upanishads* are considered a continuation of the Vedic revelation. Their teachings, in fact, conclude the Vedic revelation, and hence are known as Vedânta. The term *vedânta* means literally "*Veda's* end." All subsequent teachings, such as the knowledge contained in the *Sûtra* literature, are deemed to be no longer *shruti* or "revelation," but *smriti* or "tradition."

## The Extent of the Upanishadic Literature

Over two hundred *Upanishads* exist, and most of them have been translated into English. The earliest works, as mentioned, were composed almost four millennia ago, whereas the youngest scriptures of this genre belong to our own century. Hindu traditionalists, following the list furnished in the 500-year-old *Muktikâ-Upanishad*, generally recognize 108 *Upanishads*.

The oldest principal *Upanishads* can be arranged in rough chronological order as follows: The first group comprises the *Brihad-Âranyaka-, Chândogya-, Taittirîya-, Kaushîtaki-, Aitareya-, Kena-* (or *Talavakâra-*), and *Mahâ-Nârâyana-Upanishad*. The second group includes the *Katha-, Shvetâshvatara-, Îsha-, Mundaka-, Prashna-, Maitrâyanîya-,* and *Mândûkya-Upanishad*.

The remaining *Upanishads* are generally divided into the following five groups:

1. *Sâmânya-Vedânta-Upanishads,* which expound Vedânta in general;

2. *Samnyâsa-Upanishads,* which elaborate on the ideal of renunciation;

3. *Shâkta-Upanishads,* which disclose teachings related to *shakti,* the feminine aspect of the Divine;

4. *Sectarian Upanishads,* which expound teachings related to specific religious cults and dedicated to such deities as Skanda (God of War), Ganesha (the elephant-headed God who is invoked specifically to remove material or spiritual obstacles), Sûrya (the Sun God), or even Allah (the Moslem Creator-God), etc.;

5. *Yoga-Upanishads,* which explore different aspects of the yogic process, especially Hatha-Yoga. This category includes the *Brahma-Vidyâ-, Amrita-Nâda-Bindu-, Amrita-Bindu-, Nâda-Bindu-, Dhyâna-Bindu-, Tejo-Bindu-, Advaya-Târaka-, Mandala-Brâhmana-, Hamsa-, Mahâ-Vâkya-, Pâshupata-Brahma-, Kshurikâ-, Tri-Shikhi-Brâhmana-, Darshana-, Yoga-Cûdâ-Mani-, Yoga-Tattva-, Yoga-Shikhâ-, Yoga-Kundalî-, Shândilya-,* and *Varâha-Upanishad*. These works, all of which probably belong to the Common Era, are discussed in Chapter 15.

It should be remembered that originally all these texts—the *Vedas, Brâhmanas, Âranyakas,* and *Upanishads,* as well as the *Sûtras*—were not written down at all but memorized and transmitted from teacher to pupil by word of mouth. The Vedic corpus is what has been dubbed a mnemonic literature. To this day there are some brahmins who can recite from memory one or more Vedic *Samhitâs,* or the entire *Mahâbhârata* and *Râmâyana,* each comprising tens of thousands of verses.

While memorization was not deemed a yogic feat in itself, it helped young students acquire a rare degree of concentration that proved useful in their later spiritual work. Besides, in learning the Vedic texts by heart they were constantly exposed to the highest wisdom, which naturally opened them to the spiritual path. Today, immersed as we are in a lopsided materialistic culture, it is sometimes difficult for us to find and maintain a spiritual perspective. Fortunately, the inspired creations of ancient and modern Hindu saints, *yogins*, and sages are readily available to us in book form. We need not abandon home and work to sit at the feet of the great adepts and benefit from their vision of humanity's potential and destiny. Modern technology brings their timeless wisdom and encouragement right to our doorstep. Yet, for some of us, this only serves as preparation for a flesh-and-blood encounter with a living master of Yoga, who can unlock hidden doors in our mind so that we can experience the yogic heritage more directly and profoundly.

## II. THE BRIHAD-ÂRANYAKA-UPANISHAD

The oldest among the earliest *Upanishads* is the *Brihad-Âranyaka-* ("Great Forest") *Upanishad*, in which the meditative path is still closely connected with sacrificial concepts. This scripture begins with a set of instructions about the horse sacrifice (*ashva-medha*) interpreted as a cosmological event. The horse sacrifice was a major ceremony performed in honor of a successful king to ensure the continued prosperity of his rule. For instance, in the fourth century C.E., King Samudragupta staged this lavish ceremony after his conquest of thirteen kingdoms in southern India. On this occasion he minted gold coins depicting on one side the sacrificial horse and on the other side his favorite wife. The proud inscription on this commemorative coin reads:

"After conquering the earth, the great King of Kings with the might of an invincible hero will conquer Heaven." The last-known performance of the horse sacrifice took place in the eighteenth century at Jaipur in Rajasthan.

In the course of the horse sacrifice, the chief sacrificer's wife mimics sexual intercourse with the dead horse just before it is dismembered and cooked. The parallel to the sexual symbolism of Tantra is obvious: Like the Tantric adept during intercourse, the horse does not lose its semen during this symbolic ritual, but the "copulating" woman partakes of the animal's vital energy. In later Hindu Tantra, the yogic God Shiva is often depicted as a corpse, and his spouse Shakti is shown seated on him in a pose of sexual union.

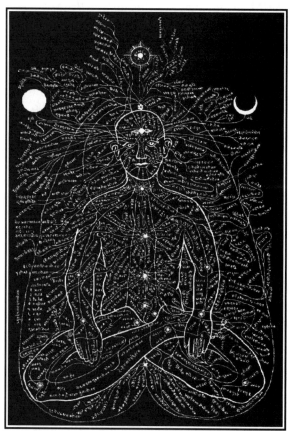

© AUTHOR

*The tree-like nature of the subtle body with its numerous conduits*

Early on, the horse came to signify the sun and, by further symbolic extension, the resplendent transcendental Self. The Self is the ultimate source of all life and yet, because of its transcendental nature, is more appropriately understood as passive (like a corpse) rather than active. It is the Self's power or *shakti* aspect, in the form of the life force animating the human personality and consciousness, that creates access to the Self. In the *Brihad-Âranyaka-Upanishad*, these symbolic associations are vaguely hinted at.

For instance, we find speculations about the origin of the world born from the Singular Being that split itself into two—male and female—thus creating the entire cosmos. Linked with this cosmogonic notion is a fundamental ethical conviction which is characteristic of the subsequent psychotechnology of liberation: Because there is essentially only the One, it is a heinous sin to cling to the multiple objects of the universe. This One is described as the true goal of humanity. Yâjnavalkya, the most outstanding figure of the early Upanishadic period, is credited with these stanzas:

As a tree, or lord of the forest,
just so, truly, is man (*purusha*):
his hairs are leaves,
his skin the outer bark.

Verily, from his skin flows blood,
as sap from the bark.
Therefore, when the skin is torn,
blood issues from him,
as does sap from a wounded tree.

His flesh is the inner bark,
the tendons the inner layer, which is
    tough.
Beneath are the bones, as is the wood.
The marrow is comparable to the pith

[of the tree].

If a tree, when felled, grows again
from its root into another,
from what root grows the mortal
    [person],
after he has been felled by death?

Do not claim, "From the seed,"
for that is generated in the living.
A tree grows indeed from seed.
After it has died, it springs forth [again].

If, however, the tree is destroyed with its
    roots,
it does not spring forth again.
From what root does the mortal grow
when he has been felled by death?

He is simply born [and then dies, you
    may argue].
No, [I say]. He is born again. Born by
    what?
The conscious, blissful Absolute (*brahman*),
the Principle of grace, the Refuge of him
    who knows
and abides in It. (3.9.28.1-7)

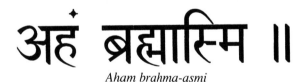

*Aham brahma-asmi*

In this marvelous passage of the *Brihad-Âranyaka-Upanishad* is intimated the higher knowledge of the mystic and *yogin*, who knows the one indivisible Ground of Being and who, like Yâjnavalkya, confidently declares: *Aham brahma-asmi* (written *aham brahmâsmi*), "I am the Absolute." The last stanza contains the key to the whole metaphor: The human "tree" is born again and again, by force of his karma, as is made clear in other passages. It is this repeated drama of birth, life, and death that, to the sensitive psyche of the *yogin*, is only pain (*duhkha*). This cycle is imaged most potently in another passage of the same scripture:

> Just as a leech when it has reached the end of a blade of grass draws itself together before making a further approach [to a different blade], so this Self, after having cast off the body and dispelled ignorance, draws itself together before making another approach [to a new body]. (4.4.3)

Clearly, there is no solace in this cycle (*samsâra*); hence, the Upanishadic sages taught the esoteric means by which the world of change can be transcended. Elsewhere in the same scripture, Yâjnavalkya proclaims:

> I have touched and found the narrow ancient path that stretches far afar. By it the wise, the knowers of the Absolute, go up to the heavenly world and are released. (4.4.8)

> He who has found and awakened to the Self that has entered this perilous and inaccessible [body-mind] is the Creator of the world, for he is the Maker of all. The world is his. He is indeed the world. (4.4.13)

> When one perceives directly the bright (*deva*) Self, the Ruler of what has become and what will be, then one does not recoil [from It anymore]. (4.4.15)

Those who know the Life (*prâna*) of life, the Eye of the eye, the Ear of the ear, the Mind of the mind, have realized the ancient, primeval Absolute. (4.4.18)

> It is to be seen by the mind alone. There is no difference in It whatsoever. He who sees difference in It reaps death after death. (4.4.19)

> It should be seen as single, immeasurable, perpetual. The Self is spotless, birthless, great, perpetual, and beyond [the subtle element of] the ether (*âkâsha*). (4.4.20)

Liberation, which is identical to immortality, is the realization of the Self in its immutable purity. This realization coincides with the transcendence of the limited mechanisms of the human body-mind and thus of conditional existence itself. What is more, Self-realization is the hidden program of the universe—what transpersonal psychologist Ken Wilber called the "Atman project." Again it is Yâjnavalkya who illustrates this point in a striking image:

> As the ocean is the single locus of all waters, as the skin is the single locus of all touch, as the nostrils are the single locus of all smells, as the tongue is the single locus of all tastes, as the eye is the single locus of all forms, as the ear is the single locus of all sounds, as the mind is the single locus of all volitions (*samkalpa*), as the heart is the single locus of all knowledge, as the hands are the single locus of all acts, as the genitals are the single locus of all pleasure (*ânanda*), as the feet are the single

locus of all movement, as speech is the single locus of all the *Vedas*—so is this [Self].

As a lump of salt, when thrown in water, dissolves in water, and no one can perceive it, because from wherever one takes it, it tastes salty—thus, my dear, this great, endless, transcendental Being is only a Mass of Consciousness (*vijnâna-ghâna*). (2.4.11-12)

Since the Self, or the Absolute, is all there is, It cannot be an object of knowledge. Therefore Yâjnavalkya argues that, ultimately, all descriptions of It are mere words. He responds to all positive characterizations of the Self by exclaiming "not thus, not thus" (*neti-neti*). This famous procedure of negation is fundamental to Vedânta spirituality: *Yogins* of this tradition are asked to constantly remind themselves of the fact that all the states and expressions of their body-mind are, in themselves, other than the transcendental Reality. No experience amounts to Self-realization. The body, as it is ordinarily experienced, is not the Self; nor are thoughts or feelings as they normally present themselves. The Self is nothing that could be pointed to in the finite world. This perpetual vigilant discernment is called *viveka*, which literally means "separating out."

Through steady application to this practice of discernment, *yogins* develop an inner sensitivity both to what is ephemeral in their nature and to the underlying eternal Ground of all their experiences. This awakens in them the will to renounce everything that they have identified as belonging to the world of change. Discernment and renunciation finally lead to the discovery of the universal Self, the *âtman*, beyond all concepts and imagery, beyond all change.

## III. THE CHÂNDOGYA-UPANISHAD

Another archaic *Upanishad* is the *Chândogya*, whose name derives from the words *chandas* or "hymn" (lit. "pleasure") and *ga* or "going," here referring to those brahmins who sang the hymns of the *Sâma-Veda* during the sacrificial ritual in Vedic times. Thus the *Chândogya-Upanishad* consists of the esoteric teachings of the *chândogas*, the Vedic chanters.

It is therefore not surprising that this scripture commences with elaborate mystical speculations about the sacred syllable *om*, the most celebrated numinous sound, or *mantra*, of Hinduism. In 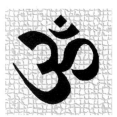 his commentary on this work, Shankara, the great propounder of Vedântic nondualism, observes that this syllable is the most appropriate name of the Divine, or transcendental Reality.

The syllable *om* has a long history that stretches back to Vedic times. It was used at the beginning and end of ritual pronouncements, just as the Christians use the word *amen*. Like all other words in the *Vedas*, *om* is regarded as divine revelation. The *yogins* of later periods have described how, in deep states of meditation, they can hear the sound *om* vibrating through the entire cosmos. This has a parallel in Pythagorean and Neoplatonic thought in the notion of the Music of the Spheres, the cosmic harmonic generated by the motion of the heavenly bodies.

In the third chapter of the *Chândogya-Upanishad*, the sacred *gâyatrî-mantra* (which to this day is recited by all pious Hindus during the morning ritual) is introduced. The text of this ancient *mantra*, which stems from the *Rig-Veda* (3.62.10), runs as follows: *Om tat savitur varenyam bhargo devasya dhîmahi dhiyo yo nah pracodayât*, or "Om. Let us contemplate that

तत् सवितुर् वरेण्यं
भर्गो देवस्य धीमहि
धियो यो नः प्रचोदयात् ॥

*The gâyatrî-mantra*

celestial splendor of God Savitri, so that He may inspire our visions." Savitri ("Stimulator") is the personification of the quickening aspect of the Vedic solar deity, Sûrya, who embodies the luminous ultimate Reality and the principle of spiritual illumination.

This chapter also contains a section (3.17) that speaks of Krishna, "son of Devakî," who is identified by some scholars as the Krishna of the *Mahâbhârata* epic. Given the new dating of the *Upanishads*, this identification now has greater credibility. Significantly, another passage (3.17.6) introduces Ghora, "son of Angiras" (after whom the *Atharva-Veda* was also named *Angirasa-Samhitâ*), as the teacher of Krishna. Here a teaching is mentioned according to which one should repeat, at the hour of death, three specific *mantras* from the *Yajur-Veda*: "You are the Undecaying! You are the Unchanging! You are the very essence of life!" This doctrine curiously resembles the teaching in Lord Krishna's *Bhagavad-Gîtâ* (8.5-6) according to which a person's final thought should be of the Divine rather than any mundane concerns, for whatever one thinks, one becomes.

In Chapter 3 we also learn that, according to Ghora, austerity (*tapas*), charity (*dâna*), rectitude (*ârjava*), nonharming (*ahimsâ*), and truthfulness (*satya*) are to be thought of as the sacrificial gift (*dakshinâ*) given to the officiating priest. In other words, it is one's way of life that is the best recompense for what one has received from one's

teachers. This notion is connected with the idea, expressed in a different passage (3.15.1), that a person—so long as he or she is a spiritual practitioner—*is* a sacrifice. In contemporary language, such a person is called a self-transcender.

The disciplines mentioned by Ghora may be understood as components of the early Upanishadic Yoga, and indeed some of them recur in the later *Yoga-Upanishads* as regular aspects of spiritual practice. Sage Ghora affords a direct link between Krishna and the tradition of the *Atharva-Veda*, and this is further strengthened by the fact that in the *Bhagavad-Gîtâ* (10.25), which is Krishna's song of instruction to Arjuna, the divine Lord exclaims that "of the great seers I am Bhrigu." The fire priest Bhrigu, founder of the Bhârgava lineage, was one of the leading lights of the Atharva tradition.

In another chapter of the *Chândogya-Upanishad*, the intriguing honey doctrine (*madhu-vidyâ*) is mentioned.

> Verily, yonder sun is the honey of the Gods. The sky is its cross-beam. The mid-region is the honeycomb. The particles of light are the brood. (3.1.1)

This peculiar esoteric psychocosmological teaching, alluded to already in the *Rig-Veda* and the *Atharva-Veda*, compares the world to a bee hive. It is clear from the phrase "honey of the Gods" that this passage should be understood metaphorically. Moreover, in another passage (3.5.1), where the upward rays are spoken of, the Absolute (*brahman*) is said to be the flower from which the honey is gathered and which drips with nectar. As we read elsewhere (3.6.3), "He who thus knows this nectar (*amrita*) . . . becomes content."

Honey (*madhu*), then, stands for the nectar of immortality, which in Tantric Yoga is thought to be secreted within the body itself. The *Chândogya-Upanishad* cryptically speaks of five kinds of nectar, which may be levels of spiritual realization. Five nectars are also known in later Tantra, which perhaps is no coincidence. Ultimately, this *Upanishad* declares (3.11.1), the knower of the Absolute "neither rises nor sets but remains alone in the center."

The same chapter (3.13) includes an exposition of the different forms of the life force (*prâna*), which are called the "divine openings" (*deva-sushi*) of the heart, the "brahmic men," and the "doorkeepers of the heavenly world." They are the gateway to the Absolute that is seated in the heart of all beings. This notion continues the speculations found already in the *Vedas* and suggests a developing knowledge of the yogic practice of breath control (*prânâyâma*).

## IV. THE TAITTIRÎYA-UPANISHAD

Third among the oldest *Upanishads* is the *Taittirîya*, which stands in the tradition of the *Yajur-Veda*, the Vedic hymnody containing the sacrificial formulas. The esoteric teachings of the *Taittirîya-Upanishad* go back to the teacher Tittiri, founder of the Taittirîya school, whose name means "partridge." The contents of this scripture are similar to that of the *Chândogya-Upanishad*. It emphasizes the mystical implications of the Vedic chants and sacrificial rituals. Of its three chapters, only the second and the third are of particular interest to the student of Yoga history.

Probably the most fascinating teaching of the *Taittirîya-Upanishad* is the doctrine, received and transmitted by Bhrigu, that everything is to be looked upon as food (*anna*). This is an early ecological idea, referring to the interlinkage of all things—the chain of life—which anticipates contemporary Eco-Yoga.[3] In the words of the *Upanishad*:

> From food, verily, creatures are produced—whatsoever [creatures] dwell on earth. Moreover, by food, in truth, they live, and into it they finally pass. (2.21)

This extends the notion, mentioned earlier, of the sacrificial nature of human existence to all forms of life. There is nothing dreadful about this thought, for, in the final analysis, life is deemed blissful. This is a most important discovery: that the Absolute is not a dry, desertlike environment but supraconscious bliss beyond description. The *Taittirîya-Upanishad* teaches that there are degrees of bliss, extending from the simple joy or pleasure of a prosperous human life to the delight on higher levels of existence (such as the realms of the Gods and forefathers), up to the immeasurable bliss of the Absolute itself—an idea that was later explored in Tantra.

> He who knows this, on departing from this world, proceeds to the self consisting of food, proceeds to the self consisting of life force, proceeds to the self consisting of mind, proceeds to the self consisting of consciousness, proceeds to the self consisting of bliss.

On this there is the following stanza:

> He who knows wherefrom words recoil
> together with the mind,
> without attaining the bliss of the Absolute,
> fears nothing at all. (2.8-9)

This passage hints at a teaching of considerable importance in later Vedânta, namely the doctrine of the five sheaths (*panca-kosha*):

1. The *anna-maya-kosha*, or sheath composed of food; that is, of material elements: the physical body.

2. The *prâna-maya-kosha*, or sheath composed of life force: the etheric body in Western occult literature.

3. The *mano-maya-kosha*, or sheath composed of mind: The ancients considered the mind (*manas*) as an envelope surrounding the physical and the etheric body.

4. The *vijnâna-maya-kosha*, or sheath composed of understanding: The mind simply coordinates the sensory input, but understanding (*vijnâna*) is a higher cognitive function.

5. The *ânanda-maya-kosha*, or sheath composed of bliss: This is that dimension of human existence through which we partake of the Absolute. In later Vedânta, however, the Absolute is thought to transcend all five sheaths.

Reaching the pinnacle of spiritual life, the sage realizes his essential oneness with the blissful transcendental Being. In his ecstasy he triumphantly proclaims:

> Oh, wonderful! Oh, wonderful! Oh, wonderful!
> I am Food! I am Food! I am Food!
> I am the Food-Eater! I am the Food-Eater! I am the Food-Eater!

I am the Maker of Poetry (*shloka*)![4]
I am the Maker of Poetry! I am the Maker of Poetry!
I am the first-born of the cosmic Order (*rita*),
prior to the Gods, [residing] in the hub of immortality!
He who gives Me [as food], he indeed has preserved Me!
I, who am Food, eat the Eater of Food!
I have overcome the whole world!
[My] effulgence is like the sun. (3.10.6-7)

The *Taittirîya-Upanishad* has preserved many archaic teachings that were part of the cultural background of those adepts who crafted the early yogic technology. It is also in this scripture (2.4.1) that we find the very first unequivocal occurrence of the word *yoga* in the technical sense, apparently standing for the sage's control of the fickle senses. However, it would take many more centuries for the Yoga tradition to fully emerge and to assume its place alongside the other paths of liberation within Hinduism.

## V. OTHER ANCIENT UPANISHADS

### The Aitareya-Upanishad

Of the three remaining *Upanishads* of the early period, the relatively short *Aitareya* is of interest because of its archaic cosmogonic material. This work, which is named after an ancient teacher, opens with a myth also found at the beginning of the *Brihad-Âranyaka-Upanishad*: "In the beginning"—that is, before the emergence of space-time—the single Self (*âtman*) decided to create, out of itself, the universe. First it created the material elements; then it created various functions (called *devas*, "divinities"), such as hearing and sight, which joined with the human form. Next the Self created food for all creatures.

As the final act of the process of world creation, the Self enters the human body through the sagittal suture (*sîman*), also known as the "cleft" (*vidriti*) and the "delighting" (*nandana*). This is the location of the *sahasrâra-cakra*, as specified in the Tantric literature. According to later teachings, the *yogin* must consciously exit through that same opening at the crown of the head at the time of death. It is quite possible that this practice was known long before the time of the *Bhagavad-Gîtâ* (8.10), in which it is hinted at.

## The Kaushîtaki-Upanishad

This scripture, titled after the old brahmin family Kaushîtaki in which it was handed down, contains a valuable detailed exposition of the doctrine of rebirth and a description of the path to the "world of the Absolute," or *brahma-loka*.[5] It also includes a long discourse on the life force as being identical with the Absolute. One passage reads as follows:

> Life is *prâna*, *prâna* is life. So long as *prâna* remains in this body, so long is there life. Through *prâna*, one obtains, even in this world, immortality. (3.2)

In a subsequent section (3.3), *prâna* is equated with consciousness (*prajnâ*). It is by means of consciousness that a person acquires true resolve (*satya-samkalpa*), the whole-body desire to transcend the finite world and thence achieve immortality. Thus, through the cultivation of the conscious life force, the sage attains the universal *prâna*, which is immortal and utterly joyous.

In the fourth chapter of the *Kaushîtaki*, we encounter the widely traveled sage Gârgya Bâlâki proudly instructing the famous king Ajâtashatru in the mystery of the *Vedas*. However, Gârgya Bâlâki's wisdom does not satisfy Ajâtashatru, who promptly proceeds to initiate the mendicant in the secret of the universal *prâna*, or life, which is consciousness and which can be known only by those who are pure in spirit. The Self, declared the king, has entered the body from head to toes and is resident in it "like a razor lies concealed in its case." This is one of a number of instances in which a member of the warrior estate instructs a brahmin.

## The Kena-Upanishad

Another archaic *Upanishad* is the *Talavakâra-* or *Kena-Upanishad*, which received its title from the opening phrase *kena*, meaning "by whom?" It starts with the question of who sent forth mind, speech, sight, and so on, thus asking for the cause of our outer-directed consciousness. To be able to answer this question, one must apperceive, as the *Upanishad* insists, the underlying unitary substratum of all experience, which is the transcendental Self (*âtman*). That which is responsible for our externalized awareness is the same Reality that is also responsible for the objects of that awareness. The transcendental Subject is the matrix of both the conditioned consciousness and the objective world.

## The Mahâ-Nârâyana-Upanishad

Although this *Upanishad* dedicated to the Divine in the form of Nârâyana (i.e., Vishnu) has often been branded as a late text containing deliberate archaisms, this scholarly judgment has

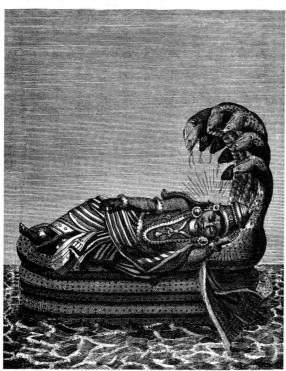

*Reproduced from* Hindu Religion, Customs and Manners

*Vishnu as Nârâyana*

been far too severe. Like other parts of the sacred canon, this *Upanishad* contains later additions or interpolations, such as the verses mentioning Pashupati, Umâ, Lakshmî, Nara-Simha, the Varâha ("Boar") incarnation of Krishna, Sadâ-Shiva, Vedânta, or *shiva-linga*. Unless we find better reasons to the contrary, however, we must count it among the earlier works of this genre standing midway between the old prose *Upanishads* and the later metric texts.

The *Mahâ-Nârâyana-Upanishad*, which belongs to the *Krishna-Yajur-Veda*, is something of a compendium of Vedic mythology and sacrificial ritual. The German indologist Jakob Wilhelm Hauer proposed that this texts consists of an older and a younger part, with the former containing archaic material about Rudra-Shiva and Nârâyana.[6] It appears that subsequently the teachings were incorporated into a more orthodox brahmanical tradition focusing on Brahma and the ideal of renunciation (*nyâsa* = *samnyâsa*),

which is praised as the highest means of realizing the Absolute (see 79.13). Thus, we really have three traditions present in this scripture: Rudra-Shaivism, Nârâyana-Vaishnavism, and Brahmanism. It is curious that despite the prominence of Rudra-Shiva ideas in the *Mahâ-Nârâyana-Upanishad*, the title of this scripture claims primacy for the Vaishnava tradition.

The text, incidentally, shares several verses with the *Shvetâshvatara-Upanishad*, which also draws on the ancient Vedic Rudra-Shiva tradition, one of the evolutionary lines in the development of Proto-Yoga. The *Mahâ-Nârâyana-Upanishad* (24.1) contains the following powerful invocation to God Rudra:

> All is verily Rudra. Let there be salutation to that Rudra. Rudra verily is the [supreme] Person (*purusha*), the glory (*mahas*) of existence. Salutation, salutation! The material universe, the manifold world, and whatever has been variously created or is being created—all that is indeed Rudra. Let there be salutation to that Rudra.

## VI. THE EARLY YOGA UPANISHADS

### The Katha-Upanishad

The *Katha-* or *Kathaka-Upanishad*, which is named after an ancient Vedic school associated with the Black *Yajur-Veda*, is widely held to be the oldest *Upanishad* that deals explicitly with Yoga. It is commonly assigned to the fourth or fifth century B.C.E., which in light of our revised chronology is too late. There is nothing in this work to conclusively suggest that it belongs to the post-Buddhist era. It could just as well have been composed in 1000 B.C.E.

This text develops its novel yogic doctrines around an old legend: A poor brahmin once offered a few old and feeble cows as a sacrificial fee to the priests. His son Naciketas, concerned about his father's afterlife, offered himself as a more appropriate reward. This roused the anger of his father, who sent him to Yama, the ruler of the after-death world. But Yama was temporarily absent, and Naciketas had to wait for three full days without food before the mighty God returned to his abode. Pleased with the boy's patience, Yama granted him three boons.

As his first gift the quick-witted young boy asked to be returned to his father alive. For his second boon he desired to know the secret of the sacrificial fire that leads to heaven. For his third boon he insisted on knowing the mystery of life after death. Yama tried to talk the boy out of the third boon, offering him all kinds of enticing substitutes—sons and grandsons, a long life, and large herds of cattle. When he failed to deter Naciketas, he proceeded to instruct him in the path to emancipation. On one level, the story is meant to portray the death-defying determination that spiritual practitioners must bring to their discipline. On another level, it depicts the initiatic process, which calls for seclusion, fasting, and confrontation with death.

# अध्यात्मयोग ॥

*Adhyâtma-yoga*

The doctrine propounded in the *Katha-Upanishad* is called *adhyâtma-yoga*, the "Yoga of the deep Self."[7] Its target is the Supreme Being, which lies hidden in the "cave" of the human heart:

The sage (*dhîra*) relinquishes joy and sorrow realizing, by means of the Yoga

of the deep Self (*adhyâtman*), the God (*deva*) who is difficult to see, hidden, immanent, stationed in the cave [of the heart], dwelling in the deep, the primordial (*purâna*). (1.2.12)

This Self (*âtman*) cannot be attained through study, nor by thought, nor by much learning. It is attained by the one whom it chooses. This Self reveals its own form. (1.2.23)

Here it is stated that the Self is not an object like other objects we can experience or analyze. It is in fact the transcendental Subject of everything. Thus there is really nothing anyone can do to acquire the Self. On the contrary, Self-realization is dependent on grace. As the *Katha-Upanishad* has it, the Self is "attained by whosoever It chooses." It is clear from the context, however, that there is something the spiritual aspirant can do: He or she can and must undergo the necessary preparation for the event of grace.

In the third chapter of this text, the anonymous composer explains that the Self is at the top of a hierarchy of levels of existence. He employs the following metaphor:

Know that the Self is the charioteer, and the body is the chariot. Know further that the wisdom faculty (*buddhi*) is the driver, whereas the mind (*manas*) is the reins.

The senses, they say, are the horses, and the sense objects are their arena. The sages call that [Self] the enjoyer (*bhoktri*) when united with the body (*âtman*), the senses, and the mind.

He whose mind is constantly unyoked, lacking in understanding—his senses are uncontrollable like the unruly horses of a driver.

But he whose mind is always yoked—his senses are controllable like the obedient horses of a driver.

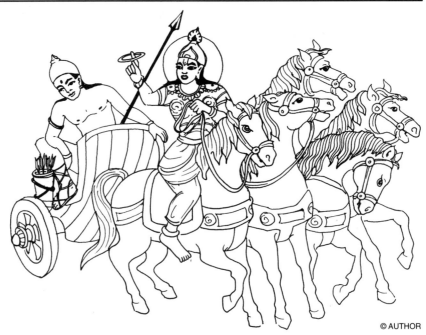

© AUTHOR

*The classic dialogue between Krishna and Arjuna occurred in a chariot*

And he who is devoid of understanding, mindless (*amanaska*), and always impure—he never attains that [lofty] goal but moves around in the cycle [of repeated births and deaths].

But he who understands, always with a pure mind, verily reaches that goal whence one is not born again.

The man who has understanding as his driver, with the mind as his [well-controlled] reins—he reaches the end of the journey, [which is] Vishnu's supreme Abode. (1.3.3-9)

The *Katha-Upanishad* understands spiritual practice as a progressive involution or retracing in consciousness, in reverse order, of the stages of the evolutionary unfolding of the world. The text distinguishes seven stages or levels that make up the Chain of Being:

1. the senses (*indriya*)
2. the sense objects (*vishaya*)
3. the lower mind (*manas*)
4. the higher mind or wisdom faculty (*buddhi*)
5. the "great self" (*mahâ-âtman*, written *mahâtman*), or "great one" (*mahat*), a kind of collective entity composed of the individuated selves
6. the Unmanifest (*avyakta*), which is the transcendental ground of Nature (*prakriti*)
7. the Self (*purusha*), the true Identity of the human being.

Only the Self is eternally beyond the dynamics of Nature in its manifest and unmanifest dimensions. Such ontological schemes, or models of the diverse modes of existence, are characteristic of the classical Sâmkhya school of Îshvara Krishna and also of the earlier Sâmkhya-Yoga schools. They were never intended as mere philosophical speculations, but they served as maps for the yogic process of involution, the climbing of consciousness to ever higher levels of being, terminating with the omnipresent Being, the Self itself.

It is the *purusha* that is the goal of the *yogin*'s psychospiritual work. But that sacred work, or self-transformative alchemy, begins very humbly with the control of the outward-going tendency of the mind. This is clear from the definition of Yoga furnished in the second chapter of this scripture, which appears to be a self-contained unit:

> This they consider to be Yoga: the steady holding (*dhârana*) of the senses. Then one becomes attentive (*apramatta*); for, Yoga can be acquired and lost. (2.3.11)

In other words, Yoga means the condition of inner stability or equilibrium that depends on one's fixity of attention. When the mind is stabilized, then one can begin to discover the wonders of the inner world, the vast horizons of consciousness. But, ultimately, as we have seen, even this exploration of inner space does not lead to liberation. It is merely a precondition for the event of grace—when the light of the transcendental Self shines through into the finite body-mind.

The teachings of the *Katha-Upanishad* represent an important breakthrough in the tradition of Yoga. In beautiful poetic form, we find expressed some of the fundamental ideas underlying all yogic practice. Better than any other scripture, this work marks the transition between the post-Vedic esotericism of the earliest *Upanishads* and the Pre-Classical Yoga of the Epic Age. With this work, Yoga became a recognizable tradition in its own right.

## The Shvetâshvatara-Upanishad

The metric *Shvetâshvatara-Upanishad*, which is appraised to be one of the more beautiful creations of this genre, is generally placed in the third or fourth century B.C.E., which seems too late. In style and content it is similar to the *Bhagavad-Gîtâ*, which belongs to the time of the Buddha. It presumably gets its mysterious name from the sage who composed it. The compound *shvetâshvatara* consists of *shveta* (white"), *ashva* ("horse"), and the superlative *tara*, and it means literally "whitest horse." According to Shankara, who wrote a learned commentary on this scripture in the early ninth (or eighth) century C.E., this is not the name but the title of a sage. He explained that *ashva* also has an esoteric significance and that in initiatic circles the term refers to the senses. Thus, the title *shveta-ashvatara* is given to someone whose senses are completely purified and under control.

Ordinarily we are at the mercy of our senses. We make this discovery quickly when we learn to meditate. At first, every sound or movement interferes with our concentration, and almost against our will we follow after every sensation that enters into our awareness. Only very gradually do we learn to disregard the input from our senses. Then we still have the overactive mind to deal with, which constantly generates thoughts. The schools of Pre-Classical Yoga and Sâmkhya regard the mind (*manas*) as a sixth sensory instrument or capacity (*indriya*). In effect, it is the relay station of the senses, where the input from the five sense organs is gathered and then forwarded to the higher mind, called *buddhi*, for further processing.

The anonymous author of the *Shvetâshvatara-Upanishad* was manifestly an adept of sensory inhibition and meditation. In his work, which is clearly informed by rich yogic experience, he expounds a Yoga that is characteristic of the panentheistic teachings of the Epic Age. The Greek-derived term "panentheism" refers to the metaphysics that sees all (*pan*) of Nature as arising in (*en*) the Divine (*theos*). In distinction to this, the better-known term "pantheism" denotes the philosophical position that simply equates Nature with God. That metaphysical equation is implicitly rejected by the sage composer of the *Shvetâshvatara-Upanishad*, who hails the Lord (*îsha, îshvara*) as dwelling eternally above his own creation.

> Following the Yoga of meditation (*dhyâna*), they perceived the self-power (*âtma-shakti*) of God (*deva*) hidden by His own qualities. He is the One who presides over all the causes connected with time and the [individuated] self (*âtman*). (1.3)

> The Lord (*îsha*) supports this universe, composed of the perishable and the imperishable, the manifest and the unmanifest. The [individuated] self, [which is] not the Lord, is bound by [its wrong notion of] being the enjoyer. But on knowing God, it is released from all fetters. (1.8)

> The foundation (*pradhâna*) [*i.e.*, Nature] is perishable. Hara [*i.e.*, God Shiva] is immortal and imperishable. The one God rules over the perishable [Nature] and the [individuated] selves. By meditating on Him, by uniting with and becoming the Real (*tattva*), there is finally the cessation of all trickery (*mâyâ*). (1.10)

> By knowing God, the falling away of all fetters [is accomplished]. Upon the waning of the afflictions (*klesha*) [*i.e.*, spiritual ignorance and its products], the falling away of birth and death [is likewise accomplished]. By meditating

on Him, there is a third [state], universal lordship, upon separating from the body. [Thus, the *yogin* becomes] the solitary (*kevala*) [Self], whose desires are satisfied. (1.11)

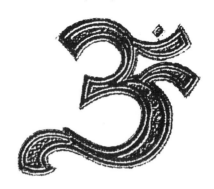

The *Shvetâshvatara-Upanishad* recommends meditation by means of the recitation of the sacred syllable *om*, called the *pranava*. The meditative process is described as a kind of churning by which the inner fire is kindled, leading to the revelation of the Self's splendor. The instructions imply knowledge of breath control (*prânâyâma*). On a more elementary level, advice is given about correct meditation posture, which should be straight, undoubtedly in order to allow the free circulation of the bodily energies. When the vital forces (*prâna*) in the body have quieted down, conscious breathing should begin as a prelude to mental concentration. This scripture even pays attention to the right environmental conditions, recommending that one should engage in Yoga practice in quiet caves and other pure places.

When the mind is stilled, all kinds of internal visions can appear, which must not be confused with God-realization. Among the first signs of successful Yoga practice are said (2.13) to be lightness, health, steadiness, clearness of complexion, pleasantness of voice, agreeable odor, and scanty excretions. This suggests, as the text claims (2.12), the transmutation of the body into a body "fashioned out of the fire of Yoga"

(*yoga-agni-mayam sharîram*). But the supreme goal of this Yoga is not any mystical vision but the realization of the transcendental Self, which releases one from all fetters. That realization is not a mere visionary state. It is not even an experience, for experience presupposes an experiencing subject and an experienced object. Rather, enlightenment or liberation is that condition of being in which the gulf between subject (mind) and object (matter) no longer exists. It is the immortal state.

The *Shvetâshvatara-Upanishad* records the following confession of its author:

> I know that great Self (*purusha*) who is effulgent like the sun beyond darkness. Realizing Him alone, one passes beyond death. There is no other way for passing [beyond the cycle of repeated births and deaths]. (3.8)

The great Being whom the wise author honors is Shiva. As on the path outlined in the *Bhagavad-Gîtâ*, where Vishnu is celebrated as the Lord of all, the *yogin* is not merely a dry ascetic but a devotee (*bhakta*), and the process of

> "May Rudra, the source and origin of the deities, the ruler of all, the great seer who watched the Golden Germ being born [at the beginning of time], endow us with auspicious wisdom."
>
> —*Shvetâshvatara-Upanishad* (4.12)

spiritual maturation and ultimate liberation is not a mechanical event but a mystery dependent on divine grace (*prasâda*). Perhaps the *Shvetâshvatara-Upanishad* was for the early Shiva worshipers what the *Bhagavad-Gîtâ* was and still is for the Vaishnava community—a sacred work of adoration of the Divine, edification of the heart, and instruction in the art of spiritual practice.

The ancient Upanishadic sages were not alone in their mystical intuitions. The era they lived in was a time of great cultural ferment, in which the warrior estate had an important part in the dissemination of wisdom. The Upanishadic sages simply gave expression to a widespread impetus for metaphysical thought and mystical experience within post-Vedic society. There were many other non-Vedic thinkers and visionaries, as well as mystics and seers who had either broken away from the Vedic mainstream more severely than the Upanishadic sages or had never been part of it. Among these radicals were Vardhamâna Mahâvîra and Gautama the Buddha. Their "heretical" teachings form the substance of the next two chapters.

"When the monk understands that he is alone . . . in the same way he should understand that the Self is likewise alone."

—*Âcâra-Anga-Sûtra*[1] 1.8.6.1

# Chapter 6
# JAINA YOGA: THE TEACHINGS OF THE VICTORIOUS FORD-MAKERS

## I. HISTORICAL OVERVIEW

The preceding chapters have outlined the gradual evolution of Hindu spirituality from the time of the *Vedas* to the emergence of the secret teachings of the first *Upanishads*. With this chapter, we interrupt our historical survey of early yogic psychotechnology within the fold of Hinduism. Here we will briefly consider a rival teaching—the great religio-spiritual tradition of Jainism.

Unlike Buddhism, Jainism has generally been looked upon by the Hindus as an offshoot of Hinduism, even a Hindu sect, rather than an independent competing tradition. There are in fact numerous parallels between the two traditions, but the fact that the Jainas form a nonthreatening minority group of little more than three million people also is significant. Of course, there also have been dark moments in the history of the interrelation between Jainas and Hindus, when the latter failed to practice the tolerance for which they are known.

Together with Hinduism and Buddhism, Jainism is one of the three major socioreligious movements to which India's spiritual genius has given birth. If we associate Hinduism with a breathtaking nondualist metaphysics and Buddhism with a stringent analytical approach to spiritual life, we find that Jainism excels in its rigorous observance of moral precepts, especially nonviolence (*ahimsâ*). It was this lofty ideal, in conjunction with an extensive teaching about the causal force (*karma*) associated with human behavior, that has exerted a lasting influence on the tradition of Yoga.

Jainism has preserved an archaic type of spirituality based on the practice of penance (*tapas*) combined with an emphasis on renunciation and a very strict code of ethics for both monks and lay followers. The ancient Jaina teachers, like the Upanishadic sages, knew of the value of the internalized ritual. In the *Uttarâdhyâyana-Sûtra* (12.44), Harikesha explains that his austerity is his sacrificial fire and that his mental and physical exertions are his ladle for the oblation. The Jaina teachers of the post-Christian era adopted many ideas and practices from Hindu Yoga, particularly as formulated by Patanjali in the second century C.E.

187

## Vardhamâna Mahâvîra

Jainism was founded by Vardhamâna Mahâvîra, an older contemporary of Gautama the Buddha, who lived in the sixth century B.C.E., when Xenophanes, Parmenides, and Zeno taught in Greece. Vardhamâna acknowledged the existence of, and his indebtedness to, previous teachers, who are known as *tîrthankaras* ("ford-makers") and *jinas* ("victors" or "conquerors"), because they have overcome the self. In fact, Jainism celebrates Vardhamâna as the twenty-fourth (and last) ford-maker, the first being the legendary Rishabha.

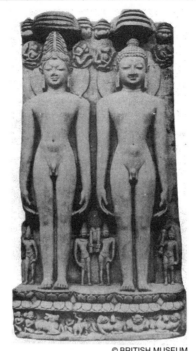

© BRITISH MUSEUM
*Vardhamâna Mahâvîra and Rishabha*

According to the traditional Jaina sources, Rishabha is said to have lived for 8.4 million years—the number 84 symbolizing completion. It is quite possible that Rishabha was a historical personage who enjoyed a long life span, though nothing is known about him apart from the later legends. There are several references to a certain seer Rishabha, son of Virat, in the *Rig-Veda* and the *Taittirîya-Âranyaka*, but there is no conclusive proof for assuming that the two were identical with the Jaina teacher of that name. It is noteworthy, however, that in the Jaina literature Rishabha is also called Keshin or "Long-hair." This possibly establishes a connection between him and such early non-Vedic religious circles as the Vrâtya brotherhoods. Also of interest is the fact that in the medieval *Bhâgavata-Purâna*, the stories given about the Hindu sage Rishabha match those in the Jaina literature, as well as the fact

that while the authors of this *Purâna* were respectful of Rishabha, they had few good words for his followers.[2]

Another legendary ford-maker, the twenty-second in line, is Arishtanemi or Neminâtha, whom Jaina tradition makes a contemporary of Krishna, the disciple of Ghora Angirasa mentioned in the *Chândogya-Upanishad*. While this connection may be completely spurious, it suggests that the earliest beginnings of Jainism are to be found outside the orthodox Vedic ritualism in the culture of ascetics, known as *shramanas*.

The life and work of the twenty-third ford-maker, Pârshva, is similarly obscured by the largely mythological accounts in the traditional literature. It is probable that he belonged, like Vardhamâna Mahâvîra, to a well-to-do warrior family, perhaps resident in Varanasi (Benares or Kâshî). It is certain that his teaching was immensely influential in the region of Bihar and beyond. One of Pârshva's most renowned disciples, who converted the king of Seyaviya, was a certain Keshin.

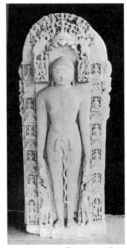

*Reproduced from*
Treasures of Jaina Bhandaras

*Pârshva*

Mahâvîra ("Great Hero") grew up under the influence of Pârshva's tradition, but did not know the man himself, who appears to have lived in the seventh century B.C.E. Mahâvîra gave Jainism its distinct shape, reforming the tradition of Pârshva. He is said to have been born at Kundagrama near Vaishalî (modern Besarh) to the north of Patna, as a member of the Naya (Jnâtâ) clan of the Licchavi tribe. His father was a local ruler. According to some traditions, Vardhamâna was married at a young age.

Most authorities are agreed that he left his worldly life behind at the age of thirty to pursue a course of rigorous austerities, which included prolonged waterless fasting, as it is still practiced in the Jaina community today.

Twelve years after setting out on his spiritual journey, he attained enlightenment. At once he started to preach the truth he had discovered for himself. He was a charismatic figure whose detachment and single-minded dedication to a self-transcending life inspired and awed many people. If his exemplary life and teaching did not make more of an impact both during his life and subsequently, it is because Jainism demands a rare degree of renunciation and self-control that holds no appeal for the masses. Vardhamâna Mahâvîra died in 527 B.C.E. at the age of seventy-two, leaving behind a small community of monks, nuns, and lay folk, numbering about 14,000 members. Today the relatively small community of Jainas include circa 2,500 monks and 5,000 nuns.

Unlike Pârshva, Mahâvîra is remembered to have walked about naked, thus declaring his uncompromising asceticism. We have encountered this practice already in connection with the long-haired ascetics of the Vedic times who, as the *Rig-Veda* (10.136) has it, were "air-clad." The issue of nudity was in fact one of the principal reasons for the split of the Jaina community into two sects, which occurred about 300 B.C.E. Whereas the Digambaras ("Space-clothed") to this day announce their renunciation of everything by going about naked, the Shvetâmbaras ("White-clothed") have opted for a more symbolic form of renunciation. For the latter, the presence or absence of garments does not make a spiritual victor. But even the Digambaras do not permit their nuns to

walk about in the nude. More than that, they deny that a woman can attain emancipation without first being reborn in a male body. By contrast, the Shvetâmbaras venerate a woman ford-maker, Malli, who was nineteenth in succession. There is one early sculpture of a nude female ascetic, which is generally held to be Malli.

When Alexander the Great invaded northern India in 327–326 B.C.E., his chroniclers reported the existence of *gymnosophistes*, or naked philosophers. Some thirteen hundred years later, the Moslem hegemonists put a stop to this practice, at least for a period of time. Naked ascetics, besmeared with ashes, can still be seen in India today. But it is not this curious custom for which Jainism should be noted. Rather, the lasting contribution of this minority religion lies in its minute examination of what constitutes a truly moral life.

## II. THE SACRED LITERATURE OF JAINISM

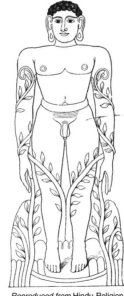

*Reproduced from* Hindu Religion, Customs and Manners

*Gomateshvara, after a monumental stone sculpture*

The history and literature of Jainism has been thus far very inadequately researched. Until recently, Western indological scholarship was curiously neglectful of Jainism, considering it a comparatively irrelevant development. Fortunately, this attitude is changing, as more information about Jainism is made available.[3]

Part of the difficulty has been that the authenticity of the Jaina canon is doubted by sections of the Jaina community itself. Thus, at the Council of Pataliputra (modern Patna) in 300 B.C.E., an attempt was made to determine the content of the fourteen *Pûrvas* ("Earlier [Teachings]"), which had until then been orally transmitted. Already at that time a faction of the community did not accept the resulting redaction. By the time the canon was actually written down, presumably in the middle of the fifth century C.E., a large portion of the original teachings of Vardhamâna and his predecessors had been irretrievably lost. The Digambaras actually deny that any of the early canonical works have survived.

According to the Shvetâmbaras, the Jaina canon consists of forty-five works in all. Because knowledge about this formidable literature is not readily available, it seems appropriate to provide at least skeletal information here:

1–12.   The twelve *Angas* ("Limbs"), which are composed in an archaic Prakrit dialect that was once spoken by the ordinary people of Magadha. They are individually listed below.

13–24.   The twelve *Upângas* ("Secondary Limbs," from *upa* and *anga*), which deal with cosmological, cosmographical, astronomical, and hagiological themes. Noteworthy among these scriptures is the *Râja-Prashnîya-Sûtra*, which records the dialogue between Sage Keshin and Prasenajit (Prakrit: Paesi), ruler of Seyavîya, in which Keshin tries to prove that the Spirit is independent of the physical body.

25–28.   The four *Mûla-Sûtras* ("Fundamental Sûtras"), which are primers for ascetics.

29–38.   The ten *Prakîrnas* ("Mixed [Scriptures]"), which contain instructions about a variety of subjects, such as prayer, conscious dying, astrology, and medicine.

39–45.   The seven *Cheda-Sûtras* ("Cutting Sûtras"), which deal with monastic rules.

To these must be added the *Nandi-Sûtra* ("Auspicious *Sûtra*"), which is a text on scriptural interpretation, and the *Anuyoga-Dvâra-Sûtra* ("Door of Disquisition *Sûtra*"), which is concerned with the nature of knowledge. They provide a scholastic context for the canon.

The twelve *Angas*, listed by their Sanskrit titles, are:

1.   *Âcâra* (Prakrit: *Âyâr*, "Conduct" ), containing important rules for Jaina monks and nuns and preserving a sacred account of Mahâvîra's life as a wandering mendicant;

2.   *Sûtra-Krita* (Prakrit: *Sûya-gad*, "Aphoristic Composition"), giving out the fundamental teachings of Jainism relative to the monastic life, and combating non-Jaina doctrines;

3.   *Sthâna* (Prakrit: *Thân*, "Receptacle"), consisting of a detailed enumeration of the key principles of Jainism;

4.   *Samavâya* ("Combination"), continuing the exposition of the *Sthâna-Anga*;

5.   *Bhagavatî-Vyâkhyâ-Prajnapti* (Prakrit: *Bhagavaî-Viyâha-Pannatti*, "Exposition of Explanations"), furnishing through its recorded dialogues a vivid picture of Mahâvîra's life and his times; this voluminous work also contains information about Gosala, an ascetic who lived with Mahâvîra for six years and who, as leader of the Ajîvika school, appears to have

attracted a large following; this work is of particular importance to the Shvetâmbara sect;

6. *Jnâtri-Dharma-Kathâ* (Prakrit: *Nâyâ-Dhamma-Kahâo*, "Stories of Knowledge and Morality"), consisting of legendary accounts that illustrate Jaina doctrines;

7. *Upâsaka-Dashâ* (Prakrit: *Uvâsaga-Dasâo*, "Ten [Chapters] on Lay Followers"), containing legends of saintly men and women from among the laity;

8. *Antakrid-Dashâ* (Prakrit: *Amta-Gada-Dasâo*, "Ten [Chapters] on End-Makers"), consisting of legends of ten ascetics who won enlightenment and brought an end to the cycle of rebirths;

9. *Anuttara-Upapâtika-Dashâ* (Prakrit: *Anuttarovavâiya-Dasâo*, "Ten [Chapters] on the Highest Risers"), containing legends of saints who ascended to the highest heavenly worlds;

10. *Prashna-Vyâkarana* (Prakrit: *Panhâ-Vâgaranâim*, "Questions and Explanations"), comprising discussions of prescriptions and proscriptions from the Jaina code of ethics;

11. *Vipâka-Shruta* (Prakrit: *Vivâga-Suyam*, "Revelation on Ripening"), containing legends that illustrate the karmic consequences of good and evil acts;

12. *Drishti-Vâda* (Prakrit: *Ditthi-Vâya*, "Instruction about Views"), comprising the fourteen *Pûrvas*, which have been lost.

The individual works of the Jaina canon are often referred to as *Âgamas*. Occasionally the number of canonical scriptures is reckoned to be eighty-four, and thirty-six *Nigamas*, which are *Upanishad*-like works, are also mentioned.

All these writings, which parallel the Vedic revelation (*shruti*), were followed by a copious and rich exegetical literature. That explanatory literature comprises ten original treatises, known as the *Nijjuttis* in Prakrit and *Niryuktis* in Sanskrit. These have their own major commentaries (Prakrit: *bhâsa*, Sanskrit: *bhâshya*), elucidations (Prakrit: *chunni*, Sanskrit: *cûrnî*), and glosses (Prakrit/Sanskrit: *tîkâ*). In addition, the sacred literature of the Jainas comprises *Purânas* (sacred encyclopedias) and *Câritras* (hagiographies), as well as a host of other instructional works.

There are also numerous extra-canonical works, such as the *Tarangâvatî*, a Prakrit poem composed by Pâdalipta Sûri, who is said to have cured King Murunda of Pataliputra of an incurable disease. An older work, dating back to perhaps 100 C.E., is the *Pauma-Carîya* of Vimala, the Jaina version of the Hindu *Râmâyana*. Around the same time lived Umâsvâti, the greatest philosopher of Jainism and author of the famous *Tattva-Artha-(Adhigama-)Sûtra*.[4] His influence within Jainism is comparable to the influence of Shankara within Hinduism.

After Umâsvâti, the most renowned Jaina philosopher, comes the Digambara scholar Kunda Kunda, whose most popular work is the *Samaya-Sâra*. He lived probably in the fourth century C.E. In the eighth century, we have Haribhadra Sûri—philosopher, logician, and artist in one person—who reputedly wrote no fewer than 1,440 works. These include several texts on Yoga, notably the *Yoga-Bindu* and the *Yoga-Drishti-Samuccaya* (an excerpt from which is given as Source Reading 7). Several centuries later lived Hemacandra, the author of the *Yoga-Shâstra*, which is also known as the *Adhyâtma-Upanishad*. Furthermore, the Jainas have composed numerous works on logic—an area where they made important contributions to Indian philosophy.

The canon of the Digambaras was created in the early post-Christian centuries. Although the Digambaras rejected the Shvetâmbara canon, they nevertheless quoted from it. Their own canon consists of two parts, the so-called *Karma-Prâbhrita* and the *Kashâya-Prâbhrita*. The former is also known as *Shat-Khanda-Âgama,*[5] or "Scripture in Six Parts." It has an extensive commentary by Vîrasena, entitled *Dhavalâ*, or "The Luminous," completed in 816 C.E. The *Kashâya-Prâbhrita* runs into a mere 233 verses, composed by Gunadhara, and also has a comprehensive commentary by Vîrasena and his disciple Jinasena.

The Digambaras also have a secondary canon, which was created in the sixth or seventh century C.E. It is divided into four subjects, which the Digambaras refer to as their "four *Vedas*": history, cosmography, philosophy, and ethics. A well-known extra-canonical work of the Digambaras is the *Svâmi-Kârttikeya-Anuprekshâ*, which deals with the twelve meditations (*anuprekshâ*) recommended for both monks and the laity. It belongs to the tenth century C.E.

Perhaps the most remarkable feature of the doctrinal world of Jainism is that, notwithstanding the scission into two sects, the differences between contending schools are minimal. In contrast to Buddhism, Jainism has succeeded in preserving its core teachings for well over two millennia. There never was a Jaina Mahâyâna, Vajrayâna, or Kalacakrayâna. Jainism portrays in extremis the kind

---

> "The sages declare that in the absence of pure experience, the suprasensuous supreme Absolute is not comprehensible even with a hundred scriptural reasons."
>
> —*Jnâna-Sâra* 203

---

of continuity that historians have observed between the ancient Indus-Sarasvatî civilization and modern Indian culture.

As is apparent from the extent of the Jaina literature alone, Jainism prospered for many centuries, even though its rather stark asceticism prevented it from achieving the same success as the Buddha's teaching. Then, in the thirteenth century, the Muslims put thousands of Jaina monks and nuns to the sword and destroyed their temples and libraries, and for a period of time severely impaired the vitality of Jaina culture. Today, Jainism is a minority religion in India but one that is by no means stagnant, as is evident from the Anuvrata movement initiated by Acarya Tulasi in Rajasthan in 1949. The movement's name, "Small Vow," is meant to suggest that even the minor vows of Jainism can bring about big changes. The history of Jainism thus continues to be an important lesson in the efficacy of vows in a life that revolves around spiritual rather than material values—an art that is all but forgotten in our Western society.

## III. THE PATH OF PURIFICATION

### The Power of Karma and Its Elimination through Morality and Meditation

Like Buddhism and Hinduism, Jaina spirituality is essentially a path to emancipation, or what is called "absolute knowledge" (*kevala-jnâna*).

That superlative condition is defined in terms of freedom from the impact of the law of moral causation, or karma. The doctrine of karma plays the same vital role in Jainism as it does in Hinduism and Buddhism. But the Jaina scholastics elaborated this doctrine more than any other. The underlying idea of karma is that the law of cause and effect applies also to the psychic or moral realm, so that a person's actions or even volitions determine his or her destiny, both in the present lifetime and future lifetimes.

There is a parallel here to modern existentialism, which argues that we are what we are because of our past decisions, and that we are free to choose what we may become, and that therefore it is in our actions that we are most truly ourselves. Another and related point of contact between existentialist philosophy and the doctrine of karma is that both understand the human condition to be one of fear (or dread). Whereas the Indian spiritual traditions teach that this condition can be wholly transcended—in the moment of enlightenment or liberation—Western existentialism, despite its frequent metaphysical formulations, is seldom so optimistic. Thus, even the German philosopher and psychiatrist Karl Jaspers, who must be counted among the more metaphysical-minded existentialists, does not concede the possibility of radical transcendence. For him, the most we can hope to accomplish is the establishment of "communication from personality to personality," so that "our relation to transcendence . . . becomes sensibly present in our encounter with the personal God."[6] From the Indian point of view, such an encounter still occurs within the conditional dimension of existence, that is to say, it falls short of liberation or enlightenment, in which the human personality as well as the personal deity is utterly transcended.

The true essence of the human individual is the Self (*âtman*). The Jainas use the terms *âtman* and *jîva* interchangeably, but whereas the former refers to the transcendental nature, the latter is the Self held in captivity by its own karma-producing actions.

In Jainism the classification into eight primary types of karma is best known, but the Jaina scholastics distinguish up to 148 different forms of karmic activity:

1. karma concealing wisdom;

2. karma concealing right insight, thus preventing the acceptance of the Jaina code of moral conduct;

3. karma leading to the experience of pleasure and pain;

4. karma causing complete delusion;

5. karma determining the length of one's life;

6. karma determining one's particular social status;

7. karma determining one's birth into a particular family;

8. karma that is generally obstructive.

From the point of view of its activity in time, karma is classified under three headings:

1. *satta-karma*, which has been accumulated in past existences; its Hindu equivalent is *sancita-karma*;

2. *bandha-karma*, which is produced in the present existence, but becomes effective only later; it corresponds to the Hindu notion of *âgâmi-karma*;

3. *udaya-karma*, which is effective now; this is the same as the Hindu idea of *prârabdha-karma*.

Furthermore, all karma is divided into two essential categories—*nikacita* (that which must be experienced) and *shithila* (that which can be avoided through the practice of Yoga). Without the latter type, life would proceed along absolutely deterministic lines. But Jainism rejects fatalism, which was one of the main points of dispute between Mahâvîra and the Ajîvika philosopher Makkhali Gosala. Gosala maintained that human beings were under the complete control of destiny (*niyati*), which he saw as an impersonal cosmic principle. Mahâvîra, however, taught that there was free will and the possibility to change and even transcend one's karmic fate. Throughout the existence of a particular animate being (*jîva*), karma is produced and experienced.

The Jainas conceive of karma as a kind of substance that can be generated, stored, and annihilated. The cycle of karma production and experience is interpreted in terms of an influx (*âsrava*) of karma, which needs to be stopped. For, as long as the inflow of karma continues, the being is bound to lifeless matter (*ajîva-pudgala*) and revolves continually in the wheel of repeated births and deaths. The concept of *jîva* comprises all animate entities, including the material elements such as water and fire. In this respect, the Jaina concept differs from the Vedântic notion of *jîva*, which is applied only to the self-conscious being.

Like the proponents of Sâmkhya, the Jainas believe in a plurality of ultimate or spiritual entities, the *âtmans*. These are, similar to the Sâmkhya *purushas* or Self-monads, essentially infinite and pure Consciousness. But they deem themselves confined to a certain form or body. Their self-limitation, which is regarded as a form of contraction of consciousness, results from the

impact of karma, and only through the reduction of karmic influences, and ultimately the total obliteration of karma, can the *jîva's* consciousness be purified and transformed into the limitless transcendental Consciousness. As Hemacandra (1089–1172 C.E.) declares in his famous *Yoga-Shâstra* (4.112a):

Emancipation [results from] the dwindling of karma, and that is achieved through self-absorption (*âtma-dhyâna*).

Acting as a receptacle of karma is the instrumental body or *karmana-sharîra*, which is the innermost of the five bodies of the human being. The remaining four are:

1. the physical human body (*audarika-sharîra*);

2. the transformation body (*vaikriya-sharîra*), which is the natural vehicle of the higher beings (i.e., deities) and which can be "acquired" by the ascetic who then is able to increase its size at will; perhaps the fantastic dimensions given for the bodies of the earlier teachers of Jainism can be explained as referring to their transformation bodies only;

3. the procurement body (*âhâraka-sharîra*), which can be temporarily created and detached from the physical body to be projected anywhere;

4. the fiery body (*taijasa-sharîra*), which is indestructible and survives death and without whose energy the lower three bodies could not operate; ascetics can use this body to burn objects.

This doctrine of the five bodies that are successively more subtle has its Hindu counterpart in the teaching of the *Taittirîya-Upanishad* mentioned in the previous chapter. But Jainism has developed its own distinct ideas about what some scholars have called subtle physiology.

According to a classification found in the Jaina canon, there are two types of animate entities: There are those who are trapped in the cosmos of dependence and suffering, called *samsârins*, and there are those who have escaped *samsâra*, the wheel of continual becoming; these are the *siddhas* or "perfected ones." The latter are without spatial location and experience the unimaginable bliss of infinite Consciousness. One of their 108 characteristics is that they can assume any shape at will, and thus are masters of the universe.

## *The Seven Categories of Existence*

The *jîvas*, or finite individuals, belong to the first of the seven basic categories known to Jainism. The second category is composed of the inanimate objects (*ajîva*). These comprise the formless dimensions of motility, space, and time, as well as the innumerable distinct forms that make up perceptible matter (*pudgala*). According to Jainism, which does not admit the existence of a supreme creator or deity, the whole creation is maintained by the interaction between the animate and the inanimate.

The third category, as already mentioned, is called influx (*âsrava*), which refers to the intake of karma, which pollutes the transcendental Consciousness to the point where it believes itself to be finite and associated, if not identical, with a physical body. Karma is attracted to a being by virtue of his or her mental and physical acts. This influx of karma is also given the name *yoga* in Jainism,

which means the "union" of the transcendental Self with physical reality; that is, the contraction of the Self around a finite material conglomerate.

The fourth category is bondage (*bandha*), whose causes are false views, attachment, negligence, passion (*kashâya*), and the association (*yoga*) with the limited body-mind. Next comes the category of "warding off" (*samvara*), which is the process of preventing the generation of karma through proper moral conduct. The central virtue of the Jaina code of morals is nonharming (*ahimsâ*), which entails the prohibition of killing animate beings for any purpose, be it for food or sacrifice, and even the mere intention of hurting another being. Jainism originally recruited its members primarily from the aristocratic families and warrior (*kshatriya*) estate. However, the strict regulations about nonharming have forced the Jaina laity into merchant careers. Ethics forms the foundation of Jaina Yoga, and it is stated that no amount of austerity or meditative practice can lead to emancipation unless it is accompanied by the careful observance of the moral rules.

The sixth category is called "exhaustion" (*nirjara*) and refers to the complete elimination of karma in the highest forms of ecstasy (*samâdhi*), brought about by extreme penance. Such penance, especially the rigorous practice of nonharming (*ahimsâ*), not only stops the flow of karma but reverses all karmic effects. From this results, as the seventh category, the transcendental state of emancipation (*moksha*), or absolute knowledge. In the ancient *Âcâra-Anga-Sûtra* (330–332), Mahâvîra declares about this state of perfect freedom:

> All sounds recoil, where reason has no
> room, nor does the mind penetrate there.
> The liberated is not long or small, round
> or triangular; he is neither black nor
> white; he is disembodied, without con-
> tact [with matter] . . . not female, male,

or neuter. Though he perceives and knows, there is no [fitting] analogy [to describe his perception or knowledge]. His being is formless. There is no condition of the Unconditioned.

The transcendental Reality, or Self, is also known as the Lord (*prabhu*). In his Sanskrit work *Âtma-Anushâsana* (266), the ninth-century teacher Gunabhadra states:

The Lord is the unborn, indestructible, formless, happy, and wise Actor and Enjoyer, [who coincides with the size of] the body only, freed from impurity, [and who] having gone upward is immovable.

In Kunda Kunda's *Niyama-Sâra* (43–46), authored in the sixth century C.E., we find the following reiteratively descriptive stanzas:

The Self (*âtman*) is free from punishment, without opposites, without mesense (*nirmama*), impartite, without [objective] support, devoid of attachment, free from defects, free from delusion, and fearless.

The Self is free from contraction (*nirgrantha*), devoid of attachment, without blemish, free from all defects, without desire, free from anger, free from pride, and without lust.

Color, taste, smell, touch, male, female,

male [or female] inclinations, etc., the [various kinds] of positions, and the [various types of] bodies—all these do not exist in the [transcendental] individual (*jîva*).

> "The Yoga teachers have said that nescience is seeing that which is eternal, pure, and the Self in the finite, impure, and non-self, and that wisdom is the perception of Reality."
>
> —*Jnâna-Sâra* 105

Know the [transcendental] individual to be tasteless, formless, without scent, unmanifest [but] conscious, unqualified, soundless, not recognizable by [any external] sign, and without describable location.

Kunda Kunda goes on to compare the true nature of the individuated self to the liberated beings (*siddha-âtman*), who know neither birth nor growth nor death. Only from the empirical (*vyavahâra*) point of view can the individuated selves be said to possess such characteristics as form and finitude, whereas from the pure (*shuddha*) viewpoint they are endowed with the same purity as those who are liberated.

## The Jaina Ladder to Liberation

At the heart of Jainism lies a carefully worked-out path that leads the faithful from the fetters of conditioned existence and suffering to absolute freedom, unsurpassable joy, and incomparable energy. Although the recommended procedure for a prosperous spiritual life is to abandon everything and to dedicate oneself completely to a life of renunciation and penance, the Jaina authorities nevertheless deem it in principle possible even for a householder to become liberated.

According to a widely accepted model, the Jaina ladder to emancipation comprises fourteen stages, known as the levels of virtue (*guna-sthâna*). This framework describes the course of a person's maturation from ordinary worldly life to spiritual liberation. It begins with the conventional state of unenlightenment, which is governed by false vision (*mithyâ-drishti*) involving the mistaken idea that one is identical with the finite body-mind. Gradually, a "taste" for right (*samyag-drishti*) appears. Now the practitioner understands that he or she transcends the skin-bound mortal frame. This knowledge grows with practice, and given steady discipline the aspirant is step by step propelled toward liberation. The fourteen stages (*sthâna*) are characterized as follows:

1. False vision (*mithyâ-drishti*): On this level an animate being is still completely unenlightened and therefore under the full sway of the forces of karma.

2. Taste for right vision (*sâsvâdana-samyag-drishti*): There is a dim understanding of what is true and false, but with long relapses into ignorance.

3. Right and false vision (*samyag-mithyâ-drishti*): An entity oscillates between truth and doubt. This stage is also called "mixed" (*mishra*).

4. Lack of self-restraint but right vision (*avirata-samyag-drishti*): At this stage right insight is no longer suppressed but control over the emotions is still a problem. Here spiritual life proper can begin, providing self-control (*virati*) is cultivated.

5. Conditional self-restraint and right vision (*desha-virata-samyag-drishti*): The importance of proper moral conduct is realized and the desire arises to renounce the world and become an ascetic; here ends the career of the householder, who must now decide either to postpone renunciation of the world or ascend to higher stages by means of asceticism.

6. Control over inattention (*pramatta-samyatâ*): The ascetic has almost completely curbed the four vices, which are anger, pride, delusion, and greed. He or she is capable of checking the tendency of the mind to slip into unconscious behavior patterns through sheer inattention (*pramâda*).

7. Controlled attention (*apramatta-samyatâ*): Through the purification of the mind, sleep is overcome, and the ascetic acquires the power for intense concentration and meditative absorption.

8. The gross struggle with cessation (*nivritti-bâdara-sâmparâyâ*): This is also called *apûrva-karana-sâmparâyâ* because of a special meditation practice by which the ascetic cultivates a joy previously not known. Moreover, the ascetic gains even greater power over himself or herself.

9. The gross struggle with noncessation (*anivritti-bâdara-sâmparâyâ*): At this stage the sexual impulses are brought under complete control and the emotional forces are equally well subdued.

10. The subtle struggle (*sûkshma-sâmparâyâ*): Now even the last trace of worldly interest is eradicated.

11. The pacification of delusion (*upashânta-mohâ*): The mistaken notion of being a separate physical entity is fully subdued and makes room for the intuition of the universal Consciousness.

12. The disappearance of delusion (*kshîna-mohâ*): Here all egoic delusion is destroyed and the ascetic, unhindered by any karma, attains full gnosis.

13. Active transcendence (*sayoga-kevalî*): This is the stage of inner isolation from all multiplicity. Should the omniscient ascetic resolve in this state to propound his newly found knowledge, he becomes a *tîrthankara* or ford-maker. This ecstatic state lasts a minimum of one *muhûrta* (forty-eight minutes) and a maximum of a little less than a *pûrva-koti* (7,056 followed by 27 zeros). The ascetic who has won through to this sublime condition is known as a transcender (*kevalin*), victor (*jîna*), or worthy one (*arhat*).

14. Inactive transcendence (*ayoga-kevalî*): In this stage of the meditative process, which lasts for no more than one *muhûrta*, even the last trace of karma is eradicated, and the ascetic emerges as a fully liberated being. This condition is attained by a *jîna* or *arhat* just prior to the death of the physical body. This stage corresponds to the *dharma-megha-samâdhi* in Classical Yoga. Beyond the fourteen stages of virtue lies liberation, the luminous Condition of the perfected being (*siddha*), free from bodily existence and karma.

It must be added that stages eight, nine, and ten hold special significance, because it is here that the spiritual practitioner gains control over the passions in their gross and subtle aspects. In order to attain the enlightened condition, the spiritual practitioner has to pass through three great inner processes. The first process, known as *yathâ-pravritti-karana*, reduces the duration and intensity of karma. By means of the second process, called *apûrva-karana*, the "knot" (*granthi*) at the heart is severed, and the practitioner becomes empowered to proceed to higher levels of meditation. This occurs in the eighth stage of the fourteenfold way of spiritual ascent. Finally, through the third process, activated in the tenth stage and known as *anivritti-karana*, the karmic material surrounding and weighing down the Self is divided into three parts: impure, pure, and mixed. Depending on which karmic parcel gets activated, the individual will either return to a worldly disposition or move on to the higher stages of meditative practice.

The main instruments governing the progression through these stages of spiritual attainment are the very intricate ethical rules laid down in the canonical literature of Jainism. As the following list of virtues bears out, there is a great similarity between Jaina, Buddhist, and Hindu ethics. Thus, in Umâsvâti's famous *Tattva-Artha-Sûtra* (9.7), written in the fifth century C.E., we find these qualifications of an ascetic, which are all considered forms of nonharming: forbearance (*kshamâ*), humility (*mârdava*), uprightness (*ârjava*), purity (*shauca*), truthfulness (*satya*), self-discipline (*samyama*), austerity (*tapas*), renunciation (*tyâga*), poverty (*akincanya*, lit. "having nothing"), chastity (*brahmacarya*). For the layman the following rules are binding: almsgiving (*dâna*), virtuous conduct (*shîla*), austerity (*tapas*), and a spiritual disposition (*bhâva*). Other scriptures contain different and often far more detailed prescriptions for the ascetics and the laity.

## *Jaina Yoga*

In its higher aspects, Jaina Yoga resembles its Hindu counterpart, and in fact the later Jaina writers like Haribhadra Sûri (c. 750 C.E.)[7] have made use of some of the codifications of Patanjali. In his *Yoga-Bindu*, Haribhadra praises Yoga as follows:

> Yoga is the best wish-fulfilling tree (*kalpa-taru*). Yoga is the supreme wish-granting jewel (*cintâ-mani*). Yoga is the foremost of virtues. Yoga is the very embodiment of perfection (*siddhi*). (37)

> Thus, it is declared to be [like] the fire [that consumes the karmic] seed of incarnation, like extreme old age in regard to aging, or fatal consumption in regard to suffering, or death in regard to death itself. (38)

> The great souls (*mahâ-âtman*)[8] accomplished in Yoga declare that even a mere hearing of the two syllables [of the word *yoga*], according to the rules, is sufficient for the removal of sins. (40)

> Just as impure gold is inevitably purified by fire, so also the mind afflicted with the taint of [spiritual] ignorance is [purified] by the fire of Yoga. (41)

> Thus, verily, Yoga is the foundation for realizing Reality (*tattva*), for this is ascertained through nothing else. There is nothing comparable [to Yoga]. (64)

> Hence, in order to realize that very Reality, the thoughtful person should always make a mighty effort. Argumentative books are of no avail. (65)

Haribhadra distinguishes between Yoga proper and what he calls preparatory service (*pûrva-sevâ*). The latter consists in the following practices:

1. Veneration (*pûjana*) of the teacher, the deities, and other beings of authority, such as one's parents and elders. In the case of the deities, this involves ritual worship with flowers and other offerings. In the case of one's elders, veneration is shown by respectful bowing and general obedience to them.

2. Proper conduct (*sad-âcâra*) involves charity (*dâna*), conformity to the social mores, the abstention from blaming others, the practice of praise and cheerfulness in adversity, as well as humility, considered speech, and integrity, observance of one's vows, the abandonment of lethargy, and refraining from reprehensible behavior even in the face of death.

3. Asceticism or penance (*tapas*) is thought to remove one's sins and should be practiced to the utmost of one's abilities. Primarily, it involves different forms of

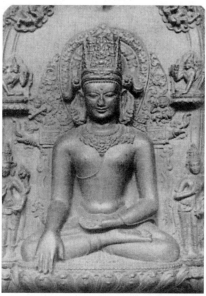

*Reproduced from Journal of Indian Art and Industry*
*A tîrthankâra*

fasting, including prolonged, month-long fasts combined with the chanting of *mantras*.

4.  Non-aversion toward liberation (*mukti-advesha*, written *muktyadvesha*) or what in the Hindu school of Vedânta is known as the desire for liberation: This disposition is essential to success in spiritual life. The desire to transcend the ego limitation must overwhelm all other desires and impulses. Haribhadra makes the point that ordinary people, under the spell of hedonism, find the ideal of liberation minimally attractive, because it does not promise the usual enjoyment. In fact, they feel threatened by the prospect of a bliss that eclipses the ego. Hence, it is important to cultivate right understanding.

This preparatory practice may be taken up by what the Jaina tradition calls the *apunar-bandhaka*, the person who, after numerous lifetimes, has grown weary of the worldly game and is embarking on his or her final embodiment. For Haribhadra, however, genuine Yoga practice is possible only for a spiritually more mature individual. He speaks of the *samyag-drishti*, the person who has correct vision or understanding, and the *câritrin*, who is firmly on the spiritual path.

The *apunar-bandhaka* is on the first of the fourteen levels of virtues described above, where the ego illusion predominates. The *samyag-drishti*, whom Haribhadra compares to the Buddhist *bodhisattva*, has attained the fourth level, where fundamental spiritual insight prevails but discipline is still a problem. The *câritrin* occupies the fifth level, which is marked by the desire to renounce the world and adopt the ascetic lifestyle.

Haribhadra speaks of five degrees of genuine Yoga, for which the *câritrin* alone is equipped:

1.  *Adhyâtman*, or *adhyâtma-yoga*, is the constant remembering, or pondering upon, one's essential nature.

2.  *Bhâvanâ*, or contemplation, is the daily concentrated observance of the essential nature (*adhyâtman*) itself, which increases the quality and time of one's dwelling in spiritually positive mental states.

3.  *Dhyâna*, or meditation, is the mind's fixation upon auspicious objects, which is accompanied by subtle enjoyment. Such meditation leads to great mental stability and the ability to influence others mentally.

4.  *Samatâ*, or "sameness," is the mood of indifference toward things that one normally would feel attracted to or repelled by. Cultivation of this attitude includes abstention from the use of psychic powers (*riddhi* or *siddhi*), and it attenuates the subtle karmic forces that bind a person to worldly existence.

5.  *Vritti-samkshaya*, or the full removal of the movements of consciousness, means the complete transcendence of karma-produced psychomental states. This leads to emancipation (*moksha*), which "is unobstructed and the seat of eternal bliss" (*Yoga-Bindu* 367).

At the core of the advanced Yoga practice is meditative absorption, which every follower of Jainism is asked to practice at least once a day for one *muhûrta* (forty-eight minutes) in the morning. The ascetic is naturally required to dedicate most of his or her time to this exercise. But lay folk can take additional vows obliging them to, say, meditate three times a day for longer periods.

There are no strict regulations about how this meditation ought to be performed; there is a choice between a variety of techniques, some of which are strongly reminiscent of Tantric exercises. In Umâsvâti's *Tattva-Artha-Sûtra* (9.27–46), meditation is explained as follows:

> Meditation (*dhyâna*) is the restraint (*nirodha*) of the single-pointed mind (*cintâ*) in [the case of one who possesses] the highest steadfastness . . .
>
> . . . up to one *muhûrta* [forty-eight minutes].
>
> [Meditation can be of four types:] disagreeable (*ârta*), savage (*raudra*), virtuous (*dharma*), or pure (*shukla*).
>
> [Only] the last two [types] are the cause of liberation.
>
> The disagreeable [meditation occurs] when upon contacting an unpleasant experience (*amano-jnâna*), [the practitioner] dwells on the memory [of that experience] in order to dissociate from it
>
> and [unpleasant] sensations,
>
> the reverse of pleasant experience,
>
> and from the "link" (*nidâna*) [which is the desire to fulfill a certain intention in a future life].

> This [disagreeable meditation occurs] in the case of the undisciplined, partly disciplined, and the lax in restraint.
>
> The savage [meditation], [which occurs] in the case of the undisciplined or partly disciplined, is for harming, lying, theft, or the preservation of possessions.
>
> The virtuous [meditation], [which occurs] in the case of the [ascetic who is] disciplined in attentiveness, is for ascertaining the revealed order (*âjnâ*) [i.e., the sacred tradition], the diminution (*apâya*) [of the Self through karma], the fruition (*vipâka*) [of karma], and the construction (*samsthâna*) [of the universe].
>
> [This meditation occurs] also in the case of those whose passions have either been pacified or vanished.
>
> [In the case of those whose passions (*kashâya*) have altogether vanished, there occur] also the [first] two pure [meditations].
>
> The latter [two pure meditations occur] in the case of the transcender (*kevalin*).
>
> [The four forms or stages of the pure meditation are:]
>
> The consideration (*vitarka*) of separateness and of singleness, absorption (*pratipatti*) in subtle activity, and the cessation of quiesced activity.
>
> This [fourfold pure meditation occurs in the case of those who respectively experience] the triple, the single, or the

[purely] bodily action (*yoga*) [as well as those who are completely] inactive.

In regard to the former [two forms, which are accompanied by] consideration, [there is] a single prop [or object of meditation].

The second [of these forms accompanied by consideration or *vitarka*] is beyond reflection (*avicâra*).

Consideration is [knowledge of what has been] revealed (*shruta*).

Reflection (*vicâra*) is the [mind's] revolving around meaning (*artha*), symbol (*vyanjana*), and activity (*yoga*).

As with all *Sûtra* compositions, this work is barely intelligible without its commentaries. In particular, aphorism 9.42 is obscure. It appears that the third degree of pure meditation (*shukla-dhyâna*) consists in bodily activity only. There is no consideration (*vitarka*) or reflection (*vicâra*) at this level. Then, in the fourth and final stage, the already calmed bodily activity is utterly transcended. The first degree of pure meditation falls into the eighth to eleventh stage of the fourteenfold path, the second into the twelfth stage, the third into the thirteenth, and the fourth coincides with the fourteenth stage and is followed by the great event of liberation.

The schema of four types or degrees of meditation is interesting, and the phraseology reminds one strongly of the *Yoga-Sûtra* of Patanjali. But Umâsvâti, the author of this Jaina work, has his own idiosyncratic interpretations of such key yogic terms as *vitarka* and *vicâra*. A similar situation pertains in Buddhism, which also offers its own interpretations, though they precede Patanjali's formulations.

Meditative absorption can be practiced either sitting or standing. The Jaina scriptures mention such postures as the "bedstead" (*paryanka*) and "half-bedstead" (*ardha-paryanka*), which are reclining postures, and the thunderbolt posture (*vajra-âsana*, written *vajrâsana*), the lotus posture (*kamala-âsana*, written *kamalâsana*), and the tailor seat or easy posture (*sukha-âsana*, written *sukhâsana*), which should be practiced at a suitable location. However, it is occasionally recommended that the place should be more disagreeable than comfortable, which reminds one of the Tantric custom of meditating on the cremation ground amidst decaying corpses—a vivid reminder of the impermanence of everything.

Some texts, like the *Yoga-Shâstra* of Hema-· candra, mention other postures (*âsana*) identical with those known in Hindu Yoga, such as the hero posture (*vîra-âsana*, written *vîrâsana*), the auspicious posture (*bhadra-âsana*, written *bhadrâsana*), and the staff posture (*danda-âsana*, written *dandâsana*). Hemacandra also refers to a certain *utkatika-âsana* (written *utkatikâsana*) and *godohika-âsana* (written *godohikâsana*), and makes the point that there are no special rules for choosing one rather than the other posture. The generic technical term for the meditative posture is *kâya-utsarga* (written *kâyotsarga*, "casting off of the body"), which is also sometimes considered a specific posture in itself. The name is meant to suggest that the purpose of such yogic postures is not so much to cultivate the body as to transcend it. In his *Niyama-Sâra* (121), Kunda Kunda gives this practice a psychological meaning:

He who, shunning the [idea of] stability in regard to other substances, such as the body, meditates without form (*nirvi-kalpa*) upon the Self cultivates the casting off of the body (*tanu*).

Hemacandra recommends breath control (*prânâyâma*) as an aid to meditation, following largely the lines of Patanjali's *Yoga-Sûtra*. However, at least one Jaina authority on Yoga, Shubhacandra, takes a different point of view in his *Jnâna-Arnava*.[9] He states that breath control is helpful in checking physical activity but interferes with concentration and is likely to produce disagreeable (*ârta*) meditation experiences. Instead, he advises the practitioner to aspire to what he calls superlative concentration (*parama-samâdhi*). This view is reinforced by Kunda Kunda, who makes the following comment in his *Niyama-Sâra* (124):

> What is the point of dwelling in the forest, chastising the body, observing various fasts, studying, and maintaining silence (*mauna*) for the renouncer (*shramana*) who lacks collectedness (*samatâ*)?

In the same work, we find this stanza:

> If you desire independence (*avashya-ka*), fix your steady thoughts upon the true nature of the Self. In this way, the

> "The highest virtue [for monks consists in] patience, humility, rectitude, purity, truthfulness, self-control, asceticism, renunciation, poverty, and chastity."
>
> —*Tattva-Artha-Adhigama-Sûtra* 9.6

quality of equanimity (*sâmâyika*) is fully cultivated in the individual. (147)

There is a certain extremism in some of the ascetic practices recommended in Jainism, like self-starvation, which do not seem to be in keeping with the ethical code of nonharming and which have therefore invited criticism from many quarters. These excesses derive from the Jainas' attitude toward physical existence, which is experienced as a source of suffering and painful limitation. The human body-mind is constantly to be chastised through fasting and other forms of penance until the human Spirit is freed from all physical bonds. Jainism, more than any other tradition, exemplifies the spirit of austerity (*tapas*), spoken of at some length in Chapter 3.

Notwithstanding this justifiable criticism, Jainism can look back on a long line of noble teachers and valiant aspirants who have demonstrated the supreme value of the yogic art of taking and keeping sacred vows. Both their spiritual resoluteness and their gentleness are an inspiration particularly to modern seekers, who do not always appreciate that spiritual life is an all-demanding transformative ordeal.

**SOURCE READING 7**

# *Yoga-Drishti-Samuccaya (Selection)*

*Translated by Christopher Key Chapple*

Haribhadra Sûri's *Yoga-Drishti-Samuccaya* ("Compendium of Views on Yoga"), which comprises 228 stanzas, is a very useful introduction to the yogic path from the Jaina perspective.

Desirous of Yoga, having bowed to the highest Jina, the strong one, [teacher of] the Yoga accessible to *yogins*, I will discourse throughout this composition on the distinctions of the Yoga system. (1)

Here indeed the essential form of the Yogas such as desire and so forth are considered, spoken for the benefit of *yogins*, out of fondness for Yoga. (2)

For the one who, although knowing the purposes of the scriptures and wanting to do them but is careless and deficient in *dharma-yoga*, there is what is called *icchâ-yoga*. (3)

*Shâstra-yoga* is known when, due to strength of intellect and speech, the powers of having no carelessness and no deficiency of faith arise. (4)

The way of beholding scripture is an excellent abode. However, due to its abundance of power, the especially highest Yoga is called exertion (*sâmarthya*). (5)

Indeed, there are different causes of the attainment of the steps called perfections; they are not always approached by the *yogins* from scriptural truths alone. (6)

There are two types of this [Yoga practice]: renunciation of *dharmas* [i.e., objects] and renunciation of Yoga. [Renunciation of] *dharmas* is complete annihilation of the desire to be active, and [renunciation of] Yoga is the [giving up of] the karma of the body and so forth. (9)

From having aligned oneself with true faith, one is considered [to hold] an "enlightened view," striking a blow against untrue [worldly] existence (*asat-pravritti*) and producing in stages true existence (*sat-pravritti*). (17)

The proper mind pays homage to the Jinas; purified, it does prostration, etc. This is the highest seed of Yoga. (23)

Endless devotion is to be followed, accompanied with the act of impeding mental activity. It is improper to have as one's intention the fruits of such action; one thus is indeed endowed with purity. (25)

This [devotion] is to be directed especially to teachers and the like; in such *yogins* arises a state of purity. Business is to be conducted according to the rules such that one has a particularly pure conscience. (26)

By nature, one's state of being becomes agitated and is thus maintained by receiving [karmic] substance (*dravya*). By injunction and by books, etc., one should resort to the final end [i.e., liberation]. (27)

When the defiled state is destroyed, a newly born hero arises. The mind is made unmanifest and there is no longer anything of importance to be done. (30)

It is declared that in the last birth of people the marks on their souls are destroyed, (31)

resulting in endless compassion for the afflicted, indifference to changes, and fitness for service, everywhere without distinction. (32)

Yoga, action, and its fruits are said to be the three authenticities (*avancaka-traya*). Depending on the highests saints is like the action of an arrow aimed at an object. (34)

This homage and so forth to the truths is the cause for firm practice, and it is the highest of causes. Then there is the diminution of impurity within one's being. (35)

Just as a sprouting seed when placed in salty water is cast away but in fresh water flourishes, so it is with a person who listens to truth. (61)

From observances people receive auspiciousness completely. One who has become well established in devotion to the *guru* brings benefit to the two worlds. (63)

Through the power of *guru* devotion, the vision of the *tîrthankaras* is seen. Through forms of meditation and so forth, one holds fast to *nirvâna* [as one's goal]. (64)

The mark of true [spiritual] endeavor (*sad-anushthâna*) is joy in exerting oneself, an absence of obstacles, proficiency in scriptures, the desire to know, and homage to the knowledgeable ones. (123)

The highest truth (*tattva*) of going beyond the world of change (*samsâra*) is called *nirvâna*. The wisdom gained from discipline is singular in truth, though heard of in different ways. (129)

That highest truth has no contradictory characteristic, is free from disturbance and disease, as well as activity. By that, one becomes free from birth, etc. (131)

Even the slightest pain to others is to be avoided with great effort. Along with this, one should strive to be helpful at all times. (150)

With faults diminished, omniscient, endowed with the fruits of all that can be accomplished, with things done now only for the sake of others, such a one attains the end of Yoga. (185)

There quickly the blessed one attains the highest *nirvâna*, from the disjunction (*ayoga*) that is the best of Yogas, having accomplished the cessation of the ailment of worldly existence. (186)

A person liberated from ailment is still in the world; just so is the [liberated person]. It is not that he is nonexistent and it is not that he is not liberated, nor that he had not been afflicted with ailment. (187)

Existence indeed is the great ailment, comprised of birth, death, and disease; it produces various forms of delusion and causes the sensation of excessive desire, and so forth. (188)

This is the chief [ailment] of the soul: giving birth without beginning to the cause of various karmas. All living beings have an understanding of this experience. (189)

When liberated from this, then one reaches the prime state of liberation. From the cessation of the fault of birth and so forth, one encounters that state of faultlessness. (190)

"Joyous is the appearance of the Buddhas. Joyous is the instruction in the true teaching (*dharma*). Joyous is the gathering of the Sangha. Joyous is the austerity of those who have gathered."

—*Dhamma-Pada* (14.16)

# *Chapter 7*

# YOGA IN BUDDHISM

## I. THE BIRTH AND EVOLUTION OF BUDDHISM

### Gautama the Buddha

Buddhism is the name given to the complex cultural tradition that has crystallized around the original teaching of Gautama (Gotama) the Buddha, who was probably born in 563 B.C.E. and died at the age of eighty. The sixth century was a time of profound cultural ferment and religious activity, particularly in the powerful kingdom of Mâgadha in southern Bihar, the homeland of early Buddhism. Mâgadha's ruling class and the population at large apparently were ill at ease with the orthodox post-Vedic priesthood. As the British historian Vincent A. Smith expressed it rather starkly:

> At that time the religion favoured by the Brahmans, as depicted in the treatises called *Brâhmanas*, was of a mechanical, lifeless character, overlaid with cumbrous ceremonial. The formalities of the irksome ritual galled

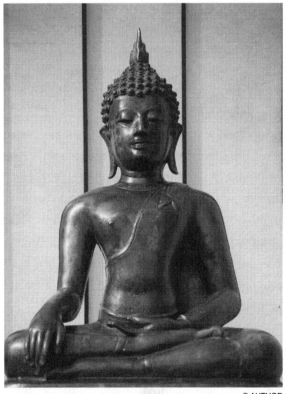

© AUTHOR

*Gautama the Buddha*

207

many persons, while the cruelty of the numerous bloody sacrifices was repugnant to others. People sought eagerly for some better path to the goal of salvation desired by all.[1]

Some of these dissenters found a haven in Jainism; others took refuge in the teaching of Gautama the Buddha. Gautama's life is only somewhat better known than that of Mahâvîra, the founder of Jainism. However, the Buddha's charismatic and benevolent personality speaks to us across the millennia in his sermons recorded in the Pali scriptures. The Buddha preached in the Mâgadhi dialect, and Pali is like Sanskrit, a sacred language that was first employed by the compilers of the Buddha's sayings and other early doctrinal works. As Christmas Humphreys, a well-known English Buddhist and popularizer of Buddhism, put it:

> His compassion was absolute . . . His dignity was unshakable, his humour invariable. He was infinitely patient as one who knows the illusion of time.[2]

Like Mahâvîra, Siddhârtha[3] Gautama was of aristocratic birth, born into the Shakya clan of Koshala, a country situated at the southern border of Nepal. After his enlightenment, he became known as the sage of the Shakyas, or Shakya-muni. Gautama grew up in the relative luxury and security of the ruling class of that period. Having become weary of his comfortable existence, he renounced the world at the age of twenty-nine and went in search of wisdom.

His quest brought him to two noted teachers who are mentioned by name in the Pali canon—Ârâda Kâlâpa (Pali: Âlâro Kâlâmo) of Mâgadha, who had three hundred disciples, and Rudraka Râmaputra (Pali: Uddako Râmaputto) of the city

of Vaishâlî, who had seven hundred disciples. The former appears to have taught a form of Upanishadic Yoga, culminating in the experience of the "sphere of no-thing-ness" (âkimcanya-âyatana). Apparently, Gautama had no difficulty entering that state, and consequently Ârâda Kâlâpa generously offered him to share the leadership of his order of ascetics. Gautama, feeling that he had not yet attained the highest possible realization, declined the offer.

Instead, he became a disciple of Rudraka Râmaputra, whose teaching promised further spiritual evolution. Again he easily achieved the state that this sage declared to be the ultimate realization—the experience of the "sphere of neither consciousness nor unconsciousness" (naiva-samjnâ-asamjnâ-âyatana), which may correspond to the Vedântic formless ecstasy (nirvikalpa-samâdhi). Gautama intuited that this exalted state also fell short of true enlightenment. Rudraka Râmaputra also offered to share with Gautama authority over his community, but the future Buddha declined and moved to Urubilvâ (Pali: Uruvelâ) on the Nairanjanâ River.

Here he resolved to practice, seated in the paryanka ("couch") posture, the deepest meditation for six years, wrestling down the passions of the body with an indomitable mind causing him to sweat profusely even during the cold winter nights. He nearly starved himself to death to assist this powerful meditation. Yet, after six long years of the fiercest self-mortification, Gautama had to admit to himself that this kind of torture, which made his limbs look like "the joints of withered creepers," was not the route to emancipation. Sensing that there must exist a middle way between uncompromising self-abnegation and the self-indulgent life of a worldling, he resumed begging for food, as had been his custom, and soon his body filled out and regained its strength. According to the mythological account given in the beautiful *Lalita-Vistara*, a well-loved Mahâyâna scripture, as soon as he had taken nourishment into his body, it started to glow in rainbow colors, manifesting the thirty-two marks (*lakshana*) of a Buddha.[4] Now confident of final success and remembering a spontaneous ecstatic experience he had enjoyed in his youth, Gautama surrendered himself to the spontaneous process of meditation.

In a single night of uninterrupted meditation, Gautama finally obtained the desired result—he became an awakened one (*buddha*). Tradition has it that he attained enlightenment on a full-moon day in May while seated under a fig tree—known as the *bodhi* or "enlightenment" tree—near the town of Uruvelâ (Bodhgayâ) in Mâgadha (Bihar). The Theravâda school of Sri Lanka recognized the full-moon day of May 1956 as the 2,500th anniversary of the Buddha's enlightenment.

For seven days Gautama the Buddha sat beneath the fig tree and applied his superb intelligence, now freed from all egoic desires and misconceptions, to understanding the mechanism of spiritual ignorance and bondage and the path to liberation. These deliberations were the foundation of his later teaching. After another seven days of silent contemplation and a short inner struggle, the Buddha resolved not to keep the newly acquired wisdom to himself but to impart it to others, to "beat the drum of the Immortal in the darkness of the world." Unfortunately, his two teachers had recently died, and so he could not share with them his great discovery. He immediately, however, sought out the five ascetics who, for a long time, had been his traveling companions but

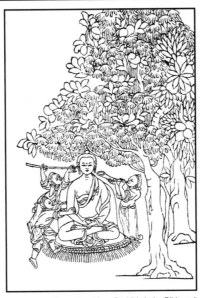

*Gautama under the fig tree*

who had left him when he abandoned his severe asceticism in favor of a meditation practice of his own design. He addressed his first sermon to them in the Deer Park of Sarnâth near modern Benares—an event remembered as the "turning of the wheel of the teaching" (*dharma-cakra-pravartana*). He spoke of his approach as the "middle way" (*madhya-mârga*), lying between the extremes of sensualism and asceticism, between world affirmation and world denial. He also disclosed the four noble truths of the omnipresence of suffering, desire as the cause of suffering, the removal of that cause, and the noble eightfold path (*ârya-ashta-anga-mârga*, written *âryâshtângamârga*).

The Buddha's teaching activity met with such rapid success that some people thought he was using magical means. Before long he was able to found monasteries from the generous funds of the royal court of King Bimbisâra of Râjagriha (modern Rajgir) and the rich merchant class, which welcomed a tolerant religion that disregarded the caste restrictions upheld by the brahmanical priesthood. For forty-five years, the Buddha wandered throughout northern India, teaching freely to anyone who came to listen to him. On one of his many tours he fell victim to dysentery. His final words, recorded in the Pali *Mahâ-Parinibbâna-Sutta* (Sanskrit: *Mahâ-Parinirvâna-Sûtra*), were:

Listen, O monks, I admonish you by saying: Composite things are impermanent. Exert yourselves with diligence! (61)

## The Spreading of the Buddha's Teaching

After the Buddha's death at Kushinâgara (Pali: Kusinârâ) in what is now Nepal, both the monastic order and the Buddhist lay community continued to prosper. The order included nuns as well, though it appears that the Buddha had been somewhat reluctant to ordain women. Then, in the third century B.C.E, during the reign of the famous emperor Ashoka of the Maurya dynasty, Buddhism was transformed from a local sect into a state religion.

The earliest record of the Buddha's teaching is the Pali canon, compiled and edited by three successive councils of the Buddhist order. The first council, which is of doubtful historicity, was convened in Râjagriha immediately after the death of the founder; the second was held in Vaishâlî about a hundred years later; and the third and most important was convened again in Râjagriha during Ashoka's reign. Soon afterward, Buddhism split into the two well-known traditions of Hînayâna ("Small Vehicle") and Mahâyâna ("Large Vehicle"), both claiming to possess the true original meaning of the Buddha's teaching. The former relied exclusively on the scriptures written in the sacred Pali language, and the latter based itself primarily on the scriptures composed in the sacred Sanskrit language. The differences between these two "vehicles" (*yâna*) increased as both schools evolved into distinct traditions.

The Hînayâna tradition, which survives today in the form of the Theravâda school of Sri Lanka, was individual oriented in so far as it placed the goal of the complete extinction (*nirvâna*) of desire above everything else. By contrast, the various Mahâyâna schools came to regard this approach as relatively barren and selfish and tried to replace it with a more holistic outlook. This included a revision of the value of the emotive and social aspects of human life and of the nature of the Buddhist goal itself. In keeping with this reorientation, *nirvâna* was no longer conceived as a goal "out there" but as the ever-present substratum underlying phenomenal existence: The famous Mahâyâna formula is *nirvâna* equals *samsâra*; that is, the immutable transcendental Reality is identical with the world of impermanence, and vice versa. What this means is that the realm of changeable forms is inherently empty (*shûnya*) and that *nirvâna* must not be sought outside *samsâra*. This fundamental proposition was first elaborated in the *Prajnâ-Pâramitâ-Sûtras* of about 200 B.C.E. and was philosophically consolidated in the fourth century C.E. by the Vijnânavâda and Yogâcâra schools, which will be discussed shortly. The best known *Prajnâ-Pâramitâ-Sûtra* is the *Hridaya-Sûtra* ("Heart *Sûtra*"), a rendering of which is given below as Source Reading 8. It emphasizes the central Mahâyâna doctrine of emptiness, or voidness.

In the fifth century C.E., Buddhism experienced a dramatic setback through the Hun invasions, during which much of its ancient heritage was destroyed. After a short period of recovery under the last native Indian emperor, Harsha, in the seventh century, a gradual decline set in. By the time of the Muslim usurpation of the kingdoms in the north of India, Buddhism had lost most of its force in India, not least because of the powerful missionary work of the Vedânta teacher Shankara, whose nondualist philosophy shows a great similarity with Mahâyâna Buddhism.

However, Buddhism fared better abroad—in Sri Lanka (Ceylon), Indonesia, China, and Japan. Already at the time of Ashoka, Buddhist monks had settled in the Far East, and in the first century C.E. Buddhism entered China, where it was destined to have a glorious future. From there the torch of Buddhist wisdom was carried to Japan in 550 C.E. Two hundred years later, Buddhism conquered Tibet and then, in the eighth century, Afghanistan.

Knowledge of Buddhism in Europe dates back to the time of Ashoka and Alexander the Great. Later, with the growing trade between India and the Mediterranean, Buddhism and also Hinduism became more influential among the European intelligentsia. Some historians have suggested, for instance, that Basilides of Alexandria owed much to Buddhist teachings. The influence of Buddhism on Christianity is perhaps best illustrated in the legend of Barlaam and Josaphat, as told by St. John of Damascus (eighth century C.E.). The legend is of Indian origin and reached the Church fathers through the circuitous route of translations into Pahlevi, Greek, and Latin. The Barlaam of the story is none other than the Buddha, and Josaphat stems from the Sanskrit word *bodhisattva* (distorted by the Arabs into *bodasaph* and, then, by the Greeks into *ioasaph*). In 1585, Barlaam was canonized, which makes the Buddha a Christian saint!

Renewed interest in Buddhism by Westerners was stimulated by the birth of the discipline of Indology (Indic studies) in the eighteenth century. It was in September of 1893, a few days after the closing ceremony of the Parliament of Religion, which had been convened in Chicago, that the first Westerner was admitted into the Buddhist order on American soil. Today there are an estimated 500,000 Buddhists in the United States alone.

## II. THE GREAT TEACHING OF THE SMALL VEHICLE— HÎNAYÂNA BUDDHISM

### The Literature of Hînayâna Buddhism

From the standpoint of the historian, the original teaching of the Buddha can no longer be identified with absolute certainty. However, considering the strong mnemonic tradition of India, there is good reason to believe that much of what has been handed down—first orally and then in written form—as the Buddha's Pali sermons (*sutta*), in fact contains the words of that extraordinary teacher. The Pali canon, upon which the Hînayâna branch of Buddhism bases itself, is known as the *Tipitaka* (Sanskrit *Tripitaka*, "Three Baskets").

The first basket, called *Vinaya-Pitaka*, contains the rules of monastic discipline (*vinaya*), which were recited from memory by Upali, the Buddha's oldest disciple, at the first council of the Sangha, shortly after the master's *parinirvâna*.

The oldest doctrinal information is contained in the *Sutta-Pitaka*, the second basket (*pitaka*) of the Pali canon, which was recited in full by Ânanda, the Buddha's cousin and personal attendant, who was blessed with a prodigious memory. It consists of the (edited) sermons or *suttas* (Sanskrit: *sûtra*) of the Buddha, which are arranged into five collections: the *Dîgha-Nikâya* (containing 34 long sermons), the *Majjhima-Nikâya* (containing 152 medium-length sermons), the *Samyutta-Nikâya* (containing 56 sermons organized by topics), the *Anguttara-Nikâya* (containing 2,308 sermons arranged according to the number of their themes), and the *Khuddaka-Nikâya* (containing 15 short works, including the famous *Dhamma-Pada*, the *Udâna*, and the *Sutta-Nipâta*).

The third basket is known as the *Abhidhamma-Pitaka*, comprising seven scholastic books, all belonging to the pre-Christian era. The original version of this basket of teachings was recited by Kassapa (Kashyapa), who presided over the first council in Râjagriha. The Pali term *abhidhamma* (Sanskrit: *abhidharma*) means "relating to the teaching" and is usually understood as signifying "higher teaching." It stands for the systematic philosophical treatment of the Buddha's *dhamma*.

The word *dhamma* (Sanskrit: *dharma*) means something like the "teaching that reflects the true law or order of the universe." For *dhamma* stands for both the teaching and the unchangeable reality, or law, expressed in it. Moreover, in Buddhism, the term can also signify an objective "thing" or a "real." In his outstanding work *A Survey of Buddhism*, the British Buddhist monk Bhikshu Sangharakshita makes this pertinent comment:

> *Dharma* (Pali: *dhamma*) is the keyword of Buddhism. So great is the frequency with which it appears in the texts, and so numerous the vitally important ideas connoted by its various shades of meaning, that it would scarcely be an exaggeration to claim that an understanding of this protean word is synonymous with an understanding of Buddhism.[5]

In addition to the canonical scriptures written in Pali, there are also numerous extracanonical texts recognized and used by the Hînayâna community. Among these works are the *Paritta* (a collection of twenty-eight texts used for magical purposes), the well-known *Milinda-Panha* (a dialogue between the Buddhist Nâgasena and the Bactrian king Milinda or Menander, who lived in the second century B.C.E.), the popular doctrinal manual *Visuddhi-Magga* of Buddhaghosa, and numerous commentaries and subcommentaries.

## The Four Noble Truths

The following discussion of Hînayâna Buddhism is based on the *Sutta-Pitaka* rather than the *Abhidhamma-Pitaka*, which some schools do not regard as giving authentic teachings of the Buddha. In this particular section, technical terms are in Pali, followed by their Sanskrit equivalents in parentheses.

The Buddha's teaching—generally referred to as the *dhamma* (*dharma*)—proceeds from the observation that life is sorrowful or *dukkha* (*duhkha*). This is the first of the four noble truths. The idea behind this insight, which the Buddhists share with the Hindus and Jainas, is this: Because everything is impermanent and does not afford us lasting happiness, our life is, in the last analysis, shot through with sorrow and pain. Thus we compete with others and even with ourselves, always in search of greater happiness, comfort, fulfillment, or security, and we feel dissatisfied even in our attainments.

In the final analysis, suffering is the tension that is intrinsic to our effort to survive as separate, egoic personalities, or individuals. But that individuality is merely a carefully maintained illusion, a convenient psychosocial convention. In truth, says the Buddha, there is no inner self. The doctrine of "no-self" or *anattâ* (*anâtman*) is fundamental to his teaching. It is probable that the Buddha emphasized the inessential nature of the human personality and of existence in general in order to counter the idealism to which the Upanishadic teachings had given rise. By insisting that the ultimate Reality was identical with the innermost core of the human being, the Self or *âtman*, the Upanishadic sages indirectly encouraged the delusion that there is, after all, an immortal personal essence. The Buddha rejected all conjectures about an immutable self-essence as futile and entertained the same position in regard to metaphysical speculations in general. However, it is evident from his recorded sayings that he occasionally availed himself of a language reminiscent of the *Upanishads*. On this point, Mahâyâna Buddhism is far more easygoing than the Buddha himself.

In any case, the Buddha's pragmatic approach exemplifies what is best in the tradition of yogic experimentalism, and it is in this spirit that the first truth, about suffering, as well as the other three truths must be understood: They must be deeply *felt* rather than merely *thought* about in abstract terms, so that they can make their point in a person's life.

The second truth is that desire, the thirst or *tanhâ* (*trishnâ*) for life—corresponding to Nietzsche's "will to live"—is the cause of the universally experienced suffering.[6] Our very cells are genetically programmed to perpetuate the biological conglomerate that we call "our" body-mind: We desire to be alive as individuals, and yet our very individuality is the factor that complicates our existence, because we separate ourselves from everything else and then look for ways to reduce or overcome the resulting sense of isolation and fear. We approach the matter from the wrong end, however. We tinker with our experiences rather than allow our understanding to penetrate to the root of our separative disposition and its accompanying survival motive. Since desire is anchored in ignorance of our true nature, the Mahâyâna teachers look upon ignorance rather than desire as the cause of suffering.

The third truth affirms that it is through the radical elimination of that innate craving, or thirst, that we can remove all experience of sorrow and win through to what is real and true. It is not enough to modify or reduce desire, because even a modified or reduced desire is still a binding force. Desire must be completely eradicated if we want to find inner peace and freedom.

The fourth truth states that the means of eradicating our craving is the noble eightfold path declared by the Buddha. That path consists in the gradual "dis-illusionment" of our egoic personality; that is, the step-by-step undermining of what we presume ourselves and the world to be, until the truth shines forth. Upon attaining the supreme condition of *nirvâna*, all suffering is transcended, because the illusory entity that is the source of suffering is fully abrogated. The force of desire is neutralized. In other words, the enlightened being is no longer an individuated person, even though the personality continues to manifest its typical (if purified) character.

Closely connected with the doctrine of the universality of suffering is the doctrine of moral causation or *kamma* (*karma*) and the correlated teaching of rebirth. Both hold a central position in Buddhist metaphysics and ethics, though the Buddha's teaching can be said to remain valid even when these are rejected. Buddhism distinguishes between two principal forms of *kamma*, namely wholesome *kamma* and unwholesome *kamma*. It is the interaction between these two types and their total effect on the individual that keep the wheel of existence in incessant rotation. As in Jainism, there is no God who could interfere in the nexus of birth and death or to whom beings are ultimately responsible. Instead, it is the mental activity of each individual, whether expressed in action or not, that alone determines his or her future through the moral law of causation inherent in the universe.

## The Doctrine of Dependent Origination

The important idea of moral causation is given formal expression in the well-known Buddhist symbol of the wheel of life or *bhava-cakka* (*bhava-cakra*), which has the following twelve links:

1. ignorance or *avijjâ* (*avidyâ*) leads to

2. action-intentions or *sankhâra* (*samskâra*), giving rise to

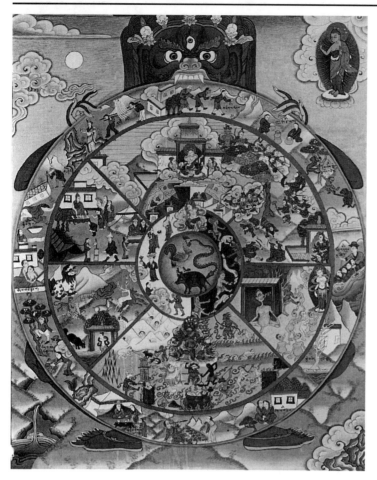

*The wheel of becoming*

9. grasping or *upâdana*, which leads to

10. becoming or *bhava*, from which results

11. birth or *jâti*, and then

12. old age and death or *jarâ-marana*.

This ancient Buddhist formula bears the name *paticca-samuppâda* (*pratîtya-samutpâda*) or "dependent origination," and it explains the relationship between the individual links of the nexus of cause and effect, which is meant to elucidate the sequence of births and deaths. It is important to realize that this whole process is thought to take place without a continuous entity, or soul, experiencing it. As I have noted, according to the Buddha, there is no abiding self that suffers repeated births. As Hans-Wolfgang Schumann puts it:

3. consciousness or *vinnâna* (*vijnâna*) from which arise

4. name and form or *nâma-rûpa*; from this originates

5. the sixfold base or *sal-âyatana* (*shad-âyatana*), that is, the objective world, which, in turn, yields

6. sense-contact or *phassa* (*sparsha*); this leads to

7. sensation or *vedanâ*, which effects

8. craving or *tanhâ* (*trishnâ*), and this gives rise to

Since there is no immortal Self which runs through the various lives like a silk thread through a string of pearls, it cannot be the same person who reaps the fruit of kammic seeds of past existences in rebirth. On the other hand the reborn person is not completely different, for each form of existence is caused by, and proceeds from, its previous existence like a flame which is lit by another one. The truth lies between identity and isolation: in conditional dependence.[7]

How this is possible becomes clear when it is understood that in Buddhism the continuous being that we ordinarily perceive ourselves or others to be is a mental construct. In reality, it is an unstable configuration of five distinct and short-lived factors or groups (*khandha, skandha*):

1.  body (*rûpa*)

2.  sensation (*vedanâ*)

3.  perception (*sannâ, samjnâ*)

4.  mental activity (*sankhâra, samskâra*)

5.  consciousness (*vinnâna, vijnâna*).

Factors 2–5 are also collectively referred to as "name" (*nâma*), which is the counterpoint to the human "form" (*rûpa*), or body. Both name and form must be transcended, which is a teaching found already in the earliest *Upanishads*.

The Buddha's denial of a transmigrating soul, or essential self, has led many students of Buddhism to the assumption that he rejected a transcendental Reality outright. This is not the case. Many passages in the Pali canon describe the ultimate condition of *nirvâna* in positive terms. It is also called "shelter," "refuge," and "security." But, more typically, the ultimate Reality, and thus also the enlightened being, is described in negative terms. In the words of the Buddha, recorded in the *Sutta-Nipâta*:

> As a flame blown out by the wind goes to rest and is lost to cognition, just so the sage (*muni*) who is released from name (*nâma*) [i.e., mind] and body (*kâya*), goes to rest and is lost to cognition. (1074)

And:

> There is no measure for him who has gone to rest, and he has nothing that could be named. When all things are abandoned, all paths of language are likewise abandoned. (1076)

Thus, the rational teaching of the Buddha terminates in the ineffable condition of *nirvâna*. Concepts and words can be helpful to spiritual seekers until they have discovered what is Real for themselves. Of course, language can also be a hindrance, because it entices us to "thingify" concepts, to treat words as if they were objective things. After enlightenment, however, language loses its fascination and is never again confused with reality.

## III. THE YOGIC PATH OF HÎNAYÂNA BUDDHISM

The description of the theoretical foundations of Buddhism may have given the impression that the teaching of the Buddha is schematic and philosophical rather than practical, but nothing could be farther from the truth. The Buddha was a dedicated *yogin* with a passion and unique gift for meditative absorption, and his teaching was primarily designed to show a concrete way out of the maze of spiritually ignorant and hence sorrowful existence.

Like Patanjali's Yoga, the Yoga of the Buddha comprises eight distinct members or "limbs" (*anga*). Hence it is known as the "noble eightfold path." The Buddha also referred to it as the "supermundane path" (*loka-uttara-magga*),[8] because it is meant for those who are seriously committed to self-transcending practice—that is, for monks and nuns. The Buddha was convinced that a person could attain enlightenment within seven days of "setting forth," that is, of taking up the life of a mendicant monk or nun.

Following are the eight limbs of the path, which should not be viewed as stages or rungs of a ladder:

1. *Samma-ditthi* (*samyag-drishti*[9]) or "right vision" is the realization of the transiency of conditioned existence and the understanding that there is indeed no self.

2. *Samma-sankappa* (*samyak-samkalpa*) or "right resolve" is the threefold resolution to renounce what is ephemeral, to practice benevolence, and to not hurt any being.

3. *Samma-vâcâ* (*samyag-vâcâ*) or "right speech" is the abstention from idle and false talk.

4. *Samma-kammantâ* (*samyak-karmantâ*) or "right conduct" consists mainly in abstention from killing, stealing, and illicit sexual intercourse.

5. *Samma-âjîva* (*samyag-âjîva*) or "right livelihood" is the abstention from deceit, usury, treachery, and soothsaying in procuring one's sustenance.

6. *Samma-vayama* (*samyag-vyayama*) or "right exertion" is the prevention of future unwholesome mental activity, the overcoming of present unwholesome feelings or thoughts, the cultivation of future wholesome states of mind, and the maintenance of present wholesome psychomental activity.

7. *Samma-sati* (*samyak-smriti*) or "right mindfulness" is the cultivation of awareness of the psychosomatic processes by means of such practices as the favorite Theravâda (Hînayâna) technique of *sati-patthâna*, consisting in the mindful observation of otherwise unconscious activities, like breathing or body movement.

8. *Samma-samâdhi* (*samyak-samâdhi*) or "right concentration" is the practice of certain techniques for the internalization and transcendence of consciousness.

The first two members of the noble eightfold path are said to deal with understanding (*pannâ*, *prajnâ*), the next three deal with behavior (*sila*, *shîla*), and the last three with concentration (*samâdhi*). The first five can also be grouped under the heading of socio-ethical regulations, while the remaining three members are specifically yogic. Exertion and mindfulness can and should be practiced throughout the entire day, but concentration (*samâdhi*) represents a special discipline for which undisturbed quiet is essential.

*Samâdhi*—in the Buddhist sense of intense mental collectedness—comprises the meditative phases from sensory withdrawal up to ecstasy, known as *jhâna* in Pali or *dhyâna* in Sanskrit. There are eight such *jhânas*:

1. *jhâna* accompanied by discursive thought and the feeling of rapturous joy (*pîti-sukha*, *prîti-sukha*);

2. *jhâna* unaccompanied by discursive thought, but still suffused with the feeling of joy;

3. *jhâna* in which the experience of joy has yielded to the subtle joy of tranquil mindfulness;

4. *jhâna* in which any kind of emotion is stopped and all that remains is utter mindfulness;

5. the mystical realization of the "sphere of space-infinity" (*âkâsa-ananca-âyatana, âkâsha-ananta-âyatana* [10]);

6. the mystical realization of the "sphere of consciousness-infinity" (*vinnâ-ananca-âyatana, vijnâna-ananta-âyatana* [11]);

7. the mystical realization of the "sphere of no-thing-ness" (*âkincanna-âyatana, âkimcanya-âyatana* [12]);

8. the mystical realization of the "sphere of neither cognition nor noncognition" (*neva-sannâ-na-asannâ-âyatana, naiva-samjnâ-asamjnâ-âyatana* [13]).

The first four are called *rûpa-jhânas* or meditations with "form" (*rûpa*), or cognitive contents, while the last four are technically known as *arûpa-jhânas* or "formless" (*arûpa*) meditations. Beyond these eight stages lies, as the *Udâna* (80) has it, *nibbâna* (*nirvâna*) itself:

> . . . a realm where there is neither the earth nor water, neither fire nor air, neither ether nor consciousness . . . neither this world nor any other world, neither sun nor moon.

The yogic nature of the Buddha's path is further evinced by the use of such techniques as posture (*âsana*) and control of the life force (*prânâyâma*).

The technical Pali term for vital force (*prâna*) in Buddhism is *kâya-sankhâra*, which means literally "bodily constituent." As opposed to the Hindu schools of Yoga, Hînayâna Buddhism does not advocate the stoppage of the vital force in the form of forced breath retention, which might do violence to the natural body. Instead, the practitioner is advised to follow the movement of the breath with the mind. This is a particular application of the technique of mindfulness (*sati*, *smriti*). This technique, known in Pali as *sati-patthâna*, is widely employed in modern Theravâda, the oldest surviving school of the Hînayâna tradition.

The most commonly adopted meditation posture is the *pallanka* (*paryanka*) seat, as depicted in innumerable seated Buddha statues. The texts emphasize erect bodily posture (*uju-kâya*), undoubtedly because experience shows that in this way both breathing and mental concentration can be considerably improved.

The *yogin* who has penetrated through all delusive phenomena by virtue of single-mindedness in the highest stage of *jhâna* enters *nibbâna*. Because the Buddha denied the notion of a continuous entity abiding within the flux of phenomenal existence, he has been accused of nihilism, but against this charge he defended himself on several occasions. When liberation is attained, it is no longer possible to say anything meaningful about the nature of the liberated or enlightened being—whether he or she exists or does not exist. Freedom is a paradox or mystery. It is to be discovered rather than talked about.

This fact, however, did not scare the Buddha's followers into silence. Over the centuries, Buddhist monastics, as well as educated lay followers, have interpreted and reinterpreted the Buddha's legacy, trying to make it accessible for their contemporaries. Not only did the Buddhist community spawn hosts of scholars, it also birthed many great *yogins* and enlightened adepts, who periodically regenerated the spiritual basis of Buddhism. Their revitalization of the Buddha's *dharma* has often had effects far beyond the sphere of Buddhism. Thus, the Buddhist teachings have exerted a significant influence on many schools of Hinduism, including the tradition of Yoga.

If the Buddha was indebted to adepts who taught an early form of Yoga, Patanjali (who gave Yoga its classical philosophical shape) in turn owed an intellectual debt to Mahâyâna Buddhism. The long historical interplay between Buddhism and Hinduism reached its peak in the sweeping cultural movement of Tantrism, starting in the middle of the first millennium C.E. It gave rise to schools that are not easily identified as either Buddhist or Hindu, as can clearly be seen in the Siddha cult, described in Chapter 17. What they all have in common, however, is a passion for personal realization, for yogic experimentation with the hidden potential of the human body-mind.

## IV. WISDOM AND COMPASSION— THE GREAT IDEALISM OF MAHÂYÂNA BUDDHISM

### The Literature of Mahâyâna Buddhism

Upon his enlightenment, the Buddha resolved not to taste the bliss of *nirvâna* to the full, thereby abandoning his human body-mind, but to compassionately reveal the path of enlightenment to others. The Buddha's decision to combine wisdom (*prajnâ*) with compassion (*karunâ*) has served many of his followers over the centuries as a guiding ideal. Mahâyâna Buddhism arose in response to the widely felt need within the Buddhist community to cultivate the feminine aspect of the spiritual path, as expressed in the virtue of compassion. It has sometimes been viewed as the

creation of lay followers, but this is mistaken. As much as Hînayâna, the Mahâyâna approach is the product of learned monks who sought to articulate the Buddha's teaching in ways accessible to their contemporaries.

The Mahâyâna teachings are enshrined in the *Sûtras*, which were composed in Sanskrit between the first century B.C.E. and the sixth century C.E. Unlike the *Sûtras* of Hinduism, which are aphoristic works, the Mahâyâna *Sûtras* are narrative scriptures. They are presented as the authentic sayings of the Buddha, corresponding to the earlier *Suttas* of the Pali canon.

Among the more important scriptures of this genre are the *Prajnâ-Pâramitâ-Sûtras*, the earliest of which is the *Ashtâ-Sâhasrikâ-Sûtra* ("The Eight Thousand") composed in the pre-Christian era, though the most popular are undoubtedly the *Hridaya-* ("Heart") and the *Vajra-Chedikâ-* ("Diamond Cutter") *Sûtras*. The longest work of this genre is the *Shata-Sâhasrikâ-Sûtra* which, as the name indicates, consists of 100,000 verses. Mention must also be made of the *Abhisamaya-Alamkâra*, an exegetical scripture attributed to the transcendental *bodhisattva* Maitreya. Lex Hixon, an American writer and spiritual teacher, said of the

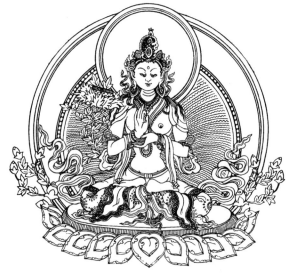

*Reproduced from* Buddhistische Bilderwelt

*Prajnâpâramitâ*

*Ashta-Sâhasrikâ* that its "teachings are fresh as a dew-covered flower—even now, after some two thousand years."[14] His comments apply to the other *Prajnâ-Pâramitâ* works as well.

Other well-known and much-loved *Sûtras*, belonging to the first centuries C.E., are the *Sad-Dharma-Pundarîka* ("Lotus of the True Teaching") and the *Lankâ-Avatâra*, commonly spelled *Lankâvatâra* ("Descent of Lankâ"). The Canadian scholar Edward Conze estimated that a mere two per cent of the Mahâyâna *Sûtras* have so far been "intelligibly translated."[15]

In addition, there are numerous secondary works produced over the centuries by thinkers and poets of the various Mahâyâna schools and in different languages, notably Sanskrit, Tibetan, and Chinese.

## *The Doctrine of Emptiness*

At the core of Mahâyâna thought lies the realization that *nirvâna* is not something that is external to the phenomenal universe, but that it is both immanent and transcendental. For the Mahâyâna adherent, suffering (*duhkha*) is not, as the followers of Hînayâna proclaim, something that can only be avoided by opting out from the world. Instead, it is an illusion that can be rectified through proper insight, and which does not call for any flight from the world. Thus, the realistic philosophy of the Hînayâna tradition is replaced by the stately nondualist conception of reality that we also meet in the Upanishads of Hinduism: There is One, which appears as many. As the author of the *Vajra-Chedikâ-Sûtra*, an old Mahâyâna text, declares:

> [Like] a star, a fault-of-vision, a lamp, an
> illusion, a dew drop, a bubble, a dream,
> a lightning flash or a cloud—thus should

the composite [phenomena] be viewed. (32)

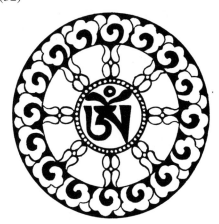

*Tibetan om symbol*

The phenomena are said to be void (*shûnya*) because they lack essence. There is only universal voidness (*shûnyatâ*), which is itself void. The Buddhist notion of voidness or emptiness is not readily grasped, and it is all too easy to dismiss it as Oriental mythologizing, whereas it is a very sophisticated philosophical notion grounded in spiritual experience. That this central Mahâyâna idea caused even Easterners some difficulty is borne out by the story of Bandhudatta, the erstwhile Kashmiri preceptor of the famous Mahâyâna teacher Kumârajîva. After his acceptance of the Mahâyâna creed, Kumârajîva naturally tried to share his newly won insight into the empty nature of things with his former teacher. But Bandhudatta would hear none of it. He deemed the doctrine of emptiness to be mere empty talk. To underscore his position, he told the following story.

A madman once asked a weaver to spin him the finest cloth possible. The weaver tried his utmost best, but the madman twice rejected his work as being too coarse. When the madman returned a third time, the weaver pointed into the air, saying that he had woven a cloth so fine that it was now invisible. The madman was delighted, paid the weaver, and picked up the invisible cloth to present it to the king.

Kumârajîva was unruffled by his teacher's hostile attitude and eventually succeeded in converting him. Emptiness is not nothingness, but no-thing-ness. When we consider phenomena most profoundly, they reveal themselves to us as illusory. But even this illusoriness is illusory, for, practically speaking, there are phenomena that form the content of our experiences. In reality, *nirvâna* and *samsâra* are both constructions of the unillumined mind, and the *yogin* must rise beyond them.

---

**SOURCE READING 8**

# *Prajnâ-Pâramitâ-Hridaya-Sûtra*

The earliest Mahâyâna *Sûtras* were composed anonymously in South India between 100 B.C.E. and 100 C.E., though according to tradition they are attributed to the Buddha himself. The most important scrip-

ture of that early period is the *Ashtâ-Sâhasrikâ-Prajnâ-Pâramitâ-Sûtra* ("Perfection of Wisdom Sûtra in 8,000 [Lines]"). Subsequently, longer and longer versions were written, which were then recondensed. The most popular of these Sanskrit condensations is the *Prajnâ-Pâramitâ-Hridaya-Sûtra*, or Heart Sûtra for short, which was perhaps composed around 300 C.E. Edward Conze, who translated several *Prajnâ-Pâramitâ* scriptures, remarked about the Heart Sûtra that it "alone can be said to have gone really to the heart of the doctrine," meaning the doctrine of emptiness.[16]

This scripture exists in two recensions, one consisting of only fifteen lines, the other of twenty-five lines (translated in this book). The shorter version appears to be the earlier one, as is attested to by the Chinese translation of Kumârajîva (c. 400 C.E.), while the longer version was translated into Chinese by Dharmacandra in 741 C.E.

The teachings of the Heart Sûtra are communicated by the transcendental *bodhisattva* Avalokiteshvara (Tibetan: Chenrezig). The doctrine of emptiness is closely associated with the *bodhisattva* ideal. Even though all things and beings are empty of essence, the *bodhisattva* nevertheless is paradoxically dedicated to liberating these phantom beings. He (or she) cannot bear to witness the suffering of others and seeks to guide them to the liberating wisdom so that

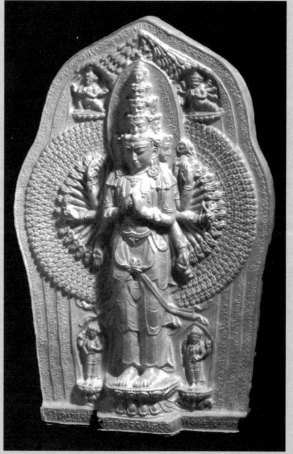

© JAMES RHEA

*Avalokiteshvara, embodiment of compassion*

they, too, may realize the ultimate Reality beyond all appearances. Even though suffering, like any finite experience, is empty, those who suffer firmly believe in their pain because their minds are clouded with ignorance. Upon enlightenment, all suffering is transcended because the deluded mind is transcended together with all phenomena. The *bodhisattva* aspires to attain enlightenment for the ultimate benefit of others.

*Om.* Homage to the Holy and Noble Perfection of Wisdom!

Thus have I heard.

At one time the Lord dwelled at Râjagriha on Vulture Peak Mountain together with a large gathering of monks and a large gathering of *bodhisattvas.*

At that time the Lord, having spoken on the course of *dharma* called "Profound Splendor," entered into concentration.

At that time also the Noble Avalokiteshvara, the great being and *bodhisattva*, was engaged in the practice of the profound Perfection of Wisdom, reflecting thus:

"The five aggregates are by nature empty," he reflected.

Thereupon the long-lived Shâriputra, through the Buddha's influence, said to the Noble Avalokiteshvara, the great being and *bodhisattva*:

"How should one teach a son of good family or a daughter of good family who wishes to practice the profound Perfection of Wisdom?"

Thus spoken to, the Noble Avalokiteshvara, the great being and *bodhisattva*, said to the long-lived Shâriputra:

"O Shâriputra, a son of good family or a daughter of good family wishing to practice the profound Perfection of Wisdom should reflect as follows:"

'The Noble Avalokiteshvara, the *bodhisattva*, engaged in the practice of the profound Perfection of Wisdom and reflected and saw that the five aggregates are by nature empty.'

"Here, O Shâriputra, form is emptiness and emptiness is form. Emptiness is not different from form, and form is not different from emptiness. That which is form is emptiness, and that which is emptiness is form. So it is also with sensations, perceptions, impulses, and consciousness."

"Here, O Shâriputra, all things are marked by emptiness, and are neither produced nor stopped, neither defiled nor immaculate, neither deficient nor complete."

"Therefore, O Shâriputra, in emptiness there is no form, no sensation, no perception, no impulses, no consciousness; there is no eye, ear, nose, tongue, body, or mind; there is no visible object, sound, smell, taste, tangible object, or mental object; there is no eye element and so on up to no mental consciousness element; there is no ignorance and no absence of ignorance and so on up to no old age and death or the absence of old age and death; there is no suffering, origination, cessation, or path; no knowledge, no attainment, and no nonattainment."

"Therefore, O Shâriputra, the *bodhisattva* is free from attainment, relies only on the Perfection of Wisdom, and lives without mental veils. Free from mental veils, he transcends misconceptions and abides having *nirvâna* as his summit."

"By relying on the Perfection of Wisdom, all the Buddhas who appear in the three times awaken to unsurpassed, complete enlightenment."

"Therefore one should know the Perfection of Wisdom, the great *mantra*, the *mantra* of great knowledge, the unsurpassed *mantra*, the *mantra* unlike any other, which alleviates all suffering and is the truth because it is free from error."

"The *mantra* of the Perfection of Wisdom is uttered thus:
TADYATHÂ OM GATE GATE PARAGATE PARASAMGATE BODHI SVÂHÂ."

# तद्यथा ॐ गते गते परगते परसंगते बोधि स्वाहा ॥

*Tadyathâ om gate gate paragate parasamgate bodhi svâhâ*

"Thus, O Shâriputra, a *bodhisattva* should be taught in the practice of the profound Perfection of Wisdom."

Thereupon the Lord emerged from his concentration and spoke approvingly to the Noble Avalokiteshvara, the great being and *bodhisattva*, thus:

"Well said, well said, O Son of Good Family! Just so, O Son of Good Family, just so should the practice of the profound Perfection of Wisdom be engaged. As you have explained it, so it is sanctioned by all the worthy *tathâgatas*."[17]

Thus spoke the Lord. The enraptured long-lived Shâriputra; the Noble Avalokiteshvara, the great being and *bodhisattva*; the monks; the *bodhisattva*s, those great beings; and the entire world with its deities, humans, demons, eagle spirits, and celestial spirits rejoiced in the Lord's speech.

Thus ends the Noble *Prajnâ-Pâramitâ-Hridaya*.

## The Bodhisattva Ideal

While the Hînayâna tradition was almost exclusively interested in the individual's salvation, the followers of the Mahâyâna school rejected this approach and sought to incorporate social values into the path to emancipation—the *bodhisattva* ideal. The spiritual hero of the Hînayâna tradition was and still is the *arhat*, the "worthy one," who has attained enlightenment. The Buddhist texts give an esoteric etymology for the designation *arhat*, deriving the word from *ari* ("enemy") and the root *han* ("to kill"). The idea behind this is that the *arhat* has killed or deadened the enemy of passion.

The *bodhisattva* ideal can be seen as an extension of the earlier *arhat* ideal, for *bodhisattvas* too are committed to transcending the self in their effort to dispel spiritual darkness

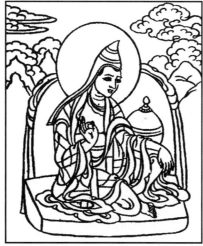

*Shântideva (from a woodblock)*

in other beings. They are the beings (*sattva*) dedicated to enlightenment (*bodhi*) for the sake of others. It is wrong to assume, as some Western writers have done, that *bodhisattvas* postpone their own enlightenment in order to help others. Rather, they make an all-out effort to attain enlightenment so that they can serve others more in their own struggle for enlightenment. Even before their enlightenment, *bodhisattvas* are motivated by compassion for all other beings—a compassion that increases infinitely once they have attained enlightenment. What *bodhisattvas* postpone is full liberation (*parinirvâna*), which would lift them out of the realms of conditioned existence where beings are suffering. In the *Bodhi-Caryâ-Avâtara*[18] of Shântideva (early eighth century C.E.), the *bodhisattva's* benign attitude is described as follows:

I am medicine for the sick. May I be their physician and their nurse until their sickness is gone. (3.7)

Having dedicated myself to the happiness of all embodied beings, may they strike me! May they revile me! May they constantly cover me with dirt! (3.12)

May they play with my body and laugh at or toy with me! Having given my body to them, why should I be concerned? (3.13)

May those who denounce, injure, and mock me, as well as all others, share in enlightenment! (3.16)

May I be a protector for those without protection, a guide for travelers, a boat, a bridge, a passage for those desiring the farther shore. (3.17)

For all embodied beings, may I be a lamp for those in need of a lamp. May I be a bed for those in need of a bed. May I be a servant for those in need of a servant. (3.18)

For all embodied beings, may I be a wish-granting gem, a miraculous urn, a magical science, a panacea, a wish-fulfilling tree, and a cow of plenty. (3.19)

There are ten stages (*bhûmi*) that *bodhisattvas* must traverse, which are understood as degrees of perfection (*pâramitâ*). They can embark on the *bodhisattva* career only after the "consciousness directed to enlightenment" (*bodhi-citta*) has awakened in them. That *bodhi-citta*, which is often misleadingly translated as "thought of enlightenment," is an empowered aspiration. It is the will to transcend everything, which is a rare thing indeed. The poet-philosopher and adept Shântideva, author of the *Shikshâ-Samuccaya* ("Compendium on Discipline") and *Bodhi-Caryâ-Avâtara* ("Entering the Conduct of Enlightenment"), compares the generation of the *bodhi-citta* to a blind person finding a jewel in a dunghill. And Shântideva marvels at the fact that the *bodhi-citta* should have arisen in his own case. The following are the ten stages of the *bodhisattva* path:

1. The joyful (*pramuditâ*) stage: After having taken the *bodhisattva* vow to be entirely dedicated to the salvation of other beings by postponing their own liberation, *bodhisattvas* then cultivate to perfection (*pâramitâ*) the virtue of open-handedness (*dâna*), that is, the liberal giving of themselves to others. This term is generally translated as "generosity."

2. The immaculate (*vimalâ*) stage: They cultivate the virtue of self-discipline (*shîla*).

3. The radiant (*prabhâkarî*) stage: Acquiring insight into the transiency of conditioned existence, they develop the supreme virtue of patience (*kshânti*).

4. The blazing (*arcishmatî*) stage: They cultivate willpower (*vîrya*).

5. The very-difficult-to-conquer (*su-dur-jayâ*) stage: They work on perfecting their meditative absorption (*dhyâna*).

6. The stage that is "present" (*abhimukhî*): They gain supreme liberation, which reveals to them the identity of phenomenal existence and *nirvâna* after death. However, they are prevented from doing so by their vow; hence they enter the "nonstatic" (*apratishtha*) *nirvâna* and continue to work for the good of all beings.

7. The far-going (*dûrangamâ*) stage: They become transcendental *bodhisattvas* freed from their human body but able to assume any shape at will. They now acquire perfection in expediency or skill (*upâya*).

8. The unshakable (*acalâ*) stage: They acquire the power to transfer wholesome karma to other beings to ease their karmic burden and speed up their spiritual growth.

9. The good-thought (*sadhumatî*) stage: They increase their effort of liberating beings as one of the great transcendental *bodhisattvas*.

10. The cloud-of-*dharma* stage: They have now fully consolidated their all-embracing knowledge (*jnâna*), and their "thusness/suchness" (*tathatâ*) radiates throughout the universe like a rain cloud shedding water. The phrase *dharma-megha*, or "cloud of *dharma*," is also found in Patanjali's Classical Yoga, where it is given a similar meaning by some interpreters.

Viewed from a Hindu perspective, the Mahâyâna path represents a synthesis between Jnâna-Yoga and Karma-Yoga, the personal cultivation of ever deeper transcending awareness (*prajnâ*) and its translation into benevolent activity for the ultimate good of all beings.

## The Doctrine of the Three Bodies of the Buddha

Mahâyâna Buddhism emerged long after the death of the historical Buddha. For the Mahâyâna followers the human Buddha was a temporary projection of the Absolute. The true Buddha is the transcendental Reality itself, which is beyond space-time. This important notion is epitomized in the Mahâyâna doctrine of the "triple body" (*tri-kâya*) of the Buddha. The three bodies are:

1. the "body of the law" (*dharma-kâya*), which is the absolute or transcendental dimension of existence;

2. the "body of enjoyment" (*sambhoga-kâya*), which is the psychic or inner dimension composed of numerous "transcendental" Buddhas;

3. the "body of creation" (*nirmâna-kâya*), which refers to the flesh-and-blood bodies of the Buddhas in human form, of which there have been many.

Thus, only in his transcendental essence is the Buddha singular. On the physical and psychic (or subtle) levels, there are many Buddhas. The next Buddha to descend into the physical realm is Maitreya ("He who is friendly"), who is now a transcendental *bodhisattva* residing in the Tushita Heaven. He and the other transcendental or celestial *bodhisattvas*—such as Avalokiteshvara and

Manjushrî—belong to the *sambhoga-kâya* of the Buddha. At the highest—tenth—level of the *bodhisattva* path, the *bodhisattva* is spiritually so elevated that some texts speak of him as a *buddha*.

These great beings (*mahâ-sattva*), whether they are called *buddhas* or *bodhisattvas*, are invoked by the followers of Mahâyâna as agents of grace. Thus, unlike Hînayâna, the Mahâyâna schools typically understand the spiritual process as a combination of self-effort and graceful intervention from the Buddhas and celestial *bodhisattvas*. Hence there is a place in the Mahâyâna approach for the discipline of meditation as well as prayer and worship, which corresponds to Bhakti-Yoga in Hinduism. This is an instance of what has been called the eclecticism of Mahâyâna—an eclecticism, however, that is a strength rather than a weakness.

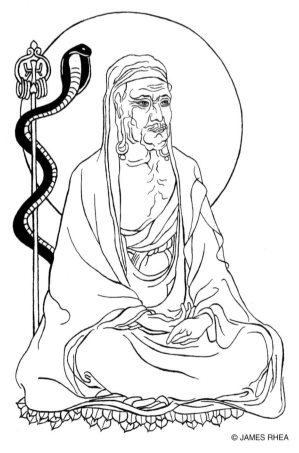

© JAMES RHEA

*Nâgârjuna*

## The Mâdhyamika School

The philosophical teachings of Mahâyâna, as found in the *Prajnâ-Pâramitâ* literature, were consolidated by the thinkers of the Shûnyavâda or Mâdhyamika school, notably Nâgârjuna (second century C.E.) and his chief disciple Âryadeva. Nâgârjuna's principal work is the influential *Mâdhyamika-Kârikâ*, on which numerous commentaries have been written. His lasting contribution to Buddhist metaphysics was his dialectics, by which he tried to demonstrate that the ultimate Reality cannot be described satisfactorily either in positive or in negative terms. For this great Buddhist thinker and adept, essentiality (*svabhâvatâ*) is that which is uncreated or unborn and which is therefore eternal. The world, by contrast, lacks such essence, and for this reason is deemed void. The transcendental Void is so called because it is empty of all possible limiting conditions.

Nâgârjuna did for Indian philosophy what Kant did for Western philosophy. Both managed to shatter metaphysical thought through strictly logical means. Yet, unlike Kant, Nâgârjuna is remembered not only as a formidable philosopher and the "father of the Mahâyâna" but also as a spiritually accomplished master (*siddha*), an alchemist, and a miracle worker about whom countless legends have been woven.[19]

**SOURCE READING 9**

## *Mahâyâna-Vimshaka of Nâgârjuna*

This short but important work on Mahâyâna philosophy is extant only in Tibetan and Chinese versions but has been reconstructed in Sanskrit by the Indian scholar Vidhusekhara Bhattacharya. The present rendering is based on this reconstruction.

Obeisance to the wise, dispassionate Buddha whose powers are inconceivable and who, out of sympathy (*dayâ*) [for all beings] has taught that which is inexpressible by words. (1)

From the transcendental perspective (*parama-artha*[20]), there is no origination (*utpâda*) and, in truth, there is no cessation (*nirodha*). The Buddha is like space (*âkâsha*), and hence also [all] beings have the one-and-the-same (*eka*) characteristic. (2)

There is no creation (*jâti*) on this or the other side. A compound-thing (*samskrita*) [simply] arises from the [existing] condition (*pratyaya*) and is, by its nature, void—the domain of the knowledge of the omniscient [Buddha]. (3)

All states (*bhâva*) are deemed by their nature to be like reflections (*pratibimba*): pure and tranquil by nature, nondual, equal, and thusness (*tathatâ*). (4)

In fact, ordinary people conceive of essence (*âtman*) in nonessence, and similarly [they wrongly imagine] joy and sorrow, indifference, passion (*klesha*), and liberation. (5)

The six [types of] birth in the world (*samsâra*),[21] supreme joy in heaven, and great suffering in hell are [likewise] not within the domain of Reality (*tattva*). (6)

Similarly [untrue are the ideas that] from inauspicious [deeds come] endless suffering, aging, illness, and death, but that by auspicious actions surely an auspicious (*shubha*) [destiny can be won]. (7)

As a painter is terrified by the image of a demon he himself has painted, so an ignoramus (*abudha*) is [riddled with] fear in the world. (8)

As some fool going to a quagmire by himself is sucked down [into it], so beings, submerged in the quagmire of imagination (*kalpanâ*), are unable to extricate themselves. (9)

The sensation of suffering is experienced by picturing existence (*bhâva*) in nonexistence (*abhâva*). [Beings] are troubled by the poison of imagining [that there is] both an object and knowledge. (10)

Seeing these helpless [beings], one should, with a mind overwhelmed with compassion, cultivate the practice of enlightenment (*bodhi-caryâ*) for the benefit of [all] beings. (11)

Having acquired merit (*sambhâra*) by this [practice] and having attained unsurpassable enlightenment (*bodhi*), one should become a Buddha, released from the bond of imagination [but remaining] a friend of the world.[22] (12)

He who understands the Real Object (*bhûta-artha*[23]) through [insight into] dependent origination (*pratîtya-samutpâda*) knows the world as void, without beginning, middle, and end. (13)

By seeing that the world (*samsâra*) and extinction (*nirvâna*) are not in reality [existent], [one realizes] the immaculate, changeless, priorly tranquil (*âdishânta*), and luminous [Reality]. (14)

The object of dream cognition is not perceived by the fully awakened [person]. [Similarly,] the world is not perceived by him who has awaked from the darkness of [spiritual] delusion. (15)

The originator (*jâtimat*) does not originate himself. Origination is imagined by worldly ones (*loka*). Both imaginings and [imaginary] beings are not conducive [to the Truth]. (16)

All this is mere mind (*citta-mâtra*); it exists like a hallucination (*mâyâ*). Hence auspicious or inauspicious action [appears to be engaged in], and from this [follows apparent] auspicious or inauspicious birth. (17)

All things (*dharma*) are restricted by restricting the mind's wheel. Hence [all] things are nonessential (*anâtman*), and thus they are pure. (18)

By presuming [that which is] eternal, essential (*âtman*), and joyous to be in things (*bhâva*) [that are] insubstantial (*nihsvabhâva*), this ocean of existence manifests for him who is enveloped by the darkness of attachment and delusion. (19)

Who can reach the farther shore of the mighty ocean of the world abounding with the water of imagination without resorting to the great vehicle (Mahâyâna)? (20)

## The Vijnânavâda and Yogâcâra Schools

A further significant development within Buddhism occurred in the fourth century C.E., which saw the emergence of the Vijnânavâda and Yogâcâra schools of the brothers Vasubandhu and Asanga, who, from one point of view, embody the perennial complementarity of theory and practice in the spiritual tradition of India. They are said to have set the "wheel of the teaching" in motion for the third time. Asanga received the teachings of the so-called Yogâcâra ("Yoga Conduct") school directly from the future Buddha Maitreya.

According to a well-known story, Asanga had exerted himself over many years to gain a vision of the celestial *bodhisattva* Maitreya. He was despairing of ever succeeding in this particular meditation. However, one day this compassionate master administered to a wounded dog by the roadside,

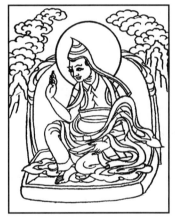

*Vasubandhu*
*(from a woodblock)*

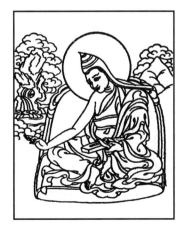

*Asanga (from a woodblock)*

forgetting his own spiritual despair. Suddenly, Maitreya revealed himself to him in the form of that dog and promptly transported Asanga to the Tushita Heaven where he taught him five great texts, notably the *Abhi-samaya-Alamkâra* and the *Mahâ-yâna-Sûtra-Alamkâra*. Dismissing this traditional story, many scholars think that the originator of the teachings contained in these works was a human teacher by the name of Maitreyanâtha.

Be that as it may, Asanga endeavored to fortify the practice of Yoga amidst a highly speculative atmosphere in Buddhist circles. According to the Yogâcâra school, the objective world is "mere mind" (*citta-mâtra*), which is also the basic position of the *Lankâ-Avatâra-Sûtra*. What this means is that our entire experience is simply that: experience, flashes of consciousness, without objective substratum. But that fleeting consciousness is, *in truth*, the ever-lasting transcendental Consciousness. This whole consideration apparently grew out of Asanga's own intense meditation practice, which taught him the spuriousness of phenomena, leading him to pure metaphysical idealism. He is also traditionally held responsible for the introduction of the Tantric approach into Buddhism.

Vasubandhu, Asanga's younger brother, was more concerned with putting the new metaphysical ideas on solid theoretical foundations. He authored the famous *Abhidharma-Kosha* and an auto-commentary (*bhâshya*) on it. His Vijnânavâda is the most popular of all the Mahâyâna schools. For him, as for the Vedânta philosophers, the ultimate Reality is pure, indeterminable, universal Consciousness (*vijnâna*). He even spoke of that Reality as the Great Self (*mahâ-âtman*, written *mahâtman*). Lower than this supreme Consciousness is what is called the "storehouse consciousness" (*âlaya-vijnâna*), which serves as the reservoir of all subconscious activators (*samskâra*) by which individual consciousnesses maintain their separateness. Even Vasubandhu's abstract formulations are intended to encourage self-transcending practice rather than mere philosophizing about Consciousness or the spiritual path.

It was Gaudapâda, the teacher of Shankara's teacher, who drank deeply from the well of wisdom

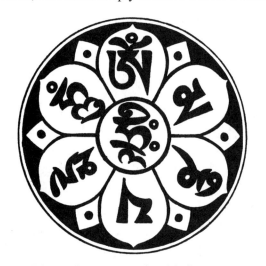

*Tibetan "om mani padme hûm" mantra*

of the Mâdhyamika and the Vijnânavâda branches of Buddhism, and both he and Shankara refer to them frequently, if critically, in their works. The similarities between Mahâyâna Buddhism and Advaita Vedânta have often been pointed out, and partly owing to Shankara's scholastic ingenuity, Advaita Vedânta rather than Mahâyâna Buddhism won out on Indian soil.

## Mantrayâna

From about the third century C.E. on, the use of *mantras*, or sacred words or formulae, came into prominence in the Buddhist tradition. The discovery that sound can have a transformative effect on the psyche goes back, however, to the *Vedas*. For millennia the brahmins have used such sacred syllables as *om* or such mantric prayers as the *gâyatrî-mantra* both to focus the mind and to invoke the higher powers. Similarly in Buddhism, *mantra*-like formulae for protecting oneself against evil, known in Pali as *parittas*, have been employed since the time of the Buddha. The Mahâsânghika school, which may have been the intermediary between the Hînayâna and the Mahâyâna traditions, possessed a special collection of *mantras* titled the *Dhâranî-Pitaka*. But in the early centuries of the Common Era some Buddhist teachers began to use *mantras* as the primary means of disciplining and transcending the mind. This came to be known as the Mantrayâna tradition, corresponding broadly to the Hindu Mantra-Yoga.

A good example of Buddhist *mantra* practice is the recitation of the famous *mantra* of the *Prajnâ-Pâramitâ* literature: *Gate gate para-gate para-samgate bodhi svâhâ*, "Gone, gone, gone beyond, fully gone beyond, enlightenment, *svâhâ*." In the *Eka-Akshari-* ("Single Letter") *Sûtra*,[24] again, the letter *a* is introduced as the sacred sound that embodies the entire *Prajnâ-Pâramitâ* literature.

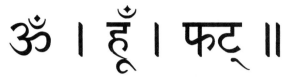

*Om, hûm, phat*

Some Buddhists texts distinguish between *mantras* and *dhâranîs*, defining the latter as "that by which something is supported" (*dhâryate anayâ iti*), the "something" being the meditating mind. *Dhâranîs* are a special category of *mantra*: They are abbreviated versions of key scriptural sayings, expressing quintessential ideas. A typical *dhâranîs* is the famous Tibetan mantric phrase *om mani padme hûm*, "*Om*, jewel in the lotus—*hûm*." The late Anagarika Govinda, a Vajrayâna initiate of German extraction, has analyzed this *mantra* in great detail.[25] The Buddhist scriptures also speak of *kavacas*, which are similar strings of sacred sounds, but are used specifically for self-protection. The word actually means "armor."

The flair for abbreviation among *mantra* creators is taken to the extreme in the case of *bîja-mantras*, which are single phonemes such as *om*, *hum*, or *phat* thought to be the "seed" for a far more complex reality and corresponding spiritual experience. They each stand for a whole cosmos of ideas. Thus *om* is the soundless sound of the absolute Reality itself, and its place in the human body is at the sacred spot between the eyebrows ("third eye"). This locus is the point of confluence between the left and the right streams of life, which then go singly to the great "door" of liberation at the crown of the head.

The Mantrayâna tradition is regarded as one of the branches or phases of Tantric Buddhism, together with the Vajrayâna, the Kâlacakrayâna, and the Sahajayâna. However, the designation Mantrayâna is also frequently applied to Buddhist Tantrism in general. Strictly speaking, however, the Mantrayâna is the introductory phase of Buddhist Tantrism, whose full flowering is present in the Vajrayâna tradition, which is discussed separately in Section V below.

## *Sahajayâna*

The Sahajayâna, which came into being in the eighth century C.E., is best understood as a reaction to, and critique of, the busy esotericism and magical preoccupations of mainstream Tantra. The Sahajayâna does not have Tantric scriptures of its own, which would almost violate its principle of spontaneity. But its teachers have left behind memorable songs, known as *dohâs* or *caryâs*, which were orally transmitted and were popular in many parts of India until the twelfth centuries C.E. The Sahajîyâ movement straddled Buddhism, Hinduism, and Jainism, and *dohâs* were composed in the languages and dialects peculiar to these traditions. Only a small number of these songs have survived, which were collected and published by the renowned Indian scholar Prabodh Chandra Bagchi.[26]

The masters of Sahajayâna taught that Reality cannot be discovered by placing unnatural restraints of one kind or another on human nature. Instead they insisted that we should follow what is the most natural in us, that is, be true to our own personal imperative. Of course, they did not preach that we should simply abandon ourselves to our passions or instincts. Rather, their natural or spontaneous approach is the way of abiding in what is inherently true of us, which is blissful freedom. Perhaps Joseph Campbell's popular phrase "Follow your own bliss" conveys something of their teaching.

The best known Buddhist *dohâs* are those of the eighth-century adept Saraha, or Saraha-pâda. His female consort (*dâkinî*)[27] was the daughter of an arrowsmith, and hence he is commonly portrayed as holding an arrow—a symbol of the penetrating power of wisdom. Saraha's name itself means "he who releases (*ha*) the arrow (*sara*)."

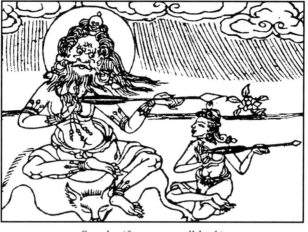

*Saraha (from a woodblock)*

While the Sahajîyâ realizers enjoyed great respect, their message was too radical to be properly understood by many. Yet, the ideal of spontaneity is of perennial value to spiritual practitioners, for it is all too easy to get caught up in a struggle for enlightenment. The *dohâs* and *caryâs* are reminders that all struggle is an egoic activity and as such a limitation on our native condition of perfect bliss.

## Kâlacakrayâna

Out of the Vajrayâna tradition emerged, some time in the tenth century C.E., the Kâlacakrayâna. The phrase *kâla-cakra* means "wheel of time" or "wheel of death" and stands for the ultimate Reality in its bipolar aspect as wisdom (*prajnâ*) and means (*upâya*), that is, the means of compassion (*karunâ*).

This tradition is associated with the wrathful deities of the Tibetan pantheon, perhaps because time itself is a destructive force. Change is inevitable and death rules supreme. The goal of the Kâlacakrayâna aspirant is to transcend time and death by manipulating his or her own microcosm, the human body-mind. As a faithful replica of the larger cosmos, the body contains all the essential features of the external world—stars, planets, mountains, oceans, and rivers. We must simply learn to decipher the hidden language of the microcosm-macrocosm parallelism.

The Kâlacakrayâna teachers emphasize the yogic path. Time or death must be outwitted particularly by means of controlling the in-breath (*prâna*) and the out-breath (*apâna*). The incessant flow of the breath of life is, to use an anachronistic metaphor, like the ticking of the clock, telling us that time is running out. *Prâna* (life) and *kâla* (time/death) are intimately linked. To stop the one is to stop the other. And this is exactly the declared purpose of the adepts of this tradition. When life and time stand still, the realization of great bliss (*mahâ-sukha*) is at hand.

Another way in which the Kâlacakrayâna teachers have expressed this is by speaking of the union of sun and moon, or *upâya* and *prajnâ* respectively. This union *is* Lord Kâlacakra. The yogic discipline (*sâdhanâ*) by which the ultimate Reality can be realized is explained in some detail in the *Kâlacakra-Tantra*, a text of the tenth century C.E.

An idiosyncratic feature of the Kâlacakrayâna is the teaching about the mystical kingdom of Shambhala, where it claims to have originated. Only great adepts are said to be able to find the secret entrances to this kingdom, which is ruled by priest-kings.

## The Ch'an or Zen School of China and Japan

The radical spirit of the Sahajayâna is present also in Japanese Zen Buddhism. Zen is the

Japanese version of the Chinese meditation (*ch'an*) tradition of Buddhism. Both Mahâyâna Buddhism and the Theravâda doctrines were introduced into China in the first century C.E., where they encountered two powerful and symbiotic religions, Confucianism and Taoism. It was the latter that supplied the masses with religious inspiration and hopes of power and immortality, and that, more than the emperor-centered Confucianism, facilitated the establishment and growth of Buddhism in China.

But Buddhism did not only flourish in China, it was also profoundly transformed, for what the Chinese found the most attractive in it was the devotional element on the one hand and the ideal of transcendental compassion on the other. They were fascinated with the figure of Amitâbha, the Buddha of infinite radiance, who reigns over the pure celestial realm known as Sukhavatî, the "Happy Land," described ornately in the smaller and the larger *Sukhavatî-Vyûha-Sûtras* and the *Amitâyur-Dhyâna-Sûtra*. These are the basic texts of what is called the "Pure Land" Buddhism of the Far East, which is the Far-Eastern Buddhist counterpart to the Bhakti-Yoga of Hinduism. The pious Buddhist hopes for reincarnation in that divine abode, or some other pure realm, such as the Tushita Heaven of the transcendental *bodhisattva* Avalokiteshvara, who ranks second to the Buddha Amitâbha (or Amitâyur, "Infinite Life"). Such a rebirth is regarded by some teachers as equivalent to attaining *nirvâna*.

The Pure Land (Chinese: Yodo-Shu) school underwent a further transformation upon arriving in Japan, where it became known as the Jodo school, founded by Honen Shonin (1133–1211 C.E.). Honen, "the superior man," felt that so many centuries had elapsed since Gautama the Buddha that no one could possibly understand his original teaching anymore. The best one could do, in his opinion, was to believe in the Buddha and pray for

his grace. Thus Honen taught a form of Mantra-Yoga, revolving around the mantric phrase *namu amida butsu*, or "Adoration to the Buddha Amida [=Amitâbha]," and otherwise requiring a minimum of disciplines. His principal disciple, Shinran Shonin (1173–1262 C.E.), turned this teaching into a pure doctrine of vicarious salvation: The Buddha Amida's grace alone suffices to raise the faithful out of conditioned existence. No self-effort (Japanese: *jiriki*) is required. The "other effort" (Japanese: *tariki*), or grace of the Buddha, who acquired inexhaustible merit through his own exertions prior to his enlightenment, is sufficient. A single invocation of the name of Buddha Amida, if done with a pure heart, is adequate to ensure one's salvation. True to his own teaching, Shinran broke his monastic vows and married a princess.

At the other end of the spectrum is the Zen tradition, which is firmly anchored in self-effort. It acknowledges Bodhidharma (470–543 C.E.), a learned South Indian monk, as its first patriarch. He arrived in China in the year 520 C.E., where he became known as Tamo (Japanese: Daruma). He inaugurated the Ch'an or meditation tradition, which was inspired by the Yogâcâra school. Bodhidharma was received by the Emperor Wu-Ti, a fervent Buddhist. When asked to define the essential principle of Buddhism, Bodhidharma laconically replied, "Vast emptiness," which disturbed the emperor greatly. After this encounter, Bodhidharma withdrew to a monastery, where he meditated in front of a blank wall for nine years. Later he observed that the mind has to become like a straight-standing wall.

His teaching attracted a growing number of monks and householders. By the time of the sixth and last patriarch, Hui-Neng (638–713 C.E.), Ch'an had become the leading form of Buddhism in China. Only half a millennium later were the Ch'an teachings brought to Japan by Eisai (1141–1215 C.E.). Zen, which has been styled "the apotheosis of Buddhism,"[28] is, like the Indian Sahajâyana, one of the most radical developments within Buddhism. Both are direct applications of the principle of voidness to daily life.

In the 1930s, Zen was introduced to the West, thanks mainly to the untiring efforts of Zen master and scholar Daisetz Teitaro Suzuki, and later through such popularizing catalysts as Alan Watts and the Beat poets and philosophers. This transplant has not always proven fruitful. As one critic, himself a Buddhist, remarked:

> Zen was designed to operate within emptiness. When coming West it is transferred into a vacuum. Let us just recollect what Zen took for granted, as its antecedents, basis and continuing background: a long and unbroken tradition of spiritual "know-how"; firm and unquestioned metaphysical beliefs, and not just a disbelief in everything; a superabundance of Scriptures and images; a definite discipline supervised by authoritative persons; insistence on right livelihood and an austere life for all exponents of the Dharma; and a strong Sangha [spiritual community], composed of thousands of mature and experienced persons housed in thousands of temples, who could keep deviations from Buddhist principles within narrow bounds.[29]

Mantrayâna and Zen demonstrate the immense plasticity of the Buddhist tradition. By comparison with the starkness of Zen, Mantrayâna is positively baroque. Zen dispenses with all gadgets and devices, seeking to force or trick the mind itself into going beyond its own illusory creations. It is comparable to a direct assault on a perpendicular rock face, relying on consciousness

alone. Tantric Buddhism is quite different. It utilizes all manners of climbing aids, and in particular appreciates the fact that we are immersed in a dimension of subtle energies that need to be harnessed for the path.

The ground for Tantric Buddhism was prepared by the rise of Mahâyâna Buddhism. Gradually, many psychotechnical devices in addition to *mantras* were introduced into the Buddhist tradition, which were meant to simplify the meditative fixing of awareness in the dark age (*kali-yuga*): The spiritual renaissance of Tantra made its appearance simultaneously in Buddhism and Hinduism. As a matter of fact, in the early Tantric teachings, Buddhism and Hinduism are peculiarly convergent. The following section introduces the salient features of Buddhist Tantra, and this will anticipate to some extent the treatment of Hindu Tantrism in Chapter 17.

## V. THE JEWEL IN THE LOTUS— VAJRAYÂNA (TANTRIC) BUDDHISM

### The Nature of Buddhist Tantra

Tantra, or Tantrism, is one of the most fascinating chapters in the long history of India's spirituality. It is, however, very difficult to define, because it so diversified that it even contains its own antithesis within itself. Thus, Tantric Buddhism, or Vajrayâna, is an esoteric ritualism that includes a vast variety of paraphernalia and the ceremonial worship and internalization of male and female deities, as well as a philosophy and practice of spontaneity (*sahaja*). Sahajayâna argues that the ultimate Reality can never be found through any external manipulations or even through disciplining of the mind, but that it is simply to be intuited as one's native Condition. In the words of Sarahapâda (eleventh century C.E.), the enlightened composer of the "Royal Song":

> When the deluded in a mirror look
> They see a face, not a reflection.
> So the mind that has truth denied
> Relies on that which is not true. (15)

> As a Brahmin, who with rice and butter
> Makes a burnt offering in blazing fire
> Creating a vessel for nectar from celestial space,
> Takes this through wishful thinking as the ultimate. (23)

> Some people who have kindled the inner heat and raised it to the fontanelle
> Stroke the uvula with the tongue in a sort of coition and confuse
> That which fetters with what gives release,
> In pride will call themselves yogis. (24)

> There's nothing to be negated, nothing to be
> Affirmed or grasped; for It can never be conceived.
> By the fragmentations of the intellect are the deluded
> Fettered; undivided and pure remains spontaneity. (35)[30]

Tantra is a practical path geared to transform human consciousness until the transmental (amanaska) Truth stands out as the obvious. What all Tantric schools have in common is the affirmation that this transcendental Truth is to be discovered in the human body itself, not somewhere else. This affirmation expresses the fundamental doctrine of the Mahâyâna tradition that the world of change (samsâra) is co-essential with the ultimate Reality, whether it be called nirvâna ("extinction") or shûnya ("void").

They also share another metaphysical credo, and that is that from the empirical point of view, the one Reality is manifested as a play of polarity—the two poles being the static male principle and the female dynamic principle: shiva/shakti or prajnâ/karunâ. This understanding is fundamental to the entire Tantric path (sâdhanâ).

Although there are a good many differences between the Buddhist and the Hindu variety of Tantrism, the basic ideas and practices are very similar. Tantra differs from the other traditions of India not because of any philosophical innovations but because of its pronouncedly syncretistic approach. As Agehananda Bharati put it, Tantra is more "value-free" than the non-Tantric traditions; that is, it permits practices that are ordinarily considered taboo in spiritual life, and some even in ordinary secular contexts.[31] Tantra is body-positive and antipuritanical. The Tantric teachers place self-experimentation above social morality, and the texts typically warn the uninitiated and the initiate alike that their teachings are radical and dangerous. But they are also insistent that they offer a shortcut to enlightenment in the present age of spiritual and moral decline.

## Sacred Gestures (Mudrâ)

The use of mantras, as already mentioned, is an important part of the Tantric psychotechnical repertoire. Even though mantras are offered as a simple route to spiritual realization, their very simplicity is deceptive. Uninformed Western imitators of Eastern wisdom tend to overlook the fact that any spiritual practice is founded in a profound commitment to self-transcendence. The mere mindless repetition of *mantras* at best leads to a trance state and at worst can induce psychosis. The admission of *mantras* into Buddhist practice opened the door for other psychotechnical devices, notably the practice of sacred gestures (*mudrâ*) and the employment of graphic representations (*mandala*) of psychocosmological events.

Just as sound has a transcending aspect, so also the positioning of the body in space can communicate or invoke primal truths. Thus the *mudrâs*, which are mostly hand gestures (*hasta-mudrâ*), are both expressive of and conducive to spiritual states. The best known Buddhist *mudrâs*, often depicted in iconography, are:

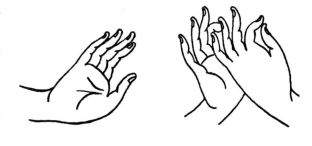

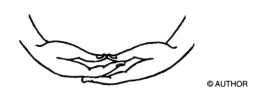

© AUTHOR

*Abhaya-mudrâ, dharma-cakra-mudrâ, and dhyâna-mudrâ*

1.  *Bhûmi-sparsha-mudrâ* or "gesture of touching the ground," which is also known as the witness gesture. The latter designation derives from the traditional biographies of Gautama the Buddha, who made this gesture when calling upon the earth to witness his success over Mâra, the spirit of evil. This *mudrâ* is executed by draping the right arm over the right knee, with palm turned inward and all fingers pointing downward, while the middle finger touches the seat or ground.

2.  *Dâna-mudrâ* or "gesture of giving," which is executed by extending the right arm over the right knee, with the palm of the right hand facing outward.

3.  *Dhyâna-mudrâ* or "meditation gesture," which is performed by having both hands, palms up, rest in the lap, the right hand on top of the left. Both thumbs touch lightly.

4.  *Abhaya-mudrâ* or "gesture of fearlessness," that is, the gesture of dispelling fear in others, which is executed with the right hand, raised to the level of the heart, with the palm turned outward and all the fingers extending upward.

5.  *Dharma-cakra-mudrâ* or "gesture of the Wheel of the Law," which is performed differently according to various traditions. In Tibet, both hands are held at the level of the chest, with the left hand in front of the right. The index fingers and thumbs of both hands form a circle and touch.

The origin of these hand gestures is not known. On one level, they are the invention of artists trying to express inner states iconographically. On another level, they undoubtedly are the products of intensive meditation practice during the course of which it is not uncommon that the body spontaneously assumes certain static as well as dynamic poses, which are known as *kriyâs* ("actions").

## *Mandala: The Geometry of Sacred Space*

In practical terms, the *mandala* ("circle") is a focusing device for the meditator. Symbolically, it is a map of the cosmos and the psyche. As the Italian Tibetologist Guiseppe Tucci explained:

It is a geometric projection of the world reduced to an essential pattern. Implicitly it early assumed profound significance, because when the mystic identified himself with its center, it transformed him and so determined the first conditions for the success of his work. It remained a paradigm of cosmic involution and evolution. Yet the man who used it no longer wanted only return to the center of the universe. Dissatisfied with the experience of the psyche he longed for a state of concentration in order to find once more the unity of a secluded and undiverted consciousness, and to restore in himself the ideal principle of things. So the *mandala* is no longer a cosmogram but a psychocosmogram, the scheme of disintegration from the One to the many and of reintegration from the many to the One, to that Absolute Consciousness, entire and luminous, which Yoga causes to shine once more in the depths of our being.[32]

The construction of the *mandala* is a meditative act in which the initiate identifies with the specific deity or deities of the *mandala* and gradually passes through the various psychic experiences and states corresponding to the different aspects of this psychocosmogram. In the end, he or she arrives at the central point (*bindu*), the symbolic seed of the manifested universe and the threshold to the transcendental Reality. If the spiritual practitioner (*sâdhaka*) is successful, this is the moment where his or her individuated consciousness dissolves, and what remains is pure Consciousness, the Absolute.

The *mandala* can be constructed either by drawing it in sand or on a piece of paper, cloth, or wood, or by picturing it in one's mind. The latter practice presumes advanced visualization abilities. In either case, the construction of a *mandala* must be preceded by appropriate purificatory rites through which the location, the materials, and not least one's body-mind are consecrated.

Typically and in greatly simplified terms, a *mandala* is composed of an outer protective surround consisting of one or more concentric circles, or walls of fire, which enclose a square structure that, in turn, contains the central point (*bindu*) or image. The square, which has four "gates," is cut by diagonal lines, yielding four triangles, each of which contains the image of a particular deity with insignia. As can be seen on any Tibetan *thanka*, or wall hanging, these *mandalas* are intricate pictorial designs, and their symbolism is still more complex, as is the liturgy associated with the *mandala* construction. By comparison, the Hindu *yantras* are relatively simple, which holds true of their symbolic content as well. They will be discussed in connection with Hindu Tantrism in Chapter 17.

## *Maithunâ: Sacred Sexuality*

*Mantras*, *mudrâs*, and *mandalas* are important Tantric devices. Another significant tool of psychic transformation, for which Tantra is best known in the West, is the practice of ritualized sexuality, which bears the technical designation of *maithunâ* and is discussed in more detail in Chapter 17 as well.

The conduct of a Vajrayâna adept is likely to be unorthodox; intent upon employing everything in life as a means to achievement, he does not except such animal processes as sleeping, eating, excreting and (if he is not a monk) sexual intercourse. The energy of passions and desires must be yoked, not wasted. Every act of body, speech and mind, every circumstance, every sensation, every dream can be turned to good account. This aspect of Tantric Buddhism has led to the great error of confounding it with libertinism. Though all things are employed as means, they must be rightly used and their right use is far removed from sensual gratification.[33]

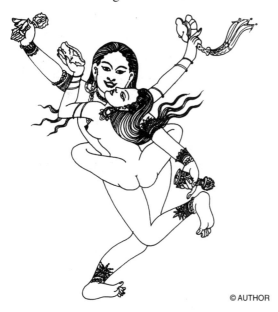

© AUTHOR

*Couple in ecstatic embrace (yab-yum)*

John Blofeld, the writer of the above quote, goes on to make the Tantric point that the use of drugs like mescaline may serve an appropriate purpose. Indeed, "psychedelic" drugs have been widely used in the spiritual traditions of the world, including the Yoga of Patanjali, though they were never advertised as ultimate keys to enlightenment, merely as stepping-stones on the spiritual path. Blofeld relates his own drug experience which plunged him into a state of ecstasy "in which dawned full awareness of three great truths I had long accepted intellectually but never experienced as being self-evident." The experience revealed to him that there was indeed a level of being on which subject and object ceased to be separate, that this condition is utterly blissful, and that everything arising to consciousness is in fact ephemeral, as is epitomized in the Buddhist doctrine of the *dharmas*, explained earlier on.

This transcendental realization of undifferentiated being is also the objective and substance of sacred sexual intercourse. It is in this practice that the "jewel in the lotus," the eternal embrace of the male and female aspect of infinite Reality, is discovered. The word *vajra* (Tibetan: *dorje*) in Vajrayâna denotes the "diamond," the substance that is so hard that nothing in the world can possibly break or even

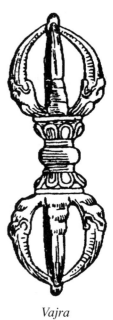

*Vajra*

chip it. In other words, it is the transcendental Reality itself. It is the supreme principle of wisdom (*prajnâ*) by which everything can be penetrated and consequently transcended. It is also the male generative force and the esoteric name of the penis.

The lotus (*padma*), on the other hand, is the symbol of spiritual unfoldment as well as of the female sex organ. Thus, sexual intercourse can be looked at from many symbolic levels. Primarily, however, the merging of the sexes in the bliss of sexual congress replicates on the human level what is forever true of existence on the transcendental level. But more of this later.

## *The Great Adepts of Tantric Buddhism*

Tantric Buddhism is the result of the contact between Indian Buddhism and the native Tibetan Bon religion. Hence we find that in the Vajrayâna tradition, more than in any other Buddhist tradition, the loftiest metaphysical doctrines are mingled with the earthiest magical practices. This becomes strikingly evident when we examine the biographies of the eighty-four *mahâ-siddhas* ("great adepts") of Tibetan Buddhism. They were not only enlightened beings but also accomplished thaumaturgists possessing all kinds of paranormal powers (*siddhi*).

Thus, prior to his spiritual conversion, Tibet's most famous *yogin*, Milarepa (1038–1122 C.E.), was wreaking havoc with his black magic. His pupilage under Marpa "the Translator" is said to have been especially hard because he had to atone for his sins during the course of his practice (*sâdhanâ*). Yet in his "Hundred Thousand Songs of Mila" (*Mila-Grubum*), Milarepa, whose name means the "cotton-clad," praises his *guru* for his great love and patience. Milarepa is the most illustrious figure of the Kagyu order, whose members usually live as hermits in mountain caves, dedicating their lives to solitary meditation. They trace their lineage back through Milarepa to Marpa the Translator (1012–1097 C.E.), who uniquely combined in himself intellectual and spiritual genius, and then to Marpa's Indian teacher Nâropa (1016–1100 C.E.). Nâropa's teacher was, in turn, Tilopa (988–1069 C.E.), who had no human preceptor but is said to have received initiation into the highest spiritual practice directly from his chosen deity (Tibetan: *yidam*,

Sanskrit: *ishta-devatâ*). Tilopa is deemed the first patriarch of the Kagyu order.

The Kagyupas are well known for their practice of *chod* ("severing"), which is a meditation in which the practitioner, through visualization and ritual, step by step dismembers his or her own body, offering it as food to deities, *dâkinîs*, and lower beings. What remains is a purified consciousness that no longer anxiously clings to the physical body or the physical realm at large.

The Kagyu order is one of the three "Red Hat" sects of Tibetan Buddhism, so called because of the color of the head dress worn by their members on ceremonial occasions. The other two are the Nyingmapa and the Sakyapa schools. The former is the oldest Vajrayâna order, which dates back to the Tibetan monastery of Samye where

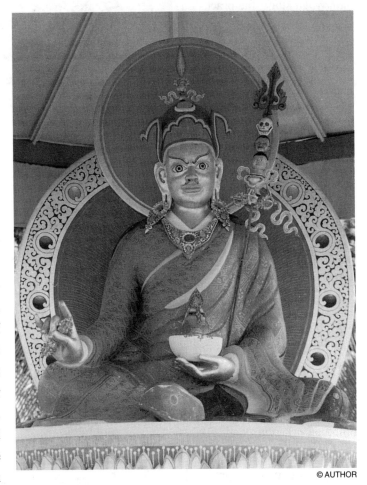

© AUTHOR

*Guru Padmasambhava (a sculpture at a Buddhist temple in Hawaii)*

the great Tantric master Buddhaguhya and over one hundred monastic scholar-translators worked on translating Sanskrit scriptures into Tibetan. An early master, who did much to spread Buddhism in Tibet and is often called the founder of the Nyingma order, is Padmasambhava, "Precious Teacher" (Guru Rimpoche), who arrived in Tibet in 747 C.E. Most Nyingmapas are married householders who are as well versed in the scriptures as they are in Tantric practices. The distinctive practice of the Nyingma order is *dzogchen*, which has become very popular among Western Buddhists. It is the practice of the highest of the three "inner" Tantras, namely (in ascending order) *mahâyoga, anuyoga,* and *atiyoga*. At the *mahâyoga* stage, the practitioner realizes that all phenomena are emanations of the mind, which is a combination of appearance and voidness (*shûnyatâ*). At the level of *anuyoga* practice, all appearances and one's own thoughts are recognized as empty (*shûnya*), and this emptiness is identified with Samantabhadrî, the feminine form of Samantabhadra, who is the embodiment of the *dharma-kâya*, the "body" of Reality. *Atiyoga* consists in the realization that all phenomena arise as a combination of appearance and emptiness. It transcends all visualization, which the Nyingmapas consider inferior to *dzogchen*. But, as

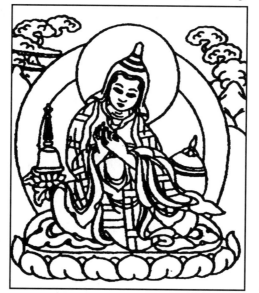

*Atîsha (from a woodblock)*

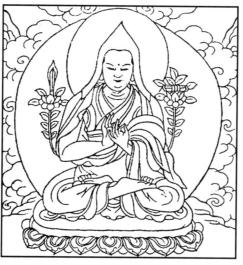

*Tsongkhapa (from a woodblock)*

many Western students tend to forget, direct perception of the empty nature of the mind and of all existence presupposes great inner calm and clarity. Thus, there is a place for other forms of meditation and visualization as an aid to achieving inner stillness.

The Sakyapas trace their lineage back to the Indian adept Virûpa and, beyond him, to Atîsha Dîpamkara Shrîjnâna (982–1052 C.E.). Atîsha was born into a royal family of Bengal, renounced the world at the age of fifteen, and became a monk (*bhikshu*) at the age of twenty-nine. After twelve years of intensive monastic study and discipline, he achieved great fame as a scholar and adept. However, when he realized the importance of generating *bodhi-citta*, the will to enlightenment, he made a thirteen-month-long journey to Indonesia to receive the teachings on *bodhi-citta* from their greatest exponent, the adept Dharmakîrti.

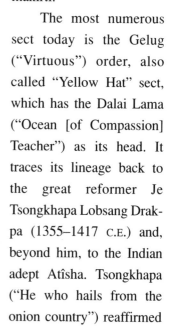

The most numerous sect today is the Gelug ("Virtuous") order, also called "Yellow Hat" sect, which has the Dalai Lama ("Ocean [of Compassion] Teacher") as its head. It traces its lineage back to the great reformer Je Tsongkhapa Lobsang Drakpa (1355–1417 C.E.) and, beyond him, to the Indian adept Atîsha. Tsongkhapa ("He who hails from the onion country") reaffirmed

Atîsha's insistence that the *Tantras* should be studied only after mastery of the *Sûtras* and their practices has been achieved. On the basis of Atîsha's "A Lamp for the Path to Enlightenment" (*Byang-chub lamgyi groma*, Sanskrit: *Bodhi-Patha-Pradîpa*), he developed the teaching of the "graduated path" (*lam rim*) on which all spiritual practices of the Gelugpas are based. This is an impressively systematic teaching of the stages (*rim*) of the path (*lam*) to liberation, serving as a syllabus of instruction.

Shortly before his death, Je Tsongkhapa asked his main disciples who among them would assume the responsibility for passing on the Tantric teachings. Only Jetsun Sherab Sengye stepped forward, and he received all the precious Tantric teachings from his *guru*. They were handed down in an unbroken line of transmission by the Segyu monastery, which, with numerous other monasteries, was destroyed during the Chinese invasion of Tibet in 1959. Only a handful of monks were able to flee to India and Nepal, where they created two new monasteries (in Kalimpong and Kathmandu respectively). Through Sherab Sengye, the Tantric teachings also were transmitted to other monasteries and now form the backbone of the Gelug tradition.

Je Tsongkhapa wrote many works, including his *magnum opus* "The Great Exposition of the Stages of the Path," his influential "The Essence of Good Explanations,"and "The Great Exposition of Secret Mantra." In 1509, at the age of fifty-two, he founded the famous Ganden Monastery,[34] which once housed around four thousand monks. He also founded the two other well-known monasteries of Drepung (1416) and Sera (1419). After their complete destruction at the hands of the Chinese communists, they were rebuilt in India.

Je Tsongkhapa's reforms were primarily aimed at restoring the monastic vows and disciplines, reintroducing clear thinking, and resuscitating pure Tantric practice among the Tibetans. He was particularly concerned about the sexual practices of those involved with higher Tantric Yoga (*anuttara-yoga-tantra*), which clashed with the monastic ideal.

## *The Six Yogas of Nâropa*

The adept Nâropa deserves our special attention, because his name is associated with the teaching of the "Six Yogas of Naro" (*naro chodrug*).[35] This practice is expounded in the Tibetan text "The Epitome of the Six Doctrines," which was translated in 1935 by Kazi Dawa-Samdup and introduced by W. Y. Evans Wentz, and contains the following:

1.  The Yoga of Psychophysical Heat (*tumo*): This practice combines visualization and breathing techniques. Utilizing the surplus of bio-energy produced through strict sexual abstinence, *yogins* visualize, among other things, one half of the letter *a* of the Tibetan alphabet, causing it to glow brightly until their entire body is filled by the blaze and then extending it to fill the cosmos. Finally,

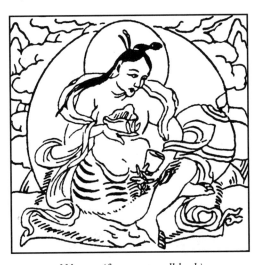

*Nâropa (from a woodblock)*

they control the blaze, gradually reducing it to a pinpoint, until it merges into the void itself. This practice generates a considerable amount of psychophysical heat, which allows the *yogins* to meditate naked for prolonged periods at temperatures well below zero in the high altitudes of the Himalayas. Several expeditions have returned with film footage documenting this extraordinary feat. This practice presupposes intimate knowledge of the "winds" (Tibetan: *lung*; Sanskrit: *prâna*, *vâyu*) and the subtle channels (Tibetan: *tsa*; Sanskrit: *nâdî*), as well as the psychoenergetic centers (Tibetan: *tsakhor*; Sanskrit: *cakra*).

2. The Yoga of the Illusory Body (*gyulu*): Meditating on the flat image of their body in a mirror, which gives the illusion of having three-dimensional depth, *yogins* proceed to experience that image as arising between the mirror and themselves. Finally, they contemplate the ultimate illusoriness, or voidness, of their own body. This leads ultimately to practitioners' identification with the "diamond body" (Tibetan: *dorje'i ku*; Sanskrit: *vajra-kâya*) of absolute Reality.

3. The Yoga of the Dream State (*milam*): In order to discover the illusoriness of the waking and the dream state, *yogins* enter the dream state at will, without sacrificing the continuity of their awareness. They carefully control the dream events. In recent years, research on what is called "lucid dreaming" has shown that it is possible to insert oneself into one's dreams consciously, and

even to control the events in them.

4. The Yoga of the Clear Light (*odsal*): This practice anticipates an experience that is said to be universal shortly after death, in which the deceased person sees momentarily the brilliant white radiance that is a form of the transcendental Reality itself. In the Yoga of the Clear Light, adepts enter into levels of awareness where that radiance can be seen, and in this way they prepare themselves for the after-death encounter with the Void in its luminous form, thus avoiding the common danger of being terrified by it and fleeing from it rather than recognizing it as their true nature.

5. The Yoga of the Transitional Realm (*bardo*): This practice is closely related to the Yoga of the Clear Light. Again adepts acquaint themselves with the after-death phenomena while they are still alive, and as a result of their "rehearsal" are able to penetrate the hallucinatory appearances that are likely to assail them in the after-death *bardo* state. Furthermore, expertise in this Yoga empowers *yogins* to decide their destiny after death, including the option to become reborn in human form into a particular environment. Generally, six *bardos* are distinguished: (a) the ordinary waking state, which lies between birth and death; (b) the dream state, which lies between deep sleep and waking; (c) the unconscious state, which is called "reality state" (*choyid bardo*) because here the mind is thrown back upon its real nature; (d) the state of

becoming (*ridpa bardo*), during which the individual in the hereafter experiences all kinds of phantasmagoric and often terrifying sights—all mental projections; (e) the state of meditation (*samtan bardo*), which is a condition of inner balance accompanied by the withdrawal of the senses from the external world; and (f) the state of birth (*kyena bardo*), which is the period from fertilization of a female egg to the moment of birth (or, rather, rebirth). These *bardos* are powered by a person's karmic tendencies. However, the first, second, and fourth *bardos* also are special opportunities for spiritual practice and growth.

6. The Yoga of Consciousness Transference (*phowa*): Through complex visualizations, combined with breath control, *yogins* conduct the bio-energy to the crown of the head. This highly secret technique is supposed to lead to actual anatomical changes. As John Blofeld observed:

> This yoga is practised for a time by nearly all initiates. At death, in accordance with their skill, they will be able to transfer themselves to realms of radiant light, into an apparitional existence or at least into a desirable incarnation. For, if they are fully successful in mastering this yoga, they will succeed in transferring the consciousness through an aperture which can be opened in the crown of the head at the sagittal suture where the two parietal bones come together or, if less skillful, from various other parts of the body, of which the mouth, anus and penis are the least desirable. The practice is performed daily until success is signalled by lymph or blood oozing from the crown of the head at the spot just mentioned. That this indeed occurs and that a small hole spontaneously opens there as a result of the yoga has been attested by numbers of reliable witnesses in China and in the Indo-Tibetan border regions.[35]

Techniques like Nâropa's Six Yogas are part of what is known as the Path of Form (*dsin-lam*). There also is a Formless Path, which consists in the moment-to-moment recognition of the manifest objects as the transcendental Reality. This Zen-like discipline is also called *gya-chenpo* (Sanskrit: *mahâ-mudrâ*, "great seal"). The attitude of seeing the absolute identity of the phenomenal world and the transcendental Reality creates an inner immunity to all fear and doubt. It establishes practitioners in their authentic being, which is sheer bliss.

This concludes our brief excursion into the heterodox traditions of Buddhism and Jainism. The next chapter picks up the historical thread within Hinduism at the time of the two great epics of India—the *Râmâyana* and the *Mahâbhârata*.

"The body knows touch; the tongue, taste; the nose, scents; the ears, sounds; the eyes, forms, but men who do not know the deep Self (*adhyâtman*)[1] do not seize that Supreme."

—*Mahâbhârata* (12.195.4)

# *Chapter 8*

# THE FLOWERING OF YOGA

## I. OVERVIEW

With this chapter we resume our delineation of the historical unfolding of Hindu Yoga, which we left off in Chapter 5. The focus of the present chapter is on the developments in the fecund period between the mysticism of the early *Upanishads* and the systematized Yoga of Patanjali. This period, which covers what I have called the Epic Age, stretches from c. 600 B.C.E. to c. 100 B.C.E.

A fair number of scriptures relevant to our study of the evolution of Yoga have survived from that period. First is the *Râmâyana*, whose epic nucleus long antedates the Buddha and even the earliest *Upanishads*. In fact, King Râma—the hero of this epic—lived during the late Vedic era, perhaps between 3000 B.C.E. and 2500 B.C.E., certainly prior to the notorious war between the Kurus and Pândavas recorded in the *Mahâbhârata*. Râma's father Dasharatha ("Ten Chariots" or "He who drives his chariot in all ten directions") was the ruler of the fabled city of Ayodhyâ. His real name was Nemi, which means "Rim" or "Circumference," this being perhaps a reference to the king's lordship over an extensive area. Scholarly consensus assigns the final redaction of the present Sanskrit version of the *Râmâyana* to c. 300 B.C.E., whereas the core of the current Sanskrit version of the *Mahâbhârata*, which includes the celebrated *Bhagavad-Gîtâ*, is generally thought to have been composed

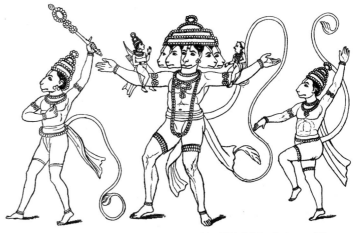

*Reproduced from* Hindu Religion, Customs and Manners

*Râma, with Sîtâ and Hanumat*

245

by c. 500 B.C.E. To be sure, these figures are largely guesswork, and we may well have to allow a far longer interval between the final redactions of these two epics.

Other survivals from the Epic Age are *Upanishads* such as the *Maitrâyanîya,* the *Prashna,* the *Mundaka,* the *Mândûkya,* the *Râma-Pûrva-Tapanîya,* and the *Râma-Uttara-Tapanîya.*[2] Their esoteric teachings go beyond the ideology of the orthodox ritualism of the brahmins. The Upanishadic sages typically rejected the idea that the brahmanical rituals inherited from Vedic and early post-Vedic times had the potency to lead to enlightenment, though they generally conceded that external rites had their proper place in religious life. Their main interest, however, was in communicating the liberating realization of the transcendental Self, and to this end they put forward more or less elaborate liberation teachings.

To the Epic Age also belongs the final redaction of the juridical-ethical literature, such as the *Dharma-Shâstra* of Manu, and the *Dharma-Sûtras* of Baudhâyana and Âpastamba, though again, their nuclei go back to late Vedic times, the period of the early *Brâhmanas.* This is certainly the case for the two *Sûtras,* but scholars think that there also may have been a *Sûtra* by Manu, which according to our revised chronology would have been created before 2000 B.C.E.

Unquestionably the most important Yoga document of the Epic Age is the *Bhagavad-Gîtâ,* which according to its colophon claims the status of an *Upanishad,* even though it forms an integral part of the *Mahâbhârata.* Before we can examine the remarkably holistic teaching of this Hindu classic, we must turn our attention to the *Râmâyana.*

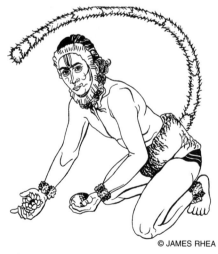

*Hanumat, the faithful servant of Râma*

© JAMES RHEA

## II. HEROISM, PURITY, AND ASCETICISM—THE RÂMÂYANA OF VÂLMÎKI

No single literary creation has been more influential in the lives of millions of people in India and Southeast Asia than the ancient poem *Râmâyana* ("Life of Râma"), which is traditionally deemed the "first poetic work" (*âdi-kâvya*). For countless generations, the tragic love story between King Râma and his beloved wife Sîtâ has served as a repository of spiritual teachings and folk wisdom. Many popular sayings derive from it, and to this day it is recited and retold during festivities. Since 1987, Indian television has broadcast a weekly serial based on the epic poem that is watched by over eighty million viewers.[3]

In its present form, the *Râmâyana* consists of around 24,000 polished verses distributed over seven chapters, with the seventh being a later addition. Although the *Râmâyana* appears to be the work of many authors, tradition acknowledges Vâlmîki as its sole composer. His name means "anthill" and is connected with a colorful story. According to legend, Vâlmîki was born a brahmin but lived as a robber for many years. Through the intervention of some well-meaning sages, he came to recognize the wrongness of his lifestyle. He repented for his transgressions by meditating while transfixed to a single spot for thousands of years, during which time ants built a hill over his body.

The drama recorded in the *Râmâyana* unfolds in the ancient country of Koshala. The story begins with the aged Dasharatha, ruler of the capital city Ayodhyâ, stating his intention to make his son

Râma successor to the throne. Kaikeyî, the youngest of King Dasharatha's three wives, whom he owed two boons, asked for her own son, Bharata, to be appointed and for Râma to be banished for fourteen years. The king had no choice; much against his will, he exiled his beloved son. Râma, son of the senior queen Kaushalyâ, received the news with stoic equanimity and promptly repaired to the forest with his brother Lakshmana and his wife Sîtâ. Sîtâ was a foundling who had been adopted by Janaka, ruler of the neighboring kingdom of Videha. Her name means "Furrow," which Janaka bestowed on her because he had found her in a furrow of the field he was tilling as part of a royal ritual.

Upon the death of his father, Bharata refused the throne and went in search of his exiled brothers. Râma, however, was intent on honoring his banishment. Instead of returning to the kingdom, he went into battle against the demons that disturbed and terrified the renouncers and sages of the forest. Râma killed thousands of demon hosts, and the chief demon, Râvana, revenged their death by abducting beautiful Sîtâ. With the help of the monkey leader Hanumat (better known by the nominative Hanumân),[4] and after many adventures, Râma managed to slay Râvana and free his wife, who had been held captive on the island of Lankâ (modern Sri Lanka, Ceylon).

The question of whether Sîtâ had been defiled by the demon ruler arose. Although she swore to her innocence, she failed to erase all doubt from her husband's mind. In the end, she insisted that Râma let the Divine decide her fate. She entered the blazing fire of a pyre that had been lighted to test her. To everyone's amazement, the flames did not singe a single hair on Sîtâ's body. Râma realized his mistake and was happy to be reunited with his brave and faithful wife. By then his exile had come to an end, and they all returned to the capital, where Râma was jubilantly welcomed.

The citizens of the capital were unconvinced of Sîtâ's innocence, however, and under public pressure Râma banished his beloved wife, ignorant of the fact that she was pregnant. While living in the remote forest hermitage of Sage Vâlmîki, Sîtâ gave birth to twin sons, Lava and Kusha. Vâlmîki composed the *Râmâyana* and taught the two children to sing the text for posterity. Râma was shocked to discover that the boys were his own children and felt great remorse at the hardship he had caused his wife. A dignified Sîtâ appeared before the assembled guests at the palace and invoked Mother Earth as witness of her purity. Promptly the ground opened up and brought forth a golden throne on which Sîtâ disappeared into the bowels of the earth. Disconsolate at the renewed loss of his beloved and faithful spouse, Râma renounced his kingdom and returned to the realm of the Gods. For the Hindus, Râma became a symbol of renunciation, equanimity, and self-discipline, whereas Sîtâ stands for the principle of womanly purity and marital fidelity.

The spirituality of the *Râmâyana* is quite archaic and reflects more the orientation of asceticism (*tapas*) than that of Yoga, the distinction between these two approaches having been made clear in Chapter 3. Râma is portrayed as wandering through enchanted forests inhabited by sages who, because of their fierce austerities, came into possession of magical powers and weapons, which they put at Râma's disposal in order to fight hosts of demons and monsters.

The *Râmâyana* introduces Râma as an incarnation of God Vishnu. At the time of the composition of the *Rig-Veda*, Vishnu was still a minor deity, but he later served as the focal point for the religious imagination and spiritual needs of a rapidly growing community of worshipers. In the Post-Vedic Era, he became the great rival of God Shiva, another minor Vedic deity who won immense popularity in later centuries. Together with God Brahma of mainline Brahmanism, Vishnu and Shiva came to form the well-known trinity (*tri-mûrti*) of popular Hinduism. Here Brahma functions as the creator, Vishnu as the preserver, and Shiva as the destroyer of the universe.

Because of his benign qualities, lovingly characterized in countless popular works, Vishnu is easily the most accessible of the three aspects of the Hindu trinity. His most striking features are his incarnations (*avâtara*), which took place in different world ages. Of his ten principal incarnations, only four were human; the others were magical animals. Vishnu's two most important human incarnations were those of Râma and Krishna.

Hindu tradition regards Râma, or Râmacandra ("Moonlike Râma"), as having lived prior to Krishna, who served as Prince Arjuna's teacher. If we place the Bhârata war around 2300 B.C.E., Râma must have lived around 2900 B.C.E., which corresponds to the first dynasty of pharaonic Egypt. Over time, a religious community sprang up that made Râma its object of worship. Râma's devotees have created several *Upanishads*, including the *Râma-Pûrva-Tapanîya* and the *Râma-Uttara-Tapanîya* mentioned earlier. Their central theological tenet is "Râma alone is the supreme Absolute, Râma alone is the supreme Reality, Shrî Râma is the saving Absolute." According to the former *Upanishad* (1.6), Râma's name is derived, among other things, from the fact that *yogins* delight (*ramante*) in him. Another great creation by a member of the Râma community is the *Yoga-Vâsishtha-Râmâyana*, which is treated in Chapter 14. This mammoth work supplies what is

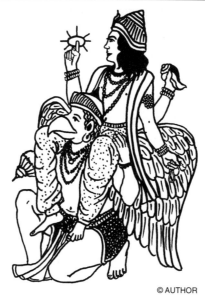

© AUTHOR

*Vishnu mounted on Garuda*

missing in the original *Râmâyana* epic, namely the whole yogic dimension. It portrays Râma as a renouncer who is discovering the truth behind the nondualist teachings of Vedânta.

The significance of the *Râmâyana* for the student of Yoga lies in the moral values it promulgates so vividly. We can regard it as a consummate treatise, in narrative form, on what are known in Yoga as the moral disciplines (*yama*) and restraints (*niyama*). It extols virtues like righteousness (*dharma*), nonharming, truthfulness, and penance. As such the *Râmâyana* can serve as a textbook for Karma-Yoga, the Yoga of self-transcending action. However, like the *Upanishads*, the *Râmâyana* favors wisdom (*vidyâ*) rather than action as the ultimate means to Self-realization. This gospel is vigorously enunciated in the *Râma-Gîtâ* ("Râma's Song"), which is a sixty-two-verse-long passage from the latter part of the *Râmâyana*, but which also circulates as an independent work, as does the *Bhagavad-Gîtâ*, which is an integral part of the *Mahâbhârata* epic. Thus in the *Râma-Gîtâ*, Mahâdeva (Shiva) instructs his divine spouse Umâ as follows:

> Hence the well-intentioned (*sudhî*) [sage] should abandon activity entirely. The combination [of wisdom and action] is not possible because [action] is contrary to wisdom. Always intent on the contemplation (*anusamdhâna*) of the Self, [the sage who practices discipline] relative to the function of all pacified senses is always intent on the contemplation of the Self. (16)

As long as the idea of a self (*âtman*) is, due to illusion (*mâyâ*), [projected] upon the body and so forth, so long must the rites [prescribed by] law be observed. Once the supreme Self has been known by the [sacred] utterance, "[The Self is] not thus (*neti*)," and having negated everything [that is finite], then [the *yogin*] should abandon action. (17)

## III. IMMORTALITY ON THE BATTLE FIELD—THE MAHÂBHÂRATA EPIC

The *Mahâbhârata* is a magnificent and invaluable treasure house of mythology, religion, philosophy, ethics, customs, and information about clans, kings, and sages throughout the ages. Not surprisingly, it acquired the title "Fifth *Veda*" or "Krishna's *Veda*." It is the grand epic of India, composed of about 100,000 stanzas (200,000 lines of primarily sixteen syllables each), which makes the *Mahâbhârata* seven times longer than the *Iliad* and the *Odyssey* combined. However, the critical edition of the epic, undertaken in the years 1933 to 1972 and consisting of nineteen volumes (plus six volumes of indexes), has only about 75,000 stanzas. In the epic's opening chapter, it is stated that the original work consisted of 24,000 verses that were subsequently expanded into approximately 600,000 verses. If true, only a sixth of its former verses have survived. Some scholars believe that the original epic consisted of only

8,800 verses, but such estimates—involving hypothetical reconstructions of the so-called *Urtext*—are hardly convincing.

The *Mahâbhârata* was definitely composed over many generations, and the final redaction of this work appears to have been made some time in the second or third century C.E., which is when the *Hari-Vamsha* ("Hari's Genealogy") was appended. The kernel of this gargantuan epic, however, easily goes back to the time after the Bhârata war, whose date is unknown. According to the inherited scholarly chronology of the nineteenth century, this eighteen-day war was fought around 600–500 B.C.E., which is clearly incorrect. Some modern researchers have therefore proposed 1500

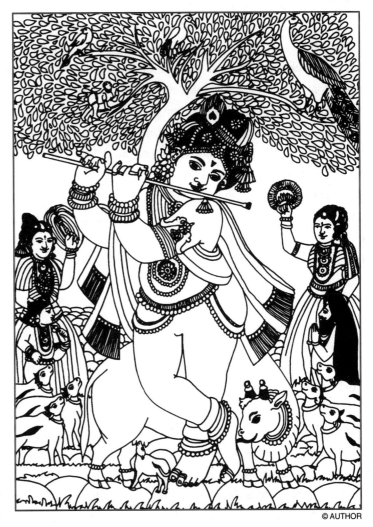

© AUTHOR

*Krishna, the only full avâtara of Vishnu, sporting with the gopîs*

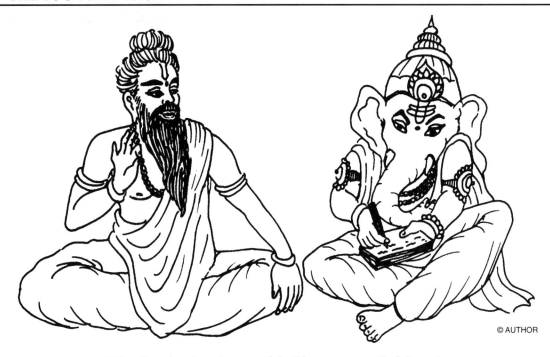

*Vyâsa dictating the epic story of the Bharata war to God Ganesha*

B.C.E. as a possible date, which apparently matches the recent archaeological data for the submerged city of Dvârakâ, described in the epic as Lord Krishna's residence. Traditional Hindu authorities, again, assign the war to around 3100 B.C.E., which is just prior to the beginning of the *kali-yuga*, but there are difficulties with both these dates. A conceivable compromise would place this work around 2000 B.C.E., which is based on the revised age of the *Brâhmana* literature.

The epic consists of eighteen books (*parvan*), to which, as mentioned above, the largely mythological account of Krishna's birth and youth—the *Hari-Vamsha*—was joined in the early post-Christian period. The number "18" occurs often in the epic and clearly has symbolic significance.[5] The narrative nucleus of the epic is the war between two old tribal kingdoms—the Pândavas (Pându's lineage) and the Kauravas (Kuru's lineage, ruled by Dhritarâshtra, the blind older brother of Pându). The compilation of the *Mahâbhârata* is attributed to the sage Krishna Dvaipâyana

("Krishna who dwells on the island"), called Vyâsa. The word *vyâsa* simply means "arranger," and no doubt was applied to a whole line of compilers. Tradition remembers Vyâsa, the individual, also as the compiler of the *Vedas* and the *Purânas*—a task exceeding the capacity of any single human being, especially since these literary genres arose over many centuries. The *Bhagavad-Gîtâ* (18.75), which is embedded in the epic, states that its existence is due to Vyâsa's grace. Thus it appears that early on the title was associated with a specific individual who was a renowned sage.

According to the epic saga, Prince Yudhishthira, one of the five sons of King Pându, lost the Pândavas's share in the kingdom, as well as his wife Draupadî, by a foul trick in a fateful game of dice—a favorite pastime since the ancient Vedic days. He and his four brothers, including Prince Arjuna (the hero of the *Bhagavad-Gîtâ*), were banished as a result. At the end of their thirteen-year exile, the five virtuous sons of Pându demanded the restoration of their paternal share in the kingdom, which was now ruled solely by King

Dhritarâshtra and his hundred sons, notably the power-hungry Duryodhana. When their lawful claim was dismissed, they went to war against the Kauravas. On the side of the Pândavas was the God-man Krishna who, though officially a non-combatant, used various divine ploys and trickery to assist the good cause of King Pându's sons. The Kauravas, though they were far more numerous, were defeated after eighteen days of the fiercest battles.

Whatever the historical realities may have been, the *Mahâbhârata* also lends itself to symbolic and allegorical interpretations. Thus, the strife between the Pândava and Kaurava cousins has often been understood as the struggle between good and evil, right and wrong, in the world and in the human heart. Beyond this, the *Mahâbhârata* puts forward a mystical point of view according to which there is an unsurpassable Condition that transcends both good and evil, right and wrong. That condition is celebrated as the highest value to which human beings can aspire. It is synonymous with freedom and immortality.

Around the epic war story, layer upon layer of instructional and legendary materials—comprising no less than four-fifths of the entire epic—have been woven over the centuries. Some scholars regard the famous *Bhagavad-Gîtâ*, found in the sixth book of the *Mahâbhârata*, as one of these additions. However, it is just as conceivable that the teachings of the *Gîtâ* were actually given in brief on the morrow of the first battle and then were elaborated on subsequently. Another expansion of the original text that is very important for our understanding of that phase in the evolution of Yoga is the *Moksha-Dharma*, which can be found in the twelfth book. In the fourteenth book of the epic, the *Anu-Gîtâ* stands out as a didactic poem. I will discuss these texts in the following sections.

For Hindus, the *Mahâbhârata* epic is a rich mine of instructive and delightful tales about heroes, rogues, renouncers, and *yogins*. For the historian of religion, it is a mosaic of ideas, beliefs, and customs of one of the most fertile eras in the intellectual history of Hinduism. The contemporary student of Yoga can fruitfully approach the epic from both these perspectives and also ponder the epic's deep symbolism.

Yoga and its cousin Sâmkhya loom large in the philosophy of the epic. As we have seen, both traditions have their roots in the pre-Buddhist era. The Yoga and Sâmkhya schools mentioned in the epic, however, appear to be post-Buddhist and thus can be placed in the centuries from 500 B.C.E. to 200 C.E.

## IV. THE BHAGAVAD-GÎTÂ—JEWEL OF THE MAHÂBHÂRATA

The *Bhagavad-Gîtâ* ("Lord's Song") is the earliest extant document of Vaishnavism, the religious tradition centering on the worship of the Divine in the form of Vishnu, specifically in his incarnation as Krishna. This tradition, which has its roots in the Vedic Age, flourished in the sixth century B.C.E. in the region of modern Mathurâ and from there spread to other parts of the Indian peninsula. Today Vaishnavism is one of the five great religious traditions of India, the other four being Shaivism (focusing on Shiva), Shaktism (focusing on Shakti, the female power aspect of the Divine), the Gânapatyas (focusing on the elephant-headed deity Ganesha or Ganapati), and the Sauras (focusing on the solar deity Sûrya).

The *Bhagavad-Gîtâ*, or simply *Gîtâ* ("Song"), is an episode of the *Mahâbhârata*, forming chapters 13–40 of the sixth book and comprising a total of 700 verses. A recension of the *Gîtâ* discovered in Kashmir contains 714 stanzas. But there also is a Balinese version of the *Gîtâ* that has only 86 stanzas, and a manuscript found in Farrukhabad has only 84 stanzas. Not a few scholars have argued that the *Gîtâ* was originally an independent text that was later incorporated into the epic. Others rightly have pointed to the seemingly flawless continuity between the *Gîtâ* and the rest of the *Mahâbhârata*. Perceiving certain inconsistencies and incongruities in the transmitted text, some scholars have tried to reconstruct the original. Thus the German scholar Richard Garbe ended up with a text comprising 630 verses, while his student Rudolf Otto was left with a mere 133 verses.[6] The American Yoga researcher Phulgenda Sinha believes he has identified the 84 stanzas of the original *Gîtâ*, largely by deleting all verses referring to what he considers to be religious dogma.[7]

The date of the *Gîtâ* is uncertain. It is generally placed in the third century B.C.E., though some scholars assign an earlier date to it, and others wrongly regard it as a post-Christian work. I accept the conclusions of the Indian scholar K. N. Upadhyaya, who, after examining all the various arguments in some depth, placed the *Gîtâ* in the period from the fifth to the fourth century B.C.E.[8] However, verses were probably added at different periods, although it seems doubtful that they can be identified with any degree of certainty. The original "Song," of course, was probably imparted by Krishna on the battlefield of *kuru-kshetra* two millennia before the Buddha.

What is certain is that the *Gîtâ* has enjoyed enormous popularity among Hindus for countless generations. This popularity is epitomized in the words of Mahatma Gandhi, who said: "I find a solace in the *Bhagavadgîtâ* that I miss even in the Sermon on the Mount . . . I owe it all to the teachings of the *Bhagavadgîtâ*."[9] The *Gîtâ*, which has been available in English translation since 1785 (in a rendering by Charles Wilkins), also has inspired many well-known Westerners, including

the philosophers Georg Friedrich Hegel, Arthur Schopenhauer, and Johann Gottfried Herder; indologist-philosopher Paul Deussen; and philosopher-traveler Hermann von Keyserling; the linguist Wilhelm von Humboldt; the writers Walt Whitman, Aldous Huxley, and Christopher Isherwood; as well as the esotericists Rudolf Steiner (founder of Anthroposophy) and Annie Besant (a leader of the Theosophical Society). The German Sanskritist and pioneering Yoga researcher J. W. Hauer summed up the sentiment of many of these personalities when he wrote:

> The *Gîtâ* gives us not only profound insights that are valid for all times and for all religious life . . . Here spirit is at work that belongs to our spirit.[10]

The *Bhagavad-Gîtâ* is a dialogue between the incarnate God Krishna and his pupil Prince Arjuna, which took place on the Kuru's battlefield (*kuru-kshetra*), located in the Gangetic plain around modern Delhi. This immortal conversation is the climax of the epic story. Its importance for the student of Yoga is obvious, since it must be regarded as the first full-fledged Yoga scripture. Indeed, the *Gîtâ* speaks of itself as a *yoga-shâstra*, or yogic teaching, restating ancient truths.

Historically speaking, the *Bhagavad-Gîtâ* can be understood as a massive effort to integrate the diverse strands of spiritual thought prevalent within Hinduism in the Epic Age. It mediates between the sacrificial ritualism of the orthodox priesthood and such innovative teachings as we have encountered in the esoteric doctrines of the early *Upanishads*, as well as in the traditions of Buddhism and Jainism. Aldous Huxley, in his introduction to the *Gîtâ* rendering by Swami Prabhavananda and Christopher Isherwood, called this ancient work "perhaps the most systematic statement of the Perennial Philosophy."[11]

## *The Mystical Activism of the Gîtâ*

The central message of Lord Krishna's Song is the balancing of conventional religious and ethical activity and otherworldly ascetic goals. The gist of Krishna's activist teaching is given in the following stanza:

Steadfast in Yoga perform actions, abandoning attachment and remaining the same in success and failure, O Dhanamjaya.[12] Yoga is called "evenness" (*samatva*). (2.48)

In order to win peace and enlightenment—so Krishna declares—one need not forsake the world or one's responsibilities, even when they oblige one to go into battle. Renunciation (samnyâsa) *of* action is good in itself, but better still is renunciation *in* action. This is the Hindu ideal of "actionless action" or inaction in action (*naishkarmya-karman*), which is the basis of Karma-Yoga. Life in the world and spiritual life are not in principle inimical to each other; they can and should be cultivated simultaneously. Such is the essence of a whole or integrated life.

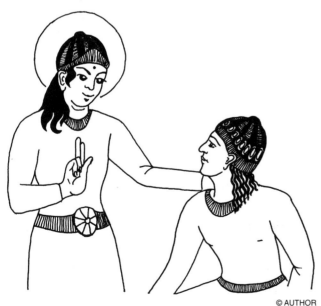

*Lord Krishna encouraging Arjuna*

Not by abstention from actions does a man enjoy action-transcendence (*naish-karmya*), nor by renunciation alone does he approach perfection (*siddhi*).

For, not even for a moment can anyone ever remain without performing action. Everyone is unwittingly made to act by the constituents (*guna*) belonging to Nature (*prakriti*).

He who restrains his organs of action but sits remembering in his mind the objects of the senses is called a hypocrite, a bewildered person (*âtman*).

But more excellent is he, O Arjuna, who, controlling with his mind the senses, embarks unattached on Karma-Yoga with the organs of action.

You must [always] do the allotted action, for action is superior to inaction; not even your body's processes can be accomplished by inaction.

This world is bound by action, save when this action is [performed as] sacrifice (*yajna*). With that purpose [in mind], O Kaunteya [i.e., Arjuna], engage in action devoid of attachment. (3.4–9)

Krishna points to himself as an example of enlightened activity:

For Me, O Pârtha [i.e., Arjuna], there is nothing to be done in the three worlds, nothing ungained to be gained—and yet I engage in action.

For, if I were not untiringly ever to abide in action, people would, O Pârtha, follow everywhere My "track" [i.e., example].

Just as the unwise perform [their deeds] attached to action, O Bhârata [i.e., Arjuna], the wise should act unattached, desiring the world's welfare (*loka-samgraha*). (3.22–25)

The secret lies in the human mind as the primary source of all action. If the mind is pure, without attachment to deeds, it cannot be defiled by them even as they are performed. Only attachment, not action as such, sets in motion the law of moral causation (or karma) by which a person is bound to the wheel of existence in ever new re-embodiments. The mind that is polished like a mirror, freed entirely of the stain of attachment, spotlessly reveals things as they truly are. And what they truly are is the Divine, the Self. The perfected *yogin* always enjoys that divine vision:

Whose self is yoked in Yoga and who beholds everywhere the same, he sees the Self abiding in all beings and all beings in the Self. (6.29)

This vision of the sameness of all things and beings is the fruit of consummate nonattachment. Nonattachment is a matter of assuming the position of the transcendental Self, the eternal witness of all processes, and of penetrating the illusion of being an acting subject, or ego. Nonetheless, actions must continue to be performed.

Acts must not only be performed in the spirit of unselfishness, or nonattachment, they also must be morally sound and justifiable. This view has not always been emphasized sufficiently in Western interpretations of the *Gîtâ*. If action

depended solely on one's frame of mind, it would be the best excuse for immoral behavior. The *Bhagavad-Gîtâ* does not propound such a crude subjectivism. For action to be "whole" (*kritsna*), or wholesome, it must have two essential ingredients: subjective purity (i.e., nonattachment) and objective rationality (i.e., moral rightness). The external factor of moral rightness or wrongness is determined by the traditional moral values and the prevalent code of behavior, as well as by the growing insight into rightness and wrongness through the practice of Yoga. The *Gîtâ* builds on the ethical foundations of the *Mahâbhârata*. The epic is, on one level, a gigantic attempt to come to grips with the nature of what is lawful (*dharma*) and what is unlawful (*adharma*). This is echoed in the following stanzas from the *Gîtâ*:

What is action? What is inaction? On this even the sages are bewildered. I shall declare to you that action which, when understood, will set you free from ill.

Indeed, [a *yogin*] ought to understand [the nature of] action (*karman*), he ought to understand wrong action (*vikarman*), and he ought to understand inaction (*akarman*). Impenetrable is the way of action.

He who sees inaction in action and action in inaction is wise among men; he is yoked, performing whole (*kritsna*) actions. (4.16–18)

The war into which Arjuna was drawn on the sagacious advice of the incarnate God Krishna was in the interest of the maintenance of a higher moral order. The Kauravas were power-hungry and corrupt rulers who had usurped the throne.

The peace-loving Pândavas, on the other hand, had the welfare of the people at heart. The *Gîtâ* portrays Arjuna's qualms about going into battle even over what is obviously right and lawful. Seeing his cousins and former teachers arrayed on the opposite side of the battlefield, he was ready to cast down his bow and surrender his claims to the throne, but Lord Krishna instructed him otherwise. His yogic teaching goes beyond both pacifism and warmongering, just as it goes beyond the mere doing of one's duty on the one hand and the neglect of one's obligations on the other. For, in the last analysis, the God-man Krishna expects his devotee to step beyond the moral realm. He makes this exhortation and solemn promise:

> Relinquishing all norms (*dharma*), go to Me alone for shelter. I will deliver you from all sin. Do not grieve! (18.66)

> The Lord abides in the heart region of all beings, O Arjuna, whirling all beings [in the cycle of conditioned existence] by His power (*mâyâ*), [as if they were] mounted on a machine (*yatra*).

> To him alone go for shelter with your whole being O Bhârata [i.e., Arjuna]! By His grace you will obtain supreme peace, the eternal Abode. (18.61–62)

> Be Me-minded, devoted to Me, sacrifice to Me, do obeisance to Me—thus you will come to Me. I promise you truly, [for] you are dear to Me. (18.65)

In the *Bhagavad-Gîtâ*, Yoga is not yet systematically outlined, as in the subsequent *Maitrâyanîya-Upanishad* and the *Yoga-Sûtra*, but all the principal elements of the path are present. For Krishna the yogic work consists essentially in the total realignment of one's daily life to the ultimate Being. Everything that is done should be done in the light of the Divine. One's whole life must become a continual Yoga. By seeing in everything the presence of the Divine and by casting off all mundane attachments, *yogins* purify their life and no longer take flight from it. With their mind immersed in the Supreme, they are active in the world, guided by the pure desire to promote the welfare of all beings. This is the well-known Hindu ideal of *loka-samgraha*, which literally means "drawing together of the world."

It is difficult to give this Yoga an appropriate label. It is not only Jnâna-Yoga and Karma-Yoga but also Bhakti-Yoga. It seeks to integrate all aspects of the human being and then to employ them in the great enterprise to reach enlightenment in this very life. For this reason, Krishna's path might best be described as a kind of early "integral Yoga" (*pûrna-yoga*).

The ethical activism of the *Bhagavad-Gîtâ* is founded on a panentheistic metaphysics: Everything exists or arises in God, while God nevertheless transcends everything. The supreme Being, Vishnu (as Krishna), is both the ultimate source of all existence and the manifest universe in its entire multiplicity. Vishnu encompasses Being as well as Becoming. Lord Krishna, the incarnate God, declares:

> By Me, unmanifest in form, this entire [universe] is spread out. All beings abide in Me, but I do not subsist in them.

> And [yet] beings do not abide in Me. Behold My lordly Yoga: My Self sustains [all] beings, yet not abiding in beings causes beings to be. (9.4–5)

Vishnu is the all-embracing Whole (*pûrna*), the One and the Many. Since the Divine is everywhere and in everything, we do not have to shun the world in order to find Vishnu, but merely need to cultivate our higher wisdom (*buddhi*), the eye of gnosis (*jnâna-cakshus*), to be able to apprehend the omnipresent Being-in-Becoming.

The *Bhagavad-Gîtâ* knows of two types of emancipation that are more accurately described as two successive stages of completeness. The first level of liberation, called *brahma-nirvâna*, is the extinction in the world-ground. Here *yogins* transcend the space-time continuum and abide in their essential nature. But this state is without outflowing love, and the divine person of Krishna remains concealed from them. The supreme Person is realized only in the higher form of emancipation when *yogins* awaken in God.

> That man who, having forsaken all desires, moves about devoid of longing, devoid of [the thought of] "mine," without ego-sense—he approaches peace (*shânti*).

> This is the state of the Absolute (*brahman*), O *Pârtha* [i.e., Arjuna]. Attaining this, one is no [longer] deluded. Abiding therein also at the end-time [i.e., at death], one attains extinction (*nirvâna*) in the Absolute. (2.71–72)

> He who has inner joy, inner rejoicing, and inner light is a *yogin*. Having become the Absolute, he approaches extinction in the Absolute. (5.24)

> Thus ever yoking the self, the *yogin* of restrained mind approaches peace, the supreme extinction that subsists in Me. (6.15)

> He who is intent on oneness (*ekatva*) and loves Me, abiding in all beings, in whatever [state] he exists—that *yogin* dwells in Me. (6.31)

Love (*bhakti*) is a key element in Krishna's teaching. On the finite plane, it is the surest mechanism by which *yogin*-devotees bond themselves

*The first stanza of the Bhagavad-Gîtâ with various commentaries*

to the Divine Person and thereby win grace. On the ultimate level, love is the very nature of the liberated condition. Thus Krishna states:

> Of all *yogins*, he who loves Me with faith and whose inner self is absorbed in Me—him I deem to be most yoked. (6.47)

How may we understand the transcendental love in which the liberated *yogin* participates? Elsewhere I proposed this answer:

> The love that flourishes eternally between God and the Self-particles who have awakened to His presence is one of ineffable divine creativity: the Whole communing with Itself. The logical mind shrinks back from this paradox. It fails to gain a foothold in that realm in which all opposites coincide. The ultimate test must be unmediated experience. This transcendental love (*para-bhakti*) is an essential part of God and can be fully realized only in and through God. This love is . . . unconditional and without object.[13]

The *Gîtâ's* teaching of the eternal love that flows from the Divine Person to the devotee and to all creation is one of the most momentous innovations in the history of Indian religiosity. The Yoga taught by Krishna, the *avâtara* (divine descent), infused Hinduism with a rare emotionality that had until then been absent from the largely ascetic efforts of the Hindu seers and sages. Suddenly the spiritual seeker was empowered to relate to the Divine in personal terms, from the heart and not merely through the exercise of the will. This had in fact been the teaching of the ancient Vedic *rishis*, but it became gradually eclipsed by the tradition of fierce asceticism (*tapas*) both within and outside the orthodox brahmanical priesthood. The *Gîtâ*, in fact, introduces Krishna not so much as an innovator but as a revivor of ancient teachings that had been lost. Tentative expressions of the same teaching can be found in the early *Upanishads*, but with the *Gîtâ* the gospel of theistic devotion entered the popular consciousness and became a vehicle for the simple spiritual aspirations of countless millions.

## SOURCE READING 10

# *Bhagavad-Gîtâ (Selection)*

Since there are numerous English renderings of the *Bhagavad-Gîtâ* available, I have abstained from bringing the full text here. However, a translation of the famous eleventh chapter in which Lord Krishna reveals his transcendental nature to his devotee Arjuna deserves to be included. This chapter is the dramatic climax of the *Gîtâ*, and Arjuna's vision of Krishna as the Divine also is the culmination of the spiritual path taught by Krishna. The vision is a classic description of the mystical state of unity in which all things coexist in eternity—a state utterly bewildering to the unillumined mind. Somewhat unprepared for Krishna's self-revelation, Arjuna, though he had prayed for it, is unable to bear the unitive vision for long and asks Krishna to resume his customary human form. This is more than a mere poetic ploy, allowing the composer to resume the metaphysical dialogue between divine teacher and human pupil, it also is a classic statement of the natural process of return from extraordinary mystical realization to ordinary life sustained by sensory awareness.

For clarification, I should add that Krishna addresses Arjuna as Pândava ("Son of Pându"), Pârtha ("Son of Prithâ [i.e., Kuntî]"), Bhârata ("Descendant of Bharata"), Dhanamjaya ("Conqueror of wealth"), and Gudâkesha ("He whose hair is gathered in a knot"). Arjuna, in turn, bestows upon Krishna various honorific epithets, such as Purushottama ("Supreme Person"), Hrishîkesha ("He whose hair is bristling from ecstasy"), and Govinda ("Cow-Finder," *go* or "cow" signifying spiritual riches).

Arjuna said:

Out of favor for me, you have declared the supreme mystery called the deep Self (*adhyâtman*) by which this confusion (*moha*) of mine is dispelled. (1)

For, I have heard of the creation and the dissolution of beings from you in detail, O lotus-eyed [Krishna], as well as of [your] immutable majesty (*mâhâtmya*). (2)

Even as you have described [Your] Self, O supreme Lord, so do I desire to see your lordly Form, O supreme Person. (3)

If, O Lord, you think it possible for me to behold that [cosmic Form of yours], O Lord of Yoga, then do reveal to me [your] immutable Self. (4)

The Blessed Lord said:

O Pârtha, behold My forms [which are] a hundredfold, a thousandfold, of varied kinds, divine, many-colored and many-shaped. (5)

Behold the Âdityas, Vasus, Rudras, Ashvins, and Maruts. Behold, O Bhârata, the many marvels never seen before.[14] (6)

Behold now, O Gudâkesha, the whole world, [with all its] moving and unmoving [things], abiding as one here in My [cosmic] body, and whatever else you desire to see. (7)

Yet never will you be able to see Me with this your [physical] eye. I will give you a divine (*divya*) eye. Behold my lordly Yoga. (8)

Samjaya [the narrator of the dialogue between Krishna and Arjuna] said:

O King [Dhritarâshtra], having spoken thus, the great Lord of Yoga, Hari, then revealed [his] supreme lordly Form to Pârtha. (9)

[His Form has] many mouths and eyes, many marvelous appearances, many divine adornments, many divine upraised weapons, (10)

wearing divine garlands and robes, anointed with divine fragrances, all-wonderful. [Behold] the God, infinite, omnipresent. (11)

If the splendor of a thousand suns were to arise at once in heaven, that would be like the splendor of that Great Self. (12)

Then Pândava saw the whole world, divided manifold, abiding in the One, there in the [cosmic] body of the God of Gods. (13)

Then Dhanamjaya, filled with amazement (*vismaya*), with bristling hair, bowing his head before the God and doing *anjali*[15], spoke [thus]: (14)

O God, in your [cosmic] body I behold the Gods and all the various kinds of beings, Lord Brahma seated on the lotus throne, and all the seers and divine serpents (*uraga*). (15)

Everywhere I behold you [who are] of endless Form, with many arms, bellies, mouths, eyes. I cannot see in you beginning, middle, or end, O All-Lord, All-Form. (16)

I behold you with diadem, mace, and discus—a mass of brilliance, flaming all round.

[Yet you are] hard to see, for [you are] entirely a brilliant radiance of immeasurable sun-fire. (17)

You are to be known as the supreme Imperishable (*akshara*). You are the supreme Treasure-Store (*nidhâna*) of all this. You are the Immutable (*avyaya*), the Guardian of the eternal law (*dharma*). You are the everlasting Person (*purusha*)—[now] I know. (18)

Without beginning, middle or end, of endless strength (*vîrya*), with infinite arms and with moon and sun as eyes: I behold you—[your] mouth a flaming offering-consumer burning up all this with your brilliance. (19)

By you alone is this interspace between Heaven and Earth pervaded, and all the quarters [too]. Seeing this marvelous, terrifying Form of yours, the triple world shudders, O Great Self. (20)

Verily, these hosts of Gods enter into you. Some, frightened, pray with the *anjali*[-gesture]. Crying out, "Hail [to you]!", multitudes of great seers (*rishi*) and adepts (*siddha*) laud you with excellent hymns. (21)

Rudras, Âdityas, Vasus, and the Sâdhyas, the Vishve[-devas], the [two] Ashvins, the Maruts, and the quaffers-of-steam, and the hosts of Gandharvas, Yakshas, Asuras, and adepts—all behold you in amazement.[16] (22)

Beholding that great form of yours, O strong-armed [Krishna], with its many mouths and eyes, arms, thighs, feet, many bellies, many formidable fangs—the worlds shudder, and so do I. (23)

Touching the sky, flaming many-colored, with gaping mouths and flaming spacious eyes—beholding you [thus], my innermost Self (*antar-âtman*) trembles, and I cannot find a hold or tranquillity (*shama*), O Vishnu. (24)

And seeing your [numerous] mouths [studded with] formidable fangs resembling the fire of time, I know not where to turn, and I find no shelter [anywhere]. Be gracious, O Lord of the Gods, O World-Home! (25)

And all these sons of Dhritarâshtra together with hosts of protectors of the earth—Bhîshma, Drona, as well as the son of Suta and also our war lords— (26)

they swiftly enter your mouths with formidable fear-instilling fangs. Some are seen sticking in between your teeth with pulverized heads. (27)

As many rivers and water torrents flow headlong into the ocean, so do these heroes (*vîra*) of the world of men enter your blazing mouths. (28)

As moths in profuse streams enter a blazing flame to be destroyed, so do the worlds in profuse streams enter your mouths to be destroyed. (29)

With flaming mouths, you lick up all the worlds, completely devouring them. Filling the whole world with brilliance, your dreadful (*ugra*) rays blaze forth, O Vishnu. (30)

Tell me who you are of dreadful form. Salutations be to you! O Best of Gods, have mercy! I wish to know you [as you were] at first. For I do not comprehend your creativity (*pravritti*). (31)

The Blessed Lord said:

I am time (*kâla*), wreaker of the matured world's destruction, engaged here to annihilate the worlds. Except for you, all these warriors arrayed in the opposed ranks shall not be [alive after this battle]. (32)

Therefore, you, arise, win glory! Conquering the enemies, enjoy a prosperous kingdom! Verily, they are already slain by Me. Be a mere tool (*nimitta*) [for Me], O Savyasâcin![17] (33)

Drona, Bhîshma, Jayadratha, and Karna, as well as the other [heroes] are [already] slain by Me. You must strike [them down]! Do not be distressed. Fight! You will conquer [all your] rivals in battle. (34)

Samjaya [the narrator] said:

Upon hearing these words of Keshava, Kirîtin [i.e., Arjuna], doing *anjali*, trembling, saluting again and bowing down, said to Krishna with stammering [voice], very frightened: (35)

Rightly, O Hrishîkesha, the world rejoices and is enraptured with your praise. The Rakshasas flee terrified in [all] directions, and all the hosts of adepts salute [you].[18] (36)

And why should they not salute [you], O Great Self, [you who are] greater even than Brahma, the primal Creator (*âdi-kartri*)? O infinite Lord of the Gods, World-Abode, you are the Imperishable, existence (*sat*) and nonexistence (*asat*) and what is beyond that. (37)

You are the primal God (*âdi-deva*), the ancient Person (*purusha*). You are the supreme Treasure-Store of all this. You are the knower and the known and the supreme Abode. By you all this is spread out, O infinite Form! (38)

You are Vâyu, Yama, Agni, Varuna, Shashânka, and Prajâpati the grandsire.[19] Salutation, salutation be to you, a thousandfold; and again and again salutation, salutation to you! (39)

Salutation to you from in front and from behind! Salutation to you from all round, O All! Endless your strength, immeasurable [your] might (*vikrama*). You complete all, hence you are all. (40)

Ignorant of this your majesty, through my heedlessness (*pramâda*), or perhaps through fondness and thinking importunately [that you are my] friend, I rashly said, "Hey Krishna! Hey Yâdava! Hey friend!" (41)

and in jest [showed] disrespect to you, while at play, reposing, sitting, or eating when alone or in the company [of others]—for that, O Acyuta, I beg forgiveness from you, the Unfathomable! (42)

You are the father of the world, [containing] moving and unmoving [things]. You are its object-of-worship (*pûjya*) and [its] venerable teacher. None is equal to you—how could there be [anything] greater in the triple world, O matchless Splendor? (43)

Therefore bowing down and bending low [my] body, I seek your grace (*prasâda*), O praiseworthy Lord. You should bear [with me], O God, as a father with a son, as a friend with a friend, or a lover with a beloved. (44)

I am thrilled at having seen what has not been seen before. But my mind is distressed with fear. [Therefore], O God, show me that [human] form [of yours]. Be gracious, O Lord of the Gods, World-Home! (45)

I wish to see you even as [before], [with your] crown, the mace, and the discus in hand. Assume that four-armed form [of yours], O thousand-armed All-Form! (46)

The Blessed Lord said:

Out of My kindness (*prasanna*) for you, O Arjuna, I have revealed this supreme Form by [My] Self's Yoga—which brilliant, all[-embracing], endless, and primeval (*âdya*) [Form] of Mine has not been seen before you by anyone. (47)

Neither by the *Vedas*, sacrifices, or study (*adhyaya*), nor by gifts, nor by rites (*kriyâ*), nor by fierce penance (*tapas*) can I be seen thus-formed in the world of men by anyone [but] you, O heroic foe (*pravîra*) of the Kurus! (48)

You [need] not tremble. Do not [succumb to] a bewildered state at seeing this terrible Form of Mine. Free from fear (*bhî*) and glad minded, you [can] behold again this My [familiar physical] form, that very [form which you know so well]. (49)

Samjaya [the narrator] said:

Having thus spoken to Arjuna, Vasudeva revealed again his [human] form, and having assumed again his pleasant [human] body, the Great Self comforted the terrified [Prince Arjuna]. (50)

Arjuna said:

Beholding [again] this pleasant human form of yours, O Janârdana,[20] I have now recovered my natural consciousness. (51)

The Blessed Lord said:

This Form of Mine, which you have seen, is very difficult to see. Even the Gods are forever eager to [be granted a] vision of this Form. (52)

In the way in which you have seen Me, I cannot be seen by [means of] the *Vedas*, nor by penance, nor by gifts, nor by sacrifice. (53)

But, O Arjuna, by love [directed to] no other, I can be seen and known in this way, and entered into in reality, O Paramtapa.[21] (54)

> He who does My work, intent on Me, devoted to Me, free from attachment, without enmity toward all beings—he comes to Me, O Pândava! (55)

## V. THE YOGIC TEACHINGS OF THE ANU-GÎTÂ

The *Anu-Gîtâ* ("After-Song"), found in the *Mahâbhârata* (14.16-50), is the earliest imitation of the *Bhagavad-Gîtâ* of which we have knowledge. "Imitation," however, is perhaps the wrong word, because it is more than a mere echo of the Lord's Song. It is intended to recapitulate the teachings given by Lord Krishna to Prince Arjuna just before the commencement of the first battle between the Pândavas and the Kauravas. After the last battle was fought and the war was won, Arjuna asked his divine teacher, the God-man Krishna, to repeat the teachings of the *Bhagavad-Gîtâ*. The *Anu-Gîtâ* is Krishna's response to this request. There are a number of other "imitation" *Gîtâs* from various periods, but none claims to be a direct recapitulation of Krishna's original song of instruction as does the *Anu-Gîtâ*.

Before giving his priceless teachings again to Prince Arjuna, Krishna rebuked his disciple for forgetting the original instructions. But Arjuna may easily be excused for this failing, given the fact that when the *Bhagavad-Gîtâ*'s wisdom was imparted to him he was in a state of dejection from having seen his friends and teachers among the ranks of the enemy.

While there are many parallels between the two *Gîtâs*, we cannot fail to note the absence of the devotional (*bhakti*) element in the *Anu-Gîtâ*. Instead this text emphasizes the element of gnosis (*jnâna*), with the Absolute (*brahman*) as the highest goal of human aspiration—not divine communion with Lord Krishna. It appears that the *Anu-Gîtâ* is an early attempt to downplay the devotionalism of Krishna's teachings—a tendency continued forcefully by Shankara, the chief proponent of Advaita Vedânta and its Jnâna-Yoga.

## VI. THE LIBERATING GOSPEL OF THE EPIC—THE MOKSHA-DHARMA

Next to the *Bhagavad-Gîtâ* and the *Anu-Gîtâ*, the most significant materials on Yoga in the *Mahâbhârata* are found in the *Moksha-Dharma* section, which comprises Chapters 168-353 of the twelfth book of the epic. Here several related but not always consonant traditions are given voice. Besides the orthodox brahmanical schools represented by Vedânta, we encounter several other traditions, notably the Pancarâtra religion (an early form of Vaishnavism), the Pâshupata religion (a form of Shaivism), Pre-Classical Sâmkhya, and Pre-Classical Yoga. These diverse teachings have sometimes been looked upon as being merely a corrupt doctrinal jumble crafted onto the nondualist metaphysics of Vedânta, but nothing could be further from the truth.

The liberation gospels present in the *Moksha-Dharma* give us important clues especially about Sâmkhya and Yoga in their "epic" forms, prior to their systematizations at the hands of Îshvara

Krishna (c. 350 C.E.) and Patanjali (c. 200 C.E.) respectively. What emerges from a careful study of the *Moksha-Dharma* is, the great similarities between Sâmkhya and Yoga notwithstanding, that these two traditions were already distinct and independent developments at the time of the final composition of the *Mahâbhârata*. This is epitomized in the following statement:

> The method of the *yogas* [i.e., *yogins*] is perception, [whereas] for the *sâmkhyas* it is scriptural tradition. (12.289.7)

"These are not the same," as the epic affirms two verses later. The distinction made here is between the pragmatic-experimental approach of the *yogins* (called *yogas*), and the reliance on traditional revelation (accompanied by rational inquiry into the nature of human existence) that typifies the followers of Sâmkhya. But Epic or Pre-Classical Yoga is not characterized simply by practice, nor Sâmkhya only by theory. Both traditions have their own specific theoretical framework and psychotechnology.

Pre-Classical Sâmkhya arose out of the Upanishadic speculations about the levels of existence and consciousness as they were disclosed in the penetrating meditations of the sages. But by the time of the *Moksha-Dharma*, Sâmkhya and Vedânta had become distinct traditions. Like some schools of Vedânta, however, Pre-Classical Sâmkhya espoused a form of nondualism.

This is also true of the epic schools of Yoga. What distinguishes epic Sâmkhya and Yoga from their classical formulations is, above all, their theistic orientation. The atheism of Classical Sâmkhya and the curious theism of Classical Yoga must be understood as deviations from a strongly theistic base, reflected in the *Upanishads*.

The reason for this shift away from the original panentheism of Sâmkhya and Yoga was a felt need to respond to the challenge of such vigorously analytical traditions as Buddhism by systematizing both Sâmkhya and Yoga along rationalistic philosophical lines. In both cases, this effort led to a metaphysical dualism that is barely

ईश्वर । बुद्ध । अबद्धिमत् ॥

*Îshvara, buddha, abuddhimat*

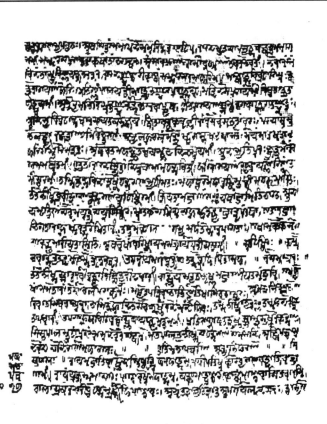

*A manuscript page of the Mahâbhârata*

convincing and that limps behind the nondualist interpretations of Vedânta.

There were important differences between the epic schools of Sâmkhya and Yoga on metaphysical-theological matters. The epic Sâmkhya teachers maintained that there is an essential identity between the individuated or empirical self, called *budhyamâna* or *jîva*, and the universal Self, called *buddha* or *âtman*. By contrast, the Yoga tradition asserted that there is more of a rift between the transcendental Self and the many empirical selves or ego-personalities. Also, according to the adepts of Yoga there is a supreme Being, or Divinity, above the collective of transcendental Selves. In comparison with that absolute Being, which is known as the "awakened" (*buddha*) principle, or as "Lord" (*îshvara*), even the liberated beings are still unenlightened or unawakened (*abuddhimat*). Thus, the epic *yogins* allowed twenty-six fundamental categories of existence, called "principles" (*tattva*), whereas the Sâmkhya followers allowed only twenty-five. These ontological principles will be discussed in Chapter 10.

The epic schools of Sâmkhya and Yoga gave rise to Sâmkhya-Yoga syncretism. For the historian of Indian philosophy and spirituality these developments, which have for so long been misunderstood, form one of the most exciting areas of inquiry. For the student of Yoga, it is important to know that Patanjali's *Yoga-Sûtra* was preceded by centuries of lively experimentation and thought about the great matter of self-transcendence. Patanjali's work, impressive as it is as a concise statement of Yoga philosophy and practice, scarcely betokens the immense ingenuity and spiritual creativity on which it was built.

When we read the *Moksha-Dharma*, we encounter all kinds of more or less elaborate and more or less abstruse teachings. In terms of actual practice, the Yoga authorities who make their appearance in the epic insist on solid moral foundations. They demand such virtues as truthfulness, humility, nonpossessiveness, nonviolence, forgiveness, and compassion, which also form the bedrock of later Yoga.

Lust, anger, greed, and fear are frequently listed as the *yogin*'s greatest enemies. There are also references to dreaming and sleep, infatuation and "mental diarrhea" (*bhrama*), as well as doubt and discontent, which are all deemed to be severe obstacles on the spiritual road. Another considerable obstruction is said to be the powers, called *siddhis* or *vibhûtis*, that can distract the *yogin* from his real concern, which is to transcend the self, or ego-personality. These powers are a natural by-product of the *yogin*'s meditation practice. Yet, as Patanjali observes in his *Yoga-Sûtra* (3.37), they are accomplishments only from the point of view of the egoic consciousness. Their exercise prevents the ecstatic state (*samâdhi*) precisely because the deployment of these powers presupposes that we pay attention to the external world and its affairs. This, in turn, means that we reinforce the habit of assuming that we are ego-personalities rather than the transcendental Self.

The *Moksha-Dharma* teachers also provide useful instructions about right diet and fasting, as well as suitable environments for yogic practice. They also knew of the value of breath control (*prânâyâma*) and distinguished between the five types of life force (*prâna*) circulating in the body. Breath control prepares the mind for the next stage of the process of gradual introversion, which is the withdrawal (*pratyâhâra*) of the senses from the external world.

Most schools of Pre-Classical Yoga subscribe to what the *Moksha-Dharma* calls *nirodha-yoga*, the "Yoga of cessation." This approach consists in the progressive disowning of the contents of consciousness—from sensations, to thoughts, to higher experiences—until the transcendental Self shines forth in its full glory. Thus, sensory inhibition, concentration, and meditation are considered the primary means of Yoga. In one section (12.188.15ff.), several degrees of meditation are distinguished that remind one of Patanjali's terminology. Thus, Bhîshma, who is not only a heroic warrior but also a wisdom teacher, speaks of the meditation stages of *vitarka* (thinking), *vicâra* (subtle reflection), and *viveka* (differentiation), though without explaining them further. These stages are called *codanâ*, since they "impel" the mind to become absorbed in the objectless condition. The *yogin* who is successful at *nirodha-yoga* enters the state of complete inner stillness, "windlessness" (*nirvâna*), which is accompanied by the total absence of sensory input. The body of such a *yogin* is said to appear to others like a stone pillar.

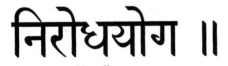

*Nirodha-yoga*

Another type of Yoga discussed in the *Moksha-Dharma* is known as *jnâna-dîpti-yoga*, the "Yoga of the effulgence of wisdom." It consists in prolonged concentration upon progressively more subtle objects. For instance, a person may first fix attention on one of the five material elements, followed by concentration on the mind (*manas*) or the higher mind (*buddhi*). Or a *yogin* may start out by concentrating on different points in the body, such as the heart, the navel, or the head, and subsequently on the Self itself. These concentration practices are called *dhârana*.

In one passage, Yoga is likened to a faultless jewel that first gathers in and then emits the bright light of the sun. The sun, of course, is a universal symbol for the Self, which is experienced as a dazzling effulgence. This metaphor describes well the essential yogic process of concentration. *Dhâranâ* gathers in the "rays" or whirls of the mind, and focuses them on the Self within, until the radiance of the Self becomes manifest in the state of ecstasy (*samâdhi*) and transforms the *yogin*'s entire being.

The fact that such teachings came to be included in the *Mahâbhârata* demonstrates their immense popularity during the period under review. In the centuries around the time of the Buddha and certainly prior to the beginning of the Christian calendar, Yoga had manifestly become a vociferous contender in the philosophical and spiritual arena of Hinduism. It was only a matter of time before an educated adept of Yoga would create a work of lasting success in which the philosophy and practice of Hindu Yoga was coherently formulated. That work was the *Yoga-Sûtra* of Patanjali to which we will turn in Chapter 9.

## SOURCE READING 11

# *Moksha-Dharma (Selection)*

The following two chapters from the *Moksha-Dharma* are in the form of a dialogue between Bhîshma and his royal pupil Yudhishthira. The first excerpt explains in some detail the impact of the three qualities (*guna*) of Nature—*sattva, rajas,* and *tamas*—upon the human mind. According to the ontological theory expounded here, these three qualities are the product of the wisdom faculty (*buddhi*), which is the first evolute of Nature (*prakriti*). Beyond the wisdom faculty, or higher mind, is the immovable eternal Witness, here called the Field-Knower (*kshetra-jna*), which is none other than the transcendental Self.

The second excerpt considers the practice of meditation (*dhyâna*), though the consideration extends only to the first of four stages. In verse 15, reflection (*vicâra*), thinking (*vitarka*), and differentiation (*viveka*) are listed as components of the first stage. This reminds one of the elements of *vicâra* and *vitarka* in the state of conscious ecstasy (*samprajnâta-samâdhi*) mentioned in Patanjali's *Yoga-Sûtra* (1.43-44).

The state of perfection (*siddhi*) to which this fourfold Yoga of meditation is said to lead is also called extinction (*nirvâna*)—a term we encounter also in the *Bhagavad-Gîtâ* (2.72; V.26). It is explained indirectly in verse 6.19 of the *Gîtâ*: "As a lamp standing in a windless (*nivâta*) [place] flickers not—that simile is recalled [when] a *yogin* of yoked mind (*citta*) practices the Yoga of the self." The term *nirvâna,* usually translated as "extinction," stems from the verbal root *vâ* ("to blow"), of which the past participle is *vâta.* The prefix *nis* (changed into *nir* before *vâna*) corresponds to the Latin prefix *ex* ("out"). The term *nirvâna* is well known from the Buddhist scriptures and has been cited by scholars as evidence that the *Gîtâ* and the *Moksha-Dharma* are post-Buddhist works. Yet, it is just as likely that the Buddha borrowed this word from already existing philosophical vocabulary.

### 12.187

Yudhishthira said:

Tell me, O grandsire, what is that which is named the deep Self (*adhyâtman*), which is considered the Self (*purusha*)? What is the inmost self and of what [nature] is it? (1)

Bhîshma said:

That deep Self that you ask me about, O Pârtha, I shall explain to you, O friend, as the most beatific joy (*sukha*). (2)

Having known that, a person finds delight (*prîti*) and joyousness (*saukhya*) in the world and obtains the fruit [thereof], which is benevolence toward all beings. (3)

Earth, wind, ether, water, and light are great elements, [which are] the origin and the end of all beings. (4)

From that [conglomerate of elements] these [beings] have been created and into that they return again and again—the great elements in beings are like the waves of the ocean. (5)

As a tortoise after extending its limbs retracts them again—similarly the elemental self (*bhûta-âtman*),[22] having created [all] beings, withdraws them again. (6)

The Creator of beings fashioned the five great elements in all beings, but the individual (*jîva*) does not see the differences in them. (7)

Sound, hearing, and the ears—[this is] the triad born from the womb of ether. From the air [come] skin, touch, and motion as well as speech as the fourth. (8)

Form, eye, and digestion are called the triple fire. Taste, moisture, and tongue are known as the three qualities of water. (9)

Scent, nose, and body—these are the three qualities of earth. The great elements are five. The mind (*manas*) is said to be the sixth. (10)

The senses and the mind, O Bhârata, are one's [means of] cognition (*vijnâna*). The seventh is said to be the wisdom faculty (*buddhi*). Furthermore, the Field-Knower (*kshetra-jna*) [i.e., the Self] is the eighth. (11)

The eye is for seeing; the mind creates doubt; the wisdom faculty is for ascertaining [the nature of things]; the Field-Knower abides as the witness [of all these processes]. (12)

He sees what is above the soles of the feet, hitherward and above. Know that by Him this entire [universe] is inwardly pervaded. (13)

The senses in man are to be completely understood. Know [also] *tamas*, *rajas*, and *sattva* as the conditions on [which the senses] are based.[23] (14)

The man who has understood this through the wisdom faculty, scrutinizing the coming and going of beings, gradually obtains the highest tranquillity (*shama*). (15)

The wisdom faculty governs the qualities (*guna*) [of Nature]. The wisdom faculty also [presides over] the senses, with the mind as the sixth [sense]. In the absence of wisdom (*buddhi*), where would the qualities (*guna*) be? (16)

Thus, this entire [universe of] mobile and immobile [things] is made of that [wisdom faculty]. It arises and is reabsorbed [into the wisdom faculty]. Hence [the universe] is declared to be so [dependent on the wisdom faculty]. (17)

That by which [the wisdom faculty] sees is the eye; [by which it] hears is called the ear; [by which it] smells is called the nose. With the tongue it recognizes flavors. (18)

With the skin it senses contacts. The wisdom faculty is passive [and] transmuted [by these processes]. That by which it desires is the mind (*manas*). (19)

The resting places of the wisdom faculty, [which have their] distinct purposes, are fivefold. They are called the five senses. The invisible [wisdom faculty] stands above these [senses]. (20)

The wisdom faculty, presided over by the Self (*purusha*), exists in the [diverse] conditions: Sometimes it obtains delight [when *sattva* is preeminent]; sometimes it grieves [when *rajas* is dominant]. (21)

Sometimes, however, it exists [in a state dominated by *tamas* in which it is] not [affected] by pleasure (*sukha*) and by suffering (*duhkha*). Thus it abides in three conditions in the human mind. (22)

That [wisdom faculty], of the essence of the conditions, transcends the three conditions, just like the wave-rich ocean, the supporter of rivers, the great boundary [is greater than its tributaries]. (23)

The wisdom (*buddhi*) that has gone beyond the conditions exists in the mind [as its] condition. However, when *rajas* is activated, [wisdom] follows that condition. (24)

Then it causes all the senses to perceive. *Sattva* is delight, *rajas* is grief, and *tamas* is delusion. These are the three [conditions in which the wisdom faculty manifests]. (25)

Whichever condition [is prevalent] in this world—they [consist in] these three combined. Thus, I have explained to you, O Bhârata, the whole nature of the wisdom faculty. (26)

And all the senses are to be conquered by the sage (*dhîmat*). *Sattva*, *rajas*, and *tamas* are always attached to creatures. (27)

Consequently a threefold sensation (*vedanâ*) is seen in all beings, O Bhârata—namely sattvic, rajasic, and tamasic. (28)

Pleasant contact [arises from] the quality of *sattva*, unpleasant contact from the quality of *rajas*. In connection with *tamas* [neither pleasurable nor unpleasant sensations] occur, [but instead there is delusion]. (29)

[That sensation] in the body or in the mind that is connected with delight is considered [evidence that] a sattvic condition exists in it. (30)

Now, [that sensation] which is connected with suffering, causing one dissatisfaction [and prompting one to] escape from it, one should consider as *rajas*-activated. (31)

Now, [that sensation] which is connected with delusion, which is like the imponderable, unknowable Unmanifest—that should be comprehended as *tamas*. (32)

Rapture, delight, bliss, joy, tranquil-mindedness—wherever they occur, the sattvic qualities [are predominant]. (33)

Dissatisfaction, distress, grief, greed, and impatience—these are viewed as signs of rajas, [and they are evident] from their causes or not [evident] from their causes. (34)

Similarly, conceit, delusion, inattention, sleep (*svapna*), and weariness (*tandritâ*)—wherever they occur, the various qualities of *tamas* [are predominant]. (35)

He who restrains well the mind, [which is] far-going, wide-roaming, of the essence of desire and doubt—he is happy here [on Earth] and in the hereafter. (36)

Behold the subtle distinction between the *sattva* [i.e., the *buddhi* or wisdom faculty] and the Field-Knower [i.e., the Self]. The one creates the qualities (*guna*), the other does not create the qualities. (37)

As the gnat and the fig tree are always connected, so also is the connection between these two. (38)

[Although] distinct by nature, they are always connected. As a fish and water, just so are these [two] connected. (39)

The qualities do not know the Self, [but] It knows the qualities all round, and the Overseer (*paridrashtri*) of the qualities always [wrongly] deems himself as their creator. (40)

But by means of the inactive, insensate senses, [the mind] and the wisdom faculty as the seventh, the supreme Self—like a lamp—performs the task of a lamp. (41)

The *sattva* [i.e., the *buddhi* or wisdom faculty] creates the qualities. The Field-Knower [merely] looks on. This is their permanent connection, of *sattva* and the Field-Knower. (42)

There is no common basis whatever for the *sattva* and the Field-Knower. [The latter] never creates the *sattva*, the mind, or the [other] qualities. (43)

When one controls the rays of those [senses] with the mind, then one's Self manifests like a [brightly] burning lamp in a pot. (44)

The sage (*muni*) whose delight is ever in the Self, who has abandoned Nature's activity, and who has become the Self of all beings—he goes the supreme course [to liberation and immortality]. (45)

Like a water-going bird is immersed [in the water but] not stained by it, just so the accomplished sage (*prajnâ*) lives among beings [without being tainted thereby]. (46)

A man should thus dissociate from the innate condition (*sva-bhâva*) by means of the wisdom faculty in this manner: He should move without grieving, without thrilling [over things], with all intoxication (*mâtsara*) gone. (47)

He who by the power of the innate condition (*sva-bhâva*) always creates the effected qualities is like the maker of a spider web. The qualities are to be known as the thread. (48)

[When the qualities] have vanished, they have not [really] disappeared. [Their total] cessation is not evident from direct perception. "[Even though it is] imperceptible, it can be established by inference." (49)

Thus have decided some, while others [argue for their total] cessation. Considering both [positions], one should decide as seems fit. (50)

Thus, this tight heart knot [i.e., philosophical problem], consisting of a difference of opinion (*buddhi*), should be loosened. [Then one will] not grieve. [Of this there is] no doubt. (51)

As dirty persons may become clean by submerging themselves in a stream, knowing full well [that they will be cleansed]—thus know wisdom (*jnâna*) as the [means of purification]. (52)

Just as someone who sees the farther shore is intimidated by a great river and therefore does not cross it—similarly those who see the deep Self (*adhyâtman*), aloneness, supreme wisdom [at first feel intimidated but then proceed to attain it]. (53)

The man who knows about this coming and going of all beings and who considers it gradually attains the Supreme by that wisdom (*buddhi*). (54)

He who has understood the triad [of the qualities of Nature] is released with the eastern light. Searching with the mind, [he becomes] yoked, truth-seeing, and desireless. (55)

The Self cannot be seen by the senses severally [or even in combination], [which are] deployed here and there and are difficult to conquer by immature persons (*akrita-âtman*).[24] (56)

Having understood this, he becomes wise (*buddha*). What other sign of wisdom [could there be]? Knowing this, the sages know they have accomplished what is to be accomplished. (57)

That which for the knowing ones no [longer holds any] fear is excessive fear for those who are ignorant. There is no higher course for anyone. Having reached the quality (*guna*) [of the supreme Self], they praise its unequaledness (*atulyatâ*). (58)

He who performs [actions] without preceding intention and who rejects that which previously was done [by him]—for him both no [longer] exist, neither the disagreeable nor the agreeable. (59)

Behold the diseased world, the grief-stricken people wailing much about this and that. Behold in this [world] the healthy and the griefless. Whoever knows both these positions knows truly. (60)

## 12.188

Bhîshma said:

Lo! I will tell you, O Pârtha, the fourfold Yoga of meditation, knowing which the great seers went to eternal perfection (*siddhi*). (1)

The *yogins*, the great seers, practice meditation as it should be done, partaking of wisdom, with the mind directed to extinction (*nirvâna*). (2)

They do not return, O Pârtha. [They are] liberated from the defects of the world-of-change (*samsâra*). The defects [arising from their] birth are gone, [and they] stand firm in their innate nature (*sva-bhâva*). (3)

[They are] beyond the opposites, abiding always in *sattva*, free, forever resorting to restraint (*niyama*) and [to things that are] free from attachment and dispute and that produce mental tranquillity. (4)

Then the sage (*muni*) should, combined with study (*svâdhyâya*), concentrate the mind on a single point, making the host of senses into a ball and sitting [immobile] like a piece of wood. (5)

He should not seek out sound with the ear. He should not know touch with the skin, nor know form with the eye, nor taste with the tongue. (6)

Also, the knower of Yoga should abandon all scents through meditation, and he should valiantly reject [all things that] agitate the group of five [senses]. (7)

Thence he should skillfully constrain the group of five [senses] in the mind, and he should settle the roaming mind together with the five senses. (8)

In the first course of meditation, the wise should settle inwardly the wandering, unsupported, five-gated (*panca-dvâra*), fickle mind. (9)

When he makes the senses and the mind thus into a ball—this I call the first degree of meditation. (10)

His mind, the sixth [sense]—fully restricted inwardly through the first [course of meditation]—will [still] quiver like a lightning flash in a cloud. (11)

Like a trembling drop of water on a leaf moves about—thus his attention (*citta*) wanders on the track of [the first course of] meditation. (12)

[Even when] the mind is momentarily somewhat controlled and stands [relatively firm] in the track of meditation, it [soon] again roams on the path of the wind [i.e., the breath] and becomes like the wind. (13)

Unresponsive [to sensory stimuli], free from affliction, free from lethargy and enthusiasm (*mâtsara*), the knower of the Yoga of meditation should renewedly settle the mind (*cetas*) by means of meditation. (14)

Reflection, thinking, and differentiation arise for the concentrating sage, beginning with the first [degree of] meditation. (15)

Even when troubled by the mind, he should perform concentration (*samâdhâna*). The sage should not become discouraged but should strive for his good (*hita*). (16)

Just as heaped piles of dust, ashes, or refuse do not [right away] become saturated when sprinkled with water, (17)

or just like dry flour, a little moistened, does not [right away] become saturated but becomes saturated gradually— (18)

just so he should, gradually, saturate the host of senses and gradually gather them. [In this manner] he will completely tranquilize [the mind]. (19)

The mind and the group of five [senses] will, O Bhârata, become tranquilized through incessant Yoga [practice], when the first degree of meditation is attained. (20)

Not by human work or by some divine [intervention] does he advance to the joy that [pertains] to him who is self-controlled. (21)

> Yoked by that joy, he delights in the practice of meditation. Thus, verily, the *yogins* go to that extinction (*nirvâna*) [which is] free from ill. (22)

## VII. THE SIXFOLD YOGA OF THE MAITRÂYANÎYA-UPANISHAD

The Maitrâyanas are mentioned already in the *Brâhmanas* and are associated with the *Krishna-* (Black) *Yajur-Veda*. They appear to have had a special connection with God Rudra, who was subsequently assimilated into Shiva of classical times. Among other works, the Maitrâyana priests created the *Shata-Rudrîya* ("Hundred [Invocations] of Rudra"), a litany that was recited for protection against evil but came to be used for meditative purposes as well. As its title indicates, the *Maitrâyanîya-Upanishad*[25] was also authored in those circles, though in much later times. While this esoteric scripture clearly contains archaic yogic lore, its extant recension was probably not composed until the fourth or third century B.C.E.[26] A section of this *Upanishad* forms an independent text going by the name of *Maitreya-Upanishad*, which appears to have been created in South India.[27]

The *Maitrâyanîya-Upanishad* opens with the story of King Brihadratha, who in the *Mahâbhârata* is remembered as an early ruler of Magadha and a faithful worshiper of Shiva. After installing his son as ruler, so the story goes, Brihadratha abandoned his kingdom to pursue austerities in the forest. After a thousand days (or years) of standing stock-still, with his arms raised high and staring into the sun, he was visited by the Self-realized adept Shâkâyanya. Finding Brihadratha worthy of instruction, Shâkâyanya

disclosed to him the mystery of the two kinds of self—the "elemental self" (*bhûta-âtman*, written *bhûtâtman*), or ego-personality, and the transcendental Self.

The elemental self is constantly suffering change until it disintegrates at death, but the transcendental Self is eternally unaffected by these changes. It can be realized through study and the pursuit of one's allotted duties, including austerities, recitation, and profound contemplation. Shâkâyanya speaks of this realization in terms of a union (*sayujya*) with the Self, the Ruler (*îshana*). Then the sage expounds the sixfold Yoga (*shad-anga-yoga*) as follows:

> The rule for effecting this [union with the Self] is this: breath control (*prânâyâma*), sense withdrawal (*pratyâhâra*), meditation (*dhyâna*), concentration (*dhâranâ*), reflection (*tarka*), and ecstasy (*samâdhi*). Such is said to be the sixfold Yoga. (6.18)

> When a seer sees the brilliant Maker, Lord, Person, the Source of [the Creator-God] Brahma, then, being a knower, shaking off good and evil, he reduces everything to unity in the supreme Imperishable. (6.19)

The *Maitrâyanîya-Upanishad* is still more specific. It mentions the central channel (*sushumnâ-nâdî*) that forms the axis of the body, along or into which the life force (*prâna*) must be forced from the base of the spine to the crown of the head and beyond. This process is accomplished by joining the breath, the mind, and the sacred syllable *om*. Next Shâkâyanya quotes two stanzas from an unidentified authority, according to which Yoga is the joining of breath and the syllable *om*, or of breath, the mind, and the senses.

This text contains many fascinating ideas, hinting at practices that suggest a further advance in the development of Yoga and that prepared the ground for Patanjali's classical formulation.

## VIII. THE INTANGIBLE YOGA OF THE MÂNDÛKYA-UPANISHAD

There are a number of *Upanishads* from the Epic Age, notably the *Îsha*, the *Mundaka*, the *Prashna*, and the *Mândûkya*,[28] which are not directly connected with the (Sâmkhya-)Yoga tradition characteristic of the Epic Age but belong to mainstream Vedântic nondualism (which is a form of Jnâna-Yoga). I will discuss here only the *Mândûkya-Upanishad*, which deserves to be singled out because it inspired the adept Gaudapâda to compose his esteemed *Mândûkya-Kârikâ*, also known by the name of *Âgama-Shâstra*. Gaudapâda was the *parama-guru* of Shankara, the most renowned philosopher of Advaita Vedânta, India's tradition of radical nondualism. The phrase *parama-guru* is not altogether clear—it could mean that Gaudapâda was the teacher of Shankara's teacher Govinda, or it could mean that he was the "root *guru*," the originator of Shankara's lineage to whom Shankara looked with great reverence. We have no reliable information about Gaudapâda. The ninth-century Vedânta scholar Ânandagiri wrote a gloss (*tîkâ*) on Shankara's commentary on the *Mândûkya-Karika* in which he mentions that Gaudapâda practiced austerities at

Bâdaraika *âshrama*, a holy site dedicated to God Nârâyana. It was Nârâyana who revealed the wisdom of nonduality to him.

Gaudapâda's date also is uncertain and depends on how we interpret the traditional phrase *parama-guru* in his case. If he was the *guru* of Shankara's teacher, then we must place him some time in the early seventh century C.E. However, according to some accounts, several teachers intervened between Gaudapâda and Shankara. It is even possible that he lived as early as the fifth century C.E., which would tally with certain Buddhist sources that apparently quote from the *Mândûkya-Kârikâ*, notably Bhâvaviveka's sixth-century *Tarka-Jvalâ* ("Conflagration of Reason").

The *Mândûkya-Kârikâ* is a brilliant philosophical exposition of the ideas found in the *Upanishad* of the same name. In fact, Gaudapâdâ's work has been considered the earliest systematic treatment of the Upanishadic metaphysics of nondualism. In the *Mândûkya-Upanishad* it is stated that if a man cannot study all 108 *Upanishads*, he can still attain liberation if he delves into the *Mândûkya*, because it contains the quintessence of Upanishadic wisdom.

The entire *Mândûkya-Upanishad*, consisting of only twelve stanzas, is a treatment of the esoteric symbolism of the sacred syllable *om*. This ancient mantra is generally thought to be composed of four units (*mâtra*)—*a*, *u*, *m*, and the nasalized echo of the *m* sound. These are symbolically related to the four basic states of

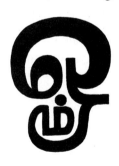

*Om symbol in South Indian script*

*The letters a, u, m, and the nâda-bindu symbol*

consciousness, which are waking, dreaming, sleeping, and the transcendental state, which is called the "Fourth" (*caturtha, turîya*). Gaudapâda's work expounds this idea further. He introduces the concept of the "intangible Yoga" (*asparsha-yoga*). The word *sparsha* means "touch" or "contact," and *asparsha* is literally "that which is free from touch or contact," in other words, that which is intangible and which does not pertain to the nexus of conditioned existence (*samsâra*). What this Yoga stands for is the radical nondualist practice of abiding in or as the Self, without contact or contamination by the so-called objective world.

From the perspective of the Self, which is one without a second, there can be no question of contact with anything. There is no outside or inside, and there are no multiple objects or beings that could be contacted through the senses. Only the unenlightened mind, which distinguishes between subject and object, thinks in terms of separation or union, disconnection or contact. It is our presumed separation from other beings and things that causes us much anxiety. Where there is no duality, there also is no fear. Gaudapâda's Yoga is the realization of that fearless Condition, the "Fourth," which is none other than the all-comprising Self. It can be attained in every moment that the mind is obliged to relinquish the illusion that there is a world of multiplicity outside itself and, instead, is brought to rest in the native state of Selfhood. In his commentary on the *Mândûkya-Kârika* (4.2), Shankara calls Asparsha-Yoga the Yoga of the nondualist vision, or *advaita-darshana-yoga*.

Asparsha-Yoga is synonymous with Jnâna-Yoga in its highest form. As such it represents the crowning achievement of the entire nondualist

tradition of the *Upanishads*. In Shankara's skillful hands it became the greatest rival of Buddhism and also of Patanjali's school of Classical Yoga.

## IX. MORALITY AND SPIRITUALITY— PRE-CLASSICAL YOGA IN THE ETHICAL-LEGAL LITERATURE

### Overview

In addition to the two epics and the *Upanishads*, elements of Pre-Classical Yoga also can be met with in a number of other semireligious works of Hinduism, notably the ethical-legal literature known as *dharma-shâstra*. Why is there this connection between ethics or morality (*dharma*) and spirituality (*yoga*)? According to an old brahmanical model of human motivation, there are four great values to which people can dedicate themselves. These are known as the human goals (*purusha-artha*): material welfare (*artha*), pleasure (*kâma*), morality (*dharma*), and liberation (*moksha*). They form a hierarchical continuum, with liberation as the highest possible value to which we can aspire. Morality and the quest for emancipation, or spiritual freedom, stand in a special relationship to each other, for the higher spiritual life can blossom only when it is securely founded on morality.

Thus, it is not surprising that we should find many references to Yoga in the manuals on ethics and law, which also regard liberation as the highest possible virtue, just as the Yoga scriptures mention all kinds of moral virtues in which the *yogin* must be established or which he must cultivate.

अर्थ । काम । धर्म । मोक्ष ॥

*Artha, kâma, dharma, and moksha*

For instance, in his *Yoga-Sûtra* (2.30-31), Patanjali lists the following five virtues that comprise the great vow (*mahâ-vrata*): nonharming, truthfulness, nonstealing, chastity, and greedlessness. These compose the first of the eight limbs (*anga*) of the eightfold path of Classical Yoga but are also an integral part of the morality espoused in the *Dharma-Sûtras* and *Dharma-Shâstras*.

The *dharma-shâstra* literature is quite extensive, and it appears that many of the original *Sûtras* were lost long ago. It is clear from even a cursory glance at the manuals on right behavior by the juristic and spiritual authorities that asceticism (*tapas*) and Yoga were an integral part of India's cultural and moral life long before the Common Era. The numerous references to *tapas* clearly point to the great age of the spiritual teachings transmitted in these works. There are comparatively few references to Yoga, and these typically connect Yoga with the discipline of restraining the senses and breath control. With the growing acceptance of Yoga into orthodox Brahmanism, this far-flung tradition was destined to play an ever more important role in the emergence of the great religious culture of so-called Hinduism. The practical orientation of Yoga proved a constant grounding force for the metaphysical flights, as well as the continuing ritual preoccupations, of the Hindu intelligentsia.

At the same time, the emphasis on personal experience in Yoga, especially such approaches as Karma-Yoga and Bhakti-Yoga, appealed to the religious-minded individual who was not born into the brahmin class with its privileged access to the sacred scriptures. Especially with the rise of Tantra around the middle of the first millennium C.E., class and caste barriers began to be torn down in the spiritual arena. In the Tantric circles, everyone—regardless of social status, education, or skin color—was at least in principle granted access to the highest teachings. The only qualification was that of spiritual readiness.

The oldest legal works are the various *Sûtras* composed by sages like Gautama, Baudhâyana, Vashishtha, and Âpastamba. Portions of them are as old as the late *Brâhmanas*, such as the *Shata-Patha*, but in the main they belong to a more recent period. These works served as the foundation for the more elaborate legal scriptures known as the *Dharma-Shâstras*, which are usually assigned to the period from 300 B.C.E. to 200 C.E. The most important of these scriptures is the *Mânava-Dharma-Shâstra*, also called the *Manu-Smriti*, which is written in the *shloka* meter. Its reputed author is Manu Vaivasvata, who is traditionally hailed as the progenitor of the present human race and the ancestor of the ruling families of Vedic India. He is mentioned in the archaic *Rig-Veda* (1.80.16) as "our father." The later *Purâna* literature speaks of Manu as the survivor of a great flood. This legend, resembling the Middle-Eastern story of Noah, is first told in the *Shata-Pata-Brâhmana* (1.8.1-6), which is over four thousand years old. The story is not found in the *Rig-Veda*, but the *Atharva-Veda* (19.39.7-9) makes reference to a golden ship stranded on the top of the Himalayan mountain range.

Ikshvâku, one of Manu's nine sons, is remembered as the founder of the solar dynasty. Manu was himself a son of the Sun God Vivasvat (hence Manu's epithet Vaivasvata). Manu's daughter Ilâ (who underwent a sex change) was the founder of the lunar dynasty, among which the Pândavas headed by Prince Arjuna, devotee of the God-man Krishna, were the most illustrious.

While Manu, if he existed at all, belongs to the earliest phase of the Vedic civilization (perhaps to the fifth millennium B.C.E.), the *Manu-Smriti* attributed to him is certainly the product of a much more recent age. Some of its ideas, however, unquestionably derive from Vedic times. Be that as it may, the *Manu-Smriti* illustrates the widespread influence of the Yoga tradition by the beginning of the Christian calendar.

## Yogic Teachings in the Legal Literature

Apart from the moral code, captured in the rules of *yama* in Yoga, the *Dharma-Shâstras* emphasize breath control as a means of expiation. Thus, in the *Manu-Smriti* (6.70ff.), there is a passage that speaks of the benefits of breath control (*prânâyâma*). It is meant to be performed with the appropriate Vedic *mantras*, especially the syllable *om*. This is considered the highest form of austerity, which "burns away" all kinds of physical and psychic blemishes.

The *Vâsishtha-Dharma-Shâstra* describes Yoga in Chapter 25, which consists essentially in the practice of breath control. Retention is defined in verse 13 as the suppression of the breath for the duration of three repetitions of the *gâyatri-mantra* together with the syllable *om*, the *vyâhritis* or "declarations" (viz. *bhûh, bhuvah, svah*), and the *shiras* ("head")-utterance ("water, fire/light, essence, immortal").[29] Breath control is said (vs. 6) to generate air, which in turn kindles the inner fire, through which water is formed. All three elements bring about the desired purification without which wisdom cannot dawn. In verse 8, Yoga is stated to be the sum of the sacred law (*dharma*) and the highest and eternal austerity.

An almost identical passage can be found, for instance, in the *Baudhâyana-Dharma-Sûtra* (4.1.23ff.), which is a much-respected work whose nucleus was presumably created during the centuries prior to the drying up of the Sarasvatî River around 1900 B.C.E.

The *Shânkhâyana-Smriti* (12.18-19), another ancient scripture dealing with Hindu law and custom, makes the exaggerated claim that sixteen daily cycles of breath control absolve even the slayer of a brahmin from his heinous sin. The *Yâjnavalkya-Smriti* (3.305) prescribes one hundred *prânâyâmas* for the expiation of all sins.

The *Manu-Smriti* and other kindred scriptures also recommend concentration (*dhârana*) as a means of atoning for one's sins, and meditation (*dhyâna*) for combating undesirable emotions like anger, avarice, and jealousy. The author of the *Âpastamba-Dharma-Sûtra* (1.5.23.3ff.), which in its extant version belongs perhaps to the third century B.C.E, quotes a verse from an unidentified work, according to which the wise person eliminates all "taints" (*dosha*) of character through the practice of Yoga. He enumerates fifteen such taints, or defects, including anger, greed, hypocrisy, and even exuberance.

The *Yâjnavalkya-Smriti* ranks in importance next to the *Manu-Smriti*, though in its available form it may have been composed several centuries later. This scripture is traditionally attributed to the illustrious Sage Yâjnavalkya, who lived at the time of the *Brâhmanas*. In one passage (3.195ff.), the entire yogic process is described—from assuming the right posture, to withdrawing the senses from the external world, to performing breath control, concentration, and meditation. This work also lists (3.202f.) several of the yogic powers (*siddhi*), such as the ability to become invisible, to remember past lives, and to see the future.

With the *Manu-Smriti* we approach the Common Era, which proved to be a most fertile phase in the evolution of the Yoga tradition. The person who gave Yoga its recognizable philosophical shape in the first or second century C.E. was a seer (*rishi*) by the name of Patanjali. We will turn to him and his famous aphorisms next.

## Part Three
# CLASSICAL YOGA

"In putting forward the *Yoga-Bhâshya*, Veda-Vyâsa explained the essence of all the *Vedas*. Therefore this is the [best] approach for those desiring liberation."

—Vijnâna Bhikshu, *Yoga-Vârttika* (1.4)

> "Yoga is a perfectly structured and integrated world view aiming at the transformation of a human being from his actual and unrefined form to a perfected form . . . It can be said that Yoga aims at freedom from nature, including the freedom from human nature; its flight is to the transcendence of humanity and the cosmos, into pure being."

—Ravi Ravindra, "Yoga: The Royal Path to Freedom,"
*Hindu Spirituality*, p. 178

# *Chapter 9*
# THE HISTORY AND LITERATURE OF PÂTANJALA-YOGA

## I. PATANJALI—PHILOSOPHER AND YOGIN

Most *yogins*, like most ordinary people, do not have an intellectual bent. But *yogins*, unlike ordinary people, turn this into an advantage by cultivating wisdom and the kind of psychic and spiritual experiences that the rational mind tends to deny and prevent. And yet there always have been those Yoga practitioners who were brilliant intellectuals as well. Thus, Shankara of the early eighth century C.E. is not only remembered as the greatest proponent of Hindu nondualist metaphysics, or Advaita Vedânta, but also as a great adept of Yoga. The Buddhist teacher Nâgârjuna, who lived in the second century C.E., was not only a celebrated Tantric alchemist and thaumaturgist (*siddha*) but also a philosophical genius of the first order. In the sixteenth century C.E., Vijnâna Bhikshu wrote profound commentaries on all the major schools of thought. He was a noted thinker who greatly impressed the German pioneering indologist and founder of comparative mythology Max Müller. At the same time he was a

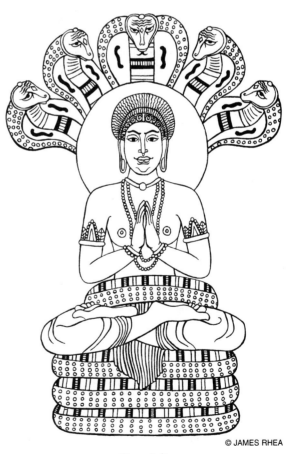

© JAMES RHEA

*Patanjali*

spiritual practitioner of the first order, following Vedântic Jnâna-Yoga.

Similarly, Patanjali, the author or compiler of the *Yoga-Sûtra*, was obviously a Yoga adept who also had a great head on his shoulders. As Yoga researcher Christopher Chapple wrote:

> Some have said that Patanjali has made no specific philosophical contribution in his presentation of the yoga school. To the contrary, I suggest that his is a masterful contribution communicated through nonjudgmentally presenting diverse practices, a methodology deeply rooted in the culture and traditions of India.[1]

The Yoga of Patanjali represents the climax of a long development of yogic technology. Of all the numerous schools that existed in the opening centuries of the Common Era, Patanjali's school was the one to become acknowledged as the authoritative system (*darshana*) of the Yoga tradition. There are numerous parallels between Patanjali's Yoga and Buddhism, and it is unknown whether these are simply due to the synchronous development of Hindu and Buddhist Yoga or are the result of a special interest in Buddhist teachings on the part of Patanjali. If Patanjali lived in the second century C.E., as is proposed here, he may well have been exposed to the considerable influence of Buddhism at that time. But perhaps both explanations apply.[2]

Disappointingly, we know next to nothing about Patanjali. Hindu tradition identifies him with the famous grammarian of the same name who lived in the second century B.C.E. and authored the *Mahâ-Bhâshya*. The consensus of scholarly opinion, however, considers this unlikely. Both the contents and the terminology of the *Yoga-Sûtra* suggest the second century C.E. as a probable date for Patanjali, whoever he may have been.[3]

In addition to the grammarian, India knows of several other Patanjalis. The name is mentioned as a clan (*gotra*) name of the Vedic priest Âsurâyana. The old *Shata-Pata-Brâhmana* mentions a Patancala Kâpya, whom the nineteenth-century German scholar Albrecht Weber wrongly tried to connect with Patanjali.[4] Then there was a Sâmkhya teacher by this name whose views are mentioned in the *Yukti-Dîpikâ* (late seventh or early eighth century C.E.). Possibly another Patanjali is credited with the *Yoga-Darpana* ("Mirror of Yoga"), a manuscript of unknown date. Finally, there was a Yoga teacher Patanjali who was part of the South Indian Shaiva tradition. His name may be referred to in the title of Umâpati Shivâcârya's fourteenth-century *Pâtanjala-Sûtra*, which is a work on liturgy at the Natarâja temple of Cidambaram.

Hindu tradition has it that Patanjali was an incarnation of Ananta, or Shesha, the thousand-headed ruler of the serpent race that is thought to guard the hidden treasures of the earth. The name Patanjali is said to have been given to Ananta because he desired to teach Yoga on Earth and fell (*pat*) from Heaven onto the palm (*anjali*) of a virtuous woman, named Gonikâ. Iconography often depicts Ananta as the couch on which God Vishnu reclines. The serpent lord's many heads symbolize infinity or omnipresence. Ananta's connection to Yoga is not difficult to uncover, since Yoga is the secret treasure, or esoteric lore, par excellence. To this day, many *yogins* bow to Ananta before they begin their daily round of yogic exercises.

In the benedictory verse at the beginning of the *Yoga-Bhâshya* commentary to the *Yoga-Sûtra*, the serpent lord, Ahîsha, is saluted as follows:

> May He who rules to favor the world in many ways by giving up His original

[unmanifest] form—He who is beautifully coiled and many-mouthed, endowed with lethal poisons and yet removing the host of afflictions (*klesha*), who is the source of all wisdom (*jnâna*), and whose circle of attendant serpents constantly generates pleasure, who is the divine Lord of Serpents: May He, the bestower of Yoga, yoked in Yoga, protect you with His pure white body.

Whatever we can say about Patanjali is purely speculative. It is reasonable to assume that he was a great Yoga authority and most probably the head of a school in which study (*svâdhyâya*) was regarded as an important aspect of spiritual practice. In composing his aphorisms (*sûtra*) he availed himself of existing works. His own philosophical contribution, as far as it can be gauged from the *Yoga-Sûtra* itself, was modest. He appears to have been a compiler and systematizer rather than an originator. It is of course possible that he has written other works that have not survived.

## Hiranyagarbha

Western Yoga enthusiasts often regard Patanjali as the father of Yoga, but this is misleading. According to post-classical traditions, the originator of Yoga was Hiranyagarbha. Although some texts speak of Hiranyagarbha as a Self-realized adept who lived in ancient times, this notion is doubtful. The name means "Golden Germ" and in Vedânta cosmomythology refers to the womb of creation, to the first being to emerge from the unmanifest ground of the world and the matrix of all the myriad forms of creation. Thus, Hiranyagarbha is a primal cosmic force rather than an individual. To speak of him—or it—as the originator of Yoga makes sense when one understands

that Yoga essentially consists in altered states of awareness through which the *yogin* tunes into nonordinary levels of reality. In this sense, then, Yoga is always revelation. Hiranyagarbha is simply a symbol for the power, or grace, by which the spiritual process is initiated and revealed.

Later Yoga commentators believed that there was an actual person called Hiranyagarbha who had authored a treatise on Yoga. Such a work is indeed referred to by many other authorities, but this does not necessarily say anything about Hiranyagarbha. The most detailed information about that scripture is found in the twelfth chapter of the *Ahirbudhnya-Samhitâ* ("Collection of the Dragon of the Deep"), which is a work of the medieval Vaishnava tradition. According to this scripture, Hiranyagarbha composed two works on Yoga, one on *nirodha-yoga* ("Yoga of restriction") and one on *karma-yoga* ("Yoga of action"). The former apparently dealt with the higher stages of the spiritual process, notably ecstatic states, whereas the latter is said to have been concerned with spiritual attitudes and forms of behavior.

There may well have been a work on Yoga of this nature, and if it did exist, it might even have antedated Patanjali's compilation. In any case, Hiranyagarbha's work is not remembered to have been a *Sûtra*, though it is quite possible that other *Sûtras* on Yoga existed prior to Patanjali's composition. It is a fact, however, that Patanjali's *Yoga-Sûtra* has eclipsed all earlier *Sûtra* works within the Yoga tradition, perhaps because it was the most comprehensive or systematic.

## II. THE CODIFICATION OF WISDOM—THE YOGA-SÛTRA

Patanjali gave the Yoga tradition its classical format, and hence his school is often referred to as Classical Yoga. He composed his aphoristic work in the heyday of philosophical speculation and debate in India, and it is to his credit that he supplied the Yoga tradition with a reasonably homogeneous theoretical framework that could stand up against the many rival traditions, such as Vedânta, Nyâya, and not least Buddhism. His composition is in principle a systematic treatise concerned with defining the most important elements of Yoga theory and practice. Patanjali's school was at one time enormously influential, as can be deduced from the many references to the *Yoga-Sûtra*, as well as the criticisms of it, in the scriptures of other philosophical systems.

Each school of Hinduism has produced its own *Sûtra*, with the Sanskrit word *sûtra* meaning literally "thread." A *Sûtra* composition consists of aphoristic statements that together furnish the reader with a thread which strings together all the memorable ideas characteristic of that school of thought. A *sûtra*, then, is a mnemonic device, rather like a knot in one's handkerchief or a scribbled note in one's diary or appointment book. Just how concise the *sûtra* style of writing is can be gauged from the following opening aphorisms of Patanjali's scripture:

*1.1:* atha yogânushâsanam (atha yoga-anushâsanam)

"Now [commences] the exposition of Yoga."

*1.2:* yogashcittavrittinirodhah (yogash citta-vritti-nirodhah)

"Yoga is the restriction of the whirls of consciousness."

*1.3:* tadâ drashthuh svarûpe'vasthânam (tadâ drashthuh sva-rûpe'vasthânam)

"Then [i.e., when that restriction has been accomplished] the 'Seer' [i.e., the transcendental Self] appears."

Of course, such terms as *citta* (consciousness), *vritti* (lit. "whirl"), and *drashtri* ("seer") are themselves highly condensed expressions for rather complex concepts. Even such a seemingly straightforward word as *atha* ("now"), which opens most traditional Sanskrit treatises, is packed with meanings, as is evident from the many pages of exegesis dedicated to it in some of the commentaries on the *Yoga-Sûtra*.

In his monumental *History of Indian Philosophy*, Surendranath Dasgupta made the following observations about this style of writing:

The systematic treatises were written in short and pregnant half-sentences (*sûtras*) which did not elaborate the subject in detail, but served only to hold before

॥ पातञ्जलयोगसूत्रम् ॥

अथ योगानुशासनम् ॥१॥
योगश्चित्तवृत्तिनिरोधः ॥२॥
तदा द्रष्टुः स्वरूपेऽवस्थानम् ॥३॥
वृत्तिसारूप्यमितरत्र ॥४॥
वृत्तय पञ्चतय्यः क्लिष्टाऽक्लिष्टाः ॥५॥
प्रमाणविपर्ययविकल्पनिद्रास्मृतयः ॥६॥
प्रत्यक्षानुमानागमाः प्रमाणानि ॥७॥
विपर्ययो मिथ्याज्ञानमतद्रूपप्रतिष्ठम् ॥८॥
शब्दज्ञानानुपाती वस्तुशून्यो विकल्पः ॥९॥
अभावप्रत्ययालम्बना वृत्तिर्निद्रा ॥१०॥
अनुभूतविषयासंप्रमोषः स्मृतिः ॥११॥
अभ्यासवैराग्याभ्यां तन्निरोधः ॥१२॥
तत्र स्थितौ यत्नोऽभ्यासः ॥१३॥
स तु दीर्घकालानैरन्तर्यसत्कारासेवितो दृढभूमिः ॥१४॥
दृष्टानुश्रविकविषयवितृष्णस्य वशीकारसंज्ञा वैराग्यम् ॥१५॥

*Sanskrit text of the first fifteen aphorisms of the Yoga-Sûtra*

the reader the lost threads of memory of elaborate disquisitions with which he was already thoroughly acquainted. It seems, therefore, that these pithy half-sentences were like lecture hints, intended for those who had direct elaborate oral instructions on the subject. It is indeed difficult to guess from the *sûtras* the extent of their significance, or how far the discussions which they gave rise to in later days were originally intended by them.[5]

Our knowledge of Pâtanjala-Yoga is primarily, though not entirely, based on the *Yoga-Sûtra*. As we will see, many commentaries have been written on it that aid our understanding of this system. As scholarship has demonstrated, however, these secondary works do not appear to have come forth from Patanjali's school itself, and therefore their expositions need to be taken with a good measure of discrimination.

Turning to the *Yoga-Sûtra* itself, we find that it consists of 195 aphorisms or *sûtras*, though some editions have 196. A number of variant readings are known, but these are generally insignificant and do not change the meaning of Patanjali's work. The aphorisms are distributed over four chapters as follows:

1   *samâdhi-pâda*, chapter on ecstasy
    — 51 aphorisms

2.  *sâdhana-pâda*, chapter on the path
    — 55 aphorisms

3.  *vibhûti-pâda*, chapter on the powers
    — 55 aphorisms

4.  *kaivalya-pâda*, chapter on liberation
    — 34 aphorisms

This division is somewhat arbitrary and appears to be the result of an inadequate reediting of the text. A close study of the *Yoga-Sûtra* shows that in its present form it cannot possibly be considered an entirely uniform creation. For this reason various scholars have attempted to reconstruct the original by dissecting the available text into several subtexts of supposedly independent origins. These efforts, however, have not been very successful, because they leave us with inconclusive fragments. It is, therefore, preferable to take a more generous view of Patanjali's work and grant the possibility that it is far more homogenous than Western scholarship has tended to assume.

As I have shown in my own detailed examination of the *Yoga-Sûtra*, this great scripture could well be a composite of only two distinct Yoga traditions.[6] On one hand there is the Yoga of eight limbs or *ashta-anga-yoga* (written *asthângayoga*), and on the other, there is the Yoga of Action (*kriyâ-yoga*). I have suggested that the section dealing with the eight constituent practices may even be a quotation rather than a later interpolation. If this were indeed correct, the widespread equation of Classical Yoga with the eightfold path would be a historical curiosity, since the bulk of the *Yoga-Sûtra* deals with *kriyâ-yoga*. But textual reconstructions of this kind are always tentative, and we must keep an open mind about this as about so many other aspects of Yoga and Yoga history.

The advantage of the kind of methodological approach to the study of the *Yoga-Sûtra* that I have proposed is that it presumes the text's homogeneity or "textual innocence" and thus does not do *a priori* violence to the text, as is the case with those textual analyses that set out to prove that a text is in fact corrupt or composed of fragments and interpolations. At any rate, these scholarly quibbles do not detract from the merit of the work as it is extant today. Now, as then, the Yoga practitioner can benefit greatly from the study of Patanjali's compilation.

## SOURCE READING 12

# *Yoga-Sûtra of Patanjali*

Every student of Yoga should, in my opinion, grapple with the *Yoga-Sûtra*. It was the very first Sanskrit text that I came across in 1965, and it has not stopped fascinating me. The following rendering of Patanjali's aphorisms is based on my own extensive textual and semantic studies. In some instances my interpretations differ from those offered in the Sanskrit commentaries. My translation is rather literal in order to convey the technical nature of Patanjali's work. All too often the popular renderings fail to do justice to the subtleties of his thought and the complexities of higher Yoga practice.

The asterisk (*) after some of the *sûtras* indicates either that they belong to what I have identified as the quoted text dealing with the eightfold path, or that they appear to have been added to Patanjali's original composition. There may be a good many more interpolated *sûtras*, especially in the third chapter, which contains lists of paranormal powers, but it does not seem particularly useful to try to identify them.

### I. Samâdhi-Pâda ("Chapter on Ecstasy")

Now [begins] the exposition of Yoga. (1.1)

Yoga is the restriction (*nirodha*) of the fluctuations of consciousness (*citta*). (1.2)

Then the Seer [i.e., the transcendental Self] abides in [its] essential form. (1.3)

At other times [there is] conformity [of the Self] with the fluctuations. (1.4)

*Comments:* In the unenlightened state, we do not consciously identify with the Self (*purusha*), but consider ourselves to be a particular individual with a particular character. This does not mean, however, that the Self is absent. Rather, it is merely obscured.

The fluctuations are fivefold; afflicted or unafflicted. (1.5)

*Comments:* The afflicted (*klishta*) states of consciousness are those that lead to suffering, while the unafflicted (*aklishta*) states are conducive to liberation. An example of the latter type is the condition of ecstatic transcendence (*samâdhi*).

[The five types of fluctuation are:] knowledge, misconception, conceptualization, sleep, and memory. (1.6)

Knowledge [can be derived from] perception, inference, and testimony. (1.7)

Misconception is erroneous knowledge not based on the [actual] appearance of the [underlying object]. (1.8)

Conceptualization is without [perceivable] object, following verbal knowledge. (1.9)

Sleep is a fluctuation founded on the idea (*pratyaya*) of the nonoccurrence [of other contents of consciousness]. (1.10)

*Comments:* This aphorism makes the point that the state of sleep, though we have no knowledge of it while it lasts, is nevertheless a content of consciousness that is witnessed by the transcendental Self. Patanjali uses the word *pratyaya*, here rendered as "idea," to signify a particular content of consciousness.

Memory is the "nondeprivation" [i.e., retention] of experienced objects. (1.11)

The restriction of these [fluctuations is achieved] through [yogic] practice and dispassion. (1.12)

Practice (*abhyâsa*) is the exertion [toward gaining] stability in [that state of restriction]. (1.13)

But this [practice] is firmly grounded [only after it has been] cultivated properly and for a long time uninterruptedly. (1.14)

Dispassion (*vairâgya*) is the certainty of mastery of [the *yogin* who is] without thirst for visible and revealed [or invisible] things. (1.15)

The higher [form] of this [dispassion] is the nonthirsting for [Nature's] constituents (*guna*), [which results] from the vision of the Self (*purusha*). (1.16)

[The ecstasy arising out of the state of restriction] is conscious (*samprajnâta*) by being connected with cogitation, reflection, bliss, or I-am-ness (*asmitâ*). (1.17)

*Comments:* Although ecstasy (*samâdhi*) implies a merging of subject and object, at the lower levels this unitive consciousness is still associated with all kinds of psychomental phenomena, including spontaneously arising thoughts, feelings of bliss, and the sense of being present as a unique entity. Patanjali calls this sense "I-am-ness." The four types of phenomena listed indicate different levels of this form of ecstasy.

The other [type of ecstasy] has a residuum of activators (*samskâra*); [it follows] the former [conscious ecstasy] upon the practice of the idea of cessation. (1.18)

*Comments:* The unitive state associated with thoughts and feelings, etc., is known as conscious ecstasy (*samprajnâta-samâdhi*). When all these psychomental phenomena have ceased to arise, then the next higher level of the unitive state is present. It is known as supraconscious ecstasy (*asamprajnâta-samâdhi*). Although in this higher state the *yogin* is no longer responsive to the environment, it must not be equated with unconscious trance.

[The ecstasy of those who have] merged with Nature (*prakriti-laya*) and [of those who are] bodiless (*videha*) [arises from the persistence of] the idea of becoming. (1.19)

[The supraconscious ecstasy] of the other [*yogins* whose path is referred to in aphorism 1.18] is preceded by faith, energy, mindfulness, [conscious] ecstasy, and wisdom. (1.20)

[The supraconscious ecstasy] is close for [those *yogins* who are] extremely intense [in their practice of Yoga]. (1.21)

Because [their intensity can be] modest, middling, or excessive, there is hence also a difference [in how close *yogins* may be to the supraconscious ecstasy]. (1.22)

Or [supraconscious ecstasy is gained] through devotion to the Lord (*îshvara-pranidhâna*). (1.23)

The Lord (*îshvara*) is a special Self [because He is] untouched by the causes-of-affliction (*klesha*), action and its fruition, and the deposits (*âshaya*) [in the depth of memory that gives rise to thoughts, desires, and so on]. (1.24)

In Him the seed of omniscience is unsurpassed. (1.25)

By virtue of [His] continuity over time, [the Lord] was also the mentor of the earlier [adepts of Yoga]. (1.26)

His symbol is the "pronouncement" (*pranava*) [i.e., the sacred syllable *om*]. (1.27)

The recitation of that [sacred syllable leads to] the contemplation of its meaning. (1.28)

Thence [follows] the attainment of [habitual] inward-mindedness (*pratyak-cetanâ*) and also the disappearance of the obstacles [mentioned in the next aphorism]. (1.29)

Sickness, languor, doubt, heedlessness, sloth, dissipation, false vision, nonattainment of the stages [of Yoga], and instability [in these stages] are the distractions of consciousness; these are the obstacles. (1.30)

Pain, depression, tremor of the limbs, and [wrong] inhalation and exhalation are accompanying [symptoms] of the distractions. (1.31)

In order to counteract these [distractions, the *yogin* should resort to] the practice [of concentrating] on a single principle. (1.32)

The projection of friendliness, compassion, gladness, and equanimity toward things— [be they] joyful, sorrowful, meritorious or demeritorious—[leads to] the pacification of consciousness. (1.33)

Or [the restriction of the fluctuations of consciousness is achieved] through expulsion and retention of the breath (*prâna*) [according to the yogic rules]. (1.34)

Or [the condition of restriction comes about when] an object-centered activity has arisen that holds the mind in steadiness. (1.35)

*Comments:* This technical-sounding aphorism contains a relatively simple idea: According to the Sanskrit commentaries, "object-centered activity" (*vishaya-vatî pravritti*) denotes a state of heightened sensory awareness called "divine perception" (*divya-samvid*). The idea is that, for instance, the heightened sensation of smell or touch focuses the mind to the point where the *yogin* may achieve the state of restriction (*nirodha*).

Or [restriction is achieved by mental activities that are] sorrowless and illuminating. (1.36)

Or [restriction is achieved when] consciousness is directed toward [those beings who have] conquered attachment. (1.37)

Or [restriction is achieved when consciousness] rests on insights [arising from] dreams and sleep. (1.38)

Or [restriction is achieved] through meditation (*dhyâna*) as desired. (1.39)

His mastery [extends] from the most minute to the greatest magnitude. (1.40)

[In the case of a consciousness whose] fluctuations have dwindled [and which has become] like a transparent jewel, [there comes about]—in regard to the "grasper," "grasping," and the "grasped"—[a state of] coincidence (*samâpatti*) with that on which [consciousness] abides and by which [consciousness] is "anointed." (1.41)

*Comments:* When the mind is completely still, it becomes translucent. Then the ecstatic state, or *samâdhi*, can occur. The underlying process of ecstasy is one in which the object of concentration looms so large in consciousness that the distinction between subject and object vanishes. Patanjali speaks of this as the "coinciding" of the experiencing subject, the experienced object, and the process of experience, which are respectively referred to as "grasper" (*grahîtri*), "grasped" (*grâhya*), and "grasping" (*grahana*).

[When] conceptual knowledge, [based on] the intent of words, [is present] in this [ecstatic state of coincidence between subject and object], [then it is called] "coincidence interspersed with cogitation." (1.42)

*Comments:* Yoga metaphysics distinguishes different levels of existence—from coarse to subtle, to unmanifest, to transcendental. The object of the ecstasy interspersed with cogitation (*vitarka-samâdhi*) belongs to the "coarse" (*sthûla*) or material realm.

On the purification of [the depths of] memory, [which has become] empty of its essence as it were, [and when] the object [of meditation] alone shines forth, [then this ecstatic state is called] "supracogitative" (*nirvitarka*). (1.43)

Thus, by this [cogitative ecstasy, the other two basic types of ecstasy]—the "reflective" (*savicâra*) and the "suprareflective"(*nirvicâra*)—are explained; [these have] subtle objects [as meditative props]. (1.44)

*Comments:* "Reflection" (*vicâra*) is a spontaneous thought process that occurs in the ecstatic state that has as its focal point a subtle (*sûkshma*) or immaterial object, such as the transcendental matrix of creation, called the Undifferentiate.

And the subtle objects terminate in the Undifferentiate (*alinga*). (1.45)

These [types of ecstatic coincidence between subject and object] verily [belong to the class of] "ecstasy with seed" (*sabîja-samâdhi*). (1.46)

*Comments:* The term "seed" refers to the remaining subliminal activators (*samskâra*) in the depths of consciousness. They give rise to future mental activity and thus to karma. When there is lucidity (*vaishâradya*) in the suprareflective [type of ecstasy, then this is called] "of the inner being" (*adhyâtma-prasâda*). (1.47)

In this [state of utmost lucidity], insight is truth-bearing (*ritam-bhara*). (1.48)

The scope [of this truth-bearing insight] is distinct from the insight [gained from] tradition and inference, [because of its] particular purposiveness. (1.49)

*Comments:* The idea expressed in this aphorism seems to be that the truth-bearing insight (*prajnâ*) reached at the highest level of conscious ecstasy (*samprajnâta-samâdhi*) is quite different from ordinary knowledge, insofar as it provides the impetus for the transcendence of all knowledge in the state of the supraconscious ecstasy (*asamprajnâta-samâdhi*), which alone leads to liberation, or Self-realization.

The activator (*samskâra*) springing from that [truth-bearing insight] obstructs the other activators [residing in the depths of consciousness]. (1.50)

Upon the restriction of even this [activator, there ensues], owing to the restriction of all [contents of consciousness], the ecstasy without seed. (1.51)

## II. Sâdhana-Pâda ("Chapter on the Path of Realization")

Asceticism (*tapas*), study (*svâdhyâya*), and devotion to the Lord (*îshvara-pranidhâna*) [constitute] the Yoga of Action (*kriyâ-yoga*). (2.1)

*Comments:* The words *kriyâ* and *karma* both mean "action," but Kriya-Yoga is different from the Karma-Yoga of the *Bhagavad-Gîtâ*. Karma-Yoga is, as we have seen, the path of "inaction in action," or ego-transcending activity. Patanjali's Kriyâ-Yoga is the path of ecstatic identification with the Self by which the subliminal activators (*samskâra*), which maintain the individuated consciousness, are gradually eliminated.

[This Yoga has] the purpose of cultivating ecstasy and also the purpose of attenuating the causes-of-affliction (*klesha*). (2.2)

Ignorance, I-am-ness, attachment, aversion, and the will-to-live are the five causes-of-affliction. (2.3)

*Comments:* The Sanskrit terms for these five sources of suffering are: *avidyâ, asmitâ, râga, dvesha,* and *abhinivesha.*

Ignorance is the field of the other [causes, which can be] dormant, attenuated, intercepted, or aroused. (2.4)

Ignorance is seeing [that which is] eternal, pure, joyful, and [pertaining to] the Self as ephemeral, impure, sorrowful, and [pertaining to] the nonself (*anâtman*). (2.5)

*Comments:* The nonself (*anâtman*) is the egoic personality and its external environment.

I-am-ness is the identification as it were of the powers of vision (*darshana*) and of the Visioner (*drik*) [i.e., the Self]. (2.6)

Attachment [is that which] rests on pleasant [experiences]. (2.7)

Aversion [is that which] rests on sorrowful [experiences]. (2.8)

The will-to-live, flowing along [by its] own inclination (*rasa*), is rooted thus even in the sages. (2.9)

*Comments:* The will-to-live (*abhinivesha*) is the impulse toward individuated existence. As such it is a primary cause of suffering and, according to Yoga, must be transcended.

These [causes-of-affliction], [in their] subtle [form], are to be overcome by the [process of] involution (*pratiprasava*). (2.10)

*Comments:* The basic building blocks of Nature (*prakriti*) are the three types of constituents (*guna*), namely the dynamic principle (*rajas*), the principle of inertia (*tamas*), and the principle of lucidity (*sattva*). Their combined interaction creates the entire manifest cosmos. Liberation is conceived as the reversal of this process, whereby the manifest aspects of the primary constituents (*guna*) resolve back into the transcendental ground of Nature. This process has the technical designation of "involution" (*pratiprasava*).

The fluctuations of these [causes-of-affliction] are to be overcome through meditation (*dhyâna*). (2.11)

The causes-of-affliction are the root of the "action deposit," and [that] may be experienced in the visible [i.e., present] birth or in an unseen [i.e., future birth]. (2.12)

*Comments:* The technical term *karma-âshaya* ("action deposit") refers to the karmic load of the individual, that is, the store of subliminal activators (*samskâra*) that give rise to and define the person.

[As long as] the root exists, [there also is] fruition from it: birth, life, and experience (*bhoga*). (2.13)

These [three] have delight or distress as results, according to the causes, [which may be] meritorious or demeritorious. (2.14)

Because of the sorrow [inherent] in the transformations (*parinâma*) [of Nature], in the pressure (*tâpa*) [of existence], and in the activators (*samskâra*) [residing in the depths of consciousness], and on account of the conflict between the fluctuations of the constituents (*guna*) [of Nature]—to the discerner all is but suffering (*duhkha*). (2.15)

*Comments:* The concept of "transformation" is crucial to Yoga philosophy. It is an elaboration of the common experience that everything undergoes constant change. Only the transcendental Self is eternally stable. For the discerning *yogin* (*vivekin*) the finite world of perpetual change is one of suffering, or sorrow, because change signals inevitable loss of what is desirable and gain of what is undesirable and hence unhappiness.

What is to be overcome is future sorrow. (2.16)

The correlation (*samyoga*) between the Seer [i.e., the transcendental Self] and the Seen [i.e., Nature] is the cause of what is to be overcome. (2.17)

*Comments:* The relationship between the transcendental Self and the world, including the mind (which is a part of Nature rather than an aspect of the Self), is experientially real enough. But it is not ultimately real. For Self and Nature are eternally distinct. The apparent correlation (*samyoga*) between the transcendental Subject and the experienced objective world is due to spiritual ignorance (*avidyâ*) and must be overcome.

The Seen [i.e., Nature] has the character of brightness, activity, or inertia; it is embodied in elements and sense organs, [and it serves] the purpose of experience (*bhoga*) or emancipation (*apavarga*). (2.18)

*Comments:* Nature, in the form of the human mind, comprises two tendencies. On one hand, it is designed for experiences, implying an egoic subject that experiences desirable or undesirable events. On the other hand, it also permits processes that lead to the transcendence of all experiences and of the ego. Why this should be so is explained through the doctrine of the three qualities (*guna*), or constituents, of Nature. While the qualities of activity (*rajas*) and inertia (*tamas*) tend to maintain the ego-illusion, the preeminence of the lucidity factor (*sattva*) creates the precondition for the event of liberation. Hence the *yogin* seeks to cultivate sattvic conditions and states.

The levels of the constituents (*guna*) [of Nature] are the Particularized, the Unparticularized, the Differentiate, and the Undifferentiate. (2.19)

*Comments:* The human body-mind is a particularized form of Nature. The sensory potentials (e.g., sound, sight, hearing, etc.), as well as the sense of individuality (Patanjali's I-am-ness, or *asmitâ*) belong to the unparticularized level of cosmic manifestation. Still more subtle is the level of the first differentiated form to emerge out of the undifferentiated ground of Nature. The most that can be said about it is that it exists and that the *sattva* constituent predominates in it. Beyond that abides the transcendental Witness-Consciousness or Self.

The Seer, [which is] the sheer [Power of] seeing, although pure, apperceives the ideas [present in consciousness]. (2.20)

The self [i.e., essence] of the Seen [i.e., Nature] is only for the sake of that [Seer, or transcendental Self]. (2.21)

*Comments:* This aphorism reiterates the point made above (2.18) that Nature serves the purposes of the Self. The realm of Nature can be used either to indulge in experiences or to catapult oneself beyond all conditional states of existence into Self-realization.

Although [the Seen] has ceased [to exist] for him whose purpose has been accomplished, it has nevertheless not ceased [to exist altogether], because [it is still] common experience (*sâdhâranatva*) for others [who are unenlightened]. (2.22)

The correlation (*samyoga*) [between the Seer and the Seen] is the reason for the apprehension of the essential form of the power of the "owner" (*svâmin*) and that of the "owned" (*sva*). (2.23)

The cause of that [correlation] is ignorance (*avidyâ*). (2.24)

With the disappearance of that [ignorance] the correlation [also] disappears; this is [total] cessation, the aloneness (*kaivalya*) of the [sheer Power of] seeing. (2.25)

The means of [attaining] cessation is the unceasing vision of discernment (*viveka-khyâti*). (2.26)

For him [who possesses the unceasing vision of discernment], there arises, in the last stage, wisdom (*prajnâ*) [that is] sevenfold. (2.27)

*Comments:* According to Vyâsa's *Yoga-Bhâshya*, the seven aspects of this wisdom are the following insights: (1) That which is to be prevented, namely future suffering, has been successfully identified; (2) the causes of suffering have been eliminated once and for all; (3) through the "ecstasy of restriction" (*nirodha-samâdhi*) complete cessation of all contents of consciousness has been achieved; (4) the means of cessation, namely the vision of discernment (*viveka-khyâti*), has been applied; (5) sovereignty of the higher mind (called *buddhi*) has been achieved; (6) the constituents (*guna*) have lost their foothold and, "like rocks fallen from the edge of a mountain," incline toward dissolution (*pralaya*), that is, full resorption into the transcendental ground of Nature; (7) the Self abides in its essential nature, undefiled and alone (*kevalin*).

Through the performance of the limbs of Yoga, and with the dwindling of impurity, [there comes about] the radiance of wisdom (*jnâna*), [which develops] up to the vision of discernment. (*2.28)

Discipline (*yama*), restraint (*niyama*), posture (*âsana*), breath control (*prânâyâma*), sense-withdrawal (*pratyâhâra*), concentration (*dhâranâ*), meditation (*dhyâna*), and ecstasy (*samâdhi*) are the eight limbs [of Yoga]. (*2.29)

Nonharming, truthfulness, nonstealing, chastity, and greedlessness are the restraints. (*2.30)

[These are valid] in all spheres, irrespective of birth, place, time, and circumstance, [and they constitute] the "great vow" (*mahâ-vrata*). (*2.31)

Purity, contentment, asceticism, study, and devotion to the Lord are the disciplines. (*2.32)

For the repelling of [unwholesome] notions (*vitarka*), [the *yogin* should pursue] the cultivation of [their] opposite. (*2.33)

[Unwholesome] notions, [such as] harming and so on, whether done, caused to be done, or approved, whether arising from greed, anger, or infatuation, whether modest, middling, or excessive—[these have their] unending fruition in ignorance (*avidyâ*) and suffering (*duhkha*); thus, [the *yogin* should devote himself to] the cultivation of their opposite. (*2.34)

When [the *yogin*] is grounded in [the virtue of] nonharming (*ahimsâ*), enmity ceases in his presence. (*2.35)

When grounded in truthfulness (*satya*), action [and its] fruition depend [on his will]. (*2.36)

When grounded in nonstealing (*asteya*), all [kinds of] treasures appear [before him]. (*2.37)

When grounded in chastity (*brahmacarya*), [great] vitality is acquired. (*2.38)

When steadied in greedlessness, [the *yogin* secures] knowledge of the wherefore of [his] births. (*2.39)

Through purity [he gains] distance (*jugupsâ*) from his own limbs, [and he also acquires the desire for] noncontamination by others. (*2.40)

298

[Furthermore,] purity of the *sattva* [constituent of his being], gladness, one-pointedness, mastery of the sense organs, and the capability for Self-vision (*âtma-darshana*) [are achieved]. (*2.41)

Through contentment (*samtosha*) unexcelled joy is gained. (*2.42)

Through asceticism (*tapas*), on account of the dwindling of impurity, perfection of the body and the sense organs [is acquired]. (*2.43)

Through study (*svâdhyâya*) [the *yogin* establishes] contact with the chosen deity (*ishta-devatâ*). (*2.44)

*Comments:* In many schools of Yoga, the practitioner is encouraged to cultivate a ritual relationship to the Divine in the form of Shiva, Vishnu, Krishna, Kâlî, or some other traditional figure, which then becomes the *yogin's* chosen deity.

Through devotion to the Lord (*îshvara-pranidhâna*) [comes about] the attainment of the [supraconscious] ecstasy. (*2.45)

Posture (*âsana*) [should be] stable and comfortable. (*2.46)

[The correct practice of posture is accompanied] by the relaxation of tension and the coinciding [of consciousness] with the infinite. (*2.47)

Thence [comes] unassailability by the opposites (*dvandva*) [found in Nature, such as heat and cold]. (*2.48)

When this is [achieved], breath control, [which is] the cutting off of the flow of inhalation and exhalation [should be practiced]. (*2.49)

[Breath control is] external, internal, or fixed in its movement, [and it is] regulated by place, time, and number; [it can be either] protracted or contracted. (*2.50)

[The movement of breath] transcending the external and the internal sphere is the "fourth." (*2.51)

*Comments:* This obscure aphorism has invited different interpretations. It probably refers to a special phenomenon that occurs in the state of ecstasy (*samâdhi*), where breathing can become so reduced and shallow that it is no longer detectable. This state of suspended breath can last for prolonged periods.

Thence the covering of the [inner] light disappears. (*2.52)

And [the *yogin* acquires] mental fitness for concentration. (*2.53)

Sense-withdrawal is the imitation as it were of the essential form of consciousness [on the part] of the sense organs by separating them from their objects. (*2.54)

Thence [results] the supreme obedience of the sense organs. (*2.55)

### III. Vibhûti-Pâda ("Chapter on Powers")

Concentration (*dhâranâ*) is the binding of consciousness to a [single] spot. (*3.1)

The one-directionality (*ekatânatâ*) of the ideas [present in consciousness] with regard to that [object of concentration] is meditation (*dhyâna*). (*3.2)

That [consciousness], shining forth as the object only as if empty of its essence, is ecstasy (*samâdhi*). (*3.3)

The three [practiced] together [in relation to the same object] are [what is known as] constraint (*samyama*). (*3.4)

Through mastery of that [practice of constraint there comes about] the flashing-forth of wisdom (*prajnâ*). (*3.5)

Its progression is gradual. (*3.6)

[In regard to] the previous [five limbs of Yoga], the three [parts of the practice of constraint] are the inner limbs (*antar-anga*). (*3.7)

Yet, they are outer limbs (*bahir-anga*) [in regard to] the seedless [ecstasy]. (*3.8)

[When there is] subjugation of the [subliminal] activators (*samskâra*) of emergence and the manifestation of the activators of restriction—[this is known as] the restriction transformation, which is connected with consciousness at the moment of restriction (*nirodha*). (3.9)

The calm flow of that [consciousness is effected] through activators [in the depths of consciousness]. (3.10)

The dwindling of "all-objectness" (*sarva-arthatâ*) and the arising of one-pointedness (*ekâgratâ*) is the ecstasy transformation of consciousness. (3.11)

Then again, when the quiescent and the uprisen ideas [present in consciousness] are similar, [this is known as] the one-pointedness transformation of consciousness. (3.12)

*Comments:* Here Patanjali tells us that the one-pointedness of the ecstatic state is due to a succession of similar contents of consciousness. Ideas flash up momentarily, and their similarity gives us the impression of continuity.

By this are [also] explained the transformations of form, time-variation, and condition [with regard to] the elements (*bhûta*) [and] the sense organs. (3.13)

*Comments:* This is a difficult aphorism. Vyâsa, in his *Yoga-Bhâshya*, offers the following illustration: The substance clay may appear as either a lump of clay or a water jar. These are its external forms (*dharma*), and the change from the one to the other form does not affect the substance (*dharmin*) itself: The clay remains the same, but the lump or jar do not have a spatial existence only, they are also placed in time. Thus, the water jar is the present time-variation of the clay. Its past time-variation was the lump of clay. Its future time-variation will presumably be dust. But, again, throughout these transformations in time, the substance remains the same. Time is a succession of individual moments (*kshana*), which imperceptibly alter the condition of the water jar; this is the well-known process of decay, or aging. The same applies to consciousness (*citta*).

The "form-bearer" (*dharmin*) [i.e., the substance] is what conforms to the quiescent, uprisen, or indeterminable form (*dharma*). (3.14)

*Comments:* The quiescent forms are those that have been, the uprisen forms are those that are, and the indeterminable forms are those that will be. In all cases, the substance is the same.

The differentiation in the sequence [of appearing forms] is the reason for the differentiation in the transformations [of Nature]. (3.15)

Through [the practice of] constraint upon the three [kinds of] transformation [comes about] knowledge of the past and the future. (3.16)

[There is a natural] confusion of idea, object, and [signifying] word [on account of an erroneous] superimposition on one another. Through [the practice of] constraint upon the distinction of these [confused elements], knowledge of the sounds of all beings [is acquired]. (3.17)

Through direct perception (*sâkshât-karana*) of activators (*samskâra*) [the *yogin* gains] knowledge of [his] previous births. (3.18)

[Through direct perception] of [another person's] ideas [in consciousness], knowledge of another's consciousness [is obtained]. (3.19)

*Comments:* Ordinary perception is a process mediated by the senses. But Yoga recognizes the existence of direct perception, which is based on the *yogin*'s conscious identification with a given object.

But [that knowledge] does not [have as its object] those [ideas] together with their [objective] support, because [that support] is absent from [the other's consciousness]. (3.20)

*Comments:* This aphorism makes the simple point that the *yogin*'s unmediated perception of the thoughts of another person does not give him knowledge of the objective realities on which those thoughts are based. Thus, if a person is fearful of the ocean, the *yogin* will perceive the person's mental image of the ocean and understand the fear connected with it, but he will not learn anything about the ocean itself.

Through [the practice of] constraint upon the form of the body, upon the suspension of the capacity to be perceived, [that is to say,] upon the disruption of the light [traveling from that body] to the eye, invisibility [is gained]. (3.21)

Karma [is of two kinds]: acute or deferred. Through [the practice of] constraint thereon, or from omens, [the *yogin* acquires] knowledge of [his] death. (3.22)

[Through the practice of constraint] upon [the virtues of] friendliness and so on, [he acquires various] strengths (*bala*). (3.23)

[Through the practice of constraint] upon the strengths, [he acquires] the strength of an elephant and so on. (3.24)

By focusing the flashing-forth (*âloka*) of [those mental] activities [that are free from suffering and illuminating upon any object, the *yogin* gains] knowledge of the subtle, concealed, and distant [aspects of those objects]. (3.25)

Through [the practice of] constraint upon the sun, [he gains] knowledge of the cosmos. (3.26)

[Through the practice of constraint] upon the moon, [he gains] knowledge of the arrangement of the stars. (3.27)

[Through the practice of constraint] upon the pole star, [he gains] knowledge of its movement. (3.28)

[Through the practice of constraint] upon the "navel wheel" (*nâbhi-cakra*), [he gains] knowledge of the organization of the body. (3.29)

[Through the practice of constraint] upon the "throat well" (*kantha-kûpa*), the cessation of hunger and thirst [is accomplished]. (3.30)

[Through the practice of constraint] upon the "tortoise duct" (*kûrma-nâdî*), [the *yogin* gains] steadiness. (3.31)

*Comments:* According to the *Yoga-Bhâshya*, the "tortoise duct" is a tubelike structure found in the chest below the "throat well." This may be one of the many pathways of the life force that comprise the subtle body.

[Through the practice of constraint] upon the light in the head, [he acquires] the vision of the adepts (*siddha*). (3.32)

Or through a flash-of-illumination (*pratibhâ*) [the *yogin* acquires knowledge about] everything. (3.33)

[Through the practice of constraint] upon the heart, [he gains] understanding of [the nature of] consciousness. (3.34)

Experience (*bhoga*) is an idea [that is based on] the nondistinction between the absolutely unblended Self and the *sattva*. Through [the practice of] constraint on the [Self's] essential purpose, [which is distinct from] the other-purposiveness (*para-arthatva*) [of Nature], [the *yogin* gains] knowledge of the Self. (3.35)

Thence occur flashes-of-illumination (*pratibhâ*) [in the sensory areas of] hearing, sensing, sight, taste, and smell. (3.36)

These are obstacles to ecstasy [but] attainments in the externalized [state of consciousness]. (3.37)

Through the relaxation of the causes of attachment [to one's body] and through the experience of going-forth, consciousness [is capable of] entering another body. (3.38)

Through mastery of the up-breath (*udâna*) [the *yogin* gains the power of] nonadhesion to water, mud, or thorns and [the power of] rising up [from them]. (3.39)

*Comments:* Early on, the *yogins* discovered that there are different aspects to the life force (*prâna*), manifesting as the breath. Each yields different paranormal powers when fully mastered.

Through mastery of the mid-breath (*samâna*) [he acquires] effulgence. (3.40)

Through [the practice of] constraint upon the relation between ear and space (*âkâsha*) [he acquires] the "divine ear" (*divya-shrotra*). (3.41)

*Comments:* Space, which is regarded as a radiant etheric medium, is one of the five elements of the material dimension of Nature.

Through [the practice of] constraint upon the relation between body and space and by coinciding [in his consciousness] with light [objects], such as cotton, [the *yogin* obtains the power of] traveling through space. (3.42)

*Comments:* Through ecstatic identification with a cotton ball, a spider's thread, or a cloud, the *yogin* is said to be able to levitate.

An external, nonimaginary fluctuation (*vritti*) [of consciousness] is the "great incorporeal" from which [comes] the dwindling of the coverings of the [inner] light. (3.43)

*Comments:* In our imagination we can reach beyond the boundaries of the body. But there is also a special yogic practice by which consciousness itself can move out of the body and gather information about the external world. This practice precedes the yogic technique of actually entering into another body. The Sanskrit commentators insist that this is not an imaginary experience.

Through [the practice of] constraint upon the coarse, the essential form, the subtle, the connectedness, and the purposiveness [of objects] [the *yogin* gains] mastery over the elements. (3.44)

Thence [results] the manifestation [of the great psychic powers], such as "atomization" (*animan*) and so on, perfection of the body, and the indestructibility of its constituents. (3.45)

Beauty, gracefulness, and adamant robustness [constitute] the perfection of the body. (3.46)

Through [the practice of] constraint upon [the process of] perception, the essential form, I-am-ness, connectedness, and purposiveness [the *yogin* gains] mastery over the sense organs. (3.47)

Thence [comes about] fleetness [as of] the mind, the state lacking sense organs, and the mastery over the matrix [of Nature]. (3.48)

[The *yogin* who enjoys] only the vision of the distinction between the Self and the *sattva* [gains] supremacy over all states [of existence] and omniscience. (3.49)

Through dispassion toward even that [exalted vision], with the dwindling of the seeds of the defects, [he achieves] the aloneness (*kaivalya*) [of the Power of seeing]. (3.50)

Upon the invitation of high-placed [beings], [he should give himself] no cause for attachment or pride, because of [the danger of] renewed and undesired inclination [for lower levels of existence]. (3.51)

Through [the practice of] constraint upon the moment (*kshana*) [of time] and its sequence [the *yogin* obtains] the wisdom born of discernment. (3.52)

Thence [arises for him] the awareness of [the difference between] similars that cannot normally be distinguished due to an indeterminateness of the distinctions of species, appearance, and position. (3.53)

The wisdom born of discernment is the "deliverer" (*târaka*), and is omniobjective, omnitemporal, and nonsequential. (3.54)

With [the attainment of] equality in purity between the Self and the *sattva*, the aloneness [of the Power of seeing is established]. End (*iti*). (3.55)

## IV. Kaivalya-Pâda ("Chapter on Liberation")

The powers (*siddhi*) are the result of birth, herbs, *mantras*, asceticism, or ecstasy. (4.1)

*Comments:* This aphorism rightly belongs to the previous chapter. Its appearance here can be explained by the fact that the commentators have misunderstood the intent of the opening *sûtras* of the present chapter.

The transformation into another species (*jâti*) [is possible] because of the superabundance of Nature. (4.2)

*Comments:* This and the following aphorisms have generally been understood to refer to the magical power of creating artificial body-minds upon which the *yogin* transfers his own karma. But a careful reading of this section suggests a more philosophical interpretation. For, it appears, what Patanjali is explaining here is the process of individuation, as it applies to the cosmos itself.

The incidental cause (*nimitta*) does not initiate the creations (*prakriti*), but [merely is responsible for] the singling out of possibilities—like a farmer [who irrigates a field by selecting appropriate pathways for the water]. (4.3)

The individualized consciousnesses (*nirmâna-citta*) [proceed] from the essential I-am-ness (*asmitâ-mâtra*). (4.4)

[Although the numerous individualized consciousnesses are engaged] in distinct activities, the one (*eka*) consciousness is the originator of [all] the others. (4.5)

Of these [individualized consciousnesses that consciousness which is] born of meditation is without [karmic] deposit. (4.6)

The karma of a *yogin* is neither black nor white; for others it is threefold [i.e., mixed]. (4.7)

Thence [follows] the manifestation of only those traits (*vâsanâ*) [in the depths of consciousness] that correspond to the fruition of their [particular karma]. (4.8)

On account of the uniformity between the [deep] memory and the activators (*samskâra*) [there is] a continuity [between the manifestation of the subliminal activators and the karmic cause], even though [cause and effect] may be separated [in terms of] place, time, and species. (4.9)

*Comments:* This aphorism explains, in a somewhat obscure fashion, that the karmic link between a person's previous existence and the present life is not arbitrary. It is preserved by the subliminal activators. Thus, nobody suffers any karmic injustice. Every individual reaps what he or she has sown in former lives.

And these [activators in the depths of consciousness] are without beginning because of the perpetuity of the primordial will [inherent in nature]. (4.10)

Because of the connection [of the traits in the depths of consciousness] with the [karmic] cause, the fruit, the substratum, and the support, [it follows that] with the disappearance of these [factors], the disappearance of those [traits is likewise brought about]. (4.11)

Past and future as such exist because of the [visible] difference in the [developmental] paths of the forms (*dharma*) [produced by Nature]. (4.12)

These [forms] are manifest or subtle and composed of the [three] constituents (*guna*). (4.13)

The "thatness" (*tattva*) of an object [stems] from the homogeneity in the transformations [of the primary constituents (*guna*) of Nature]. (4.14)

*Comments:* By "thatness" is meant the peculiar stability that gives one the impression of there being a solid object, whereas everything is constantly in a state of flux, as the Greek philosopher Heraclitus realized many centuries before Patanjali.

In view of the multiplicity of consciousnesses [as opposed to] the singleness of [perceived] objects, both [belong to] separate levels [of existence]. (4.15)

And the object is not dependent on a single consciousness; this is unprovable; besides, what could [such an imaginary object possibly] be? (*4.16)

*Comments:* This aphorism is missing in some of the Sanskrit manuscripts, and it is quite likely that it belongs to Vyâsa's *Yoga-Bhâshya*. The idea expressed here is that objects have an independent existence. This implies a rejection of the radical idealism of certain schools of Mahâyâna Buddhism.

An object is known or not known by reason of the required "coloration" (*uparâga*) of consciousness by that [object]. (4.17)

The fluctuations of consciousness are always known by their "superior," because of the immutability of the Self. (4.18)

*Comments:* The transcendental Self, which undergoes no change, is held to be superior to the changeable forms and realms of Nature, which includes the finite consciousness.

That [consciousness] has no self-luminosity because of its being seen [by the Self]. (4.19)

*Comments:* It is a common notion of Indian thought that only the Self has its own light, whereas the finite or empirical consciousness is, like the moon, illuminated by borrowed light.

And [this implies] the impossibility-of-cognizing both [consciousness and object] simultaneously. (4.20)

If consciousness were perceived by another [consciousness], [this would lead to an infinite] regress from cognition (*buddhi*) to cognition and the confusion of memory. (4.21)

When the unchanging Awareness (*citi*) assumes the shape of that [consciousness], experience of one's own cognitions [is made possible]. (4.22)

[Provided that] consciousness is "colored" by the Seer and the Seen, [it can perceive] any object. (4.23)

*Comments:* For the ordinary human consciousness to exist, there must be the presence of the transcendental Self (the Seer) and of Nature (the Seen) in its countless forms.

That [consciousness], though speckled with countless traits (*vâsanâ*), is other-purposed due to [its being limited to] collaborative activity. (4.24)[7]

*Comments:* Even though consciousness is a mechanism of Nature, it shares in the great developmental orientation of Nature, which is, ultimately, to bring about Self-realization, or liberation.

For him who sees the distinction [between the Self and the *sattva*, there comes about] the discontinuation of the projection of the [false] self-sense (*âtma-bhâva*). (4.25)

Then consciousness, inclined toward discernment, is borne onward toward the aloneness (*kaivalya*) [of the Power of seeing]. (4.26)

In the intervals of that [involuting consciousness], other [new] ideas [may arise] from the activators [in the depths of consciousness]. (4.27)

Their cessation [is accomplished by the same means] as described [in aphorism 2.10] for the causes-of-affliction (*klesha*). (4.28)

For [the *yogin* who is] always nonexploitative even in [the state of elevation, there follows], through the vision of discernment, the ecstasy called "*dharma* cloud" (*dharma-megha*). (4.29)

*Comments:* It is not clear what the precise meaning of the term *dharma* is here. Some translators have rendered it as "virtue," but at that level of ecstatic realization, it makes little sense to speak of the *yogin* as virtuous or not virtuous. He has transcended the moral categories of ordinary life. More appropriately, *dharma* could here be understood, as in certain Buddhist contexts, to refer to the primal Reality. In other words, at the consummation of the vision of discernment, the *yogin* is, as it were, enveloped by the Self. This ecstasy is a transitional phase that removes all spiritual ignorance and therefore all its fateful repercussions (such as karma and suffering), and is followed directly by the event of liberation.

Thence [follows] the discontinuation of the causes-of-affliction (*klesha*) and of karma. (4.30)

Then, [when] all coverings of imperfection are removed, little [remains] to be known because of the infinity of the [resulting] wisdom. (4.31)

Thence [comes about] the termination of the sequences in the transformations of the constituents (*guna*) [of Nature] whose purpose is fulfilled. (4.32)

Sequence is [that which is] correlative to the moment [of time], apprehensible at the extreme end of a [particular] transformation. (4.33)

*Comments:* Patanjali argues that there is a correlation between the unit of time, called "moment" (*kshana*), and the ultimate unit of the process of transformation, called "sequence" (*krama*). This atomistic conception of time foreshadows contemporary ideas about the discontinuous nature of time and of the space-time continuum.

The involution (*pratisarga*) of the constituents (*guna*), [which are now] devoid of purpose for the Self, is [what is called] the aloneness [of the Power of seeing], or the establishment of the Power of Awareness (*citi-shakti*) in its essential form. End (*iti*). (4.34)

*Comments:* Upon Self-realization, or liberation, the fundamental constituents (*guna*) of the adept's body-mind have no further purpose and so gradually resolve back into the transcendental ground of Nature. This implies that Patanjali looks upon Self-realization as coinciding with the death of the finite body-mind. What remains is the eternal Witness, the Power of Awareness, or Self (*purusha*).

## III. THE ELABORATION OF WISDOM—THE COMMENTARIAL LITERATURE

*Sûtras* were not created in the first blush of a tradition or school of thought. Rather they were authoritative summaries that drew on many generations of thinking and debating. But their conciseness proved both a stumbling block and an advantage. On one hand, the *sûtra* style gave rise to much ambiguity: As the oral transmission of the teachings became weak, the original ideas and formulations were gradually lost from sight, which encouraged the surfacing of sometimes widely divergent interpretations. For instance, the *Brahma-Sûtra* of Bâdarâyana, a key scripture of Vedânta composed perhaps around 200 C.E., has been cited in support of nondualist (*advaita*) as well as dualist (*dvaita*) schools of metaphysics. On the other hand, the inbuilt ambiguity in the *Sûtra* works allowed just such refreshing and fertile variation.

Even the most creative minds of traditional India were obliged to weave their innovative thoughts within the framework of their own tradition, whether it was Vedânta, Buddhism, Jainism, or Yoga. They had to take existing authoritative opinion into account or at least pay lip service to it. At any rate, rather than hemming in creativity, the philosophical *Sûtra* works stimulated discussion and dissent. They gave rise to commentaries, which occasioned new commentaries, subcommentaries, and glosses thereon. Patanjali's *Yoga-Sûtra*, too, inspired later generations to produce a considerable commentarial literature. There are *Bhâshyas* (original explanatory works containing much background information), *Vrittis* (original commentaries offering word-by-word explanations), *Tîkâs* (glosses on commentaries), and *Up-atîkâs* (subglosses on glosses). Typical examples of a *Tîkâ* are Vâcaspati Mishra's *Tattva-Vaishâradî*

and Vijnâna Bhikshu's *Yoga-Vârttika*—both of which are glosses on Vyâsa's *Yoga-Bhâshya*, whereas the *Pâtanjala-Rahasya* of Râghavânanda, for instance, belongs to the category of subglosses.

### The Yoga-Bhâshya of Vyâsa

The oldest extant commentary on the *Yoga-Sûtra* is the *Yoga-Bhâshya* ("Discussion on Yoga") by Vyâsa. It was probably composed in the fifth century C.E.[7] Its author is allegedly the same person who was also responsible for collecting the four Vedic hymnodies, the *Mahâbhârata* epic, the numerous *Purânas* (popular sacred encyclopedias), and a host of other works. This farfetched idea has some basis in reality, however, for the name Vyâsa means "Collector" and was presumably a title rather than a personal name, and was applied to many individuals over a long span of time. In actuality, we know as little about Vyâsa or the numerous Vyâsas as we do about Patanjali.

According to one legend, Vyâsa was the son of the sage Parâshara and the nymph Satyavatî (also called Kâlî) whom Parâshara had seduced. In appreciation of her beauty and love, the sage not only restored her virginity by magical means but also relieved her of the fishy smell that she had inherited from her mother. Vyâsa was brought up in secret on an island (*dvîpa*); hence, his epithet Dvaipâyana ("Island-born"). Because he bore the name Krishna as a child, he also came to be known as Krishna Dvaipâyana.

Sometime later, Satyavatî's beauty caught the eye of the aged king Shântanu, who promptly fell in love with her. He asked for Satyavatî's hand, which her father granted on the condition that it must be her children who would succeed to the throne, not the remaining child from the king's first marriage. Shântanu agreed after his grown son Bhîshma, whose heroic exploits are told in the

*Mahâbârata*, renounced his hereditary rights. The couple lived happily for almost twenty years and had two sons. After Shântanu's death the first-born duly ascended the throne but died during a military adventure. Then his brother, who was married to two women, was crowned. Alas, his rule was also short-lived, for he soon died of consumption. Custom demanded that since he had left no offspring the nearest male relative should sire a child with either of the two widows. Bhîshma was disqualified because he had sworn never to have children.

Satyavatî called Vyâsa to the court to perform this noble duty. The two ladies, Ambikâ and Ambâlikâ, had expected the stately Bhîshma to do the honors. They were shocked when the less-than-handsome Vyâsa, in the scant attire of a hermit, visited their chambers. Vyâsa made love first to one widow, then the other. In this way he fathered the blind Dhritarâshtra and the pale Pându. On that evening Vyâsa also sired a third child—by a maid who acted as a substitute when he wanted to repeat his duty with one of the widows. Dhritarâshtra was born blind because his mother, Ambikâ, had closed her eyes in shock upon sight of Vyâsa, whereas Pându was born pale because all blood had drained from his mother Ambâlikâ's face when Vyâsa approached her. The sage, then, is the source of the great war reported in the *Mahâbhârata*, which was fought by the sons of Dhritarâshtra and Pându respectively. We can see in this an ingenious literary device by which the creator of the *Mahâbhârata* epic inserted himself into the story, or we can assume that it may contain a kernel of historical truth.

Whoever the author of the *Yoga-Bhâshya* may have been, this Sanskrit work contains the key to many of the more enigmatic aphorisms of Patanjali's scripture. We have to use it with caution, however, since several centuries separate the two Yoga authorities. Even though Vyâsa was in all likelihood a *yogin* of considerable attainment—because he writes with great authority about rather esoteric matters—he does not appear to have been in the direct lineage of Patanjali, as some of his interpretations and terminology are at variance with the *Yoga-Sûtra*.

## Other Commentaries

From the eighth century C.E. we have the Jaina scholar Haribhadra Sûri's *Shad-Darshana-Samuccaya* ("Compilation of the Six Systems [of Philosophy]"), which includes a chapter on Patanjali's Yoga. However, strictly speaking, this is not a commentary.

The first major commentary after the *Yoga-Bhâshya* is Vâcaspati Mishra's *Tattva-Vaishâradî* ("Clarity of Truth"). Vâcaspati Mishra, who lived in the ninth century, was a pundit through and through. He wrote outstanding commentaries on the six classical systems of Hindu philosophy—Yoga, Sâmkhya, Vedânta, Mîmâmsâ, Nyâya, and Vaisheshika. But his knowledge appears to have been theoretical rather than practical. Hence, in his gloss on Vyâsa's *Yoga-Bhâshya*, he tends to expand on philological and epistemological matters, while leaving important practical considerations unexplained. A story that is told about Vâcaspati Mishra shows how much of a scholar he was. When he had completed his major work, the *Bhâmatî* commentary on the *Brahma-Sûtra*, he apologized to his wife for neglecting her for so many years by naming the commentary after her, a truly scholarly recompense. Nonetheless, his work offers many useful clues to some of the more difficult passages of the *Yoga-Bhâshya*.

From the eleventh century, we have two important works. The first is the Arabic translation of the *Yoga-Sûtra* prepared by the renowned Persian scholar al-Bîrûnî—a rather free rendering that may well have exercised a lasting influence on the development of Persian mysticism. The other work is the subcommentary known as *Râja-Mârtanda* ("Royal Sun"), or *Bhoja-Vritti*, by King Bhoja of Dhârâ, an adherent of Shaivism, who lived from 1019 to 1054 C.E. The value of this work is more historical than exegetical. Although Bhoja criticized previous commentators for their arbitrary interpretations, his own efforts are often no less capricious and perhaps less original than he made them out to be. King Bhoja was an accomplished poet and a great patron of the arts and spiritual traditions, and we must assume that his interest in Yoga was not purely theoretical either.

The next major commentary is Shankara Bhagavatpâda's *Vivarana* ("Exposition") on the *Yoga-Bhâshya*. Although this is a subcommentary, it is a remarkably original work showing the uncommon exegetical independence of a *Bhâshya*. According to some scholars, its author is none other than the famous adept Shankara Âcârya himself, who lived in the eighth century C.E. and was the greatest spokesman ever for Advaita Vedânta. The German indologist Paul Hacker was the first to propose that prior to Shankara's conversion to the nondualist philosophy of Advaita Vedânta this great preceptor had been a Vishnu devotee and an adherent of the Yoga tradition. He must then have met his teacher Govinda, who expounded to him the "intangible Yoga" (*asparsha-yoga*) of nondualism taught by Gaudapâda, the author of the *Mândûkya-Kârikâ*. It is certainly interesting that of all his writings, Shankara's commentary on the *Mândûkya-Kârikâ* contains the most references to the Yoga tradition. The British translator of the *Vivarana*, Trevor Leggett, tentatively accepted Hacker's proposal, remarking, "I have not found anything which would, as far as my knowledge goes, absolutely rule out Sankara as the author."[8]

However, this identification of Shankara Âcârya with the author of the *Vivarana* has by no means been universally accepted. In fact, recently it was seriously challenged by the Sanskrit scholar T. S. Rukmani, who has just completed a new English translation of this rare text. She judged the style of the *Vivarana* to be "un-Shankarâcârya . . . tedious, laboured, and careless."[9] Since Vâcaspati Mishra was a great Shankara scholar, his silence about the *Vivarana* is weighty and suggests a post-Vâcaspati date. Rukmani did, however, discover a single reference to the *Vivarana* in Vijnâna Bhikshu's *Yoga-Vârttika* (3.36), where the expression *vivarana-bhâshye* ("in the *Vivarana* commentary") can be found. This favors a date between the ninth and the sixteenth century for Shankara Bhagavatpâda. More specifically, Rukmani proposes that the author of the *Vivarana* was the Shankara who belonged to the scholarly Payyur family of Kerala who lived in the fourteenth century C.E. Further research is needed on this issue, though it looks increasingly probable that Shankara Âcârya had no hand in the composition of the *Vivarana*.

From the fourteenth century we also have an admirable systematic account of Classical Yoga in Mâdhava's *Sarva-Darshana-Samgraha*, which, as the title indicates, is a compendium (*samgraha*) of all (*sarva*) major philosophical systems (*darshana*) of medieval India.

From the fifteenth century stem the *Yoga-Siddhânta-Candrikâ* ("Moonlight on the Yoga System") and *Sûtra-Artha-Bodhinî*[10] ("Illumination of the Meaning of the Aphorisms"), both authored by Nârâyana Tîrtha. The former work is an independent commentary, or *Bhâshya*, while the latter text is a *Vritti*. Nârâyana Tîrtha was a scholar of the Vallabha school of Bhakti-Yoga, and his commentaries interpret Classical Yoga from the point of view of Vallabha Âcârya's Shuddha ("Pure") Vedânta. His works are of great interest not only because of their devotional element but also because they mention Hatha-Yoga and certain Tantric concepts such as the *cakras* and *kundalinî*.

In the sixteenth century, outstanding commentaries on Vyâsa's *Yoga-Bhâshya* were written by Râmânanda Yati, Nâgojî Bhatta (or Nâgesha), and Vijnâna Bhikshu. Râmânanda Yati's work, entitled *Mani-Prabhâ* ("Jewel Lustre"), comments directly on the *Yoga-Sûtra*. Nâgojî Bhatta wrote two original commentaries, the *Laghvî* ("Short [Commentary]") and the *Brihatî* ("Great [Commentary]"). The declared purpose of the latter work is to resolve the differences between (dualistic) Yoga and (nondualistic) Vedânta. He has been hailed as "perhaps the greatest learned man of the latter part of the sixteenth century."[11]

This also was the avowed goal of Vijnâna Bhikshu, who lived in the second half of the sixteenth century. He authored an elaborate commentary called *Yoga-Vârttika* ("Tract on Yoga") and the *Yoga-Sâra-Samgraha* ("Compendium of the Essence of Yoga"), which is a digest of his voluminous treatise. Vijnâna Bhikshu was a renowned scholar who interpreted Yoga from a Vedântic point of view. At the end of the nineteenth century, Max Müller spoke of him as "a philosopher of considerable grasp, [who] while fully recognising the difference between the six systems of philosophy, tried to discover a common truth behind them all, and to point out how they can be studied together, or rather in succession, and how all of them are meant to lead honest students into the way of truth."[12]

Nothing is known about Vijnâna Bhikshu, who "seems to have shunned any kind of identity

> "When a *yogin* becomes qualified by practicing moral discipline (*yama*) and self-restraint (*niyama*), he can proceed to posture and the other means."
>
> —*Yoga-Bhâshya-Vivarana* 2.29

with name and form."[13] However, some scholars have speculatively associated him with Bengal, and T. S. Rukmani, who undertook a complete English translation of the *Yoga-Vârttika*, suggested that he must have taught in or near Varanasi (Benares) because his chief disciple, Bhâvâ Ganesha (author of the *Dîpikâ*, "Torch"), resided there. Vijnâna Bhikshu is credited with the authorship of eighteen works, which include commentaries on Classical Yoga, Sâmkhya, several *Upanishads*, and the *Brahma-Sûtra*, two of which commentaries may have been wrongly attributed to him. All his works are infused with his particular type of Vedânta, which is of the epic Sâmkhya-Yoga kind and which stands in stark contrast to Shankara's *mâyâ-vâda* ("illusionism"). Vijnâna Bhikshu, in fact, often becomes quite passionate and not a little derogatory when he criticizes Shankara and his school. For him, Yoga is the preferred path to realization.

Among the later commentaries on the *Yoga-Sûtra*, mention must be made of Sadâshiva Indra's *Sudhâkâra* ("Mine of Ambrosia"), the nineteenth-century scholar Anantadeva's *Pada-Candrikâ* ("Moonlight on Words"), Râghavânanda's *Patanjala-Rahasya* ("Secret of the Pâtanjala [School]"), and Râmabhadra Dîkshita's *Patanjali-Carita* ("Patanjali's Life"), as well as Baladeva Mishra's *Pradîpikâ* ("Lamp") and Hariharânanda's *Bhâsvatî* ("Elucidation"), both composed in the twentieth century. Swami Hariharânanda (1869–1947) was the spiritual head of the Kapila Matha in Madhupur (Bihar) and an adept of Sâmkhya-Yoga.

There are a number of other, less popular works, mostly known by name only. On the whole, the secondary commentaries do not excel in originality and rely largely on Vyâsa's old scholium or one of the other commentaries. The commentarial literature of Classical Yoga tends to be dry and repetitive, scarcely reflecting the fact that Yoga has always primarily been an esoteric discipline taught by word of mouth and perpetuated through intensive personal practice rather than scholastic achievements. As Dattâtreya states in his *Yoga-Shâstra*:

> There will be success for the practitioner (*kriyâ-yukta*). [But] how can there be [success] for the nonpractitioner? (83)

> Success is never gained through mere reading of books. (84)

> Those who [merely] talk about Yoga and wear the apparel [of a *yogin*] but lack all application and live for their bellies and their dicks (*shishna*)—they cheat people. (92–93)

If the Yoga tradition, by comparison with Vedânta or Buddhism, appears somewhat weak in philosophical elaboration, it is definitely rich in experiential knowledge. For the *yogins*, perhaps more than for the adherents of the other classical Hindu systems of thought, philosophical understanding has always been only a compass to guide the initiate's inner experimentation. It was never intended to replace personal realization of the ultimate Truth, or Reality. Possibly because of their intensive preoccupation with the higher octaves of consciousness, *yogins* were extremely sensitive to the chimerical nature of conceptual thought and trusted it only up to a point. They found philosophy just for the sake of intellectual comprehension an unattractive proposition, as it cannot lead a person beyond the maze of opinion. As Sage Yâjnavalkya instructs Paingala in the *Paingala-Upanishad*[14] (4.9):

> Of what use is milk for one who is satiated with nectar? Likewise of what use are the *Vedas* when one's [innermost] Self is known? For the *yogin* who is satisfied with the nectar of wisdom there is nothing that remains to be accomplished. If there is, then he is not a knower of Reality (*tattva*).

*"The undisciplined (atapasvin) [person] does not succeed in Yoga."*

—*Yoga-Vârttika* (2.1)

# Chapter 10

# THE PHILOSOPHY AND PRACTICE OF PÂTANJALA-YOGA

## I. THE CHAIN OF BEING—SELF AND WORLD FROM PATANJALI'S PERSPECTIVE

When describing the Buddhist approach to life, the German-born Lama Anagarika Govinda ventured the following observation:

Psychology can be studied and dealt with in two ways: either for its own sake alone, i.e. as pure science, which leaves entirely out of account the usefulness or non-usefulness of its results—or else for the sake of some definite object, that is, with a view to practical application . . . [1]

These remarks apply equally to Yoga as to Buddhism. As a form of psychotechnology, Yoga deals first and foremost with the human mind or psyche. But, according to the yogic visionaries, our inner world parallels the structure of the cosmos itself. It is composed of the same fundamental layers that compose the hierarchy of the external world. Hence, the "maps" put forward by Patanjali and other spiritual authorities are psychocosmograms, or guides to both the inner and outer universe. Their principal purpose, however, is to point beyond the levels, or layers, of psyche and cosmos, for the essential nature of the human being, the Self or Spirit, is held to be utterly transcendental.

The idea of a multilayered or hierarchical cosmos is alien to the reigning paradigm of scientific materialism, yet it is a vitally important notion in ancient and modern religious and spiritual traditions.

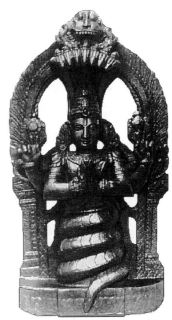

*A traditional statue of Patanjali*

317

Vast chain of being! which from God
    began,
Nature's aethereal, human, angel, man,
Beast, bird, fish, insect . . .
    . . . from Infinite to thee,
From thee to nothing. — On superior
    pow'rs
Were we to press, inferior might on
    ours;
Or in the full creation leave a void,
Where, one step broken, the great
    scale's destroy'd;
From Nature's chain whatever link
    you strike,
Tenth, or ten thousandth, breaks the
    chain alike.

Thus Alexander Pope, in his *Essay on Man*, gave poetic expression to the premodern intuition of the hierarchic connectedness of things—the chain of being. Yoga philosophy shares the same view: The cosmos is a vast structure of interlocking and nested wholes.

On one end of the "Scale of Nature" are the material forms; on the other end is the transcendental ground of Nature itself. Beyond that lies the dimension (or rather "amension") of Consciousness as the formless transcendental Selves (*purusha*). Yoga philosophy in its function as ontology—"science of being"—provides *yogins* with a map that allows them to traverse the different levels of existence until, at the moment of liberation, they leave the orbit of Nature altogether.

Various schools have devised different maps of the cosmic hierarchy. Patanjali's particular map has frequently been belittled as a mere borrowing from Classical Sâmkhya, as formulated about 350 C.E. by Îshvara Krishna in his *Sâmkhya-Karika*. The historically accurate view, however, is that Classical Yoga and Classical Sâmkhya are both extreme rationalistic expressions of divergent developments that occurred in the centuries preceding the Common Era. As we have seen in connection with the *Mahâbhârata* (notably the *Moksha-Dharma* section), it was in the period around 300–200 B.C.E. that Yoga and Sâmkhya assumed separate identities from their common Vedântic base. Moreover, the *Yoga-Sûtra* is older than the *Sâmkhya-Kârikâ*, and therefore if any borrowing has occurred it must surely be on the part of Îshvara Krishna.

There are many significant differences between Classical Yoga and Classical Sâmkhya, which can conveniently be grouped as follows:

1. *Methodology:* Classical Sâmkhya relies chiefly on the person's innate capacity for discernment (*viveka*), which is a function of the higher mind, or *buddhi*. It is through the exercise of discernment that the transcendental Self (*purusha*) is recognized as separate from the nonself, that is, the insentient world ground (*prakriti*) and its evolutes, which includes the human mind (*citta*). Discernment is followed by the renunciation of that which has been revealed as pertaining to the nonself (*anâtman*), as not constituting the essential nature of the human being. By contrast, Classical Yoga stresses the necessity for ecstatic realization, or *samâdhi*, as a vital means of transforming and ultimately transcending the world-bound consciousness. Rational knowledge alone is not deemed sufficient for exposing the false identity that is the ego-sense. Rather, true gnosis (*vidyâ*) is required to uncover the depths of the human psyche where the real roots of our habitual misidentification lie.

2. *Theology:* Classical Sâmkhya is practically atheistic in that it denies the existence of a sovereign who is superior to the many transcendental Selves. The Selves are the Divine. Classical Yoga, on the other hand, is emphatically theistic, even though the "Lord" (*îshvara*) has only a very slight role to play in the scheme of things. He is considered a *primus inter pares*, "first among many"—"a special Self," as Patanjali puts it.

3. *Ontology:* Classical Sâmkhya proposes a model of the categories of existence, or ontic principles (*tattva*), that is distinct from the model of Classical Yoga. The latter appears to be more holistic, which is best seen in the concept of *citta* comprising *buddhi, ahamkâra,* and *manas.*

4. *Terminology:* The technical vocabularies of the two schools are quite independent.

These differences appear to be primarily due to the contrasting methodologies of Sâmkhya and Yoga. The psychocosmological map put forward by Patanjali is profoundly informed by the territory he discovered in the course of his own explorations of the human psyche—the vast spaces of consciousness which are correlated to the dimensions of Nature. On the other hand, Îshvara Krishna's map gives one the impression of having been sketched on the basis of theoretical considerations and with the hindsight of many centuries of metaphysical speculations within the Sâmkhya tradition.

Both maps, of course, are intended to guide the practitioner to Self-realization. In the case of Patanjali's map, however, we have a device whose ingenuity becomes obvious only when we follow the psychoexperimental path of Yoga and begin to discover the landscapes of our own consciousness through regular meditation and (if we are so fortunate) occasional plunges into the unified condition of *samâdhi.* It is then, contrary to the atomistic ideology of scientific materialism, that we develop an appreciation for the ancient notion of the chain of being as fact, not as merely gray theory.

## The Transcendental Self and the Mind

At the apex of the hierarchy of being is the transcendental Reality, the Self or Spirit (*purusha*). For Classical Yoga, as for the other schools of Indian spirituality, the Self is the principle of pure Consciousness (*cit*), or sheer Awareness (*citi*). It is absolutely distinct from the ordinary consciousness (*citta*), with its turbulence of thoughts and emotions, which Patanjali explains as the product of the interaction between the transcendental Self (*purusha*) and insentient Nature (*prakriti*): The Self's "proximity" to a highly evolved psychophysical organism creates the phenomenon of consciousness. But Nature itself—the human body-mind on its own—is utterly unconscious.

How this absolutely transcendental Self, or pure Awareness, could have any effect at all on the ongoing processes of Nature is a philosophical conundrum that none of the spiritual traditions of the world has solved. In particular, Patanjali's metaphysical dualism does not lend itself to such a solution, and yet he tries to overcome the problem by suggesting that there is some kind of connection, which he calls "correlation" (*samyoga*), between the Self and Nature—that is, between pure Awareness and the complex of the body and personality.

That connection is made possible because at the highest level of Nature we find a predominance of the *sattva* component. The transparency of the *sattva* factor of Nature is analogous to the innate transparency or luminosity of the Self. Therefore, Nature (in the form of the psyche or mind) in its sattvic state acts like a mirror for the "light" of the Self.

Since both the Self (or, if we can trust the commentaries, the many Selves) and Nature are eternal and omnipresent, the connection between them also is without beginning. For Patanjali this correlation is the real source of all human malaise (*duhkha*), because it gives rise to the illusion that we are the individuated body-mind, or personality complex, rather than the transcendental Self. Thus, spiritual ignorance (*avidyâ*) is at the root of our mistaken identity as the finite egoic body-mind. It is, secondarily, also the source of our attachments and aversions as well as our general hunger for life (the survival instinct). Their attenuation and ultimate transcendence is the objective of the psychotechnology of Yoga.

The classical commentators assume that Patanjali believed in the existence of many transcendental Selves, yet nowhere in the *Yoga-Sûtra* itself is this clearly stated. Therefore, it is just as possible that Patanjali, true to Epic Yoga, admitted of the existence of only a single great Being containing within its infinite compass all Selves. Whatever Patanjali's position may have been, it matters little whether there are many Selves or only a single Self appearing to be manifold, because the process of realization always unfolds in the arena of duality: The witnessing Consciousness confronts the play of Nature in the form of the body-mind. If Patanjali's metaphysics should indeed stand closer to the panentheism of Epic Yoga than is generally believed, then Vijnâna Bhikshu's interpretation of the *Yoga-Sûtra* would gain greatly in credibility.

## The Yogic Concept of the Unconscious

The path to Self-realization has two main aspects. The first is dispassion (*vairâgya*), which consists in disentangling one's false identification with the nonself—that is, with everything that belongs to the various realms of Nature. The second aspect is the practice (*abhyâsa*) of identifying with the Self through repeated meditative absorption and ecstasy (*samâdhi*).

Every experience leaves its impress on the psyche, or mind. Ego-derived experiences reinforce the ego-illusion, whereas moments of self-transcendence in daily life or in the ecstatic state strengthen the spiritual impulse. The carriers of

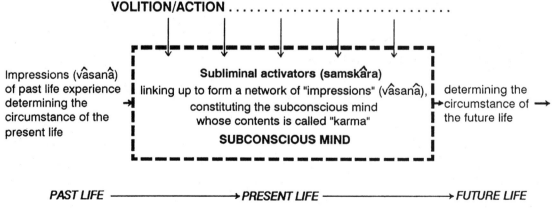

*The yogic theory of the subconscious mind*

this process of either "egoification" or "spiritualization" are traits (*vâsanâ*). These make up the depth of the human mind. If we liken the psyche to soft wax, then these *vâsanâs* are the karmic imprints left behind by our psychic activities. Every single time we sense, feel, think, will, or do anything at all, we create what the yogic authorities style a subliminal activator (*samskâra*). We can picture this as an atom that is added to a string of atoms comprising a molecule—a molecule of destiny.

The *vâsanâs*, then, are entire chains of similar karmic activators (*samskâra*). They are responsible for renewed psychomental activity in the conscious mind in the form of the five types of fluctuations or "whirls" (*vritti*) spoken of by Patanjali. The activators, combining into complex traits, are the hidden forces behind our conscious life and form the soil of our destiny. For this reason, Patanjali also uses the term "action deposit" (*karma-âshaya*), or karmic stock, for these stored impressions.

The following example will make this doctrine a little clearer: In entering this section of the book into my computer, I first of all perform the relatively complex movement of my fingers over the keyboard. In doing so, I exercise a skill acquired many years ago. I am also aware that I constantly reinforce several bad habits, such as the tendencies to tighten my shoulder muscles and squint at the screen. This is a form of karmic conditioning on the simplest level—I am likely to behave similarly the next time I sit down to write.

On a different level, I think about what I am going to write, drawing on my learning and active vocabulary. This too has its karmic aspect, for I am continually propelling my mind to think, and to think in a certain way. From a conventional point of view, this is a desirable activity because I am said to be training and refining my mind. From a spiritual perspective, however, rational thinking coincides with a particular state of being that is not altogether true of "me," because after all "I" am the transcendental Witness-Consciousness, not the contracted ego-mind-personality. "To be in one's head" means not to be present as the entire body-mind, and it is only when one is bodily present and open at the heart that the Self beyond the ego is likely to reveal itself. Therefore, when thinking becomes chronic, because of the subliminal traits set up by the constant exercise of thought, it runs counter to Self-realization.

On a further level, my actions as a writer are imbued with all kinds of spoken and unspoken expectations and motivations that generate their own karmic impressions. For a subliminal activator to be produced, I need not even be fully aware of my own feelings or moods. Thus, even sleep is not exempt from this inexorable process of karmic self-duplication.

In this theory of subliminal activators, Yoga anticipated the modern notion of the unconscious, but it went beyond the insights and goals of psychoanalysis in developing means by which the entire unconscious content can be uprooted. As we learn from the *Yoga-Sûtra* (1.50), unless the traits of subliminal activators are completely transcended through the repeated practice of supraconscious ecstasy (*asamprajnâta-samâdhi*), we are trapped in the circle of our own egoic experiences, forever alienated from the Self, which is our true identity.

## The Dimensions of Nature

The opposite pole to the multiple transcendental Selves is Nature (*prakriti*). The Sanskrit term *prakriti* means literally "she who brings forth" or "procreatrix" and refers to both the transcendental ground of the myriad manifest forms and those forms themselves. In Sâmkhya philosophy, the former also goes by the name "foundation" (*pradhâna*), which is the primordial undifferentiated continuum that potentially contains the entire universe in all its levels and categories of being. Patanjali speaks of this as the Undifferentiate (*alinga*), in which we may see a primordial field of energy.

This world ground is frequently defined as the state of balance between the constituents (*guna*) of Nature, which were introduced in Chapter 3 in the discussion of the Sâmkhya school of thought. When this primordial harmony is disturbed, the process of creation occurs. Then Nature unfolds according to a definite ground plan, whereby simpler principles give birth to ever more complex configurations (called *tattva*). This theory of cosmic evolution bears the technical name *sat-kârya-vâda* and also *prakriti-parinâma-vâda*. The former phrase implies that the effect (*kârya*) is preexistent (*sat*) in its cause, whereas the latter phrase signifies that the effect is a real transformation (*parinâma*) of Nature, not merely an illusory change (*vivarta*), as is thought in the idealistic schools of Vedânta and Mahâyâna Buddhism.

What this position implies is that whatever comes into existence is not a completely new production—out of nothing as it were—but rather the manifestation (*âvirbhâva*) of latent possibilities. Furthermore, the disappearance of an existing object does not mean its total annihilation but merely its becoming latent again (termed *tirobhâva*). This theory may well have been derived from the kind of metaphysical speculation that we find, for instance, in the *Bhagavad-Gîtâ*, where Krishna instructs Arjuna about the deathless nature of the transcendental Self. He argues that it is deathless precisely because it is never born; that is, it cannot be destroyed, for it is immune to change.

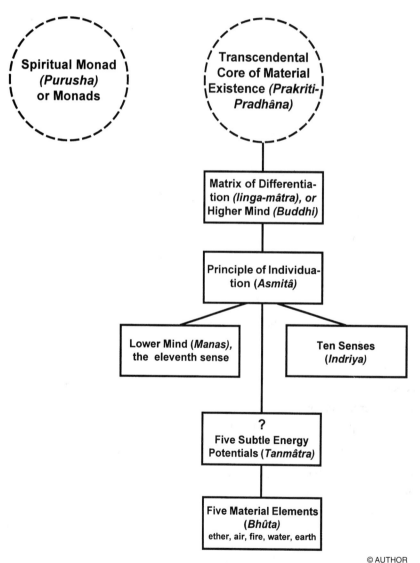

© AUTHOR

*The principles of existence according to Classical Yoga*

Of the nonexistent (*asat*) there is no coming-into-being (*bhâva*). Of the existent (*sat*) there is no nonbecoming (*abhâva*). Also, the boundary between these two is seen by the seers of Reality (*tattva*).

Yet, know as indestructible that by which this entire [universe] is spread out. No one is able to accomplish the destruction of that which is immutable.

Finite, it is said, are these bodies ["owned" by] the eternal embodier [i.e., the Self], the Indestructible, the Incommensurable. Hence fight, O Bhârata!

He who thinks of It as slayer and he who thinks [that the Self can be] slain—these both do not know. It does not slay nor is It slain.

Never is It born or does it die. It did not come-into-being, nor shall It ever come to be. This primeval [Self] is unborn, eternal, everlasting. It is not slain when the body is slain. (2.16–20)

Like the Self, the transcendental core or ground of Nature—*pradhâna* or *alinga*—also is indestructible. Yet it has the capacity to modify itself, and it does so in the process of creation, or manifestation, during which it gives birth to the multidimensional universe. Yoga reminds the spiritual practitioner, however, that even though his or her body-mind is a composite of the forces of Nature and is merely a temporary modification, it also is associated with an eternal transcendental aspect, the Self. Upon death, the material and psychic constituents of the body-mind are resolved into their hierarchically simpler forms until there is only the transcendental ground of Nature. The challenge, both during life and at the moment of death, is to awaken *as* the Self beyond all dimensions of Nature. Those who fail to do so continue to exist in simpler form on different levels of manifestation until they are reborn. At best, they merge into the transcendental ground of Nature, become "absorbed into Nature" (*prakriti-laya*), a state of pseudo-liberation. Only Self-realization is genuine enlightenment and emancipation.

## Cosmic Evolution and the Theory of the Gunas

The Self transcends the primary constituents (*guna*) of Nature. As was noted in the discussion of the relationship between Yoga and other Hindu schools of thought in Part One, the *guna* theory is one of the most original contributions of the Yoga-Sâmkhya tradition.

The *gunas*, which can be looked upon as three phases within the same homogeneous field of Nature, produce by their interplay the entire structure of the cosmos, including the psyche. Classical Yoga recognizes four hierarchic levels of existence, whose character is determined by the relative preeminence of any of the three *gunas*:

1. the Undifferentiate (*alinga*)
2. the Pure Differentiated (*linga-mâtra*)
3. the Unparticularized (*avishesha*)
4. the Particularized (*vishesha*)

The Undifferentiate is the transcendental core of Nature, which is pure potentiality. It is without any "mark" (*linga*), or identifiable characteristic. It simply *is*. Although Patanjali does not state so explicitly, the Undifferentiate is the perfect balance of the three types of *gunas*.

Out of the Undifferentiate emerges the Pure Differentiated, or *linga-mâtra*, as the first principle of manifestation or level of existence. Viewed from a psychological point of view, this is also known as Pure I-am-ness (*asmitâ-mâtra*), the cosmic sense of individuation. It has its analog in the I-maker (*ahamkâra*) or I-am-ness (*asmitâ*) on the microcosmic or individual human level. From this cosmic sense of individuation evolve the five types of fine structures (*tanmâtra*), or potentials, of sensory experience. These, in turn, give rise to the eleven types of senses (*indriya*) on one side and the five types of material elements (*bhûta*) on the other. In other words, it is the principle of Pure I-am-ness that produces both the psychomental and the physical realities.

Outside this evolutionary dynamic abide, in perfect autonomy, the numerous (or countless) transcendental Selves, which are all omnipresent and omnitemporal. But their transcendental status is not obvious to the unenlightened or ego-bound personality, which confuses the body-mind (a product of unconscious Nature) with the supraconscious Self. Yoga is a tour de force designed to undermine this confusion and guide us toward authentic existence.

In our journey toward the Self, we must inevitably cross the "ocean" of conditional reality. This passage takes place not in ordinary space-time but vertically, as it were, through the depths of our multilayered universe. The ontology of Classical Yoga provides a rough sketch of the psychocosmic geography that *yogins* can expect to encounter on their pilgrimage to the Self.

## II. THE EIGHT LIMBS OF THE PATH OF SELF-TRANSCENDENCE

Patanjali's practical spirituality comprises eight aspects, known as the limbs (*anga*) of Yoga. These are:

1. discipline (*yama*)
2. restraint (*niyama*)
3. posture (*âsana*)
4. breath control (*prânâyâma*)
5. sense-withdrawal (*pratyâhâra*)
6. concentration (*dhâranâ*)
7. meditation (*dhyâna*)
8. ecstasy (*samâdhi*)

यम । नियम । आसन । प्राणायाम । प्रत्याहार । धारणा । ध्यान । समाधि ॥

*Yama, niyama, âsana, prânâyâma, pratyâhâra, dhâranâ, dhyâna, and samâdhi*

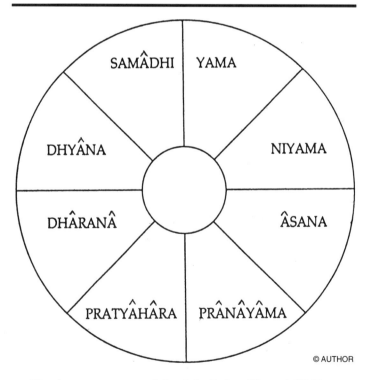

*Circular arrangement of the eight limbs of Patanjali's Yoga*

Because one limb builds upon the other, the eightfold path has sometimes been depicted as a ladder leading from the common life of self-involvement to the uncommon realization of the Self beyond the ego-personality. This progression can be looked at from a number of perspectives. Seen from one angle, it consists in the growing unification of consciousness; from another angle, it presents itself as a matter of progressive purification. Both viewpoints are present in the *Yoga-Sûtra*.

## Ethics

The foundation of Yoga, as of all authentic spirituality, is a universal ethics. Patanjali's first limb, therefore, is not posture or meditation but moral discipline (*yama*). This practice includes five important moral obligations, which can be considered the property of all major religions. These are:

1.   nonharming (*ahimsâ*)
2.   truthfulness (*satya*)
3.   nonstealing (*asteya*)
4.   chastity (*brahmacarya*)
5.   greedlessness (*aparigraha*)

Together, these constitute the great vow (*mahâ-vrata*) that, according to the *Yoga-Sûtra* (2.31), must be practiced irrespective of place, time, circumstance, or a person's particular social status. These moral attitudes are meant to bring our instinctual life under control. Moral integrity is an indispensable prerequisite of successful yogic practice.

The most fundamental of all moral injunctions is nonharming. The word *ahimsâ* is frequently translated as "nonkilling," but this fails to convey the term's full meaning. *Ahimsâ*, in fact, is nonviolence in thought and action. It is the root of all the other moral norms. The *Mahâbhârata* epic (3.312.76) employs the word *anrishamsya* ("non-maliciousness") as a synonym of *ahimsâ*.

The physician Caraka, one of the great lights of the naturopathic medicine native to India, observed that doing harm to others reduces one's own life span, whereas the practice of *ahimsâ* prolongs it because it represents a positive, life-enhancing state of mind. While this is likely to be true, the *yogin*'s motive for cultivating this virtue is a higher one: The desire not to harm another being springs from the impulse toward unification and ultimate transcendence of the ego, which is characteristically at war with itself. *Yogins* thus seek to nurture those attitudes that will gradually help them realize what the *Bhagavad-Gîtâ* (13.27) calls the vision of sameness (*sama-darshana*)—a vision that penetrates beyond the apparent differences between beings to their transcendental Self-nature.

Truthfulness, or *satya*, is often exalted in the ethical and yogic literature. For instance, in the *Mahanirvâna-Tantra* we are told:

> No virtue is more excellent than truthfulness, no sin greater than lying. Therefore, the [virtuous] man should seek refuge in truthfulness with all his heart.

> Without truthfulness the recitation [of sacred *mantras*] is useless; without truthfulness, austerities are as unfruitful as seed on barren soil.

> Truthfulness is the form of the supreme Absolute (*brahman*). Truthfulness truly is the best asceticism. All deeds [should be] rooted in truthfulness. Nothing is more excellent than truthfulness. (4.75–77)

Nonstealing, or *asteya*, is closely related to nonharming, since the unauthorized appropriation of things of value violates the person from whom they are stolen.

Chastity, or *brahmacarya* (lit. "brahmic conduct"), is of central importance in most spiritual traditions of the world, though it is differently interpreted. In Classical Yoga it is defined in ascetical terms as the abstention from sexual activity, whether in deed, thought, or words. Some authorities, like the *Darshana-Upanishad*, relax this rule for the married *yogin*. Moreover, in the medieval tradition of Tantrism, as we will see, a more sex-positive orientation came to the fore that revolutionized both Hinduism and Buddhism. But even here no unbridled hedonism is embraced. Generally speaking, sexual stimulation is thought to interrupt the impulse toward enlightenment, or liberation, by feeding the hunger for sensory experience and possibly leading to a loss of semen and vital energy (*ojas*).

Greedlessness, or *aparigraha*, is defined as the nonacceptance of gifts, because they tend to generate attachment and the fear of loss. Thus *yogins* are encouraged to cultivate voluntary simplicity. Too many possessions are thought to only distract the mind. Renunciation is an integral aspect of the yogic lifestyle.

Each of these five virtues is said to procure, when fully mastered, certain paranormal powers (*siddhi*). For instance, perfection in nonharming creates an aura of peace around *yogins* that neutralizes all feelings of enmity in their presence, even the natural hostility between animal species like the cat and the mouse or, as the Yoga commentaries put it, the snake and the mongoose. Through perfect truthfulness *yogins* acquire the power of having their words always come true. Perfection in the virtue of nonstealing brings them, effortlessly, treasures of all kinds, while greedlessness is the key to understanding their

present and former births. The reason for this, presumably, is that attachment to the body-mind is a form of greed, whereas greedlessness implies a high degree of nonattachment to material things—including the body—and this loosens the forgotten memories about former existences.

Finally, when *yogins* are established in the virtue of chastity, they gain great vigor. All Yoga scriptures are agreed that sexual abstinence does not turn *yogins* into weaklings. On the contrary, it invigorates their body and makes them especially attractive to the opposite gender—a fact that, as some *yogins* have discovered, can be either a blessing or a curse.

Some later Yoga texts mention an additional five moral precepts:

1. compassion (*dayâ*), or active love
2. uprightness (*ârjava*), or moral integrity
3. patience (*kshamâ*), or the ability to assume the witnessing consciousness and allow things to unfold as they will
4. steadfastness (*dhriti*), or the ability to remain true to one's principles
5. sparing diet (*mita-âhâra*, written *mitâhâra*), which can be considered a subcategory of nonstealing, since overeating is a form of theft from others and from Nature

In a way, the above virtuous practices are subsumed under the five categories of *yama*, or moral discipline. This creative regulation of the outgoing energies of *yogins* results in a surplus of energy, which can then be used for the spiritual transformation of the personality.

## Self-Restraint

The norms of moral discipline (*yama*) are intended to check the powerful survival instinct and rechannel it to serve a higher purpose, regulating the social interactions of *yogins*. The second limb of Patanjali's eightfold path continues to harness the psychophysical energy freed up by the regular practice of moral discipline. The constituent elements of self-restraint (*niyama*) are concerned with the inner life of *yogins*. If the five rules of *yama* harmonize their relationship with other beings, the five rules of *niyama* harmonize their relationship to life at large and to the transcendental Reality. The latter five practices are:

1. purity (*shauca*)
2. contentment (*samtosha*)
3. austerity (*tapas*)
4. study (*svâdhyâya*)
5. devotion to the Lord (*îshvara-pranidhâna*)

"Cleanliness is next to godliness," preached John Wesley, and Indic puritanism resonates with this judgment perfectly. Purification is a key metaphor of yogic spirituality, and hence it is not surprising that purity should be listed as one of the five restraints. What is meant by purity is explained in the *Yoga-Bhâshya* (2.32), which distinguishes external cleanliness from inner (mental) purity. The former is achieved by such means as baths or proper diet, whereas the latter is brought about by such means as concentration and meditation. Ultimately, the personality in its highest or *sattva* aspect must be so pure that it can mirror the light of the transcendental Self without distortion. From the *Maitrâyanîya-Upanishad* we learn about mental purity:

The mind is said to be twofold: pure or impure. It is impure from contact with desires; pure when free from desire. When one has liberated the mind from sloth and heedlessness and made it immovable and then attains to the mindless [state], this is the supreme estate. The mind should be restrained within until such time as it becomes dissolved. This is gnosis and salvation; all else is but book knowledge. He whose mind has become pure through absorption and entered the Self, he experiences a bliss impossible to describe in words and only intelligible to the inner instrument [i.e., the psyche]. (6.34)

Contentment, or *samtosha*, is a virtue praised by sages around the world. In his *Yoga-Bhâshya* (2.32), Vyâsa explains it as not coveting more than what is at hand. Contentment is thus a virtue that is diametrically opposed to our modern consumer mentality, which is driven by the need to acquire ever more to fill the vacuum within. Contentment is an expression of renunciation, the voluntary sacrifice of what is destined to be snatched from us anyway at the moment of death. Contentment is closely allied with the attitude of indifference that has *yogins* look upon a lump of earth and a piece of gold with the same coolheadedness. This allows *yogins* to experience success or failure, pleasure or sorrow, with unshakable equanimity.

Austerity, or *tapas*, is the third component of *niyama* and comprises such practices as prolonged immobilized standing or sitting; the bearing of hunger, thirst, cold, and heat; formal silence; and fasting. As discussed in Chapter 3, the word *tapas* means "glow" or "heat" and refers to the great psychosomatic energy produced through asceticism, which is often experienced as heat. *Yogins* use this energy to heat the cauldron of their body-mind until it yields the elixir of higher awareness. According to the *Yoga-Sûtra* (3.45), the fruit of such asceticism is the perfection of the body, which becomes robust like a diamond. *Tapas* must not be confused with harmful self-castigation and fakiristic self-torture, however.

In the *Bhagavad-Gîtâ*, three kinds of asceticism are distinguished, depending on the predominance of one or another of the three constituents (*guna*) of Nature:

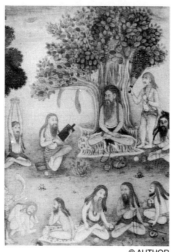
© AUTHOR
*Hindu ascetics*

> Worship of the Gods, the twice-born ones, the teachers, and the wise, as well as purity, uprightness, chastity, and non-harming—[these are] called asceticism of the body.

> Speech that causes no disquiet and is truthful, pleasant, and beneficial, as well as the practice of study (*svâdhyâya*)—[these are] called asceticism of speech.

> Serenity of mind, gentleness, silence, self-restraint, and purification of the [inner] states—these are called mental asceticism.

> This threefold asceticism practiced with supreme faith by men [who are] yoked and not longing for the fruit [of their deeds] is designated as *sattva*-natured.

> Asceticism that is performed for the sake of [gaining] good treatment, honor and reverence [from others], or with ostentation—that is called here [in this world] *rajas*-natured. It is fickle and unsteady.

> Asceticism that is performed out of foolish conceptions [with the aim] of torturing oneself or that has the purpose of ruining another—that is called *tamas*-natured. (17.14–19)

Study, or *svâdhyâya*, is the fourth member of *niyama* and a significant aspect of yogic praxis. The word is composed of *sva* ("own") and *adhyâya* ("going into") and denotes one's own delving into the hidden meanings of the scriptures. The *Shata-Patha-Brâhmana* ("*Brâhmana* of the Hundred Paths"), a pre-Buddhist work, contains the following passage, which vividly describes the extraordinary esteem in which study of the sacred lore was held:

> The study and the interpretation [of the sacred scriptures] are [a source] of joy [for the serious student]. He becomes of yoked mind and independent of others, and day by day he gains [spiritual] power. He sleeps peacefully and is his own best physician. He controls the senses and delights in the One. His insight and [inner] glory (*yashas*) grow, [and he acquires the ability] to promote the world (*loka-pakti*) [lit. "world-cooking"]. (11.5.7.1)

The purpose of *svâdhyâya* is not intellectual learning; it is absorption into ancient wisdom. It is the meditative pondering of truths revealed by seers and sages who have traversed those remote regions where the mind cannot follow and only the heart receives and is changed. The Sanskrit commentators on the *Yoga-Sûtra* take *svâdhyâya* to also mean the meditative recitation (*japa*) of the sacred texts, but King Bhoja expresses a minority opinion when he, in his *Râja-Mârtanda*, equates study exclusively with recitation.

The final component of *niyama* is devotion to the Lord, or *îshvara-pranidhâna*, which deserves our special attention. The Lord (*îshvara*), as has already been stated, is one of the multiple but coalescing transcendental Selves (*purusha*). According to Patanjali's definition, the Lord's extraordinary status among the many Selves is due to the fact that He can never be subject to the illusion that he is deprived of His omniscience and omnipresence. The other free Selves, however, have at one time experienced this loss, when they deemed themselves to be a particular egoic personality, or finite body-mind. All Selves are of course inherently free, but only the Lord is forever aware of this truth.

The Lord is not a Creator like the Judeo-Christian God, nor the kind of universal Absolute taught in the *Upanishads* or the scriptures of Mahâyâna Buddhism. This has prompted some critics to regard the *îshvara* as an "intruder" into Classical Yoga. However, the assertion that the Lord has found His way surreptitiously into the dualistic metaphysics of Patanjali's Yoga is not warranted. It overlooks the entire history of Pre-Classical Yoga, which was clearly theistic (pan-en-theistic, to be precise). A more reasonable reading of the situation would be that, in his effort to furnish a rational framework for Yoga, Patanjali gave the concept of *îshvara* a definitional twist that allowed him to incorporate it into his dualistic system. That his solution was barely satisfactory can be gathered from the many criticisms of it in other traditions and from the fact that Post-Classical Yoga returned to the pan-en-theistic conceptions of the pre-Patanjali schools.

Why did Patanjali pay any attention at all to the *îshvara* doctrine? The reason is, very simply, that the Lord was more than a concept to him and the *yogins* of his time. It makes sense to assume that the Lord, on the contrary, corresponded to an experience they shared. The idea of devotion to the Lord and grace (*prasâda*) has been an integral element of Yoga from the earliest beginnings, but especially since the rise of such theistic traditions as the Pâncarâtra, epitomized in the *Bhagavad-Gîtâ*.

The religious mind is naturally bent to worship the higher Reality. As Swami Ajaya (Alan Weinstock) remarked:

> As long as we are engrossed in our own needs, in "I" and "mine" we will remain insecure . . . Cultivating surrender and devotion replaces such self-preoccupation with a sense of our connection that sustains this entire universe. A sense of devotion and surrender opens us to experiences of being nurtured. We also learn that we have the capacity to become instruments of higher consciousness, serving and giving what we can to help others in their own awakening.[2]

Devotion to the Lord is the heart opening to the transcendental Being who for the unenlightened individual is an objective reality and force, but who upon enlightenment is found to coincide with the *yogin*'s transcendental Self. This is not spelled out in the *Yoga-Sûtra*, but it is implied in the doctrine that all the transcendental Selves, including the *îshvara*, are eternal and omnipresent; thus, even though they are spoken of as many, they must coincide with each other.

In the *Yoga-Bhâshya*, the mechanics of this process of devotion is explained as follows:

On account of devotion, [that is,] through a particular love (*bhakti*) [toward Him], the Lord inclines [toward the *yogin*] and favors him alone by reason of his disposition. By this disposition only, the *yogin* draws near to the attainment of ecstasy (*samâdhi*) and the fruit of ecstasy, [which is liberation]. (1.23

Self-restraint (*niyama*), in its five forms, is thus more than self-effort, because it entails the element of grace. *Yogins* do their utmost to understand and transcend the many ways in which the conventional ego-personality endeavors to perpetuate itself. But, in the last instance, the leap from individuated experience to ecstatic Self-realization is a matter of divine intervention.

## Posture

The first two limbs, *yama* and *niyama*, regulate the social and personal life of *yogins* in an effort to reduce the production of unwholesome volition and action, which would only increase *yogins*' karmic stock. The objective is to eliminate all karma—that is, all the subliminal activators (*samskâra*) embedded in the depths of the psyche. For this transformation of consciousness to be successful, *yogins* must create the right environmental conditions, within and without. *Yama* and *niyama* can be seen as the first steps in this direction. Posture, or *âsana* (lit. "seat"), takes this effort to the next level, that of the body.

For Patanjali, posture is essentially the immobilization of the body. The profusion of postures for therapeutic purposes

belongs to a later phase in the history of Yoga. According to the *Yoga-Sûtra* (2.46), one's posture should be stable and comfortable. By folding together their limbs, *yogins* achieve an immediate change of mood: They become inwardly quiet, which greatly facilitates their endeavor to concentrate the mind. A certain group of postures—known as "seals" (*mudrâ*)—are especially potent in altering one's mood because they have a more intense effect on the body's endocrinal system. Beginning Yoga practitioners sometimes find it difficult to detect these inner changes, perhaps because they are paying too much attention to the tensions in the musculature. With sufficient practice, however, anyone can discover the mood-altering effects of the different *âsanas*, and then the real inner work can begin. For, as Patanjali tells us, the proper execution of posture makes *yogins* insensitive to the impact of the "pairs of

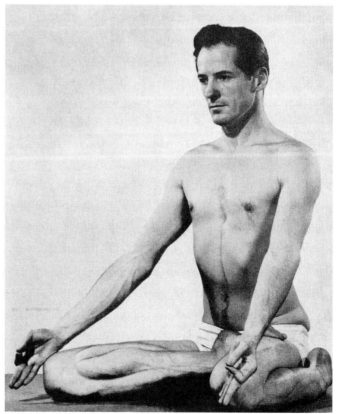

© ELEANORE MURRAY

*Hero's posture performed by Theos Bernard*

opposites" (*dvandva*), such as heat and cold, light and darkness, quiet and noise.

## Breath Control

"The whole adventure of Yoga is but a play of the Prânic force."[3] This quote spells out the signal importance of *prana*, the life force, in the process of Yoga. When *yogins* have become sufficiently aware of their inner environment and are no longer distracted by muscular tensions and external stimuli, they begin to become more and more attuned to the life force as it circulates in the body. The next step consists in energizing the inner continuum—the body-mind as it is subjectively experienced—through the practice of *prânâyâma*. *Prâna*, as has often been pointed out, is not merely the breath. Rather, the breath is only an external aspect, or a form of manifestation, of *prâna*, which is the life force that interpenetrates and sustains all life.

The technique of *prânâyâma* (lit. "extension of *prâna"*) is the most obvious way in which *yogins* seek to influence the bioenergetic field of the body. But even the practice of the moral disciplines and restraints and the techniques of sensory inhibition and mental concentration are forms of manipulating the pranic force.

Although various researchers have at different times made a case for the existence of *prâna*, their ideas have had little impact on the Western medical establishment. Some, like the Austrian physician Anton Mesmer (the *éminence grise* of hypnotism) and the American psychiatrist Wilhelm Reich (the inventor of the orgone box), were ridiculed and even persecuted for their innovative ideas. Yet, the idea of bioenergy can be found in many cultures: The Chinese call it *chi*, the Polynesians *mana*, the Amerindians *orenda*. Modern researchers speak of bioplasma. Whatever *prâna*

turns out to be—and much more research must be done before it will be accepted by modern scientists as reality—it is an experienceable fact for the practitioner of Yoga.

*Yogins* know that there is an intimate link between the life force, the breath, and the mind. The *Yoga-Shikhâ-Upanishad* declares:

> Consciousness (*citta*) is connected with the life force indwelling in all beings. Like a bird tied to a string, so is the mind.

> The mind is not brought under control by many considerations. The means for its control is nothing else but the life force. (59–60)

Through regulation of the breath, combined with concentration, the life force of the body-mind can be stimulated and directed. The usual vector is toward the head or, more precisely, the centers of the brain. This will be discussed in more detail in Chapter 17. At any rate, *prâna* is the vehicle for the ascent of attention within the body, the focusing of awareness along the bodily axis toward the brain. As the breath, or life force, rises in the body, attention ascends and leads to more and more subtle experiences. In the final stage of this process, the pranic energy is guided into the topmost psychoenergetic center (*cakra*) at the crown of the head. When *prâna* and attention come to be fixed in that spot, the quality of consciousness may change radically, yielding the ecstatic state (*samâdhi*).

## Sense-Withdrawal

The practice of both posture and breath control leads to a progressive desensitization that shuts out external stimuli. More and more, *yogins* come alive in the inner environment of their mind. When consciousness is effectively sealed off from the environment, this is the state of sensory inhibition, or *pratyâhâra*. The Sanskrit texts compare this process to a tortoise contracting its limbs. In the *Mahâbhârata*, sense-withdrawal is pertinently described thus:

> The Self cannot be perceived with the senses that, disunited, scatter to and fro and are difficult to restrain for those whose self is not prepared. (12.194.58)

> Clinging thereto [i.e., to the highest Reality], the sage should, through absorption, concentrate his mind to one point by "clenching" the host of the senses and sitting like a log.

> He should not perceive sound with his ear, not feel touch with his skin. He should not perceive form with his eyes and not taste tastes with his tongue.

> Also, the knower of Yoga should, through absorption, abstain from all smells. He should courageously reject these agitators of the group of five [senses]. (12.195.5–7)

Even though *yogins* practicing sensory inhibition are described as "sitting like a log," this does not mean they are in a coma. On the contrary, when the senses are shut down one by one, the mind generally becomes very active. This has been demonstrated in experiments on sensory deprivation, such as with the help of the so-called *samâdhi* tanks invented by John C. Lilly. Here the subject is completely immersed in salt water in a dark, insulated container, and some subjects start to hallucinate after only a few minutes. For *yogins*, of course, the challenge is not to succumb to either hallucination or sleep, but to hold the mind steady on the object of concentration.

## Concentration

As a direct continuation of the process of sensory inhibition, concentration is the "holding of the mind in a motionless state," as the *Tri-Shikhi-Brâhmana-Upanishad* (31) defines this advanced practice. Concentration, the fifth limb of the eightfold path, is the focusing of attention to a given locus (*desha*), which may be a particular part of the body (such as a *cakra*) or an external object that is internalized (such as the image of a deity).

Patanjali's term for concentration is *dhâranâ*, which stems from the verbal root *dhri*, meaning "to hold." What is being held is one's attention, which is fixed on an internalized object. The underlying process is called *ekâgratâ*, which is composed of

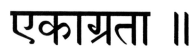

*Ekâgratâ*

*eka* ("one, single") and *agratâ* ("pointedness"). This one-pointedness, or focused attention, is a highly intensified form of the spurts of concentration that we experience, for instance, during intellectual work. But whereas ordinary concentration is mostly only a heady kind of state, accompanied by a great deal of local tension, yogic *dhâranâ* is a whole-body experience free from muscular and other tension, and therefore with an extraordinary dimension of psychic depth, in which the creative inner work can unfold.

In the *Kathâ-Sârit-Sâgara* ("River Basin of Stories"), a popular collection of stories by Somadeva (eleventh century C.E.), we find the following story which shows just how pointed concentration must be.

Vitastadatta was a merchant who had converted from Hinduism to Buddhism. His son, in utter disdain, persisted in calling him immoral and irreligious. Failing to correct his son's obnoxious behavior, Vitastadatta brought the matter before the king, who promptly ordered the boy's execution at the end of a period of two months, entrusting him to the custody of his father until then. Brooding on his fate, the lad could neither eat nor sleep. At the appointed time he was again brought to the royal palace. Seeing his terror, the king pointed out to him that all beings are as afraid of death as he. Therefore, what higher aspiration could there possibly be than practicing the Buddhist virtue of nonharming at all times, including showing respect to one's elders.

The boy, by now deeply repentant, desired to be put on the path to right knowledge. Recognizing his sincerity, the king decided to initiate him by means of a test. He had a vessel brought to him filled to the brim with oil, and he ordered the lad to carry it around the city without spilling a drop—or else he would be executed on the spot. Glad of this chance to win his life, the boy was determined to succeed. Undaunted, he looked neither right nor left, thinking only of the vessel in his hands, and at last he returned to the king without having spilled a drop. Knowing that a festival was going on in the city, the king inquired whether the boy had seen the celebrants in the streets. The boy replied that he had neither heard nor seen anyone. The king seemed pleased and admonished him to pursue the supreme goal of liberation with the same single-mindedness and passion.

This practice of concentration is difficult. At the beginning of his book *Waking Up*, psychologist Charles Tart challenges his readers to pay continuous attention to the second hand of a watch while simultaneously remaining aware of their breathing.[4] Exceedingly few people can do this without soon veering off in their thoughts. Presumably those who can maintain constant concentration for even such a relatively short span of time are skilled in meditation or a comparable practice.

But concentration is not only difficult, it is also attendant with perils, as is acknowledged in the *Mahâbhârata*:

> It is possible to stand on the sharpened edge of a knife, but it is difficult for an unprepared person to stand in the concentrations of Yoga.

> Miscarried concentrations, O friend, do not lead men to an auspicious goal, [but are] like a vessel at sea without a captain. (12.300.54–55)

The *Yoga-Sûtra* (1.30) enumerates nine obstacles that can arise in the attempt to pacify the inner world, including illness, doubt, and inattention. Yogic concentration is a high-energy state, and it is easy to see how the psychic energy mobilized in it can backfire on the unwary practitioner. As Shankara observed in his *Viveka-Cûdâmani* ("Crest Jewel of Discernment"):

> When consciousness deviates even slightly from the goal and is directed outward, then it sinks, just as an accidentally dropped ball rolls down a flight of stairs. (325)

When consciousness "sinks," it returns to ordinary preoccupations but with a higher psychic charge that can cause the undisciplined practitioner great trouble. Often it galvanizes latent obsessions, notably those related to sexuality and power. In this regard, the number of fallen *yogins* is legend. All esoteric traditions warn neophytes that once they take the first step on the path the only safe direction is forward.

## Meditation

Prolonged and deepening concentration leads naturally to the state of meditative absorption, or *dhyâna*, in which the internalized object or locus fills the entire space of consciousness. Just as one-pointedness of attention is the mechanism of concentration, "one-flowingness" (*ekatânatâ*) is the underlying process of meditation. All arising

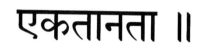

*Ekatânatâ*

ideas (*pratyaya*) gyrate around the object of concentration and are accompanied by a peaceful, calm emotional disposition. There is no loss of lucidity, but, on the contrary, the sense of wakefulness appears to be intensified, even though there is no or little awareness of the external environment.

In his original work *A Map of Mental States*, the British psychologist John H. Clark aptly characterized *dhyâna* thus:

> Meditation is a method by which a person concentrates more and more upon less and less. The aim is to empty the mind while, paradoxically, remaining alert.

> Normally, if we empty our minds, as we do when we settle down to sleep—for instance, "counting sheep" to narrow our thoughts—we become lethargic and eventually go to sleep. The paradox of meditation is that it both empties the mind and, at the same time, encourages alertness.[5]

The initial purpose of yogic meditation is to intercept the flux of ordinary mental activity (*vritti*), which comprises the following five categories:

1. *pramâna*—knowledge derived from perception, inference, or authoritative testimony (such as the sacred scriptures)
2. *viparyaya*—misconception, perceptual error
3. *vikalpa*—conceptual knowledge, imagination
4. *nidrâ*—sleep
5. *smriti*—memory

The first two kinds of mental activity are disposed of by the practice of sense-withdrawal. The tendency toward conceptualization gradually diminishes as meditation deepens. Sleep, which is due to a preponderance of the *tamas* constituent, is overcome by maintaining a state of wakeful attentiveness in the practice of concentration and meditation. Memory, the source of the mechanically arising thought fragments or imagery that are so troubling to the beginner, is the last to be blocked out. It is still active in the lower ecstatic states, where it generates presented ideas (*pratyaya*) of the nature of spontaneous insights, and is fully transcended only in the highest type of ecstatic realization, which is known as *asamprajnâta-samâdhi*. In this sublime condition of temporary identification with the Self, the subliminal activators (*samskâra*) responsible for the externalization of consciousness are uprooted. Memory can be said to have two aspects, a gross one, which is effectively disabled through meditation, and a subtle one which is neutralized through the supraconscious ecstasy.

The process of restriction (*nirodha*) has three major levels:

1. *Vritti-nirodha*, which is the restriction of the five categories of gross mental activity in meditation mentioned above.

2. *Pratyaya-nirodha*, which is the restriction of the presented ideas (*pratyaya*) in the various types of conscious ecstasy (*samprajnâta-samâdhi*). Thus, *yogins* must go beyond the spontaneously arising insights or thoughts (*vitarka*) in the ecstatic state of *savitarka-samâpatti* described in the next section, just as they must go beyond the feeling of bliss (*ânanda*) in the ecstatic state of *ânanda-samâpatti*, also described below.

3. *Samskâra-nirodha*, which is the restriction of the subliminal activators in the supraconscious ecstasy (*asamprajnâta-samâdhi*). In this elevated state, *yogins* disable the depth memory itself, whose traits (*vâsanâ*) constantly generate new psychomental activity.

## Ecstasy

In the same way in which concentration, when sufficiently acute, leads to meditative absorption, the ecstatic state (*samâdhi*) ensues when all the "whirls" or "fluctuations" (*vritti*) of the ordinary waking consciousness are fully restricted through the practice of meditation. Thus concentration, meditation, and ecstasy are phases of a continuous process of mental deconstruction or unification. When this process unfolds in relation to the same internalized object, it is called "constraint" (*samyama*) by Patanjali.

The ecstatic state, as the culmination of a long and difficult process of mental discipline, is as elusive as it is crucial to a proper appraisal of

Yoga. It has often been interpreted as a self-hypnotic trance, a relapse into unconsciousness, or even an artificially induced schizophrenic state. But these labels are all inadequate. What is seldom understood is that, first, *samâdhi* comprises a great variety of states and, second, those who have actually experienced this unified condition in its various forms unanimously confirm that mental lucidity is one of its hallmarks. Yoga psychologists are well acquainted, however, with pseudo-ecstatic states that can rightly be understood as relapses into unconsciousness (*jâdya*).

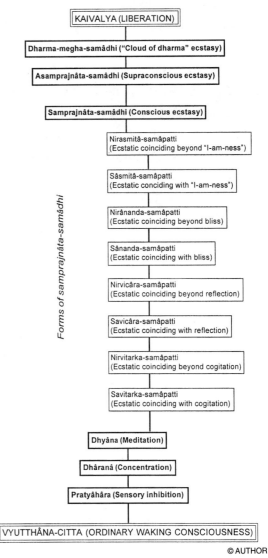

*The states of ecstasy (samâdhi)*
*according to Classical Yoga*

© AUTHOR

Genuine *samâdhi*, though, is always accompanied by suprawakefulness—a point that C. G. Jung, for instance, failed to appreciate, and his erroneous views on this subject are still being echoed by others.[6] Even if one were to consider it impractical or undesirable to cultivate the various *samâdhi* states, one must not deny that they are stations on a road leading not to a diminution of consciousness or of the human being but to a greater reality and good. The major significance of India's psychotechnology for our age lies precisely in its having amassed evidence for the existence of a condition of being—namely the condition of Self-Identity or transcendental Being-Consciousness—which is barely recognized in our Western spiritual heritage and about which modern science is ignorant.

For this reason, we must be cautious about passing summary judgment on yogic states, ideas, and practices unless we have tested them in the unbiased manner for which science prides itself. As Mircea Eliade, world-renowned authority on the history of religion, cautioned in his groundbreaking work on Yoga:

> Denial of the reality of the yogic experience, or criticism of certain of its aspects, is inadmissible from a man who has no direct knowledge of its practice, for yogic states go beyond the condition that circumscribes us when we criticize them.[7]

Although it is possible to define *samâdhi* formally, no amount of description can fully convey the nature of this extraordinary condition for which there is no reference point in our everyday life. Its most momentous component is undoubtedly the experience of complete fusion between subject and object: The *yogin*'s consciousness assumes the nature of the contemplated object.

This identification is accompanied by acute wakefulness, a mood of bliss, or the sense of pure existence, depending on the level of ecstatic unification.

In his *Yoga-Sûtra*, Patanjali has elaborated a phenomenology of *samâdhi* states that is distilled from millennia of yogic experience. He distinguishes between two major species of *samâdhi*, namely conscious ecstasy (*samprajnâta-samâdhi*) and supraconscious ecstasy (*asamprajnâta-samâdhi*). These correspond to the Vedânta distinction between formative ecstasy (*savikalpa-samâdhi*) and formless ecstasy (*nirvikalpa-samâdhi*) respectively.

Whereas the supraconscious ecstasy is of a single type, conscious ecstasy has a variety of forms. These forms also bear the technical designation of "coincidence" (*samâpatti*), because subject and object coincide. The simplest form is *vitarka-samâpatti*, which is ecstatic unification in regard to the coarse (*sthûla*)

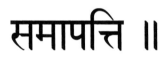

*Samâpatti*

aspect of an object. For instance, if the object of contemplation is a particular deity—say, the blue form of four-armed Krishna—*yogins* entering *samâdhi* now become one with Krishna's image. That image is vividly experienced as a living reality, so that *yogins* experience themselves as the blue-skinned Krishna. Their unified experience is interspersed with all kinds of spontaneous (nondiscursive) thoughts, but, unlike during meditation, these do not disrupt their ecstatic enjoyment. Upon the cessation of all ideation (*vitarka*), *yogins* enter the supracogitative ecstasy (*nirvitarka-samâdhi*).

The next higher or deeper level of ecstatic unification occurs when *yogins* identify with the subtle (*sûkshma*) aspect of their object of contemplation. In our example, they would experience themselves as Krishna on progressively less differentiated planes of existence, until there is only the irresoluble matrix of Nature left. This condition, again, has two forms, depending on the presence or absence of spontaneous thoughts. The first is known as "reflective ecstasy" (*savicâra-samâdhi*), the second as "suprareflective ecstasy" (*nirvicâra-samâdhi*).

According to Vâcaspati Mishra's interpretation of the *Yoga-Sûtra*, as found in his *Tattva-Vaishâradî*, there are four additional levels of subtle unitary experience: *sa-ânanda-samâpatti* ("coincidence with bliss," written *sânandasamâpatti*), *sa-asmitâ-samâpatti* ("coincidence with I-am-ness," written *sâsmitâsamâpatti*), *nirânanda-samâpatti* ("coincidence beyond bliss"), and *nirasmitâ-samâpatti* ("coincidence beyond I-am-ness"). The first type consists in the experience of pervasive bliss. The second type is simply the overwhelming sense of being present, in our case as the very essence of Krishna. There is a sense of "I," or individuated existence, but no longer any role identity. The I is expanded infinitely. It is rather difficult to gain even an intuitive sense of the content of the third and the fourth types. We may question whether the scholar Vâcaspati Mishra actually experienced these additional types of ecstasy for himself or whether they were merely inferred by him. At any rate, Vijnâna Bhikshu, who was a Yoga adept, explicitly rejected the last two types of ecstatic experience.

All these types are forms of conscious ecstasy (*samprajnâta-samâdhi*). They are experiential states in which the ego-personality is partially transcended. From one perspective, they can even be regarded as means of obtaining knowledge about the universe through the capacity of the human consciousness for chameleon-like identification with the object of contemplation.

Radically distinct from these ecstatic states is the supraconscious ecstasy (*asamprajnâta-samâdhi*), which coincides with temporary Self-realization. Here, for the duration of the experience, *yogins* transcend the realms of Nature and identify with their authentic being, the Self (*purusha*). This presupposes a total turnabout, or *parâvritti* (Greek: *metanoia*), in their consciousness, a complete transformation of the body-mind. It cannot be accomplished through sheer exertion of will. Rather, *yogins* must empty and open themselves to the higher Reality beyond the ego-personality. Since this is not something they can initiate at will, the moment of radical opening is often described, as we have seen, in terms of the intervention of grace.

*Asamprajnâta-samâdhi* is the only avenue to recover conscious awareness of the transcendental Self-Identity and its eternal freedom. In this supraconscious ecstasy, there is neither an object of contemplation nor a contemplating subject. To the ordinary mind it appears as a state of frightening voidness. When maintained over a sufficiently long period of time, the fire of this ecstasy gradually transmutes the unconscious, obliterating all the subliminal activators (*samskâra*) that spawn renewed ego-conscious activity and the resultant karma.

## III. LIBERATION

At the peak of this ecstatic unification, *yogins* reach the point of no-return. They become liberated. According to the dualistic model of Classical Yoga, this implies the dropping of the finite body-mind. The liberated being abides in perfect "aloneness" (*kaivalya*), which is a transmental state of sheer Presence and pure Awareness. Some schools of Vedânta, which hold that the ultimate Reality is nondual, argue that liberation does not have to coincide with the death of the physical body. This is the ideal of "liberation in life" (*jîvan-mukti*). Patanjali, however, does not appear to have subscribed to this ideal.[8] For him, the *yogin*'s greatest good lies in severing himself completely from the round of Nature (*prakriti*) and abiding merely as the attributeless Self, one among many and, as we must assume, intersecting with all other Selves in eternal infinity. This is also the ideal of Classical Sâmkhya.

It is difficult for the ordinary person to imagine what such untarnished Selfhood would be like, even when one has had glimpses of ego-transcendence during deep meditation. What is clear is that, by definition, it is not an experience, because there is neither a subject nor an object left to give rise to the knowledge connection. But neither is it

a state of unconsciousness. All realizers agree that it is an utterly desirable condition, worthy of our absolute commitment.

The laborious path of Yoga leads thus beyond itself. Yogic psychotechnology is merely a ladder that the spiritual practitioner climbs, only to cast if off in the last moment. Patanjali's formulations are useful only to the degree that they can guide us to that instant of recognizing our inherent freedom, which gives us the authority and power to see Reality in its nakedness and go beyond all formulations, creeds, dogmas, models, theories, or points of view.

## Part Four
# POST-CLASSICAL YOGA

"When shall my yearning for devotion—

The highest state of knowledge and

The highest state of Yoga—

Become fulfilled, O Lord?"

—Utpaladeva, *Shiva-Stotra-Avalî* (9.9)[1]

"There is no other happiness here in this world
Than to be free of the thought
That I am different from you.
What other happiness is there?
How is it, then, that still this devotee of yours
Treads the wrong path?"

—Utpaladeva's *Shiva-Stotra-Avalî* (4.17)[1]

# *Chapter 11*

# THE NONDUALIST APPROACH TO GOD AMONG THE SHIVA WORSHIPERS

## *I. OVERVIEW*

Everything is only the Absolute (*brahman*). There is no other. I am That. Verily, I am That. I am only That. I am only That. I am only the everlasting Absolute.

I am only the Absolute, not the worldling (*samsârin*). I am only the Absolute. I have no mind. I am only the Absolute. I have no wisdom (*buddhi*). I am only the Absolute, and not the senses.

I am only the Absolute. I am not the body. I am only the Absolute, not the "cow-pasture" [*i.e.*, the field of cosmic existence]. I am only the Absolute. I am not the psyche (*jîva*). I am only the Absolute, not differentiated existence.

I am only the Absolute. I am not unconscious. I am the Absolute. There is no death for me. I am only the Absolute, and not the life force (*prâna*). I am only the Absolute, higher than the highest. (6.31–34)

Everything is only the Absolute. The triple world is pure Consciousness, the pure Absolute. There is nothing but bliss, supreme bliss (*parama-ânanda*). (6.42)

The experience of ecstatic unity expressed in the above passage from the *Tejo-Bindu-Upanishad* is at the heart of the Upanishadic wisdom tradition. The sages of the early *Upanishads* were the first to speak of this grand realization explicitly and with unbridled enthusiasm. Their nondualist insights were

341

echoed by the later sages of Vedânta in various ways. For them, as for their predecessors, metaphysics was an attempt to find a rational explanation for what was a living experience for them—the realization of the singular Being, called *âtman* or *brahman*.

This mystical realization of all-embracing unity (*ekatva*) is not characteristic of Patanjali's Yoga, which distinguishes sharply between Spirit (*purusha*) and Nature (*prakriti*). It is possible, however, to accommodate certain levels of the unitary mystical realization even within the dualistic framework of Classical Yoga, for Patanjali accepts that Nature includes a transcendental dimension that is the source of all manifest forms. Merging with that transcendental aspect of Nature—a state known as *prakriti-laya*—can be considered a form of mystical union. For Patanjali, though, such merging with the ground of the world is not equivalent to gaining liberation. As he sees it, there can be no ultimate salvation within the province of Nature. True liberation involves going beyond all of Nature's dimensions, including its transcendental basis (*pradhâna*).

Only the realization of the transcendental Self (*purusha*), or Spirit, amounts to genuine everlasting freedom. This, however, is not a matter of union but of simple identity. Self-realization is the awakening of *yogins* to their authentic or essential being, which abides forever beyond the orbit of Nature, vast as it is.

Patanjali did not accept the Upanishadic or Vedantic equation of the transcendental Self (*âtman*) with the transcendental ground of the objective world, called *brahman*. Even though the eightfold path of the *Yoga-Sûtra* became very influential, Patanjali's dualistic metaphysics has always been considered an oddity within the fold of Hinduism. Most Yoga schools during his time and in subsequent periods espoused one or another form of nondualism (*advaita*), which can be traced all the way back to the *Rig-Veda*. The Yoga teachings that succeeded Patanjali but that did not adopt his dualistic metaphysics can be referred to collectively as Post-Classical Yoga.

The literature of Post-Classical Yoga is even more diversified and richer in content than the literature of Pre-Classical Yoga. First of all, there are the Yoga teachings of the *Samhitâs* ("Collections"), the religious works of the Vaishnavas of both the north and south of the Indian peninsula, as well as the numerous works dependent on them. This voluminous literature is briefly discussed in Chapter 12. Like the *Âgamas* ("Traditions") of the Shaivas and like the *Tantras* ("Looms") of the Shakti worshipers, the *Samhitâs* have barely been researched. Their teachings are incredibly intricate, and I can do no more here than scratch the surface of what amounts to an ocean of works in Sanskrit and the vernacular languages. Another rich mine of yogic teachings is the *Purâna* literature, which is introduced in Chapter 13. The core of this literature was created in the Vedic Era, but in their present form even the oldest *Purânas* barely date back before the closing centuries of the first millennium B.C.E. The *Purânas* ("Ancient [Teachings]"), as we will see, are popular encyclopedias that, among other things, contain brief treatments of Yoga and numerous fascinating stories about aspirants and masters.

A post-classical work that deserves to be singled out for special treatment is the tenth-century *Yoga-Vâsishtha*. Its radical idealism has for centuries been an unfailing inspiration particularly to Hindus of the Himalayan region. I will introduce this remarkable poetic creation in Chapter 14.

The most significant texts of Post-Classical Yoga are the so-called *Yoga-Upanishads*—a designation invented by Western scholars. These are scriptures from various epochs and geographical areas that represent various points of view within the Yoga tradition, though all have a nondualistic slant. They will be discussed in more detail in Chapter 15.

An important phase of Post-Classical Yoga, covering the period from approximately the seventh to the seventeenth centuries C.E., is represented by the schools belonging to the tradition of "body culture" (*kâya-sâdhana*), such as the Siddha movement and Nâthism. These include orientations like Hatha-Yoga that seek to approach Self- or God-realization by probing the spiritual potential of the human body. These schools will be discussed separately, in Chapters 17 and 18, because of their significance for the development of Hinduism and because of the growing attention they receive in the West.

We will start this review of Post-Classical Yoga with the more extreme sects of the ramified Shaiva tradition, which has its root in the Vedic Era. Some of the Shaivite practices are rather radical, inasmuch as they severely challenge conventional morality. They are considered to be "left-hand" schools, because they champion the literal enactment of the ultimate truth of nonduality, while the "right-hand" schools, by and large, condone only the symbolic expression of that truth. The difference between these two approaches is best epitomized in their contrasting attitudes to sexuality. While the adherents of the right-hand schools generally see sexuality as a threat to spiritual growth, the followers of the left-hand path within Shaivism employ sexuality for their spiritual transformation.

In India, as in many other parts of the world, the left side is associated with inauspiciousness or pollution, and the right side with auspiciousness, purity, and what is good. The Sanskrit term *vâma-âcâra* ("left conduct," written *vâmâcâra*) has negative connotations in conventional contexts, but it is used by the left-hand schools themselves, though not because they admit to being partial to evil. Rather, in their exploration of our spiritual

potential, they acknowledge the existence of the dark or shadow aspects of the human personality and of life in general. More than that, they actively associate with that which the "normal" person fears, avoids, or represses. The reason for this eccentric approach is partly to reclaim the repressed aspects of human existence and partly to demonstrate that life can and should be lived, under all circumstances, from the point of view of the ultimate truth of nonduality: If there is only the singular, all-comprising Being, then, to put it bluntly, it must also be the essence of genitals, death, and garbage.

## II. THE LEFT-HAND FOLLOWERS OF SHIVA—"SKULL-BEARERS," "PHALLUS-WEARERS," AND OTHER ASCETICS

In their quest for ultimate security and happiness, the spiritual seekers of India have at times, as have those of other countries, ventured into territory that lies well outside the social establishment. There were and still are individuals and small groups whose lifestyle or practices look extreme, even bizarre, to the conventional mind. In his book *Sadhus: India's Mystic Holy Men*, the Dutch psychologist, photographer, and traveler Dolf Hartsuiker has recorded in word and image some of the unusual manifestations of India's otherworldly saints.[2] The photographs depict naked ascetics whose bodies are completely covered with ashes or are laden with beads and flower garlands and painted in bright colors, or who dress and behave like women in honor of Goddesses Sîtâ and Râdhâ. Then there are those who wear a chastity belt or who stand on one leg or with an upraised arm withered from years of neglect.

Hindus have the reputation of being exceptionally tolerant in matters of religion, and indeed no culture on Earth has produced so much variety in its religious practices and ideas as Hinduism. When we as Westerners look a-skance at some of the expressions of religious fervor and spiritual aspiration in Hinduism, we must remember that our vision is defined by the powerful biases current in our own highly secular-ized modern culture. It is particu-larly important to remember this in the following discussion of some of the more unusual mani-festations of Hindu spirituality.

In the *Mahâbhârata* epic (12.337.59), five religious tradi-tions are mentioned as being prominent: the sacrificial religion of the *Vedas*, Yoga, Sâmkhya, Pâncarâtra, and Pâshupata. We will next turn to the Pâshupata tradition, which is a particular phase in the development of the reli-gious community of Shaivism that identifies the Absolute with God Shiva.

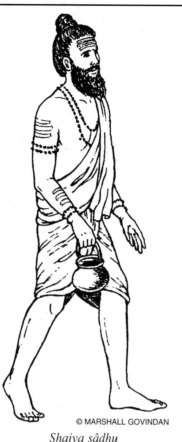
© MARSHALL GOVINDAN
*Shaiva sâdhu*

## The Pâshupata Tradition

The religious order of the Pâshupatas is com-monly thought to have been founded by a certain ascetic named Lakulîsha, who may have lived in the second century C.E. However, Shiva wor-shipers included ascetics already in the pre-Buddhist period, so the Pâshupatas can be regard-ed as a comparatively late development within Shaivism. We know of Lakulîsha only through legends. The name means literally "Lord of the Club" and is explained by the fact that the Pâshupatas carried a club (*lakula*) as one of their sectarian insignia. Lakulîsha, or Lakulin ("Club

Carrier"), was venerated as an incarnation of God Shiva himself.

According to the *Kâravana-Mâhâtmya*, a relatively recent work, Lakulin was born into a brahmin family of what is now Gujarat. He was an extraordinary child, possessing all kinds of superhuman powers, but died in his seventh month. His grieving mother cast his tiny body into the river. A group of tortoises carried it to the holy site of Jaleshvara-Linga, where the life force reen-tered his limbs. He was brought up as an ascetic and later became a renowned teacher. According to some accounts, Lakulin died after a life of severe austerities and Shiva entered his body to reani-mate it so that the Pâshupata doc-trine could be disseminated in the world. His fol-lowers regarded him as the last incarnation of Shiva.

Lakulin is said to have had four principal dis-ciples—Kushika, Gârgya, Kurusha, and Mai-treya—to which sometimes the name of Patanjali is added as a fifth. But this is doubtful, since nowhere in the *Yoga-Sûtra* or the commentarial literature is there any suggestion of Patanjali con-doning the kind of extreme practices for which the Pâshupata sect was notorious. The connection between Patanjali and Lakulîsha, however, is not without historical interest because it strengthens the traditional claim that Patanjali (the grammari-an who is identified with the Yoga master) be-longed to the tradition of Shaivism. The same Pat-anjali, who is assigned to the second or third cen-tury B.C.E., refers in his *Mahâ-Bhâshya* (5.2.76) commentary on Pânini's grammar to itinerant ascetics who were draped in an animal skin (*ajina*) and carried an iron lance (*lauha-shûla*) and staff (*danda*).

Hindu iconography typically depicts Lakulin seated in the lotus posture, with a citron in his right hand and a club in his left and his penis stiff with life force. We may see in the club and the citron the symbols of the male and female aspects of the Divine respectively, though undoubtedly they have other esoteric significances as well. The erect penis suggests not sexual licentiousness but the mastery of the sexual drive and the conversion of semen into the mysterious *ojas*, or subtle vitality, that is an important part of the alchemical processes occurring in the body of the Yoga adept.

What was so controversial about the Pâshupatas was their insistence on shocking the public with their eccentric behavior, such as babbling, making snorting sounds, imitating the walk of a cripple, pretending to suffer from tremor of the limbs, making foolish statements, and making sexual gestures in the presence of women. With these escapades they sought to court public disapproval, which would test their capacity for humility and self-transcending practice. In his commentary on the *Pâshupata-Sûtra*, Kaundinya observes:

> He should appear as though mad, like a pauper, his body covered with filth, letting his beard, nails, and hair grow long, without any bodily care. Thereby he cuts himself off from the estates (*varna*) and stages of life (*âshrama*), and the power of dispassion is produced. (3.1)

But there was a further purpose to this strange practice. The Pâshupatas thought that by attracting censure they absorbed the bad karma of others, while transferring their own good karma to them, thereby enhancing their impulse toward total transcendence of the realm of good and bad.

This curious practice is known as the *pâshupata-vrata* or "Pâshupata vow."

As is evident from the *Pâshupata-Sûtra*, ascribed to Lakulîsha, the earlier schools of this tradition were heavily ritualistic, and philosophy played only a secondary role. The ritual Yoga of the Pâshupatas included many ecstatic practices, such as singing, dancing, and laughter. But these were only engaged in the "unmanifest" (*avyakta*) or concealed state, when the initiates were amongst themselves, whereas the above-mentioned eccentric behavior was displayed in the "manifest" (*vyakta*) or public state, when they removed all identifying sectarian marks and behaved like complete outcasts.

The Pâshupatas were surprisingly successful, and their order grew rapidly in size and influence. By the sixth century, Pâshupata temples were scattered throughout India. There are two possible explanations for the success of this sectarian movement. The first is that it offered a sense of belonging that was not based on the prevalent caste hierarchy. The second is that the movement promised active participation in simple religious rituals, as well as an emotion-based experience of the sacred.

The philosophical elaboration of the Pâshupata sect began with Kaundinya, who composed his *Panca-Artha-Bhâshya*[3] ("Commentary on the Five Topics [of the *Pâshupata-Sûtra*]") sometime in the fifth century C.E. A further level of philosophical sophistication is present in the *Gana-Kârikâ*, attributed to a certain Haradatta, which has a fine commentary, called *Ratna-Tîkâ* ("Jewel of Exposition"), by the famous tenth-century logician Bhâsarvajna.

In brief, the Pâshupatas are theists. For them the Lord (*îshvara*, *îsha*) is the creator, sustainer, and destroyer of the world. He comprises a manifest and an unmanifest aspect, and is utterly independent of the world. He has unlimited power of knowledge (*jnâna-shakti*) and unlimited power of action (*kriyâ-shakti*). One of the most controversial dogmas of the Pâshupatas is the notion that the Lord's will is entirely independent of the karmic law. He can, theoretically, reward evildoers and punish the good. The consummate state of liberation, which is called the "end of suffering" (*duhkha-anta*, written *duhkhânta*), is entirely a gift of grace (*prasâda*). This is explained as a state of undiminished attention (*apramâda*) on Reality.

Prior to liberation is the accomplishment of the condition of Yoga, which is defined as "the union of the self (*âtman*) with the Lord." As is made clear in the *Pâshupata-Sûtra* (5.33) itself, this union is not a complete merging of the self with the ultimate Reality, as in nondualistic Vedânta, but a form of transcendental bonding, which Lakulîsha gives the technical designation of *rudra-sâyujya*, "alliance with Rudra," Rudra being Shiva. Here the *yogin's* body-mind is constantly informed by the Divine, and his practice consists in continual surrender to Shiva.

The liberated being shares in most of the transcendental capabilities of the Lord, such as freedom from fear and death, and lordship over the universe. As in Classical Yoga, the relationship between the liberated beings and the Lord is a curious one: Although they are absolutely one with God, God is at the same time something more than those liberated beings, either individually or collectively. Whereas Patanjali rejected the deistic idea of the Lord as Creator, Lakulîsha celebrated Shiva as Pashupati, the "Lord of Beasts." The "beasts" (*pashu*) are none other than the fettered souls that, in birth after birth, are forever recycled in the great ecology of Nature—unless they experience the grace of Shiva.[4]

Pâshupatism shares none of the gender-positive attitudes of Tantra. For the Pâshupata ascetics, women are, in the words of Kaundinya's commentary (1.9), "horror and illusion incarnate." They can entice and delude men even at a distance and therefore are to be avoided at all cost. This kind of misogynism is quite characteristic of what I have called mythic or verticalist Yoga, which in its drive for total transcendence succumbs to seeing the cosmos as inherently hostile and dangerous. Many schools of Mediterranean Gnosticism committed the same error, and whenever bodily existence is rejected, the denigration of the female gender is never far behind.

## The Kâlâmukha Order

Lakulîsha was venerated also by the Kâlâmukhas, a well-organized sect that developed out of the Pâshupata tradition. None of their scriptures have survived, and we know of their beliefs and practices only from the writings of their critics. The Kâlâmukha order may have originated in Kashmir. It thrived, together with the Pâshupata order, in the southeast of the peninsula between the eleventh and thirteenth centuries C.E. It appears that there may have been an actual migration of Lakulîsha adherents from north to south at the beginning of the eleventh century, perhaps because they had lost patronage in Kashmir.

The name *kâlâmukha*, meaning "black-faced,"[5] probably derives from the fact that these ascetics wore a striking black mark on the forehead, indicating their renunciation. They existed in two big divisions, known as the "power assembly" (*shakti-parishad*) and the "lion assembly" (*simha-parishad*) respectively, each of which had its own subdivisions. We may speculate that the former were in practice and theory oriented more toward the feminine or power aspect of the Divine, whereas the latter's orientation was more toward the masculine or Shiva aspect of the transcendental Reality.

The Kalâmukhas were fond of learning and had a special relationship with the Nyâya school of thought, a traditional system of logic. Thus, according to one epigraphic record, Someshvara, a renowned teacher of the Kâlâmukha order, received in 1094 C.E. a generous donation from his township in recognition of his great yogic accomplishments and his equally great learning in the arts and sciences. As is clear from many other temple inscriptions, the Kâlâmukhas laid great store by the careful observance of the moral virtues codified by Patanjali under the categories of moral discipline (*yama*) and self-restraint (*niyama*).

The epigraphic evidence does not bear out the widespread belief that the Kâlâmukhas practiced revolting and obscene rituals. It appears that they were commonly confused with another Shaiva order, the infamous Kâpâlikas, who definitely did not belong to mainstream Shaivism but were Tantric in character.

## The Kâpâlikas

The early history of the Kâpâlikas ("Skull Bearers"), also called Mahâvratins ("Great-Vowed"), is unknown. They got their name from the occult custom of carrying around a human skull, which served as a ritual implement and an eating utensil. References to skull bearing are found already in works belonging to before the Common Era, but it appears that the Kâpâlika order originated only toward the middle of the first millennium in the south of India. Certainly by the sixth century C.E., the Kâpâlikas were frequently referred to in

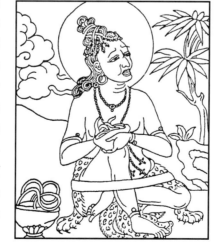

*The adept Kâpâla (from a woodblock)*

the Sanskrit literature.

As in the case of the Kâlâmukhas, no Kâpâlika scriptures have come down to us, and the little we know of them stems largely from the opponents of this extreme form of asceticism, though we also have a few positive (or at least neutral) accounts. For the most part, these descriptions seem accurate, since to this day the small group of surviving Kâpâlikas in Assam and Bengal engage in the practices for which they have been notorious for many centuries.

In his *Harsha-Carita*, a beautifully crafted but incomplete Sanskrit biography of the seventh-century king Harsha, the celebrated court poet Bâna describes an encounter between King Pushpabhûti and the Kâpâlika adept Bhairava. The ascetic accepted the king into pupilage and soon asked him to participate in the kind of nocturnal rite for which the Kâpâlikas were famous. After anointing a corpse with red sandalwood, Bhairava, painted black and wearing only black garments and ornaments, seated himself on its chest. Then he lit a fire in the corpse's mouth and offered black sesame seeds into it, while reciting magical incantations. Suddenly the ground before them split open and a fierce-looking spirit entity emerged and attacked Bhairava, the king, and three other disciples who were present. Bhairava managed to disable the entity but refused to kill it and was later rewarded for his mercy by Goddess Lakshmî. At any rate, the ritual proved successful, and Bhairava acquired the status of a *vidyâ-dhâra* or "possessor of wisdom."

That not all Kâpâlikas were such relatively benign individuals is brought home by another story found in the *Dasha-Kumâra-Carita* ("Biography of the Ten Princes") by the renowned seventh-century poet Dandin. According to this story, Mantragupta, one of the ten princes, overheard a husband and wife complain that they had constantly to do chores for their teacher, and thus they had no time for each other. They called their *guru* a black magician (*dagdha-siddha*)—literally "burnt adept." Curious about it all, the prince surreptitiously followed them back to their teacher's hermitage.

Soon Mantragupta spotted the adept seated at a fire. He was smeared with ashes and wore a necklace of human bones, and his appearance was quite frightening. Then the prince heard the magician sternly order his hapless servants to sneak into the palace and abduct the king's daughter, which they did. The prince remained in hiding. Then, to his horror, he saw the magician swing his sword to decapitate the princess. Just in time, Mantragupta jumped forward, seized the sword, and beheaded the magician instead.

In Mâdhava's *Shankara-Dig-Vijaya* ("Shankara's World Conquest"), a fourteenth-century hagiography of Shankara, the great teacher of nondualistic Vedânta, there is another fascinating story. One day, so the legend goes, a cruel-hearted Kâpâlika approached the venerable Shankara, praising him as a true adept who has realized the Self and begging him for mercy. Shankara listened to him openheartedly but with sublime indifference. The Kâpâlika explained that he had been performing austerities already for a hundred years to win Shiva's favor. He wanted to ascend into Shiva's heavenly domain with the physical body, and Shiva promised to fulfill this desire if he were to offer him the head of a king or an all-knowing sage. Having

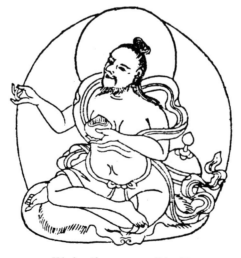

*Kânha (from a woodblock)*

failed to procure the head of a king, the Kâpâlika now asked for Shankara's head. He had gauged the great adept correctly, for Shankara agreed without a moment's hesitation. He fixed a time and place where the transaction could take place without the knowledge of Shankara's disciples, who would surely try to prevent the decapitation. At the appointed hour, Shankara entered into the state of formless ecstasy (*nirvikalpa-samâdhi*), patiently awaiting the sword blow to his neck.

The Kâpâlika approached him with eyes rolling wildly from alcohol intoxication. He raised his trident to lop off Shankara's head. In that moment, Padmapâda, one of Shankara's main disciples, saw in his mind's eye what was about to happen. He uttered an invocation to his chosen deity, Nri-Simha, the Man-Lion incarnation of God Vishnu. Instantly the faithful disciple assumed the God's leonine form, flew through the air, and arrived at the secret hiding place. Just as the Kâpâlika swung his trident, Padmapâda jumped on him and tore open his chest. Shankara returned to his ordinary consciousness and, seeing the mutilated body of the Kâpâlika and the blood-drenched shape of Nri-Simha before him, begged the God to withdraw his terrific aspect and manifest mercy instead. Thereupon Padmapâda regained his ordinary consciousness and form and promptly prostrated himself at his teacher's feet.

There undoubtedly were villains and psychotics among the Kâpâlikas, but most were probably content with wearing skulls stolen from cemeteries where they practiced their strange magical rituals. And there were a few genuine masters, like the Buddhist adept Kânha, of the eleventh century C.E., who in his songs calls himself a skull bearer (*kâpâlin*). He speaks of mating with, and then killing, the licentious washerwoman (*dombî*), who here stands for the feminine aspect of the transcendental Reality. To murder Shakti means to transcend her.

Kânha's statement also contains a reference to the sexual practices of the Kâpâlikas. Though renunciates, they gathered every spring and autumn for a big orgiastic ceremony. In the course of the ceremony they performed the "Five M's" for which Tantrism achieved notoriety: the consumption of liquor (*madya*), meat (*mâmsa*), fish (*matsya*), and parched grain (*mudrâ*), which is thought to have aphrodisiacal properties, as well as the performance of ritual intercourse (*maithunâ*) with specially prepared women.

The Kâpâlikas, like the Pâshupatas and Kâlamukhas, were worshipers of Shiva—but Shiva in his terrifying aspect as Bhairava. The purpose of all the Kâpâlika rites was to achieve communion with God, through which the practitioner acquired both superhuman powers (*siddhi*) and liberation. They offered human flesh in their ceremonies and have been accused—probably rightly—of occasionally performing human sacrifice. The practice of human sacrifice (*purusha-medha*) was already known in ancient Vedic India, but for the seers (*rishi*) was a purely symbolic ritual. They understood that the real *purusha* sacrifice is the archetypal self-offering of the cosmic Person, without which the universe could not have come into existence. Over the centuries, however, actual human sacrifice continued to be resorted to by some extremist sects and overzealous kings as a means of propitiating the Divine. In 1832 the British Raj finally outlawed this custom.

From the perspective of the evolution of human consciousness, this gruesome Kâpâlika practice must be regarded as a terrible regression from the high moral sensibility achieved in the Buddhist and Jaina communities, which celebrate the virtues of nonviolence and compassion. From a yogic point of view, it was likewise a step back into unfortunate literalism, for the Upanishadic sages had already understood that sacrifice was a matter of the renunciation of the ego, not of animal slaughter or human murder. By the fourteenth century the Kâpâlika order was virtually extinct, perhaps brought down by the cumulative karma of those who failed to grasp that Yoga consists in the metaphorical sacrifice of the self.

## The Aghorî Order

The Kâpâlikas were replaced by the Aghorî order. The word *Aghorî* derives from *aghora*, meaning "nonterrible," which is one of the names of God Shiva in his terrific aspect. Presumably, only the initiate who knows how to propitiate Shiva is not fearful of the God's dread-instilling or wrathful aspect. The Aghorîs, who are both venerated and feared by the villagers of India to this day, aspire to obliterate all human-made institutions in their way of life. Thus, they live in cremation grounds or on dunghills, drink liquor or urine as readily as water, and break all social conventions by eating meat and the flesh of human corpses.

Recently, an outstanding book was published that documents the life and teachings of a modern Aghorî master, Vimalananda (d. 1983), who said about himself, "Either I must be mad or everyone else is; there are no two ways about it."[6] The author of the book, who was a close disciple of Vimalananda, comments about his teacher's extremist approach:

> Aghora is not indulgence; it is the forcible transformation of darkness into light, of the opacity of the limited individual personality into the luminescence

of the Absolute. Renunciation disappears once you arrive at the Absolute because then nothing remains to renounce. An Aghorî goes so deeply into darkness, into all things undreamable to ordinary mortals, that he comes out into light.[7]

The Aghorî does more than encounter his own shadow, as it is called in Jungian terms. He encounters the shadow of his society, possibly of humanity as such, for he pushes himself to the very edge of human existence. In doing so, he certainly comes to the brink of madness, and not a few explorers of this path of negation have succumbed to insanity. The Aghorîs put into radical practice the philosophy of challenging all values for which the nineteenth-century German philosopher Friedrich Nietzsche achieved fame. Incidentally, Nietzsche himself, who was a mere theoretician in such matters, died in an insane asylum. The Aghorî lifestyle demands a rare fortitude and a level of renunciation that is natural to few individuals.

## The Lingâyata Sect

Another Shaiva sect that achieved great popularity after the decline of the Kâpâlikas is the Lingâyata tradition, so called because its members worship Shiva in the form of a phallic symbol (*linga*), standing for the creative process in the Divine. They carry a miniature stone *linga* in a small box attached to a necklace. Twice a day, the faithful sit quietly in meditation with the *linga* in the

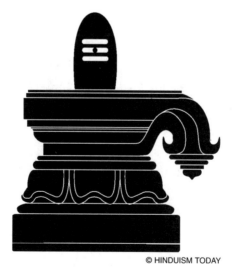

© HINDUISM TODAY

*Linga in a yoni base*

left hand, performing the various rituals. The Lingâyatas are also known as Vîra-Shaivas, "Heroic Followers of Shiva." This sect originated in the twelfth century C.E., though its adherents believe that the roots of their faith reach back into the hoary past and that the adept Basava ("Bull"), or Basavânna (1106–1167 C.E.), merely reorganized their tradition.

Six stages (*sthâla*) of meditation are distinguished:

1. *Bhakti*, or love-devotion, which is expressed in ritual worship at the temple or in the home.

2. *Mahesha*, "Great Lord" (from *mahâ* and *îsha*), is the phase of disciplining one's mind, with all the trials this entails.

3. *Prasâda*, or grace, is the peaceful stage in which the devotee recognizes the Divine working in and through everything.

4. *Prâna-linga*, or "life sign," is the stage in which the devotee is certain of the Lord's grace and now begins to experience the Divine in the consecrated temple of his or her own body-mind.

5. *Sharana*, or "[going for] refuge," is the phase in which the devotee becomes a fool of God, where he no longer identifies with the body-mind, but is also not yet completely at one with the Divine; he longs for Shiva as does a woman for her absent lover.

6. *Aikya*, or "union," with the Divine: Here formal worship is at an end, because the devotee has *become* the Lord; the pilgrim has arrived at his destination and found that he was never apart from it.

The devout Lingâyatas aspire to see Shiva in everyone and everything. As Basava expressed it so beautifully in one of his poems:

The pot is a God. The winnowing
fan is a God. The stone in the
street is a God. The comb is a
God. The bowstring is also a
God. The bushel is a God and the spouted
cup is a God.

Gods, Gods, there are so many
there's no place left
for a foot.

There is only
one God. He is our Lord
of the Meeting Rivers.[8]

The popularity of the Lingâyatas was largely due to the fact that they championed greater social equality—favoring, for instance, the removal of caste distinctions, the remarriage of widows, and late marriage. This more moderate sect affords a convenient bridge to Âgamic Shaivism, another conservative religious movement, which will be discussed next.

## III. THE POWER OF LOVE—THE SHIVA WORSHIPERS OF THE NORTH

By no means do all devotees of God Shiva follow the perilous path of the Kâpâlikas and Aghorîs described in the previous section. Indeed, most of them cultivate a far more moderate approach to God-realization, though it may well include such Tantric rites as sexual intercourse with a consecrated partner.

Both mainstream and left-hand Shaiva beliefs and practices are found codified in the vast *Âgama* literature of the North and the South. We will look at the northern branch of Âgamic Shaivism first because it appears to be marginally older. The *Âgamas*—the word means simply "tradition"—understand themselves as a restatement of the ancient wisdom of the *Vedas* and are therefore often called the "Fifth *Veda*" (as are the *Purânas* and the *Mahâbhârata*). They purport to be for the spiritual seeker of the "dark age" (*kali-yuga*), who lacks the moral fiber and the mental concentration necessary to pursue the path of liberation by the more traditional means. The same intent is expressed in the *Tantras*, which are *Âgama*-like scriptures that have Shakti (the feminine counterpart of Shiva) as their metaphysical and practical focus. However, mainline brahmins, who accept the revelatory authority of the *Vedas*, reject both the *Âgamas* and *Tantras* as false revelations.

The Âgamic canon is traditionally said to comprise twenty-eight "root" (*mûla*) scriptures and 207 secondary scriptures (called *Upâgamas*).[9] In his *Pratishtha-Lakshana-Sâra-Samuccaya*, the Bengali prince Vairocana (early ninth century C.E.) mentions no fewer than 113 works, many of which are *Tantras*. In his *Tiru-Mantiram* (63), the great Tamil adept Tirumûlar refers to a group of nine *Âgamas*. Since he is generally placed in the seventh century C.E., these must all have been creations of the preceding period. It is thought that the earliest of these works were authored in the sixth century C.E. in the north of India but proliferated rapidly in the subsequent centuries, though they could have been in existence several hundred years before then. These scriptures increasingly incorporated the notion of *shakti*, and for this reason later on merged imperceptibly with the *Tantras*.

According to tradition, Shiva taught four groups of *Tantras* with four of his faces: Garuda (issuing from the Sadyojâta face), Vâma (from the Vâmadeva face), Bhûta (from the Aghora face), and Bhairava (from the Tatpurusha face). The twenty-eight *Âgamas*, however, are said to have issued from Shiva's Îshana face.[10] Sometimes they are said to have been taught by all five faces of Sadâ-Shiva.

The names of the most important works of the principal *Âgamas* are the *Kâmikâ* (comprising 12,000 verses, of which 357 are lost), *Karana* (16,151 verses), *Ajîta*, *Sahasra*, *Suprabheda* (4,666 verses), *Raurava*, *Makuta*, *Mâtanga*, and *Kirana* (1,991 verses). The most important works of the secondary *Âgamas* are the *Mrigendra*, *Vâtula-Shuddhâkhya*, *Paushkâra* (800 pages long), *Kumâra*, and *Sârdha-Trishati-Kâlottara*.

It is impossible to do justice to the complexity of the history and the philosophy of the *Âgama* literature in the context of this volume. To simplify matters, we can say that the southern and the northern schools of Shaivism found vindication in the *Âgamas* for their own distinct positions. Southern Shaivism—also known as Shaiva-Siddhânta—favors a qualified monism that, in practice, is polarized, with Lord Shiva on one side and the devotee (*bhakta*) on the other. This is epitomized in the devotionalism of such great saints as Tiruvalluvar, Sundarar, and Mânikkavâcakar. By contrast, northern Shaivism leans toward an idealist, or a radically nondualist, interpretation of reality, similar to Advaita Vedânta.

## Northern Shaivism

One of the earliest expressions of Shiva worship in Northern India was the Krama system of Kashmir, which was in vogue by the seventh century C.E. This system consists of two branches of practice. One has Shiva as the ultimate principle of existence; the other revolves around the worship of the Goddess Kâlî as the Divine, par excellence. Their practical method roughly coincides with Râja-Yoga, although moral discipline (*yama*), self-restraint (*niyama*), and posture (*âsana*) are not listed as separate "limbs" (*anga*), whereas reasoning (*tarka*) is counted as a separate category of spiritual practice. Significantly, the Kâlî branch of the

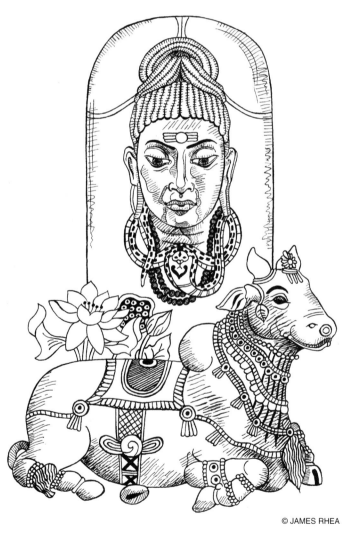

© JAMES RHEA

*Shiva and Nandi*

Krama system involves left-hand practices such as the literal use of wine, meat, and sexuality during the Tantric rituals.

The Kashmiri tradition of Shaivism flourished in the pristine form of the Trika ("Triadic") system. Its name is derived from the fact that it acknowledges the interdependence of the following three aspects of the Divine: Shiva (the male pole), Shakti (the female pole), and Nara (the conditional personality seeking liberation). The Trika tradition comprises the original doctrines of the *Âgamas* with their preeminently dualistic orientation, the teachings of the Spanda or "Vibration" school, and the doctrines of the Pratyâbhijna or "Recognition" school.

At the beginning of the ninth century C.E., the Kashmiri adept Vasugupta "discovered" the *Shiva-Sûtra*, rather like hidden spiritual treasures (Tibetan: *terma*) are discovered by masters of the Nyingma order of Tibetan Buddhism. The *Shiva-Sûtra* is a digest of the earlier *Âgama* teachings that had the declared intention to bring to light the nondualist approach of these doctrines. According to Kshemarâja, author of a tenth-century commentary on the *Shiva-Sûtra*, God Shiva appeared to Vasugupta in a dream. He revealed to him the secret location in which the *Shiva-Sûtra* could be found inscribed in rock. Upon waking, Vasugupta promptly went to the place shown to him in the dream and found Shiva's seventy-seven aphorisms.

Even though the word *yoga* is nowhere used in the *Shiva-Sûtra*, this scripture is a unique treatise on Yoga. It distinguishes four levels of yogic means (*upâya*):

1. *Anupâya* ("nonmeans"): The practitioner realizes the Self spontaneously, without effort, as a result of the teacher's transmission of the teaching.

2. *Shâmbhava-upâya* ("Shambhu's means"): Shambhu is another name for Shiva. This level of Yoga is also known as *icchâ-upâya* or "means of the will." When the mind is perfectly still, the transcendental Shiva-Consciousness flashes forth spontaneously, without exertion on the part of the practitioner.

3. *Shâkta-upâya* ("Shakti's means," written *shâktopâya*): The *shâmbhava-upâya* calls for a degree of spiritual maturity that few possess. Most people find it impossible to go beyond conceptualization (*vikalpa*) and to simply rest in perceptual awareness. The very effort to outwit the conceptual mind merely tends to produce new conceptual content. Therefore, Vasugupta put forward an alternative—to attach attention to what he calls "pure" (*shuddha*) concepts. By this he means such intuitions as the following: Our true identity is not the ego-personality but the transcendental Self, and the knowable universe is not external to us but a manifestation of our transcendental Power. In this way, we can remove the ingrained illusion of duality between subject and object.

4. *Ânava-upâya* ("limited means"): The *shâkta-upâya* seeks to trick the mind into a new way of looking at its own nature and the nature of the apparently external world. Vasugupta particularly recommended Mantra-Yoga for this process, since the dwelling of the mind on the hidden meaning of such *mantras* as "I am Shiva" (*shivo'ham*) ultimately blots out the distinction between the *mantra* and the mind, and so forms a

foundation for the revelation of Shiva-Consciousness. At the level of *ânava-upâya*, the practitioner resorts to such common yogic practices as breath control, sense-withdrawal, concentration, and meditation. Ultimately, the practitioner has to transcend this level and discover the transcendental "I"-Consciousness through the more direct means of *shâkta-upâya* and then *shâmbhava-upâya*.

> "One should always remain fully awake, viewing the 'pasture' [i.e., the world] through wisdom. One should superimpose everything upon the single [Self]. Then one cannot be troubled by another."
>
> —*Spanda-Kârikâ* 3.12

The commentaries on the *Shiva-Sûtra* contain invaluable materials on the technique of breath control or *prânâyâma*, which is more sophisticated than that expounded in the *Yoga-Sûtra*. Especially interesting is the teaching that associates different forms of delight, or bliss (*ânanda*), with the contemplation of the various types of life force (*prâna*) in the body. The doctrine of the "ascent" (*uccâra*) of the life force as subtle vibration is connected to complicated speculations about the mystical sound "matrices" (*mâtrika*), which are the root of all *mantras*.

This and other forms of the *ânava* discipline are found, for instance, in the *Vijnâna-Bhairava*, a much-loved scripture probably composed in the seventh century C.E.. This text has been called an initiatory manual for those advanced *yogins* who desire to explore the Yoga of delight (*camâtkâra*), the play of Consciousness within itself. Bhairava ("Fear-Inspiring") is another name of Shiva, who fills the sinner with dread and the mystic with awe.

A further developmental stage of the tradition of Northern Shaivism is present in the *Spanda-Sûtra* and its commentarial literature. The *Spanda-Sûtra*, also called *Spanda-Kârikâ*, is generally ascribed to Vasugupta as well, though some traditions name his disciple Kallata as its composer. The technical term *spanda* is explained as "a quasi-movement." It is not successive motion as we encounter it in space-time, but an instantaneous vibration in the transcendental Reality itself, which is the source of all manifest movement—perhaps what physicist David Bohm styled "holo-movement."

*Spanda* is the ecstatic throbbing of the Shiva-Consciousness. This notion is in striking contrast to the static interpretation of Selfhood in Classical Yoga, where the Self is merely an eternally disinterested watcher of events in the body-mind. This new dynamic concept was no doubt invented to account more adequately for the higher realizations experienced by the adepts of Shaiva Yoga.

## The Pratyâbhijna School

The third phase or camp of Northern Shaivism is represented by the Pratyâbhijna or "Recognition" school, founded by Somânanda (ninth century C.E.), a disciple of Vasugupta. The two key scriptures of this school are the *Pratyâbhijna-Sûtra* of Utpala, a pupil of Somânanda, and the several commentaries of Abhinava Gupta, a tenth-century adept who was also a remarkably prolific writer. Abhinava Gupta composed some fifty works, including his *Tantra-Âloka*[11] ("Light on Tantra"), a work of encyclopedic proportions on the philosophy and ritual of Âgamic Shaivism. Madhurâja Yogin, a pupil of Abhinava Gupta, left us this devotional portrait of his *guru*:

His eyes are rolling with spiritual bliss. The center of his forehead is clearly marked with three lines, made with ashes. His luxuriant hair is tied with a garland of flowers. His beard is long, his body rosy. He is dressed in silk, white like the rays of the moon, and is seated in the heroic posture on a soft cushion placed on a throne of gold. He is attended by all his pupils, with two female devotee-messengers standing by his side.[12]

Local tradition has it that, after completing his final commentary on the Pratyâbhijna system, Abhinava Gupta, accompanied by 1,200 disciples, entered the Bhairava cave near the Kashmiri village of Magam and was never seen again. He is remembered even today as a fully realized adept (*siddha*). Abhinava Gupta and many of the other great masters of Northern Shaivism are wonderful illustrations that mystical aspiration and philosophical acuity can be successfully combined.

One of the most popular manuals of the Pratyâbhijna school is the *Pratyâbhijna-Hridaya* ("Heart of Recognition"), written by Râjanaka Kshemarâja, a disciple of Abhinava Gupta. It is evident from this and Abhinava Gupta's own writings, as well as other related scriptures, that the Pratyâbhijna practitioners were well acquainted with Yoga, not least Kundalinî-Yoga. They are important sources for our understanding of the early developmental phase of Hatha-Yoga.

The Pratyâbhijna school gets its name from its principal doctrine that liberation is a matter of "recognizing," or remembering, that our true identity is not the limited body-mind but the infinite Reality of Shiva. In their analysis of existence, the Pratyâbhijna masters arrived at the following thirty-six categories or principles (*tattva*):

1. *Shiva*, the ultimate Reality, which is pure Being-Consciousness.

2. *Shakti*, the power aspect of the ultimate principle, which is not really separate from Shiva but merely appears so from the unenlightened point of view. Shakti is the transcendental source of the entire manifest and unmanifest cosmos. The *yogin* experiences Shakti as bliss (*ânanda*).

3. *Sadâ-Shiva* ("Eternal Shiva"), or Sadâkhya ("Ever-Named," from *sadâ* or "ever" and *âkhya* or "named"), is the will aspect of the One Being. In the scale of yogic realizations, this elevated principle is the ecstatic experience of "I am this," in which Consciousness encounters itself vaguely as an object.

4. *Îshvara* ("Lord"), is a further progression of the psychocosmic evolution, where the objective or "this" (*idam*) side of the universal Consciousness is still more accentuated. The ecstatic experience on this level is now "This am I" rather than "I am this."

5. *Sad-Vidyâ* ("Being-Knowledge") or Shuddha-Vidyâ ("Pure Knowledge") is ecstatically experienced as a perfect balance between the subject ("I") and the objective ("this") aspect of the universal Consciousness.

6. *Mâyâ* ("Illusion") is the first of the so-called "impure" (*ashuddha*) principles, because it relativizes existence through the agency of its five functions, known as "jackets" (*kancuka*). They

are referred to as "jackets" because of their concealment of the truth that there is only the One Being-Consciousness, which is Shiva. These five functions are (7–11):

7. *Kalâ*[13] ("Part"), which stands for secondary, or partial, creatorship.

8. *Vidyâ* ("Knowledge"), which signifies limited knowledge as opposed to omniscience.

9. *Râga* ("Passion"), which is desire for limited objects rather than universal bliss and satisfaction.

10. *Kâla*[14] ("Time"), which stands for the reduction of eternity to the temporal order, divisible into past, present, and future.

11. *Niyati* ("Destiny"), which refers to the law of karma as opposed to the eternal freedom and independence of the Divine.

12. *Purusha* ("Male"), which is the individuated being, the source of subjective experience, resulting from the activity of the *mâyâ-tattva*. The *purusha* is here different from the *purusha* of Classical Yoga, which Patanjali conceives as being utterly transcendental.

13. *Prakriti* ("Nature"), which is the matrix of all objective aspects of manifestation. Unlike Classical Yoga and Classical Sâmkhya, Kashmiri Shaivism proposes that every *purusha* has its own *prakriti*.

14-36. The remaining principles are identical to the twenty-four principles (*tattva*) known in the Sâmkhya tradition, namely the higher mind or, as I prefer to call it, the wisdom faculty (*buddhi*), the I-maker (*ahamkâra*), the lower mind (*manas*), the five cognitive organs (*jnâna-indriya*, written *jnânendriya*), the five conative organs (*karma-indriya*, written *karmendriya*), the five subtle elements (*tanmâtra*), and the five coarse elements (*bhûta*).[15]

Yoga is understood as a gradual ascent to the transcendental Source, which involves the progressive penetration of the various layers of illusion that are created by the *mâyâ* principle. While success on the spiritual path depends on the guidance of a realized master, ultimately it is the grace of Shiva that bestows liberation on the deserving practitioner.

The mysticism of northern Shaivism holds great attraction for the Westerner interested in India's wisdom because it is well argued in rational language. In recent years, northern Shaiva teachings have been brought to Europe and America by the late Swami Muktananda, an adept of the Siddha tradition. He empowered numerous Westerners through the method of *shakti-pâta* ("descent of power"), either through his touch or his mere glance. Joseph Chilton Pearce reported the following incident:[16]

A young heart surgeon from Florida, who was disturbed by the hard emotional attitude in his profession, met Swami Muktananda during a meditation intensive. Muktananda grabbed him by the bridge of the nose and held on. In that instant, the young doctor experienced himself as a "body of blue energy."

Then he had a visionary experience of his right arm clinging tightly to the branch of a tree. He felt his fingers being pried loose from the branch. Then something snapped inside him. He experienced himself entering Muktananda's head. In his words, "there I found myself in an immense vacuum—an infinite space. A wave of emotion swept up from my belly and I wept for fifteen minutes or more." Afterward, he felt "cleaned out" and peaceful. Pearce called this a "classical account of Shaktipat," which turned the young surgeon's life around, granting him the empathy for his patients he had been hoping for.

## *Lallâ—Love Poetess Extraordinaire*

In addition to the various schools of Shaivite philosophical mysticism, Kashmir also produced a small number of Shiva-worshiping poets. Foremost among them is the woman mystic Lallâ (or Lal-Ded), who lived in the fourteenth century C.E. On the metaphysical basis of the Trika system, Lallâ pursued the discipline of Laya-Yoga, which revolves around the awakening of the occult *kundalinî-shakti*, or serpent power. The method by which she achieved complete surrender to Shiva was the well-tried path of meditative recitation of the sacred syllable *om* combined with breath control and concentration. In one of her verses, written in melodious Kashmiri, Lallâ hints at having accomplished the process of Kundalinî-Yoga:

> After crossing the six forests [i.e., psychoenergetic centers of the body], the lunar part was trickling down. Nature was sacrificed with the breath/wind (*pavana*). With the fire of love I scorched my heart. Thus I attained Shankara [i.e., Shiva]. (38)

Other verses in her *Lallâ-Vâkya* suggest the same: Lallâ was a Self-realized adept who knew firsthand the secrets of Laya-Yoga, which culminates in the dissolution (*laya*) of the individuated self into the transcendental Self. Thus in one stanza (51) she speaks of having recognized the Self, Shiva, within herself: "When I saw Him dwelling within me, I realized that He is everything and I am nothing."

Although Lallâ speaks of her longing for Shiva in the days prior to her realization, she eschews emotional language and prefers to use the lofty metaphors of metaphysics. We know nothing about Lallâ's life, though tradition remembers her as having wandered naked in the cold climate of her homeland. This is hardly credible, since in her poetry Lallâ herself speaks of the necessity for clothing and feeding the body properly. Perhaps the nudity attributed to her is a symbol of her profound surrender to Shiva, which stripped her of all egoic motivation.

**SOURCE READING 13**

## *Shiva-Sûtra of Vasugupta*

According to the Shaiva tradition of Kashmir, the *Shiva-Sûtra* was discovered by Vasugupta, who probably lived in the latter half of the eighth century C.E. There are different accounts of how the secrets of this *Sûtra* were revealed to Vasugupta, but they all mention that he was instructed in a dream. We know from Patanjali's *Yoga-Sûtra* (1.38) that *yogins* take their dreams seriously. The *Shiva-Sûtra* is the fountainhead of the sacred literature of Kashmiri Shaivism.

### Book I

The Self (*âtman*) is [pure] Consciousness (*caitanya*). (1.1)

[Finite] knowledge is bondage. (1.2)

The source [of the manifest world together with its] collocation [of manifest effects] is embodied in [limited] activity (*kalâ*). (1.3)

*Comments: Kalâ* (to be carefully distinguished from the word *kâla* or "time") is finite or conditional activity, which is one of the five "coverings" or "jackets" (*kancuka*) of *mâyâ*, the power of world illusion. The others are *vidyâ* (limited knowledge), *râga* (attachment), *kâla* (time), and *niyati* (causality). By contrast to finite activity, the creativity of the Self is absolute and incomprehensible to the unenlightened mind.

The matrix [of sound] is the foundation of [conditional] knowledge. (1.4)

*Comments:* The Sanskrit word *mâtrikâ* ("matrix" or "little mother") refers to the Sanskrit alphabet with its fifty letters, which are thought to be primal sounds.

The [spontaneous] flashing-forth (*udyama*) [of the transcendental Consciousness] is Bhairava. (1.5)

*Comments:* Bhairava is God Shiva, here in the sense of the absolute Reality underlying phenomenal or conditional existence.

Upon [ecstatic] union with the "wheel" (*cakra*) of powers, [there comes about] the abolition of the universe [as a distinct object of consciousness]. (1.6)

[Even] during the differentiation [of consciousness into the three modes of] waking, dream sleep, and deep sleep, [there is continuous] emergence of enjoyment of the Fourth [i.e., absolute Reality]. (1.7)

The waking state (*jâgrat*) [consists in conditional or finite] knowledge (*jnâna*). (1.8)

Dream sleep (*svapna*) [consists in] imagination (*vikalpa*). (1.9)

Deep sleep (*saushupta*) [corresponding to] illusion (*mâyâ*) [consists in complete] unawareness (*aviveka*). (1.10)

The heroic lord [i.e., the enlightened being] is the [conscious] enjoyer of the triad [of waking, dream sleep, and deep sleep]. (1.11)

*Comments:* The Sanskrit commentaries explain the word *vîra*, here translated as "heroic," as referring to the senses, so that the *vîresha* (*vîra-îsha*) is metaphorically the lord over the senses. Indeed, the enlightened being, who identifies with supreme Consciousness, is the master of the senses and the mind. This spiritual attainment is referred to as *svacchanda-yoga* or "union with the self-dependent [Reality]."

The stages of Yoga are a wonder (*vismaya*). (1.12)

The power of will (*icchâ-shakti*) [of the enlightened being] is Umâ [or] Kumârî. (1.13)

*Comments:* Umâ is the divine Consort, or transcendental Power, of the Absolute, Shiva. Kumârî, the "Virgin," is the same Power in its playful aspect as the creatrix or destroyer of the universe. The meaning of this aphorism is that the enlightened adept's will coincides with the divine Will, wherefore he is capable of all kinds of extraordinary feats.

[In the state of ecstatic union] the world (*drishya*) [becomes the adept's] body. (1.14)

Through the confinement (*samghâta*) of the mind (*citta*) in the heart, [there comes about the transcendental] vision of the world [and its] sleep [i.e., the void]. (1.15)

*Comments:* The word *svâpa*, or "sleep," stands here for the absence of all objects. Even this void becomes transcendentally illumined or "animated" by the enlightened adept, as is made clear in aphorism 3.38.

Or through [conscious] union with the pure Principle (*tattva*), [the enlightened adept becomes] free from the power [that restricts] the "beast" (*pashu*) [i.e., the fettered personality]. (1.16)

Self-knowledge [consists in] awareness (*vitarka*). (1.17)

*Comments:* Here the term *vitarka* is a technical expression denoting the adept's transconceptual awareness. The word has a different meaning in Patanjali's *Yoga-Sûtra*.

[For the enlightened adept] worldly bliss is the delight of ecstasy (*samâdhi*). (1.18)

Upon [ecstatic] union with the [transcendental] Power [as explained in aphorism 1.13, the enlightened adept obtains the capacity for] the creation of [any kind of] body. (1.19)

[Other paranormal abilities that may spontaneously appear in the enlightened adept are:] combining the elements or separating the elements, and compacting the universe [as a whole]. (1.20)

Through the emergence of pure wisdom, [the adept acquires] the power of lordship over the "wheel" [of all other powers]. (1.21)

Through [ecstatic] union with the "great lake" [i.e., the transcendental Reality, the adept gains] the experience of the potency (*vîrya*) of *mantras*. (1.22)

### Book II

The mind [of the adept] is a *mantra*. (2.1)

*Comments:* The adept's mind is continuously potentized and polarized relative to the transcendental Reality, Shiva. Therefore it can be said to be analogous to a *mantra*, which esoterically is explained as "that which protects (*tra*) the mind (*man*)."

[Spontaneous] application is efficacious. (2.2)

*Comments:* Constant abidance in and as the Real is the means of realization, or enlightenment, just as the constant repetition of a *mantra* leads to success.

The secret [hidden in all] mantras is the Being (*sattâ*) embodied in wisdom. (2.3)

Expanding the mind relative to the "womb" (*garbha*) [i.e., the finite world, amounts to no more than] a dream lacking differentiated knowledge. (2.4)

Upon the [spontaneous] emergence of wisdom, [there occurs a great "seal" (*mudrâ*) known as] *khecârî*, [which is] the state of Shiva. (2.5)

*Comments:* The term *khecârî* means literally "she who moves in the space [of supreme Consciousness]."

The teacher (*guru*) is the means [of ultimate realization]. (2.6)

Insight into the "wheel" [i.e., spectrum] of matrices [of sound is obtained through the teacher's instruction]. (2.7)

[The adept's] body is an oblation [poured into the fire of the transcendental Reality]. (2.8)

[Finite] knowledge is [merely] food. (2.9)

*Comments:* The meaning of this aphorism is that finite knowledge is instrumental on the phenomenal plane but of no ultimate usefulness. Wisdom, however, guides adepts to enlightenment and they use their finite being—the body-mind—as an oblation that is offered up in a final gesture of self-transcendence.

Upon the recession of wisdom [in the case of an aspirant], the vision [of the world is like] a dream arising from that [wisdom]. (2.10)

*Comments:* Even after wisdom recedes, there is an afterglow that continues to inform the *yogin's* vision or experience of the world.

## Book III

The [phenomenal] self (*âtman*) is the mind (*citta*). (3.1)

[Finite] knowledge is bondage. (3.2)

*Comments:* This aphorism reiterates aphorism 1.2.

*Mâyâ* is nondifferentiation (*aviveka*) about the principles [of existence (*tattva*)], such as [limited] activity (*kalâ*). (3.3)

Dissolution of the parts (*kalâ*) [should be achieved] in the body. (3.4)

*Comments:* According to Kshemarâja's commentary, the *kalâs* in question are the various ontological principles or categories (*tattvas*), such as the elements, the subtle elements, and the mind.

Dissolution of the currents (*nâdî*) [of the life force], conquest of the elements, isolation from the elements, and separation from the elements [are accomplished through yogic contemplation]. (3.5)

[Paranormal] power (*siddhi*) [results] from a veil of delusion (*moha*). (3.6)

Through the conquest of delusion, through infinite enjoyment (*âbhoga*) [of the Real, there comes about] the conquest of spontaneous wisdom. (3.7)

[The enlightened adept is always] awake; [for him] the second one [i.e., the world of duality] is a ray-of-light. (3.8)

*Comments:* The world is a "ray-of-light" (*kara*) because the enlightened adept experiences it as identical with the divine Reality.

The self (*âtman*) [of the enlightened adept is like] a dancer. (3.9)

*Comments:* The meaning of this obscure aphorism is that enlightened adepts, though they may engage in all kinds of activities, are only play-acting so to speak. They are not really involved in their actions, because they have ceased to identify with the limited body-mind and its functions.

The inner self (*antar-âtman*) [of the enlightened adept is like] a stage. (3.10)

*Comments:* This aphorism, which continues with the dramatic metaphor of *sûtra* 3.8, emphasizes that the enlightened adept is pure witness. He is constantly and continuously aware of the contents of his own mind, which no longer has the power to delude him.

The senses are [like] spectators. (3.11)

Through the force of [transcendental] insight (*dhî*), power over *sattva* [is obtained]. (3.12)

*Comments:* The term *sattva*, or "realness," stands for the luminous aspect of Nature. It is one of the three primary constituents of phenomenal existence. The compound *sattva-siddhi* also can be understood in the sense of "perfection of luminosity." Both senses are applicable.

[Thus] the condition of independence (*sva-tantra*) [or liberation] is accomplished. (3.13)

As [the adept accomplishes transcendental independence, or liberation] in [regard to] this [body], so [does he accomplish perfect independence in regard to] all else. (3.14)

Attentiveness (*avadhâna*) to the "seed" (*bîja*) [i.e., the Source of the world, should be cultivated]. (3.15)

He who is established in the seat (*âsana*) [of the transcendental Consciousness] easily plunges into the "lake" [i.e., the ultimate Reality]. (3.16)

He effects creation by his own measure. (3.17)

*Comments:* Since the enlightened adept is one with the divine Reality, he or she also is the absolute creator of everything.

While wisdom prevails, the elimination of [future] birth [is certain]. (3.18)

Maheshvarî and so forth, [residing] in the classes [of letters of the alphabet] beginning with *ka*, are the mothers of "beasts" (*pashu*) [i.e., fettered beings, but they have no power over the enlightened adept in whom wisdom blossoms.] (3.19)

The Fourth [i.e., the ultimate Reality] should be poured like oil into the three [conditional modes of consciousness, namely waking, dream sleep, and deep sleep]. (3.20)

He should enter [into the Fourth] by immersing himself with his mind (*citta*). (3.21)

Upon the equalization of the life force (*prâna*), [there comes about] the vision of sameness. (3.22)

*Comments:* When the breath is no longer erratic and the body's energies are harmonized, the mind too is balanced. Then everything reveals itself as the same One.

In the interim, [there occurs] the generation of inferior [states of consciousness]. (3.23)

*Comments:* The *yogin*, who has not yet fully and stably realized the ultimate Reality, experiences intermittently lower states of consciousness, which lack full awareness of the fundamental sameness of all things.

Upon [ecstatic] union between the self-concept (*sva-pratyaya*) and objects (*mâtra*), [the *yogin* brings about] the reemergence of the vanished [vision of sameness]. (3.24)

He becomes like Shiva. (3.25)

[Retaining] the functioning of the body [for the sake of others is his only] vow. (3.26)

[His] conversation is recitation. (3.27)

Self-knowledge is [his] gift [to others]. (3.28)

And he who is established in Avipa is a cause of [higher] knowledge (*jna*). (3.29)

*Comments:* In Kshemarâja's tenth-century commentary, the difficult compound *avipastha* is explained as "established in the protector (*pa*) of animals (*avi*)," that is, "established in those who protect the finite beings." Thus, it is taken to refer to the Goddesses that preside over the letters of the Sanskrit alphabet.

For him the universe is an extension of his [innate] power. (3.30)

The maintenance and absorption [of the universe are likewise an extension of his innate power]. (3.31)

Despite such activity [as the maintenance and absorption of the universe, there is] no discontinuity owing to [the enlightened adept's] condition as witness. (3.32)

[The adept] considers pleasure and pain as external. (3.33)

Free from these, he is indeed alone (*kevalin*). (3.34)

However, the dynamic [or karmic] self [i.e., the unenlightened personality] is afflicted by delusion. (3.35)

Upon the eclipse of differentiation [based on the unenlightened mind, the adept acquires] the capacity for [bringing forth] other creations. (3.36)

The power of creation [is well established] on account of one's own experience [in dreams and meditation, etc.]. (3.37)

[There should be] animation of the three states [of unenlightened consciousness] by the principal [State, which is Reality itself]. (3.38)

As with the [various] states of consciousness, [there should also be animation by the ultimate Reality] in regard to body, senses, and external [objects]. (3.39)

For the "confluent" (*samvâhya*) [unenlightened individual, there is constant] extroversion (*bahir-gati*) because of desire. (3.40)

*Comments:* Driven by desire, the consciousness of the unenlightened person habitually flows out toward the external world. This externalizing flux of attention is captured well in the rare word *samvâhya*, denoting the individual who "flows together" with objects.

For him who is in the condition of being rooted in that [Fourth, or ultimate Reality, there results] termination of individuality (*jîva*) owing to the ending of that [desire for contact with objects]. (3.41)

Then, he who has the elements for his covering is released, mighty, supreme, and the same as the Lord [i.e., Shiva]. (3.42)

The connection with the life force (*prâna*) is natural. (3.43)

*Comments:* The meaning of this aphorism appears to be that even though finite life depends on the connection of the life force with a particular consciousness, in the case of the enlightened adept, this is not an intrinsic limitation. In fact, *prâna* is a manifestation of the ultimate Reality. Ultimately, *prâna* is the universal Life itself.

Through constraint (*samyama*) [i.e., through ecstatic identification with] the innermost center of the nose, how [can the ultimate Reality not be realized] in the left, the right, and the central [channels of the life force]? (3.44)

*Comments:* This is another obscure aphorism carrying a wealth of esoteric information. The innermost center (*antar-madhya*) of the nose (*nâsikâ*) is really the core of the life force or consciousness. By practicing successively concentration, meditation, and ecstasy relative to that subtle central point, the adept is able to abide as the ultimate Reality, regardless of whether the life force flows through the left channel, the right channel, or the central channel. In Tantrism and Hatha-Yoga, these channels through which the life force circulates are respectively known as *idâ-nâdî*, *pingalâ-nâdî*, and *sushumnâ-nâdî*. The *Shiva-Sûtra* uses the word *saushumna* for the last, which is the most important, since it is the conduit for the awakened *kundalinî-shakti*, the psycho-spiritual power that brings about a total alchemical transmutation of the human body-mind.

[In the case of the *yogin*] let there be repeatedly the opening-and-closing [of the vision of sameness]. (3.45)

*Comments:* The phrase *pratimîlana* is a technical expression of Kashmiri Shaivism. Here rendered as "opening-and-closing," it literally means "counter-closing." It refers to the high yogic art of seeing the ultimate Reality, Shiva, both within oneself and in the outer world. This practice comprises both subjective ecstasy (as epitomized in the closing of the eyes, or *nimîlana*) and objective ecstasy (as epitomized in the opening of the eyes, or *unmîlana*). This condition is otherwise known as spontaneous ecstasy, or *sahaja-samâdhi*.

## IV. FOR THE LOVE OF GOD— THE SHIVA WORSHIPERS OF THE SOUTH[17]

During the period between the seventh and the ninth century C.E., Âgamic Shaivism also gained momentum in the South. The Tamil-speaking Shaivas deny that their *Âgamas* hailed from the North. Be that as it may, they produced a vast and beautiful literature whose doctrines are known as Shaiva-Siddhânta. The metaphysics of this tradition, as already mentioned, is a form of qualified nondualism: Shiva is the One Reality, and the insentient (*acit*) world of multiplicity is no mere illusion but a product of Shiva's power (*shakti*). This is an important distinction from the northern

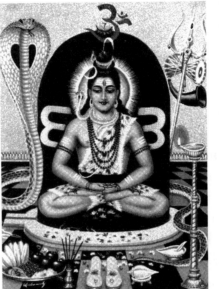

*Contemporary poster image of Shiva*

tradition, which favors an illusionist interpretation of the world. In both traditions, however, liberation is dependent on grace (*prasâda*).

Rejecting the *Vedas*, the Tamil Shaivas have their own sacred corpus, the *Tiru-Murai*, also often referred to as the "Tamil *Veda*." This collection of ancient hymns in praise of God Shiva was put together by Nambi-yândâr Nambi, who lived toward the end of the eleventh century C.E. These hundreds of hymns are arranged into eleven chapters, of which the tenth is the best known— the famous *Tiru-Manti-ram* of the adept-bard Tirumûlâr (seventh century

C.E.). It consists of more than three thousand verses. Tirumûlâr's teaching is a mixture of devotionalism, yogic technique, and gnosis (*jnâna*).

We may see in Tirumûlâr an early master of the widespread Siddha tradition, which will be addressed shortly. In one stanza (1463), he defines a *siddha*, or adept, as someone who has experienced the divine light and acquired power (*shakti*) through yogic ecstasy. For the historian of Yoga, the most important part of Tirumûlâr's work is the third section, consisting of 333 verses, where he explains the eight-fold limbs of the Yoga path à la Patanjali, and the fruits of correct Yoga practice, including the eight great supernormal powers (*mahâ-siddhi*). He also introduces several Tantric practices, notably the *khecârî-mu-drâ*, which is defined in verse 779 as the "simultaneous arresting of the movement of breath, mind, and semen." The *Tiru-Mantiram* is as important to southern Shaiva Yoga as the *Bhagavad-Gîtâ* is to the northern Vaishnava Yoga tradition.

The Tamil-speaking South still revers its great saints, the Nâyanmârs, who lived between the sixth and the tenth centuries C.E. Tradition knows of sixty-three Nâyanmârs ("Leaders"), whose saintliness and spiritual heroism is still annually celebrated in the Aravattu-Muvar-Ula festival. Their largely legendary life stories are preserved in Cekkilâr's

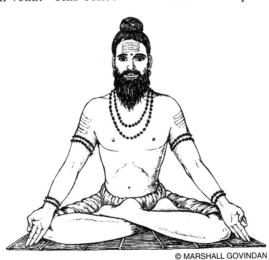

© MARSHALL GOVINDAN

*Tirumûlâr*

*Peria-Purânam*, an eleventh-century compilation. This popular work is as edifying to read as are the Christian hagiographies, providing we put ourselves in a spiritually receptive mood and are willing to ignore cultural differences. For the human heart speaks a universal language. The *Peria-Purânam* is filled with samples from the poetic outpourings of the saints, in which they glorify the Divine Lord, asking for nothing but to be devotees, forever absorbed in contemplating Him.

The four most revered saints of southern Shaivism are Appar, Sambandhar, Sundarar, and Mânikkavâcakar. Appar, who lived in the seventh century C.E., is generally deemed the first of the Nâyanmârs. He was born into the Jaina tradition, but after he was miraculously cured from a painful stomach ailment when praying in a Shiva temple, he converted to the Shaiva faith. Wandering from temple to temple where he performed menial services, Appar sang his love poetry in honor of God Shiva. His songs were widely influential. In one of them, he speaks of himself as a fool who fails to appreciate Shiva's constant proximity.

Like am I
to the profitless fool
who milks a dry cow

in a darkened room!

Fool that I am
trying to warm myself
by the twinkle
of a glow-worm
when a bright fire
is at hand!

As vain
as seeking alms
in a deserted village!

Is it not futile
to bite at an iron rod
when a piece
of sugarcane
is close at hand![18]

Appar, who saw himself as Shiva's humble servant, dismissed conventional religious practices like pilgrimage, penance, or study of the sacred scriptures, teaching instead that a profound love for Shiva is sufficient to achieve freedom and lasting happiness. His message caused great rancor among his old Jaina community. Legend has it that he was brought before the Jaina ruler Gunabhâra (alias Mahendravarman Pallava) at Kanchipuram, who asked him to renounce his new faith. When Appar refused, the king had him thrown into a lime kiln, but the saint was kept alive by his continuous chanting of the *mantra nama-sivaya* (Sanskrit: *namah shiv-âya*). When even poison, a mad elephant, and drowning could not end the saint's life, the ruler finally capitulated in shame and became Appar's disciple.

*Reproduced from* Slaves of the Lord

*Fresco of Nâyanmârs*

Another luminary of southern Shaivism is Sambandhar, whose poems open the sacred canon. He was a younger contemporary of Appar, with whom he traveled for several months, visiting temples and singing songs of praise that touched the hearts of many. Some traditional authorities believe that he is obliquely referred to in Nârada's *Bhakti-Sûtra* (83), where he is called Kaundinya (which is indeed Sambandhar's *gotra* or lineage name).

In his songs, Sambandhar often glorifies both Shiva and his divine spouse Pârvatî, and unlike his more ascetic counterparts he freely extolled the beauty of the female gender and of Nature. Sambandhar also is remembered as a worker of miracles, and according to a well-known legend he even revived a young girl who had already been cremated. He himself indicates in one of his hymns that the Lord blessed him with certain powers, including the power to drop his body at will.

A third much-loved poet-saint is Sundarar, who lived in the early part of the eighth century C.E. The mood of his songs is strikingly different from

ஐந்து கரத்தன ஆன முகத்தனே
இந்து இளம்பிறை போலும் எயிற்றனே
நந்தி மகன்தனே, ஞானக் கொழுந்தினைப்
புந்தியில் வைத்தடி போற்றுகின் றேனே.
திருமூலர் திருமந்திரம்

*A verse from the Tiru-Mantiram*

the poetry of his predecessors and the other Nâyanmârs, for Sundarar considered himself not a slave or servant of Lord Shiva but his friend. Because of the extreme familiarity with which he addresses God in his hymns, Sundarar came to be known as the "insolent devotee" (Tamil: *van tontar*). In his lyrical poems, he calls Shiva a madman, teasing the God for his strange attire. He even dares to ask for Goddess Pârvatî's hand in marriage, which all-benevolent Shiva grants to this impudent devotee.

Later, Sundarar fell in love with a beautiful girl by the name of Sangili who made flower garlands for the temple, and he asked Shiva to bring about their marriage as well. The request was granted on the condition, stipulated by the girl

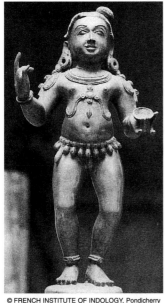

*Sambandhar*

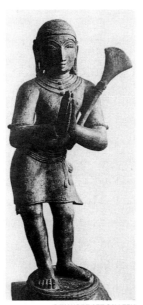

*Appar*

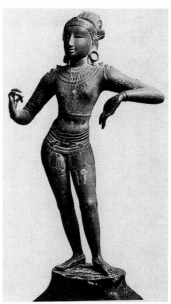

*Sundarar*

herself, that Sundarar would never leave her. After a few years of marital bliss with Sangili, the eccentric saint longed to be reunited with his first wife, Pârvatî. Upon breaking his vow, Sundarar promptly lost his eyesight. Now he traveled from temple to temple, reproaching Shiva for punishing him with blindness. He chided the Lord for depriving him of his eyesight, given that he, Shiva, has three eyes—the third eye being located on his forehead. Taking pity on his wayward devotee, Shiva restored the sight in one eye, and when Sundarar continued to lament his fate and blame the Lord for his misfortune, even healed the other eye.

Though not counted among the Nâyanmârs, Mânikkavâcakar ("He whose utterances are rubies") is remembered as one of four Nalvars, or great Shaiva saints, together with Appar, Sambandhar, and Sundarar. Mânikkavâcakar lived in the middle of the ninth century C.E. and was the prime minister of King Varaguna Pândya of Madurai. While on a royal mission to purchase horses, Mânikkavâcakar encountered a charismatic teacher—Shiva in disguise—who set his spirit on fire so much that the young minister

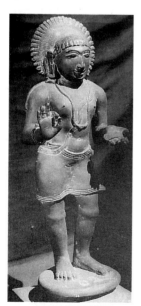

© PUDUKOTTAI MUSEUM, India

*Mânikkavâcakar*

spent the king's purse on building a Shiva temple at Perunturai. The ministerial saint was swiftly thrown into prison and was released only after the intervention of Lord Shiva himself.

Many of Mânikkavâcakar's exquisite love songs tell of his mad passion for Shiva and the mood of uncontrollable ecstasy that often overwhelmed him. In one composition he sings:

While unperishing love melted my bones,
    I cried
I shouted again and again,
      louder than the waves of the
      billowing sea,
I became confused,
    I fell,
    I rolled,
    I wailed,
Bewildered like a madman,
Intoxicated like a crazy drunk,
    so that people were puzzled
    and those who heard wondered.
Wild as a rutting elephant which cannot
    be mounted,
    I could not contain myself.[19]

For Mânikkavâcakar, God is ever merciful, and his grace knows no bounds. The path to God is intense love-devotion (*bhakti*), accompanied by deep meditation upon the Lord. The poet-saint sees no greater good than to be united with Shiva, the divine lover, clinging to him lost in ecstasy. Mânikkavâcakar's poetry is found in the *Tiru-Vâcakam*, the eighth book of the *Tiru-Murai*, which is sung daily in numerous temples and homes of Tamilnadu.

The southern Shaiva saints were ascetics of the heart, for in their external lives it would have been difficult to distinguish them from their neighbors. Most of them were married and had children, work to accomplish, and properties to care for. But they had inwardly renounced everything and become humble servants of Lord Shiva, ennobling their entire culture by their own love and humility. The age-old Shaiva community thus continued to cherish and perpetuate the spirit of Bhakti-Yoga and the ideal of *loka-samgraha*, or benefiting the world.

"Krishna, [who is called] Govinda,
is the supreme Lord *(îshvara)*, the embodiment
of Being, Consciousness, and Bliss,
without beginning and end, cause of all causes."

—*Brahma-Samhitâ* (5.1)

# Chapter 12

# THE VEDANTIC APPROACH TO GOD AMONG THE VISHNU WORSHIPERS

## I. GOD IS LOVE

When the heart is open it tends to burst into song and poetry. The ecstatic literature of the Shiva worshipers, especially of the southern part of the Indian peninsula, is a lasting testimony to this fact. And so is the great devotional literature of the Vishnu community to which we will now turn.

The five hymns dedicated to God Vishnu in the *Rig-Veda* were early blossoms on the Vaishnava tree of wisdom. Many centuries went by before the next great work of Vaishnavism saw the light of day. This was the *Bhagavad-Gîtâ* ("Song of the Lord"), the most popular of all Yoga works. Composed in its present version some 2,500 years ago, it inspired later generations of mystics to compose such incomparable devotional works as the poetry of the Âlvârs and Bauls, the *Bhâgavata-Purâna*, and the *Gîtâ-Govinda*, all of which will be introduced shortly. The *Bhagavad-Gîtâ* even served other poets as a model for similar didactic songs, and over one hundred Sanskrit *Gîtâs* are known. Thus there is, for instance, an *Anu-Gîtâ* (a recapitulation of the *Bhagavad-Gita* found in the *Mahâbhârata* itself), an *Uddhâva-Gîtâ* (embedded in the *Bhâgavata-Purâna*), a *Ganesha-Gîtâ* (in honor of the elephant-headed deity Ganesha), and a *Râma-Gîtâ* (in honor of Râma, an incarnation of Vishnu). Nearly one hundred other *Gîtâs* are known, at least by name.

The sacred literature of the Vaishnava community is as vast and complex as that of the Shaiva community, which I have touched on in the previous chapter. The early post-Christian centuries saw the creation of the *Samhitâs* ("Collections"), which are the Vaishnava equivalent to the Shaiva *Âgamas* and the *Tantras* of the Shakti worshipers.[1] Tradition speaks of 108 *Samhitâs*, though more than two hundred works of this genre are known. They belong to the Pancarâtra branch of Vaishnavism, which is mentioned already in the *Mahâbhârata*.

The oldest *Samhitâs* appear to be the *Sâtvata* (apparently referred to in the *Mahâ-Bhârata*), *Paushkara, Varâha, Brahma,* and *Padma.* Other important texts of this genre are the *Ahirbudhnya* and

371

the *Jayâkhya*. Like their Shaiva counterparts, the *Samhitâs* in principle organize their material into four sections, which are respectively known as *jnâna-pâda* (dealing with wisdom teachings or metaphysics), *yoga-pâda* (introducing yogic techniques), *kriyâ-pâda* (concerned with the building of temples and creation of sacred images), and *caryâ-pâda* (dealing with religious or ritual practices).

The anonymous composers of these scriptures were all familiar with Yoga practice, and their understanding of what this entails is roughly similar. The emphasis of their teachings is not so much on achieving mystical states of inwardness as on ritual worship and a moral way of life, interspersed with philosophical considerations, yet the declared ultimate goal is union with the Divine in the form of Vishnu (in the form of Nârâyana, Vasudeva, etc.)

The *Vishnu-Samhitâ* (chapter 13), which is typical of this genre of sacred literature, introduces a sixfold Yoga (*shad-anga-yoga*), which it styles *bhâgavata-yoga*. But many other works of the Vaishnava canon recommend Patanjali's eightfold Yoga. This is true of the *Ahirbudhnya-Samhitâ*, for instance, whose author clearly was aware of the *Yoga-Sûtra*. The text (31.15), however, defines Yoga in consonance with medieval Vedânta as "the union of the individual self with the transcendental Self." This work also mentions a variety of Yoga postures (including *kûrma-*, *mayûra-*, *kuk-kuta-*, and *go-mukha-âsana*) and recommends their practice for maintaining good health. The emphasis, however, is on the spiritual aspect of Yoga, without which none of these practices would be of lasting benefit.

## II. THE ÂLVÂRS

In contrast to the Pancarâtra *Samhitâs*, which are primarily theological and ritual works, the Âlvârs ("Deep-diving ones"), who flourished in the eighth and ninth centuries C.E., created a body of inspirational poetry, some of which is still sung in South India. The Âlvârs are a group of twelve adepts of Bhakti-Yoga, whose compositions are gathered in the *Nâlâyira-Tivyap-Pirapantam* (Sanskrit: *Nâlâyira-Divya-Prabandha*), which is given the same respect as the sacred *Vedas* of the brahmins. Their poems sparkle with passionate love for the Divine, and their archetypal symbolism touches us deeply even in translation. Most of the four thousand poems, or hymns, in this collection were composed by Tirumankai and Namm Âlvâr. The latter is the most popular of these saints, and his *Tiruvâymoli* (included in the *Pirapantam*) is given a status comparable to that of the *Sâma-Veda*. Namm Âlvâr is said to have been born absorbed in yogic ecstasy and to have crawled into a hollow tree trunk, where he remained in ecstatic absorption (*samâdhi*) for sixteen years until the man who was destined to become his chief disciple arrived. In his *Tiruvâymoli* (1.1.1) he declared:

"Who is He who is the
    highest good
diminishing all other
    heights?
Who is He who bestows
    wisdom and love
dispelling ignorance?
Who is He who rules the
    immortals beyond
    sorrow?
Worship his radiant feet that
    end all sorrow."

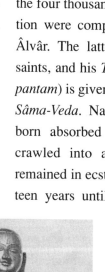

© FRENCH INSTITUTE OF INDOLOGY, Pondicherry

*Namm Âlvâr*

The Âlvârs were steeped in Krishna mythology: Krishna, the youthful cowherd, a full incarnation of the Divine Vishnu, at play with the cowgirls, the *gopîs.*

In the spiritual experiences of these Âlvârs we find a passionate yearning after God, the Lord and Lover . . . the emphasis is mostly on the transcendent beauty and charm of God, and on the ardent longings of the devotee who plays the part of a female lover, for Krishna, the God . . . The rapturous passions are like a whirlpool that eddies through the very eternity of the individual soul, and expresses itself sometimes in the pangs of separation and sometimes in the exhilaration of union.

The Âlvâr, in his ecstatic delight, visualizes God everywhere, and in the very profundity of his attainment pines for more. He also experiences states of supreme intoxication, when he becomes semi-conscious, or unconscious with occasional breaks into the consciousness of yearning . . . The Âlvârs were probably the pioneers in showing how love for God may be on terms of tender equality, softening down to the rapturous emotion of conjugal love.[2]

The twelve holy Âlvârs included only a single woman mystic, Ântâl, who lived soon after 800 C.E. Ântâl ("She of fragrant tresses"), who worshiped God Vishnu primarily in the form of the beautiful Krishna, authored two works. The first is the popular *Tiruppâvai* ("Sacred Vow"),

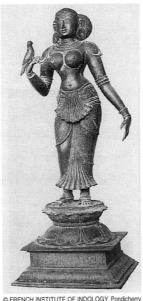

© FRENCH INSTITUTE OF INDOLOGY, Pondicherry

*Ântâl*

consisting of only thirty Tamil verses, which are still sung by young women wishing for a happy marriage. The second work, written after the *Tiruppâvai,* is the *Nâcciyâr-Tirumoli* ("Sacred Song of the Lady"), consisting of fourteen hymns with a total of 143 verses, of which only the sixth hymn is widely known. The latter. work extols the path of the unmarried saint, and it is rich in the beautiful imagery of bridal mysticism. Here Ântâl expresses her pining for Krishna, who melts her soul and tortures her heart with yearning until he graces her with a glimpse of his lovely face. She describes herself growing pale and losing weight—a maiden desperately in love, restless with longing, who has lost all sense of shame and proportion over her lover. In one hymn, Ântâl speaks of having her dream fulfilled: She beheld Krishna's radiant face glowing like the rising sun. In the same hymn, this great *bhakti-yoginî* promises that those who meditate on her verses will cure their heart's pain and find eternal peace at the feet of the Lord.

The experience of separation (*viraha*) from the Divine is among the devotee's most vauable allies, for it deepens devotion. This is captured nowhere more powerfully than in the traditional figure of Râdhâ and the other cowgirls of Vrindâvana, whose love for Lord Krishna was boundless.

## III. THE BHÂGAVATA-PURÂNA

The theme of erotic spirituality is fully explored, if not exploited, in the *Bhâgavata-Purâna,* also known as the *Shrîmad-Bhâgavata,* which depicts the God-man Krishna as husband to

16,108 women, each of whom bore him ten sons and one daughter. The *Bhâgavata-Purâna* is a magnificent tenth-century work that has been called "the richest treasure hidden in the bosom of the liberated, the incomparable solace to the disturbed soul."[3] No other scripture, with the exception of the *Bhagavad-Gîtâ*, has enjoyed such widespread popularity through the centuries. Numerous commentaries have been written on this work, which holds aloft the great ideal of love-devotion (*bhakti*) to the Lord (*bhagavat*).

Central to the *Bhâgavata-Purâna's* gospel of devotion to the Divine is the rich metaphor of the *râsa-lîlâ*—the playful dance of beauteous love. One night, the lovesick *gopîs* stole away from their homes in the village to be with their beloved Krishna. Seeking to kindle their passionate longing for him, he played his magical flute, whose unearthly sounds held them spellbound.

At the climax of Krishna's love play with the maidens, he danced a dance of ecstatic abandon with them, giving each girl the impression that he was dancing with her alone. So all-consuming was their passion for him that they were completely oblivious of the other girls—a perfect metaphor for the psyche absorbed in devotion to the Lord.

The idea of the *râsa-lîlâ* can be traced back to Chapter 63 of the *Hari-Vamsha* ("Hari's lineage"), which is an appendix of 18,000 stanzas to the *Mahâbhârata*. This appendix is generally dated to the first few centuries C.E.

Yoga is mentioned in many passages of the *Bhâgavata-Purâna*. In one such place (11.20.6), three approaches are distinguished, namely the path of wisdom for those who are weary of rituals, the path of action for those who are still inclined toward worldly and sacred activity, and the path of devotion for those who are fortunate enough to be neither weary of actions nor overly inclined to them, but simply have faith in the Lord and his power of salvation. The *Bhâgavata-Purâna* accepts Patanjali's eightfold path but rejects his dualist philosophy. Also, the eight limbs of the yogic path are defined somewhat differently from the *Yoga-Sûtra*. This is most apparent in the delineation of the constituent practices of moral discipline (*yama*) and self-restraint (*niyama*). Where Patanjali lists five practices for each set, the *Bhâgavata-Purâna* (11.19.33ff.) has twelve. But always it is devotion that is recommended as the supreme means of reaching liberation. The adept Kapila, who is remembered as the founder of the Sâmkhya tradition and is identified with God Vishnu, is credited with these pertinent words:

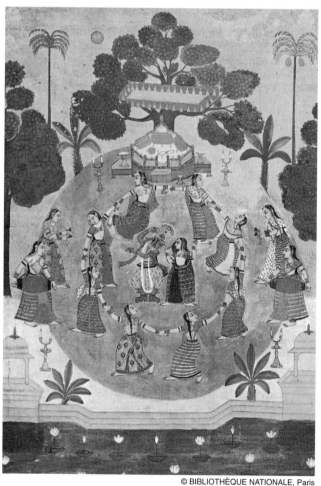

*The rasa-lîlâ*

When the mind is firmly fixed on Me by intense Bhakti-Yoga, it becomes still and steady. This is the only way for attaining the highest bliss in this world. (3.25.44)

On the path of devotion, concentration is always the fixing of attention upon the divine Person, whereas meditation is the contemplation of the Lord's form, as depicted in iconography: with a four-armed, garlanded dark-blue body; a serene expression on his kind face; holding a conch, a disc, and a mace in his hands; wearing a crown on his head and the magical *kaustubha* jewel around his neck; and bearing the *shrî-vatsa* ("blessed calf") mark on his chest. The dark-blue hue of Krishna's body is the result of his drinking the poisoned milk of the female demon Pûtanâ who suckled him. The implements in his hands are all instruments of war, and their use destroys the enemy—the ego—and leads to liberation. The magical jewel was created during the churning of the world ocean at the beginning of time. The mark on Krishna's chest is one of the signs of his superior birth and of his principal vocation as a cowherd (*gopa*), a protector of cattle and of human souls.

Liberation is thought to be of different degrees, depending on the devotee's level of proximity to, or identification with, the Lord. At the lowest stage, the devotee dwells in the divine location—Vaikuntha Heaven—in the Lord's company. This is called *sâlokya-mukti*. When the devotee's power and glory equals that of the Lord, it is known as *sârishti-mukti*. When he or she is abiding in close proximity to the Lord, it is called *sâmîpya-mukti*. The penultimate level of liberation is *sârûpya-mukti*, in which the devotee attains perfect conformity with the Lord. Finally, there is *ekatva-mukti*, or the "liberation of singleness," in which the last trace of difference between the devotee and the Divine is lifted.

Of particular interest for the Yoga student are Chapters 6–29 of the eleventh book of the *Bhâgavata-Purâna*. This section is known as the *Uddhava-Gîtâ*, after the sage Uddhava, to whom the God-man Krishna expounds the Yoga of devotion. This "Song," which is sometimes referred to as Krishna's last message, praises love-devotion above all other means:

Just as fire that is ablaze with flames reduces wood to ashes, so devotion to Me removes all sin, O Uddhava. (11.14.19)

Neither through [conventional] Yoga nor Sâmkhya, nor righteousness (*dharma*), nor study, nor austerities, nor renunciation (*tyâga*) does he reach Me as [readily as he does through] devotion (*bhakti*), or the worship of Me. (11.14.20)

I, the beloved Self of the virtuous, am realized through singular devotion, through faith. Devotion established in Me purifies even [outcastes] like the "dog-cookers" (*shva-pâka*) from their [lowly and impure] birth. (11.14.21)

The devotee of Krishna is portrayed as an individual capable of deep emotion, worship, and renunciation as follows:

He whose speech is interrupted by sobs, whose heart (*citta*) melts, who unabashedly sometimes laments or laughs, or sings aloud or dances—[such a person] endowed with devotion to Me purifies the world. (11.14.24)

Faith in the nectar-like stories about Me, constant proclamation of My [greatness], deep reverence (*parinishthâ*) in worshiping [Me], and praising Me with hymns; (11.19.20)

delight in service [to Me], making prostrations [before Me], rendering greater worship to My devotees, and considering all beings as Me; (11.19.21)

doing bodily activities for My sake, reciting My qualities in sayings, offer-ing the mind to Me, and banishing all desires; (11.19.22)

renouncing things, pleasure, and enjoyment for My sake, [undertaking] whatever sacrifice, gifting, oblation, recitation, vow, and penance for My sake— (11.19.23)

by such virtues, O Uddhava, self-surrendered people acquire love-devotion (*bhakti*) for Me. What other task remains for such a one? (11.19.24)

## SOURCE READING 14

# *Uddhava-Gîtâ (Selection)*

The following is a translation of Chapter 13 of the *Uddhava-Gîtâ*, which speaks of the householder who has retired to the forest in order to pursue his quest for the Divine. The description of the hermit's life drives home the single-mindedness with which the serious practitioner must cultivate the yogic path.

The Blessed Lord said:

He who wishes to withdraw into the forest should live peacefully in the forest in the third quarter of his life, entrusting his wife to his sons or [taking her] with him. (1)

He should subsist on bulbs, roots, fruits, and wild plants and wear bark, cloth, grass, leaves, or a hide. (2)

He should let his hair, body hair, nails, and beard grow dirty and not clean his teeth. Three times [a day, at sunrise, noon, and sunset,] he should immerse himself in water and sleep on the ground. (3)

In the summer he should practice austerity with the five fires [i.e., four fires around him and the sun overhead]. During the rains he should expose himself to the downpours. In winter he should immerse himself up to his neck in water. In this fashion he should practice penance (*tapas*). (4)

He should eat [food] cooked over a fire or [food that has] ripened over time, crushing it with a rock in a mortar, or even with the teeth as a mortar. (5)

Understanding the power of the [right] place and time, he should gather all means of subsistence himself, and he should not eat [food] offered by others or what has been discarded. (6)

The forest-dweller should worship Me [Krishna] with pleasing sacrificial cakes from wild plants, not with animal [sacrifices prescribed] by the scriptures. (7)

The expounders [of the sacred tradition] prescribe for the sage (*muni*) the four-month [disciplines], and the [daily] fire ritual, as well as the new-moon and the full-moon [observances] as previously [mentioned]. (8)

By thus performing asceticism (*tapas*), the sage who is steady in his duty (*dharma*) and worships Me by asceticism reaches Me from the world of the seers (*rishi-loka*). (9)

But what greater fool is there than he who undertakes this great, unexcelled asceticism practiced with [immense] difficulty for [the sake of realizing] insignificant desires? (10)

When he is unable to [follow these] rules because of congenital tremors from old age, he should project [i.e., visualize] the [sacred] fires within himself, and with his mind intent on Me, he should enter the fire [of the Spirit]. (11)

When he is running out of time in the worlds [driven by] action (*karma*) and its fruition, he should adopt dispassion (*virâga*), and having completely abandoned the fire [rituals], he should go forth [as a renouncer]. (12)

Sacrificing to Me according to the injunctions and giving all that is his to the [offici-ating] priests, as well as placing his own life-breath (*prâna*) into the fires, he should go forth [feeling] carefree. (13)

For the sage (*vipra*) intent on renunciation, the Gods, [fearing] that he may really tran-scend them and reach the Supreme, create obstacles in the form of his wife and other [loved ones]. (14)

If the sage wants to retain a [second] piece of cloth, it should be no larger than the loin-cloth (*kaupîna*). Having abandoned [everything], he should have nothing but his staff and bowl, except [during times of] distress. (15)

He should place his foot after purifying [the ground] with his gaze and drink water purified with a cloth. He should utter words purified by truth and conduct [his life] with a purified mind. (16)

Silence (*mauna*), inactivity, and breath control (*anila-âyâma*)[4] are the restraints of speech, body, and mind. He who does not have these, O friend, cannot become an ascetic (*yati*) by [carrying around] a staff. (17)

He should go to the four estates (*varna*) for alms, except to the sinful. He should go to seven houses unannounced and should be content with whatever is given. (18)

Going to a water tank outside [the village] and bathing there, he should, with speech restrained and apart [from other people], eat the purified remnant [of food left over after making proper offerings to the deities], leaving no remnant himself. (19)

He should roam alone over the earth, unattached and with the senses controlled, delighting in the Self, playing in the Self, Self-possessed, seeing the same [Self in everything]. (20)

Sheltering himself in a secluded and protected [spot], his pure intention (*âshaya*) [focused] upon My being (*bhâva*), the sage should contemplate the singular Self as nondistinct from Me. (21)

He should consider the Self's bondage and liberation through the cultivation of wisdom. Bondage is distraction (*vikshepa*) through the senses, and liberation is the control of these [senses]. (22)

Therefore the sage, restraining the six types [of senses, including the lower mind or *manas*], should roam [over the earth] with his intention (*bhâva*) on Me. Finding great delight in the Self, [he should be] dissociated from [all] lowly desires. (23)

He should roam over the earth abounding in virtuous countries, rivers, mountains, forests, and hermitages, entering cities, villages, herdsmen's stations, and caravansaries [only] for the purpose of begging [alms]. (24)

He should go for alms mainly to places with hermitages of forest-dwelling [ascetics]. By [eating] grains or herbs, he achieves a pure mind (*sattva*), free from delusion. (25)

He should not perceive this [world], seeing that it perishes. With unattached mind, he should abstain from [all] purpose in this [world] and the next. (26)

"This world, mind, speech, and the group of life forces are all illusions (*mâyâ*) [superimposed] upon the Self." By reasoning thus and relying on himself, he should abandon [these illusory phenomena] and not consider them [anymore]. (27)

Pursuing wisdom, without attachment, devoted to Me, unconcerned, he should roam about, free from rules, having abandoned the stages of life (*âshrama*) with their [respective] characteristics. (28)

[Even though he is] wise (*budha*), he should play like a child; [though] skillful, he should behave like a fool; [though] learned, he should talk like a madman; [though] educated (*naigama*), he should behave in cowlike fashion. (29)

He should not be fond of debating the *Vedas*, nor be a heretic, nor an arguer. He should not at all take sides in controversies over useless statements. (30)

The sage (*dhîra*) should not be agitated by people nor should he agitate people. He should be forbearing about insults and never harass anyone. In regard to the body, he should feel enmity to no one, like [peaceful] cattle. (31)

The singular supreme Self alone is in [all] beings, just as the [one] Moon is reflected in [many] vessels. [All beings] dwell in the Self, and [all] beings are of the [same] Self. (32)

Cultivating steadiness and relying on destiny, he should not be sad when he does not get food, nor be delighted when he does get some. (33)

He should desire food, [because] this is appropriate for the maintenance of life. By means of it one can reflect upon the truth, knowing which one is liberated. (34)

The sage should accept whatever food comes to him by fate, excellent or otherwise; similarly, [he should accept] whatever clothes and bedding are provided. (35)

The knower (*jnânin*) should practice cleansing, sipping [of water to rinse his mouth], bathing, and other disciplines, but not because of [any scriptural] prescriptions, just as I, the Lord, [do everything] as play. (36)

For him there is no so-called misconception and, [if he has any], it is removed by seeing Me. Until the termination of the body, [he enjoys] a certain vision [of Me]. Thence he is united with Me. (37)

The Self-possessed (*âtmavan*) who is disgusted with actions producing suffering [but who] has not inquired into My teaching (*dharma*) should go to a sage [who can serve him as a] teacher (*guru*). (38)

Intent on Me as the teacher, he should practice devotedly, with faith, and uncomplaining until he realizes the Absolute (*brahman*). (39)

The charioteer of the unruly senses, however, who has not restrained the six types [of senses, including the lower mind], who is without wisdom and dispassion, and [yet who] lives [the life of an ascetic carrying] the triple staff . . . (40)

. . . he, a destroyer of virtue (*dharma*), cheats himself and the deities (*sura*), as well as Me residing in himself. With his taints (*kashâya*) "uncooked" (*avipakva*), he is deprived of our [world] and the next. (41)

The lifestyle (*dharma*) of a monk [includes] tranquillity (*shama*) and nonharming, of a forest-dweller asceticism and [pure] vision (*îkshâ*), of a householder protection of beings and sacrifice (*ijyâ*), of a twice-born [brahmin] service to the preceptor. (42)

Chastity, asceticism, cleanliness, contentment, and kindness to beings are also a householder's duties. Worshiping Me is desirable for all. (43)

He who worships Me thus constantly by [performing] his duties, and is devoted to none other and intent on Me in all beings, soon finds My love. (44)

O Uddhava, by unswerving devotion, he comes to Me, the great Lord of all the worlds, the Absolute, the [ultimate] cause, the origin and end of all [beings and things]. (45)

With his being (*sattva*) thus cleansed by [the performance] of his duties, knowing My state, endowed with wisdom and knowledge, he soon attains Me. (46)

Associated with devotion to Me, this duty (*dharma*) relating to the estates (*varna*) and stages of life (*âshrama*) [and which is] marked by [proper] conduct, verily, is conducive to the highest (*nihshreyasa*), the Supreme. (47)

I have disclosed this to you, O friend, [which is] what you asked Me: how a devotee (*bhakta*) disciplined in [the performance] of his duties attains Me, the Supreme (*para*). (48)

## The Alchemy of Hatred

Perhaps the most extraordinary teaching of the *Bhâgavata-Purâna* is the "Yoga of hatred" (*dvesha-yoga*), according to which a person who thoroughly hates the Divine can achieve God-Realization as readily as one who deeply loves the Lord. Sage Nârada, a frequent spokesman for the Bhâgavata religion, expresses it thus:

> All human emotions are grounded in the erroneous conception of "I" and "mine." The Absolute, the universal Self, has neither "I"-sense nor emotions. (7.1.23)

> Hence one should unite [with God] through friendship or enmity, peaceableness or fear, love or attachment. [The Divine] sees no distinction whatsoever. (7.1.25)

Nârada goes on to mention Kamsa, who reached God through fear, and Shishupâla, king of the Cedis, who reached God through hatred. In fact, Shishupâla's hatred was cultivated over several incarnations. He was the demon king Hiranyakashipu ("Gold-Cloth"), who tortured his son Prahlâda for his devotion to Vishnu, but was disemboweled by the God who assumed the form of Nara-Simha ("Man-Lion"). In another birth Shishupâla was the demon Râvana who was slain by Râma, an incarnation of Vishnu.

The idea that hatred can turn out to be a pathway to God, shocking as it is to conventional sensibilities, is a logical consequence of the ancient esoteric doctrine that we become whatever we meditate upon. The intense hatred that Shishupâla entertained toward Lord Vishnu had the effect that he thought about the Divine incessantly, and therefore ultimately became absorbed in it. This brings home the fact that the spiritual process is a matter of the play of attention. Of course, for such a powerful negative emotion to have a liberating effect, there must exist the right karmic preconditions as well. Absolute hatred is as impossible for an ordinary individual as absolute love.

## The Devî-Bhâgavata

In connection with the great *Bhâgavata-Purâna*, at least brief mention must be made of the *Devî-Bhâgavata*. Although it is a prominent Shâkta work, it is modeled on the *Bhâgavata-Purâna*, and it illustrates the vital tradition of devotion among those who worship the Divine in its feminine aspect. This secondary *Purâna* was composed perhaps in the twelfth or thirteenth century C.E.

## IV. THE GÎTÂ-GOVINDA

While the *Bhâgavata-Purâna*, true to its syncretistic Puranic character, deals with all kinds of theological, philosophical, and cosmological matters besides telling the story of Krishna's heroic life, the somewhat later *Gîtâ-Govinda* ("Song of Govinda") is solely dedicated to celebrating Lord Krishna's love of his favorite shepherdess, Râdhâ. The name Govinda is one of Krishna's many appellations. It means literally "cow-finder" and refers to the God-man's occupation as cowherd in the Vrindâvana region. There is an esoteric significance to the name as well, since the Sanskrit word *go* not only means "cow" but also stands for "wisdom." Thus, Govinda is the finder of gnosis (*jnâna*).

This Sanskrit poem by the twelfth-century Bengali writer Jayadeva is a profound allegory of the love between the personal God and the human self, which has strong erotic overtones. It is expressive of a new trend in the Vaishnava devotional movement, coinciding with its expansion to the North of the Indian peninsula. Suddenly, great prominence was given to the figure of Râdhâ as an embodiment of the feminine principle of the Divine. Confiding in a friend, Râdhâ recounts her love adventure with Krishna thus:

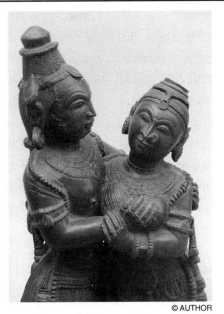
© AUTHOR
*Krishna and Râdhâ in loving embrace*

Secretely at night I went to his home in a concealed thicket where he remained in hiding. Anxiously I glanced in all directions, while he was laughing with an abundant longing for the delight (*rati*) [of sexual union]; O friend! Make the crusher of [the demon] Keshin love me passionately. I am enamored, entertaining desires of love! (2.11)

I was shy at our first union. He was kind toward me, [showing] hundreds of ingenious flatteries. I spoke through sweet and gentle smiles, and he unfastened the garment around my hips. (2.12)

He laid me down on a bed of shoots. For a long time he rested on my breast, while I caressed and kissed him. Embracing me, he drank from my lower lip. (2.13)

I closed my eyes from drowsiness. The hair on his cheeks bristled from my caresses. My whole body was perspiring, and he was quite restless because of

his great intoxication with passion. (2.14)

Râdhâ pines for her lover, as the awakened heart yearns for God. Reflecting the radical spirit of Tantra, the *Gîtâ-Govinda* extensively employs sexual metaphors to convey the bodily passion that the devotee feels when he or she contemplates God. In its erotic explicitness it surpasses the comparable literature of the bridal mystics of medieval Christendom.

## V. THE BHAKTI-YOGA OF THE VAISHNAVA PRECEPTORS

The ecstatic devotionalism of the Âlvârs attracted not only the illiterate masses, who were moved by the Âlvârs' strong sentiments of love, but also stimulated the intelligentsia to develop sophisticated philosophical doctrines revolving around the ideal of love (*bhakti*). The first of these learned Vishnu devotees was Nâthamuni, who lived in the tenth century C.E. He is said to have often walked about naked, chanting the sacred name of God Vishnu. Some scholars identify him with Shrî Nâtha, the author of several works, including the *Yoga-Rahasya* ("Secret Doctrine of Yoga"). Another important figure among the so-called "preceptors" (*âcârya*) of Vaishnavism was Yâmuna, the grandson of Nâthamuni. He wrote six works, of which the *Siddhi-Traya* ("Triad of Perfection") is the most significant. According to tradition, Yâmuna, who described himself as a "vessel of a thousand sins," learned the eightfold Yoga from Kuruka Nâtha. It was

Nâthamuni who had entrusted Kuruka Nâtha with this teaching for the benefit of his grandson. Interestingly, the modern Yoga master Tirumalai Krishnamacharya, who died in 1989 at the age of 101, traced his lineage back to Nâthamuni. Shrî Krishnamacharya passed his teachings on to T. K. V. Desikachar (his son), B. K. S. Iyengar (his brother-in-law), Indra Devi, and Pattabhi Jois, who all have become great teachers in their own right.[5]

The most influential preceptor was unquestionably Râmânuja (1017–1137 C.E.), who sought to unite the Vaishnavism of the South and the North, and to some degree succeeded in doing so. Yâmuna, who had expressed a keen interest in meeting the brilliant Râmânuja, was dead by the time Râmânuja came to pay homage to him. Three of Yâmuna's fingers were curiously twisted, and Râmânuja took this to be a final message to him.

He understood it to mean that he should preach the Vaishnava doctrine of unconditional surrender, or *prapatti*, and write a commentary on the *Brahma-Sûtra*, as well as on many other works championing the Vaishnava faith as taught by the Âlvârs.

The visit to Yâmuna occurred after Râmânuja had been asked to leave the *âshrama* of his own teacher, Yâdavaprakâsha, who was a learned but irascible man. His discipleship had been stormy, because he begged to differ from his *guru* on several doctrinal issues. Whereas Yâdavaprakâsha avowed a strictly nondualistic interpretation of the Vaishnava scriptures, Râmânuja was at heart a qualified nondualist, believing that the Divine is not a mere distinctionless One but comprises infinite differentiation.

Râmânuja lived a long and eventful life, and his many works expounding the philosophy of Vishishta-Advaita formed the foundations of a comprehensive exegetical literature that offered the most serious challenge to the radical nondualism of Shankara's school.

Râmânuja and his followers oppose Shankara's notion that the experienced world of multiplicity is unreal. They place no faith in the doctrines of *mâyâ* ("illusion") and *avidyâ* ("ignorance"), by which the Shankara camp seeks to explain the fact that, even though there is only the Absolute, we actually experience distinctions. If there were such an agent as ignorance, the followers of Râmânuja argue, it could not be located in the omniscient transcendental Reality. But if it is not located in the Absolute, it would form an alternative reality to it, which would completely undermine the idea of radical nondualism.

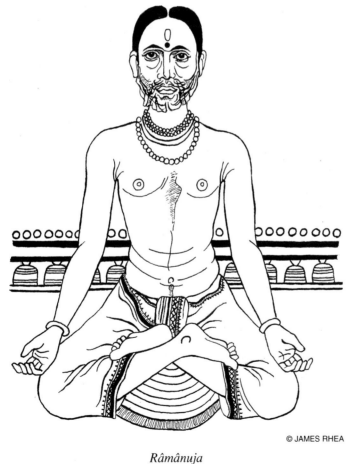

© JAMES RHEA

*Râmânuja*

Râmânuja was an eager protagonist of Yoga, which he understood as Bhakti-Yoga. For him, the purpose of meditation is to generate love for the divine Person. He was consequently rather critical of Patanjali's Yoga, which is not only dualistic but also aims at stilling the mind rather than turning the heart to God. Râmânuja was similarly wary of Jnâna-Yoga, as taught by Shankara, because in the beginner it tends to lead to intellectualism and self-delusion. In preparation for meditation, or the contemplative remembrance of the Divine, one should instead engage in Karma-Yoga.

From Râmânuja's point of view, liberation is not the annihilation of the self but rather the removal of its limitations. The liberated being attains the "same form" as the Divine, though this does not imply the obliteration of all distinctions. Rather, liberation is conceived as a kind of fellowship with and in the divine Person—a condition of continuous love-devotion—but whereas the divine Person is infinite and the absolute creator of the universe, the liberated devotee is finite and has no power of creation. For Râmânuja, liberation occurs only after death. Love is the means and the goal, and it can and should be cultivated throughout one's life on Earth or in any of the higher realms of existence.

Yogic teachings also played a role in the schools of the other four great Vaishnava preceptors—the Vedântic dualist Madhva (1238–1317 C.E.), the theologian of duality-in-nonduality Nimbârka (mid-twelfth century C.E.), the pure nondualist Vallabha (1479–1531 C.E.), and the ecstatic Krishna Caitanya (1486–1533 C.E.), who argued that the true nature of Reality is imponderable. These teachers and their

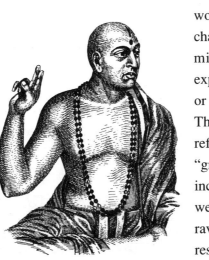

*Madhva*

numerous adherents all enlist the capacity for self-transcending love and surrender as the principal means of liberation. It is here that psychospiritual technology is the most artful and the least in danger of degenerating into crude manipulation of the body-mind, as is characteristic of some schools of Hatha-Yoga. Of course, the path of the heart, or Bhakti-Yoga, has its own risks, such as rampant irrationalism and unbridled emotionalism. It appears, however, to be inherently more conducive to a balanced approach by integrating the intellect with the feeling aspect of the psyche. The heart (*hrid*, *hridaya*) has from ancient times been acknowledged as a primary focus of the spiritual process. "The heart," says a modern sage, "is the cradle of love."[6] And it is at the heart that, according to many schools and traditions, the great awakening occurs.

The *bhakti* movement gives feeling precedence over the intellect. This emphasis is best seen in the notion of *bhâva*. In the context of ordinary life, the term *bhâva* signifies "sentiment" or "emotion," which includes aesthetic appreciation. According to the Sanskrit dramatists, there are nine predominant emotions: love, joy, sorrow, anger, courage, fear, disgust, surprise, and renunciation.

In a spiritual context, the word *bhâva* denotes feeling-charged ecstasy or the ultimate mind-melting love-devotion experienced in the presence of, or in union with, the Divine. This elevated state is often referred to as *mahâ-bhâva*, or "great mood," whose symptoms include spontaneous laughter, weeping, singing, dancing, and raving. At times, *mahâ-bhâva* resembles madness, and not a few Vaishnava ecstatics have called themselves madcaps because of the irrational behavior engendered by the intense emotion experienced during the ecstatic state.

A closely related concept in the Vaishnava tradition is that of *rasa*, a term which means literally "taste" or "essence" and here refers to the basic mood of a person or situation. Thus Vishnu devotees experiencing ecstasy are said to enjoy the mood of love (*bhakti-rasa*). The term was first introduced in connection with the dramatic arts, where it conveys the principal mood that integrates the various elements of a dramatic composition. Whereas *rasa* represents an objective sentiment, *bhâva* refers more to a subjective, personal mood. Just as there are nine types of *bhâva*, there also are nine corresponding types of *rasa*, which can be subjectively experienced through the *bhâvas*.

## VI. JNÂNADEVA AND OTHER SAINTS OF MAHARASHTRA

One of the great Vaishnava adepts of the path of devotion, tempered by wisdom, is Jnânadeva (1275–1296 C.E.). He was the second of four children born to pious but poor brahmin parents who lived in the village of Alandi near Pune (Poona) in Maharashtra, a country that has spawned many fine saints and sages. His older brother, Nivritti Nâtha, was a disciple of Gahini Nâtha, who belonged to the tradition of Goraksha Nâtha, the great Hatha-Yoga master and *mahâ-siddha*. He had been initiated at the tender age of seven, and in turn initiated Jnânadeva when he

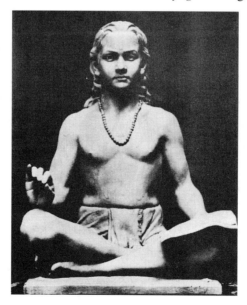

*Jnânadeva*

was still very young, definitely before his fifteenth year.

It was at age fifteen that Jnânadeva composed, in honor of his *guru* and brother Nivritti Nâtha, his famous poetic Marathi commentary on the *Bhagavad-Gîtâ* that has been treasured as much for the depth of its wisdom as its stylistic beauty. This extensive commentary of nearly nine thousand verses was delivered orally spontaneously by him chapter after chapter and was only subsequently written down. It has two titles: *Bhâva-Artha-Dîpikâ* ("Light on the Original Meaning," written *Bhâvârthadîpikâ*) and, more simply, *Jnâneshvarî* (from the words *jnâna* or "wisdom" and *îshvarî* or "female ruler"). Jnânadeva's friend and disciple Nâmadeva of Pandharpur, the author of many devotional works, spoke of the *Jnâneshvarî* as "a wave of brahmic bliss."

At the behest of his brother-*guru*, he also composed the *Amrita-Anubhava* ("Experience of Immortality," written *Amritânubhava*), which has been called the greatest philosophical work in the Marathi language. Another work, the *Changadeva-Pâsashthi*, was composed as an instructional poem for the *yogin* Changadeva, who had been proud of his magical powers but had discovered humility when sitting at Jnânadeva's feet. Additionally, there are about nine hundred devotional hymns (*abhanga*) attributed to Jnânadeva.

Jnânadeva was not only a realized master and poetic genius but also a miracle worker, who, among other things, is said to have made a buffalo recite verses from the *Rig-Veda* and to have brought the saintly

Saccidânanda Bâbâ back to life. Yet, such feats meant nothing to him compared with his love for the Divine and his teacher. At only twenty-one years of age, he had himself buried alive to exit this world while immersed in deep meditation. His *samâdhi* site in Alandi continues to attract pilgrims.

His *Jnâneshvarî* (6.192–317), among other things, includes a remarkable description of the *kundalinî* process as taught in early Nâthism. For him, the awakening of this formidable power locked in the human body was intimately connected with *guru-yoga*, the spiritual discipline of honoring the teacher as an embodiment of the Divine. He begins Chapter 15 with the following words:

> Now I shall place my *guru*'s feet on the altar of my heart. (1)

> Pouring my senses as flowers into the cupped hands of the experience of union with the Supreme, I offer a handful of these at his feet. (2)

Jnânadeva's philosophy was firmly rooted in his personal spiritual realization. He rejected Shankara's *mâyâ-vâda* (which regards objective reality as illusory), and instead taught that the notion that the world's appearance is due to ignorance (*avidyâ*) is itself illusory. Rather, he tells us, the world is divine play, and its cause is none other than the Supreme itself. Instead of being merely an illusion that deludes people, the universe is an expression of divine love. Similarly, the individuated psyche (*jîva*) is not, as Shankara insisted, "mere appearance" but a necessary manifestation of the ultimate Reality, which experiences its own delight in the mirror of creation. Consequently, for Jnânadeva, the purpose of human life is not liberation—in the sense of escaping from a merely illusory world—but

moment-to-moment realization of the presence of the Divine in and as one's body-mind.

Another celebrated Maharashtrian saint is Eka Nâth (1533 or 1548–1599 C.E.), who was orphaned at an early age and brought up by his grandparents. At the age of twelve, following an inner voice, he secretly left his home to become a disciple of Janârdana Svâmin, with whom he lived for six years. Later he was married, but he maintained a rather formal relationship with his wife and insisted that one should keep a distance from all women other than one's wife. He was a man of tremendous self-control and patience and had a keen sense of the equality of all people. He created a voluminous spiritual literature, including commentaries on the eleventh chapter of the *Bhâgavata-Purâna* and on the first forty-four chapters of the *Râmâyana*, as well as numerous devotional hymns.

Eka Nâtha was a true *bhakta* who shed tears of joy in the state of ecstatic union with the Beloved. In one of his *abhangas*, he speaks of having discovered the "eye of the eye" and his entire body being endowed with vision. His love for the Divine was inseparable from his love for his *guru*, and in all his songs of praise he joins his own name to that of Janârdana to honor the eternal bond between them. For him, a God-realized sage, all distinction between worshiper and worshiped had ceased. There was only the One.

In the seventeenth century, the Maharashtrian *bhakti* movement produced the saintly figure of Tukârâma (1598?–1650? C.E.), who was born into a poor family of farmers. He experienced every conceivable hardship, for which he was, however, grateful, as it kept him humble and open to the Divine. According to one traditional account, he ascended to heaven in Christlike fashion.

He was greatly influenced by Jnânadeva but reflected more the emotional approach of Nâmadeva, which is expressed in his many popular *abhangas.* His inspired poetic creations were on everyone's lips, but his success among the ordinary people filled the local intelligentsia with envy. One of his enemies went so far as to throw all his *abhangas* into the river. Distraught by this callous act, Tukârâma started a rigorous fast to learn directly from the Beloved whether he was to desist from composing further songs. After thirteen days of abstaining from both food and water, he was granted the assuring vision. His troubles in the village continued, however. One of his revilers even poured boiling water on him, which caused him great agony but did not deter him from practicing forgiveness and patience. As fate would have it, sometime later the same man suffered from a seemingly incurable and very painful illness. In the end, he had to ask for Tukârâma's help, which was promptly given. The saint composed a special *abhanga* for the sinner, which immediately healed him.

Tukârâma observed only two vows: to fast on *ekâdashî* day and to always sing God's praise. Tukârâma, who lived during troubled times, exhorted his disciples to become heroic warriors on the spiritual battlefield. He had many disciples who were distinguished for their own spiritual realization and literary creativity.

Another great Maharashtrian saint is Râmadâsa (1608–1681 C.E.), who practiced twelve years of severe austerities before he had his longed-for vision of Râma. He had numerous disciples, including King Shivajî, who carried the *bhakti* tradition into the eighteenth century.

## VII. THE MINSTREL-SAINTS OF MEDIEVAL BENGAL

Ever since the time of the Buddha, Bengal has been a country of spiritual, intellectual, and artistic creativity. In medieval times, Bengal was an unparalleled melting pot for both Tantra—notably in the form of the Sahajîyâ mysticism—and the movement of devotionalism (*bhakti-mârga*). One of its great scions was Jayadeva, the twelfth-century author of the *Gîtâ-Govinda* mentioned above. Two centuries later, it produced the ecstatic poet Candîdâs, who is considered the father of Bengali poetry. His love songs featuring Lord Krishna and his beloved Râdhâ are sung in the Bengali villages to this day.

Candîdâs is also still famous for the scandal he caused when he, a brahmin by birth, fell head over heels in love with the low-born washer maid Râmî. It was this passionate human love that fueled Candîdâs's spiritual poetry, making his poems masterworks of Bhakti-Yoga. He sings of Râdhâ's overwhelming love for Krishna, who makes her tremble with excitement and whose divine flute produces such enchanting music that she cannot seal her ears or shield her heart from the notes. Râdhâ is, of course, a symbol of the poet's own intense passion for the Divine.

In the fifteenth century, Shrî Caitanya, who is counted among the five great preceptors of Vaishnavism, preached the gospel of ecstatic love throughout Bengal. His missionary travels even took him to the extreme South of the Indian peninsula. Though renowned as a Vedânta scholar, Caitanya left a mere eight verses of devotion and instruction to his followers—a composition known as the *Shiksha-Ashtaka.* Caitanya's teaching is the foundation for the contemporary Krishna Consciousness movement, which was established in America in 1965 by the then seventy-year-old Shrila Prabhupada, also known as A. C. Bhaktivedanta Swami (1896–1977).

Shrila Prabhupada belonged to the Bengali Gaudîya lineage that traces its origin back to Madhva and even to early Vedic times. After Madhva and Caitanya, who infused it with the lifeblood of spiritual realization, the greatest luminary of this lineage was his chief disciple, Jîva Gosvâmin. He authored the *Shad-Sandarbha*, which seeks to explain the *Bhâgavata-Purâna* from an esoteric point of view, and the *Tattva-Sandarbha*, which is a philosophical introduction to the former work, as well as twenty-three additional books. The Gaudîya lineage has produced many other works, all of which extol the ideal of *bhakti*.

Many other devotional poets followed in the footsteps of Caitanya and his predecessors. Among them are the Bauls of modern Bengal, who consider themselves madmen (*kshepa*). The name Baul is said to derive from the Sanskrit term *vâtula*, meaning "madness." The Bauls' madness is of the ecstatic variety, and their only concern is to inwardly delight in the presence of the Divine and to outwardly give witness to their love-devotion through song and dance. The Bauls include women ecstatics, notably the twentieth-century "mothers" Anandamayi Ma, Arcanapuri Ma, Lakshmi Ma, and Yogeshvari Ma. The contemporary Western teacher Lee Lozowick also has modeled his lifestyle and teaching after the love-mad eccentric ways of the Bauls.[7]

In India there is also a group of Moslem Bauls, who are known as Auls (from the Arabic word *awliya*, meaning "proximity" to God). The distinction between the Hindu and the Muslim Bauls (who are Sufis) is very

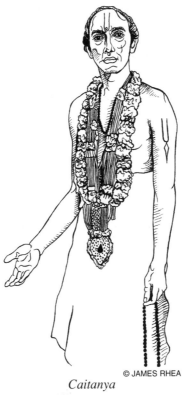

© JAMES RHEA
*Caitanya*

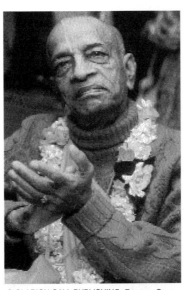

© CLARION CALL PUBLISHING, Eugene, Oregon
*A. C. Bhaktivedanta Swami (Shrila Prabhupada)*

fluid and is even denied altogether by some of them—a fitting demonstration of the essential truth of the *bhakti* movement that the Lord is one and exists for all people.

## VIII. POPULAR LOVE MYSTICISM OF THE NORTH

A portrayal of the *bhakti* movement, however brief, would be incomplete without mentioning the North Indian saints Kabîr, Mîrâ Bâî, Tulsî Dâs, and Sur Dâs, who inspired many generations of pious Hindus with their mystical poetry.

Kabîr, the son of a Muslim weaver, spent his youth in the sacred Hindu city of Benares (Varanasi). His date of birth and year of death are uncertain. Some scholars favor 1398 to 1448 C.E., while others espouse 1440 to 1518 C.E. or similar dates.

Early on, Kabîr cherished recitation (*japa*) of the divine name of Râma, which angered both his fellow Muslims and his Hindu contemporaries. In time, however, Kabîr became a lasting symbol of tolerance. According to one tradition, Kabîr was a disciple of Râmânanda, who was a pupil of the famous South Indian master Râmânuja. It is clear from his poetry, however, that he also was greatly influenced by Sufism, which had taken firm root in India by the beginning of the thirteenth century C.E. This influence is best seen in Kabîr's rejection of all religious images.

Kabîr was a spirited spokesman for simple and direct devotion to the Divine who never failed to point out the inherent limitation of all external or conventional religious forms. He regarded himself as "Râma's wife" or "God's bride," yet he was eager to emphasize that Râma (Hindi: Râm) was not an exclusively Hindu deity. Hence, he used many other names for the Divine in his poetry. For him God was undefinable and unknowable, beyond the reach of doctrines and dogmas. Kabîr insisted, however, that God could be realized within oneself when one knows how to "turn the key to the tenth door." The "tenth door"—as opposed to the nine portals (openings) of the human body through which consciousness flows outward—is located in the middle of the head. This locus also is known as the "third eye."

Kabîr's poetry, written in Hindi, is unsophisticated, yet powerful and penetrating. A large number of his poems and utterances were compiled in 1570 C.E. by one of his followers under the title *Bîjak*. Many of these creations were included in the *Âdi-Granth*, the sacred scripture of the Sikhs, whose spirituality is briefly introduced in Chapter 16.

Another great and much-loved poet-saint of that era is Mîrâ Bâî, a Rajput princess, who probably lived from 1498 to 1546 C.E. Her spiritual aspiration was awakened by the death of her parents and husband in short succession. It led her to adopt the itinerant life of a *bhakti* minstrel. Her chosen deity was Lord

Krishna, in whom she put her faith completely. She pictures herself sporting with him in the mystical region of Vrindâvana as one of his shepherdesses (*gopî*). Rich in imagery and metaphor, Mîrâ Bâî's songs of love-devotion are highly lyrical and designed to awaken in others the same intense longing for Krishna.

A generation later, Tulsî Dâs (1532–1623 C.E.) sang the glory of God in the form of Râma. Followers of Râmânanda rescued him from the life of a street urchin, and he became a much-loved composer of many popular Hindu poems in honor of God Râma. He created a much-celebrated vernacular version of the *Râmâyana* epic, known as the *Râma-Carita-Mânasa* ("Lake of Râma's Life").

A contemporary of Tulsî Dâs and rivaling him in fame was Sur Dâs. Like the Greek Homer he was born blind, yet his love poetry dedicated to Krishna bespeaks his visionary genius. His poetic creations have been collected in the *Sur Sâgar* ("Sur's Ocean"), a massive work containing over five thousand poems in one edition, though several thousand more bear his name. Tradition remembers Sur Dâs as a truly inspired and prolific poet, yet undoubtedly not all the poems ascribed to him are actually from his pen.

Northern India has produced many other poet-saints representing the passionate path of Bhakti-Yoga revolving around the worship of God Vishnu in one of his manifestations—too many inspired poet-saints to mention here individually.

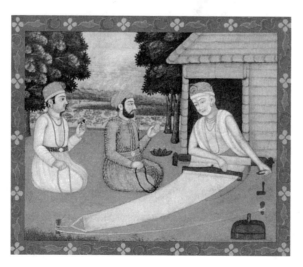

*Kabîr*

> "One should fortify the *Veda* by means of the *Itihâsas* [popular story collections] and the *Purânas*, for the *Veda* shrinks back from the untutored who might damage it."
>
> —*Vâyu-Purâna* (1.201)

# Chapter 13

# YOGA AND *YOGINS* IN THE PURÂNAS

## I. THE NAKED ASCETIC

One upon a time, God Shiva, in the youthful guise of the skull-carrying naked ascetic Kâlabhairava, was wandering in the Devadâru forest. He was accompanied by his spouse Satî and God Vishnu in human form. The forest was inhabited by many saints, seers, and sages and their families. Wherever Kâlabhairava went, the women became so infatuated with him that they ripped off their clothes, touched him, embraced him, and followed him around. The young men were similarly affected by him. The holy men, however, were infuriated by the stranger's outrageous demeanor and his magical effect on their women and sons. They demanded that he cover his genitals and start doing real penance (*tapas*). Using their store of psychic power gathered over decades of fierce austerities, they repeatedly cursed Kâlabhairava. Yet their curses bounced back "like starlight falling upon the sun's brightness," without doing any damage whatsoever. Furious about their failure, they started to beat the naked ascetic with sticks, and he had to flee.

Then Kâlabhairava and his entourage arrived at the hermitage of Sage Vashishtha, where he begged for alms. The sage's wife, Arundhatî, approached the visitor with great reverence, wanting to feed him. But again Kâlabhairava was driven away by the holy men of the area. They shouted after him that he should tear out his penis so that it could not offend people any longer. Without hesitation, Kâlabhairava tore out his genitals—and instantly vanished. Suddenly the entire world was plunged into darkness, and the earth quaked.

At last it dawned on the seers and sages that Kâlabhairava was none other than God Shiva himself, and they were overcome with shame and terror. Upon the advice of Brahma, the Creator of the universe, they sought Shiva's forgiveness by worshiping his symbol (*linga*), the principle of creativity. In due course, Shiva returned to the forest and revealed to the penitent sages the secrets of the Yoga of the Lord of Beasts (*pâshupata-yoga*).

391

This story, which is told in the *Kûrma-Purâna* (chapter 2), is typical of the legendary materials with which the *Purâna* literature abounds. These stories were intended for the ears of the rural folk, and they never failed to entertain and edify, as well as to explain the sacred practices and ideas of those who had dedicated their lives to the pursuit of liberation or paranormal powers, as the case may be.

## II. YOGIC TEACHINGS IN THE PURANIC ENCYCLOPEDIAS

The *Purânas* are popular encyclopedias in the rambling style of the *Mahâbhârata* epic, though they are somewhat more structured. The word *purâna* itself simply means "ancient" and here denotes an age-old narrative; it refers to the contents of these narratives, which deal with the origins of things—from genealogies of royal families to the genealogy of the universe itself. The *Purânas* are a mixture of myth and history, tradition and innovation.

The Puranic lore extends back to Vedic times, when the *Purânas* were still memorized and orally transmitted rather than written down. However, a reference in the *Atharva-Veda* (11.7.24) suggests that already at that early time there might have been written works going by the name of *Purâna*. They are sometimes regarded as a fifth *Veda*, which indicates the high esteem in which they were once held. Originally they were transmitted by storytellers (*suta*) outside the brahmanical orthodox circles, but over the centuries became increasingly the property of brahmin families specializing in their recitation. In some respects, the *Purânas* were to the general public what the *Vedas* and *Brâhmanas* were to the Vedic priestly families. Their mythology depended to some degree on Vedic mythology but followed its own course of evolution; and today, while traditional Hindus scarcely remember the myths and legends of the *Veda*, they are steeped in the richly imaginative world of the Puranic legends.

None of the earliest compositions of this literary genre have survived, but very probably some of their ancient teachings are remembered in the eighteen great *Purânas* that are extant today. The oldest of these texts, however, appear to have been created only in the early centuries of the first millennium C.E. Some—like the important *Bhâgavata-Purâna*—are still later compositions. All of these works undoubtedly contain material from various periods, and all are traditionally said to have been authored by Sage Vyâsa ("Arranger"), who also is credited with having collected the four Vedic *Samhitâs*. According to the *Vishnu-Purâna* (3.6), Vyâsa compiled the so-called *Purâna-Samhitâ* from various ancient tales and then passed it on to his disciple Romaharshana. He, in turn, imparted it to his disciples Kashyapa, Sâvarni, and Shâmsapâyana, each of whom created his own text.

The eighteen *Mahâ* ("Great")-*Purânas*, each of which consists of tens of thousands of verses, are the *Brahma-* (also sometimes referred to as the *Âdi*, "Original")-, *Padma-*, *Vishnu-*, *Vâyu-*, *Bhâgavata-*, *Nârada-*, *Mârkandeya-*, *Agni-*, *Bhavishya-*, *Brahma-Vaivarta-*, *Linga-*, *Varâha-*, *Skanda-*, *Vamâna-*, *Kûrma-*, *Matsya-*, *Garuda-*, and *Brahmânda-Purâna*.

In addition to the *Mahâ-Purânas*, there are also eighteen *Upa* ("Secondary" or "Minor")-*Purânas*, as well as a number of local compositions bearing the title *Purâna*. One of the most significant of these secondary texts is the *Devî-Bhâgavata-Purâna*, which is dedicated to the worship of the great Goddess.

All these works seek to instruct the faithful of the various religious traditions, and they have been most influential in the education of the masses. They purport to deal, ideally, with five principal themes. Usually they start with a mythological account of the creation (*sarga*) of the world. This is followed by a treatment of the world's re-creation (*pratisarga*) after its destruction at the end of a cycle (*kalpa*). A third major topic is the genealogies (*vamsha*) of the seers and deities. Next in sequence of treatment is a mythological account of the cosmic eras called *manvantara* ("Manu interim"). These are the great cycles of existence, each of which has its own Manu, who, like the Hebrew Adam, gives birth to humankind. Lastly, the *Purânas* are supposed to deal with the genealogical histories (*vamsha-anucarita*[1]) of the royal dynasties.

Few *Purânas* conform to this traditional ideal of what are called the "five characteristics" (*panca-lakshana*), and most contain much extraneous matter, including brief treatments of yogic teachings. The types of Yoga discussed differ greatly, but they all tend to be integrally connected with the worship of particular deities, primarily Vishnu and Shiva. Not surprisingly, therefore, most of these teachings have a ritual character, though some texts offer a more contemplative type of Yoga.

The *Brahma-Purâna* deals with Yoga in Chapter 235 (stanzas 4–29). Here we can read that practitioners should first lovingly venerate their teacher and study the yogic scriptures as well as achieve competence in the *Vedas, Purânas,* and *Itihâsas* (histories). Then, after acquainting themselves with the dietary rules, the proper time and place for practice, and the faults (*dosha*) on the yogic path, they should begin the practice of Yoga (*yoga-abhyâsa*), transcending greed and the pairs of opposites (*dvandva*).

Practitioners are advised to avoid practicing with a distracted mind or when they are weary or hungry, or when it is too cold, too hot, or too windy. They should also avoid places that are too noisy or too close to water or fire, a dilapidated cow pen, crossroads, a place infested with crawling creatures, a cemetery, a river bank, a monastery, an anthill, a well, a spot covered with dry leaves, or an otherwise dangerous place. Those who ignore this advice are warned that they might encounter a variety of difficulties, including deafness, blindness, heaviness, loss of memory, dumbness, sluggishness, and fever. Suitable locations are a hermitage (*âshrama*), a vacant building in a quiet town free from fear, or an isolated, pure, and delightful temple.

The best times for practicing Yoga are said to be the morning, noon, or the first or last *yâma* (three hours) of the night. Practitioners are further advised to sit on a seat that is neither too high nor too low, and facing east. At all times, they should keep the body from head to toes in an even posture. The recommended posture is the lotus posture (*padma-âsana*, written *padmâsana*), which entails gazing at the tip of the nose with half-closed eyes. The eyes should be closed for meditation, however, and the favored procedure is meditation by means of the sacred syllable *om*. This involves placing the organs of action, the cognitive organs, and the five elements in the "knower of the field" (*kshetra-jna*), which is the universal Self as it resides in the finite body-mind (called the "field" or *kshetra*).

Those who become competent at this will be able to withdraw their senses as a turtle withdraws its limbs. Success in Yoga comes to those who abandon all sense objects and find the supreme Absolute, which is the pure *purusha-uttama* (written *purushottama*), the unsurpassable Spirit. This is also called the "fourth" (*turya*), which transcends the three states of waking, dreaming, and sleeping. In stanza 235.28, Yoga is defined as "the union of the mind and the senses [with the Self]" (*manasash ca indriyânâm ca samyogah*).

The *Padma* ("Lotus")-*Purâna*, for instance, has an appendix to its last book, entitled "The Essence of the Ritual Yoga" (*Kriyâ-Yoga-Sâra*), which recommends that Vishnu should be worshiped not through meditation (*dhyâna*) but through prayers and sacrificial rites. In contrast, the *Vishnu* ("Pervader")-*Purâna*, which deals with Yoga in its short sixth book, understands Yoga as the path of meditation. The only object fit to be contemplated is Vishnu, who alone grants eternal freedom.

The *Vâyu* ("Wind")-*Purâna*, in its concluding chapters, introduces Yoga as a means of attaining "Shiva's city" (*shiva-pura*), which corresponds to the Vaishnava notion of *vaikuntha*, Vishnu's heavenly domain. Its particular approach is styled *mâheshvara-yoga*, meaning "Yoga of the great (*mahâ*) Lord (*îshvara*)." It consists of five elements (*dharma*): breath control (*prânâyâma*), meditation (*dhyâna*), sensory inhibition (*pratyâhâra*), concentration (*dhâranâ*), and recollection (*smarana*). Breath control, again, is of three degrees. The mild variety involves breath retention of twelve units (*mâtrâ*), the middle variety twenty-four, and the superior variety thirty-six. Full control of the life force obliterates all sins and bodily imperfections. Breath control leads to peace (*shânti*), tranquillity (*prashânti*), luminosity (*dîpti*), and clarity-grace (*prasâda*). Peace washes away the sins of one's fathers; tranquillity neutralizes personal sins; luminosity refers to vision of the past, present, and future; clarity-grace is the state of perfect contentment obtained through pacification of the senses and the mind, together with the five kinds of life force in the body. Sensory inhibition is here understood as the control of one's desires, by which the influence of the external reality is overcome. Meditation reveals oneself to be as luminous as the sun. It produces the various supernormal powers, which are called "obstacles" (*upasargas*) and should be avoided. Everything in the realm of Nature can become an object of meditation, and the *yogin* is advised to meditate on the seven categories of existence one after the other and then leave them behind. The seven categories consist of the five elements, the lower mind (*manas*), and the higher mind (*buddhi*). Through the nonattachment gained from this practice, the *yogin* becomes able to focus exclusively on the Lord, Maheshvara, and thereby achieve the ultimate goal of liberation (*apavarga*).

The *Bhâgavata-Purâna*, which is replete with yogic materials, was briefly discussed in Chapter 2 in connection with Bhakti-Yoga, and was more fully treated in Chapter 12. Its *Uddhâva-Gîtâ* (see Source Reading 14) is an inspiring Yoga text for those pursuing the path of devotion.

The *Linga* ("Distinguishing Mark")-*Purâna* introduces yogic concepts in Chapters 7–9. The term *linga* is often translated as "phallus," but really it stands for the cosmic creative principle, which is the distinguishing mark of the Divine in the form of Shiva. According to legend, when Brahma and Vishnu sought to determine the extent of Shiva's *linga*, they could not find its beginning or end. As Shiva himself explains in the *Linga-Purâna* (1.19.16), the *linga* is so called because at the end of time everything becomes dissolved (*lîyate*) in it.

In the eighth chapter of this *Purâna*, the eightfold Yoga, as first outlined by Patanjali, is said to arise from wisdom (*jnâna*), which is given by grace. Discipline (*yama*) is defined as abstention by way of austerity. Under self-restraint (*niyama*), the following ten practices are listed: cleanliness (*shauca*), sacrifice (*ijyâ*), asceticism (*tapas*), charity (*dâna*), study (*svâdhyâya*), control of the sexual organ (*upastha-nigraha*), ritual (*vrata*), fasting (*upavâsa*), silence (*mauna*), and bathing (*snâna*). Alternatively, self-restraint is said to consist in noncraving (*anîhâ*), cleanliness, contentment (*tushti*), asceticism, recitation (*japa*) of Shiva's name, and postures (*âsana*).

Sensory inhibition, again, is explained as dedication (*pranidhâna*) to Shiva in body, mind, and speech and unflinching devotion to one's preceptor, as well as withdrawal of the senses from the external world. Concentration is fixation of the mind on an appropriate locus, while meditation is a natural product of concentration. Ecstasy is the state in which the supreme Consciousness alone shines forth as if there were no body.

> "By means of exhalation in conjunction with the syllable *hûm*, the teacher [should gently] strike [the disciple's] chest with a flower and enter into the disciple's body."
>
> —*Agni-Purâna* 83.12

Breath control is regarded as the root of the higher states. The mild degree of breath control is defined as twelve moments forming a single "stroke" (*udghâta*), the middle degree two such "strokes," and the superior degree three. At each level of practice, breath control causes various symptoms, including sweating, shivering, dizziness, horripilation, and even levitation. As in many medieval Yoga texts, breath control is described as being of two basic types: *sagarbha* and *agarbha*, or "with seed" and "without seed." Here the term *garbha* refers to *mantra* recitation.

In its ninth chapter, the *Linga-Purâna* gives a long list of obstacles and omens. The former include the paranormal powers (*siddhi*), which manifest when Yoga practice is pursued with vigor. Chapter 88 offers a review of this *pâshupata-yoga*; the author of the *Linga-Purâna* claims that only this type of Yoga can yield the eight great paranormal powers, here called *aishvarya*.

The *Kûrma* ("Tortoise")-*Purâna*, named after Vishnu's incarnation as a tortoise, contains many fascinating myths about Vishnu, but also about Shiva. In its second part, we find two well-known *Bhagavad-Gîtâ* "imitations"—the *Îshvara-Gîtâ* and the longer *Vyâsa-Gîtâ*. The former didactic song has a detailed commentary by the philosopher-*yogin* Vijnâna Bhikshu, who even felt that since this text contains all the salient ideas of the *Bhagavad-Gîtâ*, he could dispense with a commentary on it.

The *Agni* ("Fire")-*Purâna*, a massive but late work that is more encyclopedic in character than the other *Purânas*, contains extensive information about rituals, including *mantra* recitation, *mudrâs* (hand gestures), the construction of *yantras* (mystic diagrams similar to the circular *mandalas*), and *prânâyâma* (ritual breath control). Patanjali's eightfold Yoga is explained in Chapters 352–358.

An important place is assigned to Yoga in the *Garuda* ("Eagle")-*Purâna*, which dedicates three whole chapters (viz. 14, 49, and 118) to the eightfold path. This Vaishnava scripture was probably created in its present form around 900 C.E. It defines *tapas* as sense control rather than penance, and it mentions only two meditation postures: the lotus posture and the bound lotus posture (*baddha-padma-âsana*[2]). Concentration, again, is said to be of the duration of eighteen cycles of breath control, whereas meditation is twice that long, and the unbroken chain of ten cycles of concentration leads to ecstasy (*samâdhi*). This text also refers to Bhakti-Yoga and to Tantric Yoga.

The voluminous *Shiva-Purâna* deals with Yoga in different places. Thus, in Chapter 17 of the first book, the Yoga of mantric recitation is introduced. 1,080,000,000 repetitions of the sacred *mantra om* are said to lead to the mastery of "purified Yoga" (*shuddha-yoga*), which is synonymous with liberation. The text further explains that *shiva-yogins* are of three types. First there is the *kriyâ-yogin*, who engages in sacred rites (*kriyâ*), and then there is the *tapo-yogin*, who pursues asceticism (*tapas*). Last there is the *japa-yogin*, who observes the practices of the other two types, but who in addition constantly recites the holy five-syllabled *mantra* "Om, obeisance to Shiva" (*om namah shivâya*).

Yoga makes its appearance again in Chapters 37–39 of the concluding book of the *Shiva-Purâna*, where it is defined as the restraint of all activities, and mental concentration upon Shiva. Five types or degrees are distinguished:

1. Mantra-Yoga is the focusing of attention by means of the sacred five-syllabled invocation of Shiva (mentioned above).

2. Sparsha-Yoga ("Contact Yoga") is Mantra-Yoga coupled with the control of the life force (*prânâyâma*).

3. Bhâva-Yoga ("Yoga of Being") is a higher form of Mantra-Yoga, where contact with the mantra is lost and consciousness enters a subtle dimension of existence.

4. Abhâva-Yoga ("Yoga of Non-being") is the practice of meditation upon the universe in its entirety, associated with the transcendence of object-related awareness.

5. Mahâ-Yoga ("Great Yoga") is the contemplation of Shiva without any restricting conditions.

The *Mârkandeya-Purâna*, which derives its name from Sage Mârkandeya, a central figure in this narrative, belongs to the fourth or fifth century C.E. and is deemed one of the oldest texts of this genre. It speaks of Yoga in Chapters 36–43 and addresses in detail the qualities of an individual suited for Yoga, and also the environmental conditions necessary for success in its practice. The body is recognized as an important instrument on the spiritual path. This *Purâna*, moreover, offers an original measure for assessing yogic perfection: There should be no fear in the *yogin* toward other beings, and other beings should not fear him.

*Yogins* are subdivided according to the prevalence of one of the three primary constituents (*guna*) of Nature. They are also distinguished by their achievement on the path. Thus, at the *bhrama* ("roaming") stage, the *yogin*'s mind is fickle, impeding his progress. At the *prâtibha* ("understanding") stage, the *yogin* comprehends all the sacred scriptures and other branches of knowledge. At the *shravana* ("listening") stage, he understands the significance of the different realms of existence. At the *daiva* ("divine") stage, he perceives higher beings, such as the deities (*deva*).

Lastly, the *Devî-Bhâgavata-Purâna* of the Vaishnavas, which almost resembles a *Tantra*, is a repository of spiritual wisdom relating to Goddess worship. It too includes sections about Yoga. What makes this work, which was probably composed in the thirteenth century C.E., particularly interesting is its high appraisal of the female gender. This is given the authority of tradition in a legend according to which Brahma, Vishnu, and Shiva had to be transmuted into women before they could behold Devî in her supreme form. As is known from the context of actual Tantric ritual, female initiates (called *bhairavîs*) once played a signal role in the transmission of Tantric teachings.

Indeed, from one perspective, the *kundalinî-shakti* can be seen as an internalized symbol of the initiatory function of these female adepts. The technical term *kundalinî* is, in fact, a feminine word, and so is the term *sushumnâ*, which refers to the axial pathway through which the *kundalinî* power surges upward into the psychoenergetic center at the crown of the head. According to the *Devî-Bhâgavata*, like other Tantric scriptures, the seven psychoenergetic centers strung like pearls on the axial pathway are all associated with female deities. The Yoga of this *Upa-Purâna*, not surprisingly, integrates love and devotion with the psychotechnology characteristic of the Tantric approach.

Thus, the *Purânas* contain records of, and references to, a variety of yogic schools. Some of these schools follow, more or less strictly, Patanjali's model of the eightfold path, though occasionally they interpret the eight limbs differently from that great Yoga authority. What distinguishes them most markedly from Patanjali's tradition, however, is that they all propose a single ultimate principle, the Self or God.

Puranic Yoga has been little researched, though fortunately all the major *Purânas* are available in more or less reliable English translations, and other texts of this literary genre continue to be rendered into English under the Indian Translation Series program, which is jointly sponsored by the government of India and UNESCO. When completed, the "Ancient Indian Tradition & Mythology Series," translated by a board of scholars and published by Motilal Banarsidass in Delhi, will comprise one hundred volumes. The fund of myths and legends preserved in these scriptures is a perennial inspiration to the Yoga student.

---

**SOURCE READING 15**

## *The Mârkandeya-Purâna (Selection)*

The following excerpt is from the fortieth chapter of the *Mârkandeya-Purâna*, where Sage Dattâtreya instructs his disciple Alarka. It conveys a sense of the ritualized nature of this yogic teaching.

He should set his foot only after [the path in front of him] has been purified by the eye. He should drink only water filtered through cloth, only utter words purified by truth, and only think of what has been purified completely by wisdom (*buddhi*). (4)

The knower of Yoga should nowhere be a guest, and he should not participate in ancestor worship, sacrifices, pilgrimages to [the shrines of] deities, and festivals. He also should not mix with the crowd for purposes of demonstration. (5)

The knower of Yoga should wander about begging [his daily sustenance] and live off what he finds in the refuse. [He should beg] at places where no smoke arises [from the hearth], where the coal is extinguished, and among all those who have already eaten, but also not continually among these three. (6)

Since the crowd despises and mocks him because of this, the *yogin* should, yoked [in Yoga], tread the path of the virtuous, [so that he might] not be tarnished. (7)

He should seek alms among the householders and the huts of mendicant monks: Their mode of life is considered the foremost and best. (8)

The ascetic (*yati*) should furthermore also always stay [close to] the pious, self-controlled, and magnanimous householders versed in the *Vedas*. (9)

In addition [he should stay close to] the innocent and non-outcastes. Begging among the casteless is the lowest mode of life that he could wish. (10)

The begged food [may consist of] gruel, diluted buttermilk or milk, barley broth, fruit, roots, millet, corn, oil-cake, or groats. (11)

And these are pleasant eatables that support the *yogin*'s [struggle for] perfection (*siddhi*). The sage should turn to them with devotedness and highest concentration (*samâdhi*). (12)

After first having drunk water, he should collect himself silently. Then he should [offer] the first oblation to the [life force] called *prâna*. (13)

The second [oblation] should be to *apâna*, the next to *samâna*, the fourth to *udâna*, and the fifth to *vyâna*. (14)[3]

After having completed one oblation after the other, [all the while practicing] the restraint of the life force (*prâna*) [through controlled breathing], he may then enjoy the remainder to his heart's content. Taking again water and rinsing, he should touch his heart [i.e., chest]. (15)

Nonstealing, chastity, dispassion, absence of greed, and nonharming are the five most important vows of the mendicant (*bhikshu*). (16)

Absence of wrath, obedience toward the teacher, purity, moderation in eating, sustained study—these are the five well-known [forms of] self-restraint (*niyama*). (17)

Above all, [the *yogin*] should dedicate himself to knowledge that leads to the goal. The multiplicity of knowledge as it exists here [on Earth] is an obstacle to Yoga. (18)

He who seized-by-thirst (*trishita*) dashes along [in the belief that he must] know this or that will not even in a thousand eons obtain that which is to be known, [namely the ultimate Reality]. (19)

Abandoning society, curbing wrath, eating moderately, and controlling the senses, he should block the gates [of the body] by means of wisdom (*buddhi*) and let the mind come to rest in meditation. (20)

That *yogin* who is yoked incessantly should always practice meditation in empty rooms, in caves, and in the forest. (21)

Control of speech, control of action, and control of the mind—these are the three [masteries]. He who [practices] these restraints unfailingly is a mighty "triple-restraint" ascetic. (22)

"Upon hearing, considering, and understanding this [*Yoga-Vâsishtha*], asceticism, meditation, and recitation are superfluous. What more does a man require for the attainment of liberation?"

*—Yoga-Vâsishtha* (2.18.36)

# *Chapter 14*
# THE YOGIC IDEALISM OF THE YOGA-VÂSISHTHA

## *I. OVERVIEW*

Whatever is in this [book] is also [to be found] in others, but what is not in it will also not [be found] elsewhere. Hence the learned know this [work] as the treasury of all philosophical learning. (3.8.12)

Thus announces proudly the composer of the *Yoga-Vâsishtha-Râmâyana*, a philosophical work of about 27,687 verses (though tradition mentions a total of 32,000) written in the finest poetic Sanskrit. The author—whom tradition fancifully identifies with Vâlmîki, the creator of the *Râmâyana* epic—is poet, philosopher, psychologist, and *yogin* in one person. In the form of an imaginary dialogue between the ancient hero Râmacandra and his teacher Vashishtha,[1] Vâlmîki presents an abundance of ideas, stories, and experiences that show a rare depth and universality of outlook.

The original and now lost version of the *Yoga-Vâsishtha* was probably composed in the eighth century C.E., and in the ninth century it was fashioned into the still extant *Laghu* ("Small")-*Yoga-Vâsishta* by Gauda Abhinanda, consisting of 4,829 verses (though tradition speaks of 6,000 verses). The full version was created some time in the tenth century C.E. In its various forms, Vâlmîki's work has exercised considerable influence on Yoga and Vedânta theory and practice. It has been translated into a number of Indian vernaculars, notably Hindi and Urdu, and it also has several commentaries and summaries. Thus, the fourteenth-century Vedânta philosopher Vidyâranya quotes no fewer than 253 verses from it in his famous *Jîvan-Mukti-Viveka*, and he also compiled the *Yoga-Vâsishtha-Sâra-Samgraha*, which consists of some 2,300 verses. There also is a 225- or 230-verse abridgment known as the *Yoga-Vâsishtha-Sâra* by an unknown authority. The modern saint Ram Tirtha called the *Yoga-Vâsishtha* "one of the greatest books, and the most wonderful according to me, ever written under the sun . . . which nobody on earth can read without realizing God-consciousness."[2]

## II. MIND ONLY— THE IDEALISTIC APPROACH

The philosophy of the *Yoga-Vâsishtha* is radically nondualist. The fundamental thesis of this scripture, reiterated innumerable times, is that there is only Consciousness (*citta*). This Consciousness is omnipresent, omniscient, and formless. Sage Vashishtha also refers to it as the Absolute (*brahman*), stating that just as the mind of a painter is filled with numerous images of a great variety of objects, so the pure Consciousness is suffused with the images of the multiple forms of Nature—an idea that we also encounter in the teaching of the Christian mystic Meister Eckehart. Vashishtha defines the Absolute as follows:

> It is the Self (*purusha*) of volition (*samkalpa*), devoid of physical form such as earth [and the other material elements]. It is singular (*kevala*), Consciousness only, the essential cause of the existence of the triple universe.[3] (3.3.11)

The phenomenal world is but a reflection of that universal Mind. It *is* that Mind. The experienced objects are simply an idea (*kalpanâ*) conjured by the Mind, as are the objects populating our dreams. Space and time, too, are imaginary products of the Mind. We fail to realize this truth merely on account of spiritual ignorance (*avidyâ*), which has us in its grip. When the *yogin* enters the unifying state of ecstasy (*samâdhi*), space evaporates and time stands still.

The world is neither real nor unreal. It is situated in Consciousness but appears to the unenlightened mind as something external. It is like a dream, or a bubble rising in the absolute Consciousness. Once it is understood that the world we perceive is "our" world, "our" creation, and that bondage and freedom are states of mind, the next step is to break down the habit of wrong conceptualization. The mind (*manas*) itself must be transcended.

This philosophy is best characterized as a form of idealism in which Brahma, standing for the Cosmic Mind, is the generator of all ideas under whose spell we fall as long as we do not recognize our true nature as the singular Self.

The spiritual path outlined in the *Yoga-Vâsishtha* is essentially that of Jnâna-Yoga, and it has great similarity with the Buddhi-Yoga taught in the *Bhagavad-Gîtâ*, wherein action and knowledge are blended harmoniously. Vashishtha disdains the kind of asceticism that is performed with an empty mind or that is attended with pain. The genuine *yogin*, according to him, is free from the push and pull of passionate attraction on the one side and hostile rejection on the other. Such a *yogin* looks at a lump of gold and a pile of rubbish with the same unperturbed mind.

According to Vashishtha, it is the human mind alone—spellbound by the Mind of the Creator-God—that creates the illusion of bondage or the reality of liberation. There is, therefore, no point in external renunciation. Rather, what is needed is a total *inner* reorientation. He calls this doctrine "mental liberation" (*cetya-nirmuktatâ*). Yoga is variously defined by him as "the restriction of the fluctuations of the mind," "nonemotionality" (*avedanâ*), and "separation from the effects of the poison of passion." In contrast with the teaching of the God-man Krishna, which emphasizes our emotional capacities in the form of devotion (*bhakti*), Vashishtha stresses the cognitive side of our psychic life. He has little patience, however, with those who are merely interested in intellectual gyrations without proper application in life. The knowledge he deems useful is wisdom, or real insight, that leads to illumination.

Thus, the author of the *Yoga-Vâsishtha* seeks, in ever new ingenious phrases and metaphors, to evoke in his readers the conviction that they are absolutely in charge of their own destiny, if only they can see the trick the human mind is playing on them. Destiny (*daiva*) is a formidable force, but human effort (*paurusha*)—literally "manliness"—is superior to it.

According to one passage (6.13), Yoga consists of both Self-knowledge (*âtma-jnâna*) and the restriction (*samrodha*) of the life force (*prâna*). The former is the path of meditative absorption; the latter approach may be identified with Kundalinî-Yoga, involving the arousal of the Consciousness-Energy hidden in the body.

Both the mind and the life force are said to be most intimately associated. The stoppage of the one leads to the cessation of the other. By "mind" (*manas*), Vashishtha means the ego-consciousness, which projects its own world through the process of imaginative volition (*samkalpa*), propelled by the force of root desire (*vâsanâ*). He compares the mind to a madman with a thousand hands, who constantly beats himself, inflicting pain on his body. The mind is galvanized by the vibration (*spanda*, *parispanda*) of the life force circulating in the body, while the life force is impelled by primal desire (*vâsanâ*). Control of the quivering of the life force is the most direct means of quieting the mind and transcending the compelling force of desire. But Vashishtha also recommends concentration and meditation as superb aids for taking charge of the mind.

## III. THE YOGIC PATH

Vashishtha's Yoga comprises the following seven stages (*bhûmi*):[4]

1. *Shubha-icchâ* ("desire for what is good," written *Shubheccâ*): A person becomes aware of his or her spiritual ignorance and state of suffering and begins to desire to know the truth through the study of the traditional lore.

2. *Vicâranâ* ("consideration"): Through the deepening of study and contact with holy people, the practitioner's conduct improves, and his or her desire for liberation is kindled.

3. *Tanu-mânasâ* ("refinement of thinking"): This stage is characterized by a growing sense of indifference to the things of the world.

4. *Sattva-âpatti* ("attainment of being," written *sattvâpatti*): The practitioner becomes capable of getting in touch with pure Consciousness through meditation.

5. *Asamsakti* ("nonattachment"): By virtue of true illumination, the mature practitioner becomes perfectly indifferent to the world, which is recognized as being a mere production of the mind.

6. *Pada-artha-abhâvanâ* ("nonimagining of external things," written *padârthâbhâvanâ*): The world is recognized to be unreal like a dream.

7. *Turya-gâ* ("abiding in the Fourth"): The *yogin* transcends everything and remains perpetually in pure Consciousness, which is called the "Fourth" (*turya*, *turîya*, *caturtha*), as in Upanishadic Vedânta, since it transcends the

states of waking, sleeping, and dreaming.

*Yogins* who have realized the Fourth, or the Self, are liberated even while the body-mind continues to exist. This is the ideal of "living liberation" (*jîvan-mukti*). Because they are no longer ensnared by the ego-illusion, they can be all things to all people, reflecting people's own states of mind, but themselves living in perpetual bliss.

Enlightenment is ego-transcendence in every moment, regardless of whether the body-mind is active or in a state of repose. Vashishtha relates the story of King Bhagîratha, who abandoned his kingdom in order to dedicate himself to spiritual life. After years of meditation at a remote place, Bhagîratha attained enlightenment. One day he happened to wander through his former kingdom, and when the people recognized him they begged him to accept the throne again, as his successor had just died. Because nothing can bind a Self-realized adept, Bhagîratha accepted and for many years ruled over his people, bringing justice and wisdom into their lives.

The *Yoga-Vâsishtha* is a truly remarkable creation, which has had a strong influence on the more literate community of Yoga and Vedânta practitioners of medieval India. It is a lasting monument to the wisdom of nondualism.

---

**SOURCE READING 16**

## *Yoga-Vâsishtha (Selection)*

The following is a complete rendering of Chapter 53 of the sixth book of the *Yoga-Vâsishtha*. Chapters 53–58 form what is known as the *Brahma-Gîtâ*, which is modeled on the *Bhagavad-Gîtâ*. The context is the same as that given in the *Bhagavad-Gîtâ*: Arjuna is facing his kinfolk on the battlefield. He is despondent and refuses to fight lest he kill his relatives and teachers on the enemy's side. But the God-man Krishna, Arjuna's teacher and charioteer, reprimands him for this faulty attitude. He argues that Arjuna's dilemma springs from spiritual ignorance (*avidyâ*), on account of which he experiences himself as a limited egoic being rather than the omnipresent Self.

Krishna insists that Arjuna should fight because he is fighting for the maintenance of the moral order of the universe, and because it is his duty as a member of the warrior estate to do so. Death, Krishna declares, only affects the body. Our true nature is immortal. The transcendental Self (*âtman*) cannot be slain. It is the only Reality there is. All objects that appear to the unenlightened mind actually arise in and as that singular Being-Consciousness.

The Blessed Lord [Krishna] said:

Arjuna! You are not the slayer [of your kinfolk]. Give up the impurity of the self-will (*abhimâna*). You are the eternal Self itself, free from senescence and death. (1)

He who has no ego-sense (*ahamkrita-bhâva*) and whose mind (*buddhi*) is not stained, even if he were to destroy the worlds, he does not slay nor is he bound. (2)

Whatever arises in consciousness, that is experienced within [as pleasure or pain]. Give up the inner consciousness of "I am he, this, that." (3)

O Bharata [i.e., Arjuna]! [The thought] "I am connected with such-and-such" or "I have lost [such-and-such]" [merely] torments you, subjecting you to joy and sorrow all round. (4)

Performing actions severally through [the force of] the constituents (*guna*) [of Nature] and with [only] a fragment (*amsha*) of the Self, the Self deluded by the "I-maker" (*ahamkâra*) [begins to] think "I am the doer." (5)

Let the eye see, the ear hear, the skin sense, and the tongue taste [of things]: This is the state [in which one asks] "What is there?" and "Who am I?" (6)

When there is a prompting for action or for pleasure in the mind of a great-souled [adept], there is no "I" (*aham*) in this. What is your [ego] in [your present] share of trouble (*klesha*)? (7)

O Bhârata! [Action], which is accomplished by a combination of many [factors], is [the product] of the plight (*duhkha*) of a single self-will (*abhimâna*) and is performed for pleasure. (8)

Shunning attachment, *yogins* perform actions [without self-investment, but] merely with the body, the mind (*manas*), the wisdom faculty (*buddhi*), or the isolated senses, and for the purification of the self. (9)

Those whose body is not subdued by the antidote [lit. "nonpoisonous powder"] to the "I" while they are acting or even slaying—they cannot [cure their malady of spiritual] indigestion. (10)

[For him who is] defiled by the impure [idea of] "mineness" toward the body, Consciousness (*cit*) does not shine forth. Even though he may be wise and very learned, he is like an ill-bred person. (11)

He who is patient, devoid of [the idea of] "mine" and "I," the same in joy and sorrow, he, though performing obligatory and nonobligatory [actions], is not stained [by his deeds]. (12)

O Pândava [i.e., Arjuna]! The excellent innate duty (*sva-dharma*) of the warrior, though [apparently] cruel, is for your highest good, joy, and prosperity. (13)

Though [you may deem it] a blameworthy as well as an unlawful course of action, it is [really] the best for you. Be the immortal here [on Earth], just as [you carry out your allotted] work. (14)

[To do] one's duty is good even for the ignorant, how much more for the truly understanding [person]. The understanding [person, from whom] the "I-maker" has slipped away, is not stained even on failing [to do his duty perfectly]. (15)

Abiding in Yoga, perform actions while giving up [all] attachment, O Dhanamjaya! When you perform actions as necessary, while remaining unattached, you are not bound [by them]. (16)

With the body [subdued like] the tranquil Absolute (*brahman*), perform actions conforming to the Absolute. [When your] conduct is an offering to the Absolute, you become the Absolute in an instant. (17)

With every purpose (*artha*) offered up to the Lord (*îshvara*), having the Lord as [your very] Self, free from ill, [recognize] the Lord as the Self of all beings—thus be an adornment to the surface of the earth. (18)

With all volition (*samkalpa*) cast off, an equable, tranquil-minded sage, performing [actions] with the self yoked through the Yoga of renunciation—thus cultivate a liberated mind. (19)

Arjuna said:

O Lord! What is the nature of abandoning attachment, of offering [one's actions] to the Absolute, of the form of offering to the Lord, and of renunciation in general? (20)

Likewise, [what is the nature] of wisdom and Yoga? O Lord, this relate to me step by step to remove my great delusion (*moha*) [about reality]. (21)

The Blessed Lord said:

When all volition is appeased, the mass of desires (*vâsanâ*) are pacified as well. The form (*âkâra*), [for which there is] no conception (*bhâvanâ*) whatsoever, is known as the supreme Absolute. (22)

Application (*udyoga*) toward That the mature-minded (*krita-buddhi*) know to be wisdom and Yoga. "The Absolute is the whole world as well as the 'I' (*aham*)"—[this realization] is known as the offering to the Absolute. (23)

Like the chest of a stone[-sculpture], which is void inside and void outside, [the Absolute] is tranquil, lucid as the vault of the sky, neither to be seen nor beyond vision. (24)

The slight bulge [of the hollow statue] appears as other [than what it is]: It is the reflection of the world that, like the ether-space (*âkâsha*), is [mere] voidness (*shûnyatâ*). (25)

*Comments:* This somewhat obscure stanza tries to make the point that the apparent external world is void, that is, the formless transcendental Reality.

What is this [idea that] "I exist"? Every single [being and thing] has arisen from Consciousness (*citi*). Who is the "recipient" (*pratigraha*) who is, as it were, a minutest[5] fragment [of the Absolute]? (26)

This [ego-"recipient"] is not a separate entity [apart from the Absolute], [although] it appears to be a separate entity. Separation cannot be a [real] limitation, [and hence] one realizes that there is no "I." (27)

As with the "I," so it is with a pot, etc., or even a monkey, or the ocean, or one's desires. What about the "recipient" of egoism? (28)

When conceptual distinctions, whether manifold through variety or singular, are presented to the Self, [which is of] the essence of Consciousness (*samvid*), how can there be a grasper? (29)

Thus [comes about] the cessation of the apperceived distinctions in one's mind. Casting off the fruit of one's actions the sages know as renunciation (*samnyâsa*). (30)

Casting off the nets of volition is called nonattachment, or the contemplation (*bhâ-vanâ*) of the one Lordship (*îshvaratva*) of the whole net of [Nature's] promptings. (31)

[The mind] shining forth without duality is [what is meant by] offering up to the Lord. By the force of the unillumined (*abodha*) [mind], the Consciousness-Self is named [i.e., conceived] differently. (32)

It is said that the meaning of the words "awakened self" is undoubtedly the one world. The "I" is space; the "I" is the world; the "I" is oneself, and also the "I" is activity (*kar-man*). (33)

The "I" is time; the "I" is dual and non-dual; the "I" is the world. Be devoted to Me, love Me, worship Me, salute Me. Having thus restrained the self by being dedicated to Me, you will seek Me out. (34)

*Comments:* Here Vâlmîki switches to a transcendental perspective. The "Me" is not the finite ego but the "I Am" of the Divine.

Arjuna said:

O Lord! You have two forms, a higher and a lower one. When and to which form shall I resort [in order to attain ultimate] perfection? (35)

The Blessed Lord said:

O sinless one! Know that there are indeed two forms of Me, a common and a higher one. The common [form is that which] is endowed with hands, etc., holding the conch, discus, and club. (36)

My higher form is infinite. It is single, free from ill. This is designated by the words "Absolute," "Self," "supreme Self," etc. (37)

As long as you are unenlightened and occupied with knowledge about the nonself [i.e., the world], you should be fond of worshiping God in his four-armed shape. (38)

In this way you become fully enlightened. Then you will know that higher [form of Mine]. [Through the realization] of My infinite form, one is not born again. (39)

O crusher of the enemy! That condition where the Unknowable is known, that is My Self. Quickly resort to the Self and for the Self! (40)

When I say "I am this [world] and this [world] is me," then I teach you this [from the viewpoint] of the Self's reality in order to instruct you. (41)

I deem you wide awake. You are reposing in the Condition [of Truth]. You are free from [all] volitions. Realize that you are of the nature of the one true Self! (42)

Behold the Self abiding in all beings and all beings in the Self. You are the Self [which is ever] yoked in Yoga, seeing the same everywhere. (43)

He who worships the Self abiding in all beings as the singularity (ekatva) of the Self, even though variously active, he is not born again. (44)

The [true] meaning of the word "all" is "singularity"; the [true] meaning of the word "one" is [the "oneness"] of the Self. For him who has swiftly vanished in [the Self], that Self neither exists nor does not exist. (45)

He who shines as the [luminous] space (loka) between the "minds" of the three worlds, he surely ascends to the experience "I am the Self." (46)

Comments: Here the transcendental Self is likened to the radiant interstices between the worlds of earthbound existence, the psychic "ether," and the heavenly realms. The metaphor of space is common among the Hindu mystics. The word loka, standing for "world" or "space," is probably derived from the stem ruc, meaning "to shine, be resplendent."

He who, in the three worlds, is the "taste experience" of the milk of cows and sea creatures, he is this Self, O Bhârata! (47)

Comments: Milk is considered a highly desirable food by yogins. The transcendental Self is here compared to the delicious taste of milk, since it nourishes and sustains all.

He who is the subtle experience in all bodies, by which one is to be released, he is this omnipresent Self. (48)

Just as there is butter in every [kind of] milk, similarly the Supreme abides in the bodies of all things. (49)

Just as the luster of all [kinds of] gems and treasures of the sea [shines] within and without, so I am in [all] bodies, abiding [in them, and yet] seemingly not abiding [in them]. (50)

Just as space is inside and outside thousands of pots, so I abide as the Self in the bodies of the three worlds. (51)

Just as a thread strung with a mass of hundreds of pearls [is concealed but nevertheless present], so does this invisible Self abide in the visible bodies [of all beings]. (52)

That which is the universal Being (*sattâ*) in the multitude of things—from [the Creator-God] Brahma down to a blade of grass—know that to be the unborn Self. (53)

[The Creator-God] Brahma is a slightly vibrating form of the Absolute (*brahman*), [which emerges] because of delusion (*bhrama*) by a process [that establishes] the egoity (*ahamtâ*), etc., as well as the world (*jagattâ*), etc. (54)

Since the Self is of the form of this [entire] world, what can destroy it, and [what can] it destroy here? How can one, O Arjuna, be defiled by the misery of the world, by good or evil? (55)

Abiding as a witness, [the Self is] like a mirror toward its reflections. He who sees that it is indestructible among destructible [things], he [truly] sees. (56)

I explain that I am this [world] and yet also not this [world]: Thus I am the Self. Know Me to be the Self of everything, O Pândava. (57)

All these processes of creation and dissolution occur in the Self. The egoity (*ahamtâ*) abiding in the [finite] consciousness (*citta*) is like the water moving in the ocean. (58)

Like the solidity of stones, or the hardness of Earth's trees, or the liquidity of waves, so is the Selfhood (*âtmatâ*) of things. (59)

He who sees the Self abiding in all beings and all beings in the Self, and [who sees that] the Self is not an [egoic] agent, he [truly] sees. (60)

Just as the water of waves of different shapes [is always the same], so, O Arjuna, is the Self in a [desert] caravan, etc., or in the beings of the golden [Himalayas]. (61)

Just as multitudes of different waves roll in the [same] ocean, similarly the beings in the golden [Himalayas] or in the caravans, etc., [have their subsistence] in the supreme Self. (62)

The totality (*jâta*) of things and beings, including the great [Creator-God] Brahma, O Bhârata, know everything as one. There is not even the least separateness. (63)

How can the modifications of states in the three worlds be recognized as that? Where are they? What is the world [apart from the Self]? Why are you [still] uselessly bewildered? (64)

"I am ever of the form of the unborn [ultimate Reality]. I am dispassionate and untainted. I am pure. I am awakened. I am eternal. I am mighty."

—*Tejo-Bindu-Upanishad*[1] (3.42)

# Chapter 15

# GOD, VISIONS, AND POWER: THE YOGA-UPANISHADS

## I. OVERVIEW

"That art thou" (*tat tvam asi*). "I am the Absolute" (*aham brahma-asmi*, written *aham brahmâsmi*). "All this is the Absolute" (*sarvam brahma asti*, written *sarvam brahmâsti*). These are the three great metaphysical maxims of the ancient Upanishadic sages. What they seek to communicate is that Reality is singular and, therefore, that we are in truth only that all-encompassing single Being, which is unsurpassably blissful and superconscious. The *Upanishads* call it by many names, but the most common designations are the "Absolute" (*brahman*) and the "Self" (*âtman*). These didactic maxims are far more than pious affirmations. Throughout the over two hundred extant *Upanishads*, we find scattered testimonies to the fact that for their composers and transmitters the nondual Being-Consciousness-Bliss was a living reality, not merely an abstract hypothesis or a belief.

Patanjali's philosophical system was (at least apparently) among the few schools within the Yoga tradition to break with the Vedântic metaphysics of nondualism, and to boldly assert a plurality of transcendental Selves (*purusha*). This led to a great deal of controversy and debate, from which the proponents of nondualist Vedânta emerged as final victors, for the basic tenor of Hindu Yoga is distinctly nondualist. Even in Bhakti-Yoga, which favors an I-Thou relationship between the devotee and the Divine, the unity of the Godhead is affirmed. As a result, Patanjali's compilation of Yoga aphorisms, though widely respected, came to be exploited more for its practical contents than its philosophy. We find that many later Yoga authorities refer to his definitions of the eight limbs of the yogic path but virtually ignore his metaphysics, unless they criticize it.

This also is the situation in the so-called *Yoga-Upanishads*, which all promulgate a Vedântic type of Yoga. These are works modeled on the earlier *Upanishads* but belonging, for the most part, to the post-Patanjali era. They have not yet been critically edited or studied, and therefore their interrelationships and dates are still uncertain. However, they contain very important expositions of the yogic path,

413

and practitioners of Yoga can certainly benefit from a close reading of these works, which are all available in reasonably reliable translations.

The following sections provide brief summaries of the contents of twenty *Yoga-Upanishads*.[2] I will start with the five so-called *Bindu* ("Point")-*Upanishads*: the *Amrita-Bindu-*, *Amrita-Nâda-Bindu-*, *Tejo-Bindu-*, *Nâda-Bindu-*, and *Dhyâna-Bindu-Upanishad*, which make use of *mantras* as a means of focusing and ultimately transcending the mind. Sound also plays an important role in the teachings of the *Hamsa-*, *Brahma-Vidyâ-*, *Mahâ-Vâkya-*, and *Pâshupata-Brahma-Upanishad*. These works are followed by the *Advaya-Târaka-* and *Mandala-Brâhmana-Upanishad*, which expound a Yoga of light phenomena. Then there is the short but highly instructive *Kshurikâ-Upanishad*, which epitomizes the essence of all forms of Yoga. The concluding category comprises those *Upanishads* that tend to be more comprehensive and textbook-like treatments of Kundalinî-Yoga, namely the *Yoga-Kundalî-*, *Darshana-*, *Yoga-Shikhâ-*, *Yoga-Tattva-*, *Yoga-Cûda-Manî-*, *Varâha-*, *Tri-Shikhi-Brâhmana-*, and *Shândilya-Upanishad*.

## II. SOUNDING OUT THE ABSOLUTE

The world is sound. It sounds in pulsars and planetary orbits, in the spin of electrons, in the quanta of atoms and the structure of molecules, in the microcosm and in the macrocosm. It also sounds in the sphere between these extremes, in the world in which we live.[3]

This is how Joachim-Ernst Berendt, a well-known German producer of radio programs and musicologist, begins one chapter in his fine book *Nada Brahma*. His excursion into the mystery of what he calls primal sound, the transcendental sound that gives rise to all manifestation, shows that religio-spiritual traditions around the world have explored sound as part of their quest for the transmutation of consciousness.

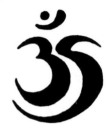

In India, undoubtedly the oldest and most sacred sound or word (*mantra*) is the syllable *om*, symbolizing the Absolute. It is pronounced with a strongly nasalized or hummed *m*, which is indicated in Sanskrit by a dot (called *bindu* or "seed-point") under the letter *m*. Whereas the syllable *om* by itself is said to represent the creative or manifest dimension of the Divine, the echo, or *bindu*, of the sound *m* is thought to represent the Divine in its unmanifest dimension. Shyam Sundar Goswami, a modern practitioner of Laya-Yoga, explained the esoteric significance of the *bindu* as follows:

> *Bindu* is a state in which power is at maximum concentration. When mental consciousness is in the bindu state, diversified mental powers are collected and highly concentrated as mental dynamism . . . *Bindu*—the power point—is a natural and indispensable condition associated with power in its operation. *Bindu* occurs both in the mental and material fields. The atom is the *bindu* of matter; the nucleus the *bindu* of a protoplasmic cell; and *samâdhi* consciousness the *bindu* of the mind.[4]

Thus, the *bindu* is latent concentrated power—whether it be of consciousness or of sound, or of Nature itself. The five *Bindu-Upanishads*,[5] which espouse a form of Mantra-Yoga, build upon the age-old Vedic speculations about this sacred sound. The German Yoga researcher Jakob Wilhelm Hauer even thought that these scriptures were composed not too long after the emergence of Buddhism, but this seems unlikely. They are definitely minor *Upanishads*, which were not commented on or cited by the great Vedântic teacher Shankara, and therefore were probably composed after him. Shankara is generally thought to have lived between 788 and 820 C.E., but Hajime Nakamura has made a good case for the earlier date of 700–750 C.E.[6] Since all the *Bindu-Upanishads* are named in the list of 108 *Upanishads* furnished by the *Muktikâ-Upanishad*,[7] they were obviously composed prior to this text. However, the date of the *Muktikâ-Upanishad* is also uncertain, though we know that it is quoted in the *Jîvan-Mukti-Viveka* written by the famous Vedânta scholar Vidyâranya who was born around 1314 C.E. In fact, in the same work he either cites or refers repeatedly to the *Amrita-Bindu-* and the *Amrita-Nâda-Bindu-Upanishad*.

The esoteric notion of *bindu* appears to belong to the vocabulary of Tantra, and therefore it is reasonable to assign these texts to the heyday of the Tantric tradition, perhaps between 900 and 1200 C.E. As a matter of fact, even in its more conventional sense of "drop [of water]," the word *bindu* does not occur in any of the early *Upanishads*, and is first found in the relatively late *Maitrayanîya-Upanishad* (3.2).

## Amrita-Bindu-Upanishad

The *Amrita-Bindu* ("Immortal Point")-*Upanishad*, also known as the *Brahma-Bindu-Upanishad*, is a short work of only twenty-two stanzas. It makes a distinction between the practice of the tonal (*svara*) syllable *om* and the higher practice of the nontonal or unsounded (*asvara*) syllable, as perceivable only by yogic means. They are also respectively referred to as the lettered/perishable (*kshara*) and the nonlettered/imperishable (*akshara*) aspects of this great *mantra*. By meditating upon the latter aspect, the spiritual practitioner is assured of finding peace of mind. To this end, he or she also is advised to dispense with all book knowledge, just as one winnows the husk from the grain. The ultimate realization of this Mantra-Yoga is identification with the Absolute in the form of Vasudeva ("All-God"). A complete rendering of this scripture is given as Source Reading 3.

## Amrita-Nâda-Bindu-Upanishad

With a total of thirty-eight stanzas, the *Amrita-Nâda-Bindu* ("Immortal Sound-Point")-*Upanishad* is only slightly longer than the previous work. But it makes several important points about Mantra-Yoga. First of all, it treats *mantra* meditation as part of a sixfold (*shad-anga*) Yoga, consisting of sense-withdrawal, meditation, breath control, concentration, reflection (*tarka*),[8] and ecstasy—in that order.

Breath control (*prânâyâma*) is defined as the triple recitation of the *gâyatrî-mantra* with a single breath. This famous Vedic *mantra* was introduced in Chapter 5 when discussing the *Chândogya-Upanishad*. This *mantra* includes the sacred syllable *om*. The regulation of the breath in the above manner causes a switch in consciousness whereby attention becomes more and more focused. This enables the *yogin* to contemplate the transcendental Self in the practice of concentration (*dhâranâ*), which consists in merging the desire-filled mind with the Self. One full cycle of *prânâyâma* as described is known as a "measure" (*mâtrâ*). Concentration is said to be seven or eight such measures long, whereas the condition of union (*yoga*), that is, ecstatic realization (*samâdhi*), is reckoned to be twelve such measures long.

Of interest is the doctrine of the "seven gates" (*sapta-dvâra*) that can lead the *yogin* to liberation. These are respectively called "heart gate" (*hrid-dvâra*), "wind gate" (*vâyu-dvâra*), "head gate" (*mûrdha-dvâra*), "liberation gate" (*moksha-dvâra*), "cavity" (*bila*), "hollow" (*sushira*), and "circle" (*mandala*). They refer to diverse anatom-ical structures, though the author does not divulge anything about them. The last four are probably all esoteric loci in the head. These technical terms hint at the fact that the composer of this *Upanishad* was steeped in esoteric lore that was far more sophisticated than the text of his own composition. The *yogin* who diligently follows this Yoga, sketched with such tantalizing brevity, is promised liberation (*kaivalya*) in six months.

---

**SOURCE READING 17**

## *Amrita-Nâda-Bindu-Upanishad*

Although the meaning of this text is not always entirely clear because its Sanskrit is in part defective, it nonetheless makes many interesting statements that deserve to be considered by students of Yoga. Tradition counts this scripture as the twenty-first in the catalogue of 108 *Upanishads*.

Having studied the scriptures (*shâstra*) and repeatedly practiced [their teachings] again and again, the sage who understands the supreme Absolute should then discard them as [he would cast aside] a torch [after the rising of the sun]. (1)

Mounting the chariot of the sound *om* and making Vishnu the charioteer, he who desires a place in Brahma's world and who is eager to worship Rudra [who is a form of Shiva] (2)

should steer the chariot [to the Absolute], providing he is on the chariot's track. Stopping at the end of the chariot's track and abandoning the chariot, he goes [to the Absolute]. (3)

*Comments:* The metaphor of the chariot is a Hindu favorite. It is used already in the *Bhagavad-Gîtâ* to represent the body. Here it refers to the sound *om*, which is introduced as the vehicle to the Divine. Today we might use an elevator to illustrate the same point: We use it to get to the top floor, but once we are there, we leave it behind.

Having abandoned the state of the [three] symbols of the measures, and disengaging from vocal expression, he goes [forward into] the subtle State by means of the unsounded sound *m*. (4)

*Comments:* The three manifest parts (or morae) of the sacred syllable *om* are the vocalized sounds *a, u*, and *m*. After the waning of the audible nasalized sound *m*, the inaudible sound *m*, i.e., its mental "echo," is used as a vehicle for concentration. This fourth "sound" is the *bindu* ("seed-point").

He should regard the five [types of] sense objects, such as sound, and the exceedingly restless mind as his reins: That is called sense-withdrawal. (5)

Sense-withdrawal, meditation, breath control, concentration, reflection (*tarka*), and ecstasy (*samâdhi*) are called the Yoga with six limbs. (6)

Just as the impurities of mountain ore are smelted, similarly the defects (*dosha*) caused by the sense organs are burned by "breath concentration" (*prâna-dhâranâ*). (7)

*Comments:* The defects spoken of here are inner states like anger, sorrow, jealousy, etc., which are engendered by our outgoing consciousness.

One should burn the defects by means of breath control and guilt (*kilbisha*) [i.e., the karmic deposits of negative emotions] by means of concentration. Having done away with guilt, one should consider [practicing] the retention [of the breath]. (8)

Retention (*rucira*), exhalation, and inspiration of air (*vâyu*) are said to be the triple breath control; [they are also called] emptying, filling, and holding (*kumbhaka*). (9)

With prolonged breath (*âyâta-prâna*), one should thrice recite the *gâyatrî* together with the formulas (*vyâhriti*), the *pranava* [i.e., the sacred syllable *om*], and the "crest" (*shiras*)—that is called breath control. (10)

*Comments:* There are several technical terms in this stanza that call for an explanation. As stated earlier, the *gâyatrî* is the famous Vedic mantra *tat savitur varenyam bhargo devasya dhîmahi dhiyo yo nah pracodayât*, "Let us contemplate that celestial splendor of God Savitri so that He may inspire our visions." The introductory formulas are *bhûh*, **bhuvah**, and *svah*, standing for earth, mid-region, and heaven respectively. The "crest" is the invocation *paro rajase'savad om,* "who is beyond all darkness—*om,*" which is often affixed to the *gâyatrî-mantra.*

Ejecting the air into the ether, making void the extrinsic (*nirâtmaka*) [breath], one should force it into a condition of voidness: Such is the description of exhalation. (11)

As a man would suck up water with the mouth by means of a [hollow] lotus stalk, similarly the air should be seized: Such is the description of inhalation. (12)

One should neither breathe out nor breathe in, nor should one move the limbs. Thus should one force the condition: Such is the description of retention. (13)

To see things as would the blind, to hear sounds as would the deaf, and to look upon the body as a log: Such is the description of the pacified [condition]. (14)

Considering the mind is volitional, the wise casts it into the Self and thus concentrates on the Self: This is proclaimed as concentration. (15)

Inference (*ûhana*) in consonance with the tradition is called reflection (*tarka*). That which, when obtained, is deemed the same [in everything] is called ecstasy (*samâdhi*). (16)

[Seated] on the ground on a seat of *darbha*-grass in a pleasant [location] free from any defects, guarding oneself mentally and reciting the "chariot" [i.e., the sacred syllable *om*] and the "wheels" (i.e., the formulas and the "crest" mentioned in verse 10), (17)

assuming the Yoga posture (*yoga-âsana*), the lotus posture (*padmaka*), the auspicious (*svastika*) [posture], or even the blessed posture (*bhadra-âsana*), and facing properly toward the north, (18)

one should—having drawn up the air (*marut*) while blocking one nostril with a finger—focus on the [inner] fire and contemplate only the sound [*om*]. (19)

*Om* is the one-syllabled Absolute. This *om* should not be exhaled. One should [practice] repeatedly by means of the divine *mantra* for release from [all] impurity. (20)

Thereafter, the *mantra*-knowing sage (*budha*) should gradually, as explained before—and proceeding above the navel—contemplate the coarse and the subtle, commencing with the coarse. (21)

The greatly thoughtful (*mahâ-mati*) [*yogin*] who gives up glancing sideways, up, or down and who abides steady and immobile should constantly practice Yoga. (22)

And the duration of concentration is the immobilization (*vinishkampa*) for the measure of a [hand] clap. However, [the ecstatic state of] Yoga is known as restraint for the period of twelve measures (*mâtrâ*). (23)

That which is without soft consonants, without consonants, without vowels, without palatals, gutturals, labials, and nasals, and which also lacks the semivowels and both sibilants: That is the imperishable [sound *om*] that never ceases. (24)

He who sees the path [to the Absolute], his life force (*prâna*) approaches [It]. Hence one should always practice that [Yoga] which is for traveling on the path [to Freedom]. (25)

[*Yogins*] know the gate of the heart, the gate of the wind, the gate of the head, and likewise the gate of liberation, as well as the "cavity" (*bila*), the "hole" (*sushira*), and the "circle" (*mandala*). (26)

Fear, anger, sloth, excessive sleep, excessive wakefulness, excessive eating, and non-eating: These the *yogin* should always avoid. (27)

When practiced constantly, gradually, and correctly according to the rules, wisdom arises of itself undoubtedly within three months. (28)

The Gods are seen within four [months]; within five the process is extended [to the level of the Creator]; in six months, [the *yogin*] undoubtedly reaches liberation (*kaivalya*), as desired. (29)

The earthy [contemplation] is of five measures, the watery of four measures; the fiery is of three measures, and the windy is two-measured. (30)

The ethereal [contemplation] is of one measure. But one should [really] contemplate the nonmeasure (*amâtrâ*): Having made the connection with the mind, one should contemplate the Self within oneself. (31)

The life force is thirty and a half digits [in length as it leaves the body with the breath], where it is transferred to the [different] *prânas*. This is known as the life force transcending the external life force. (32)

The breath (*nishvâsa*) calculated for a day and a night [is said to be] 13,180 and 100,000 [exhalations and inhalations]. (33)

*Comments:* The total figure 113,180 must be divided by five, since the five *prânas* are involved. This gives us 22,636 respirations in twenty-four hours, or 15.7 per minute. In other scriptures, the idealized number of respirations is given as 21,600. In either case, this approximates the average number of respirations for an adult person.

The first [form of the life force known as] *prâna* is in the heart place; *apâna*, however, is in the anus; *samâna* is in the navel region; *udâna* is situated at the throat; (34)

*vyâna* always abides pervading all the limbs. Now the colors of the five [kinds of life force] such as *prâna* in [their proper] order: (35)

The *prâna* wind is known to resemble a blood-colored gem. The *apâna* in the middle of this [body] is like the cochineal insect. (36)

The *samâna* in the middle between both [i.e., between the *prâna* and the *apâna*] resembles white cows' milk. And the *udâna* is pale, whereas the *vyâna* is like a flame. (37)

He whose [life force], having broken through this region (*mandala*) of the wind, rises to the head, wherever he may die, he will not be born again; he will not be born again. (38)

*Comments: Yogins* use both recitation of the syllable *om* and their breath as a means of focusing their awareness, which leads to the ascent of attention coupled to the life force. The idea is to guide the life force upward toward the crown of the head, until it breaks through the fontanel (called *brahma-randhra* or "brahmic fissure") and rushes beyond the head into blissful infinity. In Tantra, the life force is thought to kindle the far more potent *kundalinî-shakti*, which by means of *prâna* is enticed to enter the axial pathway and ascend to the psychoenergetic center at the crown of the head where it merges with the infinity of Consciousness personified as Shiva.

## Nâda-Bindu-Upanishad

The *Nâda-Bindu* ("Sound-Point")-*Upanishad* comprises fifty-six stanzas. It starts with an exposition of the esoteric meaning of the sacred syllable *om*, which is said to consist of three and a half "measures" (*mâtrâ*), namely the sounds *a*, *u*, *m*, and the "half-measure" (*ardha-mâtrâ*), which is the nasalized echo of *m*, elsewhere referred to as the "seed-point" (*bindu*). This *mantra* is called the *vairâja-pranava*, that is, the "resplendent humming." In one place (stanzas 9–16), twelve such measures are spoken of, as well as the states of consciousness correlated with them.

There also is a passage describing the practice of the inner sound (*nâda*), which can be located in the right ear during meditative absorption. Through repeated practice this sound can become so prominent that all external sounds are drowned out by it. It also gives rise to a variety of other inner sounds resembling those produced by the ocean, a water fall, a kettle drum, a bell, a flute, and so on. The inwardly perceived sound becomes increasingly subtle, until the mind becomes so completely one with it that the individual forgets himself or herself. The mind undergoing this process is compared to a bee that is only interested in the nectar of a flower, not the scent that attracted it. The end state is one of total mental repose, perfect indifference to worldly existence. The *yogin* who has achieved this sublime state is described as being a *videha-mukta*, or one who has reached disembodied liberation.

## Dhyâna-Bindu-Upanishad

The *Dhyâna-Bindu* ("Meditation Point")-*Upanishad*, which has 106 verses, expands on the mystical speculations of the *Nâda-Bindu-Upanishad*. Employing an old Upanishadic metaphor, it likens the syllable *om* to a bow, with oneself as the arrow and the Absolute as the target. The individual who truly *realizes* the ultimate import of this metaphor is liberated even while being embodied. Meditation on the lotus of the heart—that is, the esoteric center at the heart—is recommended, and prescriptions for its visualization are given.

From verse 41 on, which lists the limbs of a sixfold Yoga, the text changes gear and reads like a Hatha-Yoga work. Thus, we find a description of other principal psychoenergetic centers (*cakra*) of the body, including the "bulb" (*kânda*) in the lower abdomen where the 72,000 currents or pathways (*nâdî*) of the life force are said to originate. This is followed by a discussion of the ten types of life force animating the body and how the life force relates to the dynamics of the psyche (*jîva*).

हंस । सोऽहम् ॥

*Hamsa, so'ham*

The psyche, it is stated, continually recites what is called the *hamsa* ("swan")-*mantra*. The sound *ham* (pronounced like "hum") is associated with inhalation, the sound *sa* with exhalation. The sequence *hamsa-hamsa-hamsa* can also be heard as *so'ham-so'ham-so'ham*, which has the esoteric meaning of "I am He." That is to say, "I am the Divine." Thus, the body itself is constantly affirming its own true essence. This spontaneous recitation, effected by the automatic breathing process, is known as the *ajapa-gâyatrî*, or the "unrecited *gâyatrî*." The *yogins* of yore calculated that we normally inhale and exhale around 21,600 times in the course of a day. The *yogin's* task is to aid this natural process through controlling the breath and thus the mind.

This six-limbed Yoga is clearly a form of Kundalinî-Yoga. The "serpent power" (*kundalinî-shakti*) is sought to be awakened by a variety of means, including "locks" (*bandha*) applied to the anal and abdominal muscles and the throat, and such practices as the famous "space-walking seal" (*khecârî-mudrâ*) and the "great seal" (*mahâ-mudrâ*), which will both be explained in Chapter 18. Again, the goal of this Yoga is the state of aloneness (*kaivalya*), or liberation. The term *kaivalya* is borrowed from Patanjali's *Yoga-Sûtra*, but in the present context it means merging with the Divine rather than perfect separation from Nature.

## Tejo-Bindu-Upanishad

The *Tejo-Bindu* ("Radiance Point")-*Upanishad* has six chapters with a total of 465 verses. Chapters 2–4 and Chapters 5–6 appear to have once been two independent texts. Only the first chapter and the beginning of the fifth chapter somewhat justify the title of this *Upanishad*, while the remaining sections are expositions of Vedânta nondualism and have nothing to do with the practice of Mantra-Yoga.

The reader is exhorted to meditate on the "swan" (*hamsa*), by which here is meant the transcendental Self beyond the three states of consciousness—waking, dreaming, and sleeping. The anonymous composer of this work puts forward a fifteen-limbed (*panca-dasha-anga*, written *pancadashânga*) Yoga, consisting of the following:

1. Discipline (*yama*), which is defined as the "restraint of the senses by means of the knowledge that everything is the Absolute" (1.17).

2. Self-restraint (*niyama*), which stands for "application to the innate [Self] and dissociation from what is alien" (1.18);

what is "alien" is everything that is perceived to be other than the Self.

3. Renunciation (*tyâga*), which is explained as the "abandonment of the phenomenal world as a result of beholding the true superconscious Self" (1.19).

4. Silence (*mauna*), which in this context is not so much ritual silence as the quieting of mind and mouth in virtue of the awe felt when the transcendental Self appears on the horizon of the meditative consciousness.

5. Place (*desha*), which is esoterically explained as "that by which this [world] is eternally pervaded" (1.23)—that is, the transcendental Space of Consciousness.

6. Time (*kâla*), which is likewise explained in mystical rather than conventional terms.

7. Posture (*âsana*), which is specified as the adept posture (*siddha-âsana*, written *siddhâsana*).

8. "Root lock" (*mûla-bandha*), which is a Hatha-Yoga practice that is here given a new, occult significance, for the author interprets it as "the root of the world" (1.27).

9. Bodily balance (*deha-sâmya*), which is explained as a merging with the Absolute; the conventional interpretation of this term, as the practice of standing like a tree, is explicitly rejected.

10. Steadiness of vision (*drik-sthiti*), which is seeing the world as the Absolute rather than the common yogic practice of fixing one's sight on the spot between the eyebrows where the "third eye" is situated.

11. Breath control (*prâna-samyama*), which is defined as "the restriction of all fluctuations [of consciousness]" (1.31).

12. Withdrawal (*pratyâhâra*), which is understood here not as sensory withdrawal but as the mental state of locating the Self in the objects of the world.

13. Concentration (*dhâranâ*), which is defined as having the vision of the Absolute wheresoever the mind may wander.

14. Contemplation of the Self (*âtma-dhyâna*), which yields supreme bliss.

15. Ecstasy (*samâdhi*), which is defined as "the complete forgetting of the fluctuations [of consciousness] by repeatedly [assuming] the form of the Absolute, the unchanging fluctuation [of transcendental Consciousness]" (1.37).

The *Tejo-Bindu-Upanishad* (1.42) makes the further point that the ecstatic state entails the realization of the Absolute as fullness (*pûrnatva*), whereas the experience of emptiness (*shûnyatâ*) is considered an obstacle on the path. This is a dismissal of the Mahâyâna Buddhists, who speak of the ultimate Reality as the Void.

The subsequent chapters are more formulaic, giving us hundreds of variations on the great dictum of nondualism—"I am the Absolute." In Chapter 4, the ideal of living liberation (*jîvan-mukti*) is referred to. The Self-realized adept, who experiences his or her perfect identity with the Divine while being embodied, is called a *jîvan-mukta*. By contrast, the *videha-mukta* is described as having abandoned even the knowledge of being identical with the Absolute.

The whole group of *Bindu-Upanishads* demonstrates the high level of sophistication in yogic psychotechnology and metaphysical speculation characteristic of the post-Patanjali Yoga tradition, which was greatly influenced by Tantra.

## III. SOUND, BREATH, AND TRANSCENDENCE

Unless we are for some reason deliberately seeking to regulate our breath, we are ordinarily quite unaware of breathing. However, as soon as we begin to meditate, we become awkwardly conscious of the sound produced by the two bellows in our chest. For beginners this can be a disturbing experience; for *yogins*, however, this rhythmic sound is music to their ears, because they can fasten their attention on it until the mind itself is transcended and they enter the soundless domain of the transcendental Reality.

*Yogins* regard the breath, which is technically known as *hamsa* ("swan"), as a manifestation of the transcendental Life, or Self, which also is referred to as *hamsa*. As we have seen in the preceding section, the two syllables of the word—*ham* and *sa*—stand for the ingoing and outgoing breaths, as well as the ascending and descending currents of the life force. They contain a great secret, for the continuous sound of the breath conveys the message, "I am He, I am He, I am He." In other words, the breath is a constant reminder of the absolute truth that we are identical with the great Life of the cosmos, the Absolute, or transcendental Self. This creative idea is at the core of the teaching of the *Hamsa-Upanishad*,

## *Hamsa-Upanishad*[9]

This short work consists of twenty-one verses. Those who are incapable of contemplating the Self directly are advised to resort to the craft of silent *hamsa* recitation, which involves the conscious observation of the spontaneous "prayer" of the breath. In this way, the text states, all kinds of internal sounds (*nâda*) are generated. Ten levels are distinguished, and the practitioner is asked to cultivate only the tenth and most subtle level of the internal sound, which resembles that of a thundercloud. It leads to identification with the Self, the realization of Sadâ-Shiva, the "Eternal Shiva," who is the refulgent, peaceful Ground of all existence.

## *Brahma-Vidyâ-Upanishad*[10]

A more elaborate treatment of this Hamsa-Yoga is found in the *Brahma-Vidyâ* ("Knowledge of the Absolute")-*Upanishad*, a work of 111 stanzas. The practice of *hamsa* recitation and meditation is recommended for both householders and forest anchorites, as well as mendicant *yogins*. It is said to lead to both spiritual perfection and paranormal powers. This form of Hamsa-Yoga is combined with practices designed to awaken the serpent power and conduct it to the highest psychoenergetic center at the crown of the head.

> "He is lauded as a swan (*hamsa*) who knows the swan that is stationed in the heart and endowed with the unstruck sound, the self-luminous Consciousness-Bliss."
>
> —*Brahma-Vidyâ-Upanishad*
> 20b-21a

## *Mahâvâkya-Upanishad*[11]

Like the *Tejo-Bindu-Upanishad*, the *Mahâvâkya* ("Great Saying")-*Upanishad*, a tract comprising twelve passages, speaks of the goal of the yogic process as fullness. This condition, it states, is not merely ecstasy (*samâdhi*), yogic perfection, or the dissolution of the mind. It is, rather, perfect identity (*aikya*) with the Absolute.

## *Pâshupata-Brahma-Upanishad*[12]

The *Pâshupata-Brahma-Upanishad* is a Shaiva work of seventy-eight verses distributed over two chapters. It derives its name from the followers of God Pashupati, who is none other than Shiva, the Lord of the "beasts" (*pashu*), or souls, which are in bondage. This scripture is grounded in the sacrificial symbolism of the brahmins and introduces the practice of the *hamsa-mantra* as a form of internal or mental sacrifice. This process is also called *nâda-anusamdhâna* or "application to the [inner] sound"—a term particularly associated with the Kânphata *yogins*. It is connected with an esoteric notion according to which there are ninety-six "solar beams" in the heart. These are rays, or links, originating in the transcendental Self through which the Divine can be creative in the human body-mind. "This occult fact about the Absolute is not disclosed anywhere else," states the text (1.25). It is further said that liberation is possible only for the *yogin* who is able to meditate on the identity of the *hamsa* as sound with the *hamsa* as the transcendental Self.

On the philosophical question of how the singular transcendental Reality can give rise to the world of multiplicity, the anonymous composer suggests silence as the wisest disposition. Because of his radical nondualist philosophy, he can even declare that liberation is sought only by those who feel themselves bound. For the same reason, dietary restrictions do not apply to the liberated sage, for, as the ancient *Taittirîya-Upanishad* teaches, the released being is always both food and the consumer of food: The transcendental Self is forever devouring itself in the form of the multiple objects of the phenomenal world.

## IV. PHOTISTIC YOGA

Mysticism is universally associated with experiences of light, even more than with sound. In fact, the transcendental Reality is frequently described as utter brilliance and as such is compared to the sun, or is called the sun beyond the sun. Liberation also is widely referred to as enlightenment or illumination. As the authors of *The Common Experience* note:

> The enlightened are bathed in light. Likewise they irradiate light, which is represented by the aura that surrounds the heads of saints and *bodhisattvas* in Christian and Buddhist art. There is a subtle form of light that strikes the inward eye and suffuses the body. Enlightenment is no metaphorical term.[13]

One of the most memorable passages of the *Bhagavad-Gîtâ* is the description of Arjuna's vision of Lord Krishna as the ultimate Being (see Source Reading 10). Awed by Krishna's self-revelation, Arjuna exclaims:

Without beginning, middle or end, of endless strength, with infinite arms, and moon and sun as eyes, I behold you—[your] mouth a flaming offering-consumer burning up all this with your brilliance. (11.19)

Prince Arjuna, who at the time of his vision had not yet undergone the full yogic process, was ill prepared for this sudden encounter with the God-man Krishna in his transcendental aspect. He thus begged Krishna to have his ordinary consciousness restored to him so that he could once again behold Krishna's familiar human body. It is always fear—the fear of losing oneself—that prevents the ultimate event of enlightenment even in those who are advanced on the spiritual path. Thus, in the *Tibetan Book of the Dead*—the *Bardo Thödol*—the person preparing for the great transitional process of death is specifically instructed not to be afraid of the Clear Light that he or she will perceive in the after-death state.

Experiences of inner light occur well before the *yogin* has reached the point of spiritual maturity where the encounter with the transcendental Light takes place, and to which the only viable response is self-surrender. These experiences, known as photisms, can be looked upon as dress rehearsals for the great experience of the Light of lights. They can be quite spectacular internal fireworks, though more often they are simpler experiences of localized or sometimes diffused nonphysical light or lights. The experience of the "blue pearl" (*nîla-bindu*), often talked about by Swami Muktananda in his autobiography *The Play of Consciousness*, is such a preliminary manifestation of the Ultimate.

Just as Mantra-Yoga or Nâda-Yoga make use of the vibrations of sound to internalize and transcend the ordinary consciousness, Târaka-Yoga avails itself of the higher vibrations of both white and colored light. Moreover, it includes aspects of the practice of the inner sound (*nâda*).

The word *târaka* means literally "he who crosses" or "deliverer." It denotes the ultimate Reality, which is the true liberating agency. The term is found already in the *Yoga-Sûtra* (3.54), where it refers to the liberating wisdom (*jnâna*) that results from continuous discernment (*viveka*) between the transcendental Subject and the objective world, including the mind. In Vedânta scriptures, the term can also stand for the *om-kâra*, that is, the sound *om*. Later, *târaka* came to stand for photistic Yoga, which appears to have been fairly widespread in India during the medieval period, and may have exercised considerable influence on Chinese Taoism.

## *Advaya-Târaka-Upanishad*[14]

Târaka-Yoga is specifically dealt with in the *Advaya-Târaka* ("Nondual Deliverer")-*Upanishad*, which is a compact text of only nineteen passages. The "nondual deliverer" is the transcendental Consciousness, which reveals itself to the *yogin* in a "multitude of fires"—similar to the way in which Paul of Tarsus was visited by a "blinding light" on the road to Damascus in an experience that changed his entire life. The photistic manifestations are seen as a means of reaching the unmanifest supreme Light. They are significant only as signs along the way.

This *Upanishad* appears to have served as model for the more elaborate *Mandala-Brâhmana-Upanishad*. Unlike the latter scripture, the *Advaya-Târaka-Upanishad* makes no attempt to integrate the Yoga of light phenomena with Hatha-Yoga techniques. Verses 14–18 may have been interpolated.

**SOURCE READING 18**

# *Advaya-Târaka-Upanishad*

Presently we would like to expound the secret doctrine of the nondual Deliverer for [the benefit of] the ascetic (*yati*) who has subdued the senses and is filled with the six virtues, namely quiescence and the rest. (1)

*Comments:* The six virtues praised in Vedântic circles are quiescence (*shama*), restraint (*dama*) of the senses, cessation (*uparati*) of desire or worldly activity, endurance (*titik-shâ*), collectedness (*samâdhâna*), and faith (*shraddhâ*).

Always realizing "I am of the nature of Consciousness (*cit*)," with eyes completely shut or else with eyes somewhat open, by looking inward above the eyebrows—he, beholding the Absolute, the Supreme, in the form of a multitude of fires of Being-Consciousness-Bliss, assumes the appearance [of luminosity]. (2)

[This secret doctrine is known as] Târaka-[Yoga] because [it enables the *yogin*] to overcome (*samtârayati*) the great dread of the cycle of conception, birth, life, and death. Realizing the psyche (*jîva*) and the Lord (*îshvara*) to be illusory, and abandoning all differentiation as "not this, not that" (*neti-neti*)—that which remains is the nondual Absolute. (3)

For the attainment of that [nondual Absolute] careful attention (*anusamdhâna*) should be paid to the Three Signs. (4)

In the middle of the body there exists the *sushumnâ*, the "channel of the Absolute," of the form of the sun and of the luminosity of the full moon. Originating at the root-prop (*mûlâdhâra*), she [i.e., *sushumnâ*, the central channel] extends to the "brahman fissure." In the center of that [*sushumnâ*] is the famous *kundalinî*, with a radiance equal to myriads of lightning flashes and subtle-membered like the thread of a lotus fiber. Having beheld it with the mind, a person is liberated because of the obliteration of all sin (*pâpa*). If he incessantly beholds the splendor (*tejas*) [of the *kundalinî*] by virtue of the flashing-forth of Târaka-Yoga in a specific area (*mandala*) on the forehead (*lalâ-ta*), he is an adept. Then the sound *phû* is produced in his two ear holes, [which should be] blocked with the tips of his forefingers. Then beholding in [an elevated] state of mind that region [in the form of] a blue light located in the middle of the eyes, by looking inward, he attains unexcelled bliss. Thus does he perceive in his heart. Such is the perception of the Internal Sign to be practiced by the seekers after liberation. (5)

Now [follows] the perception of the External Sign. If he perceives in front of the nose, at [a distance of] four, six, eight, ten, and twelve thumb breadths in succession the space (*vyoman*) that is doubly endowed with gleaming yellow color [and again] in the semblance of blood-red [color], [which at times] is like blue radiance or dark [blue-]ness, he is a *yogin*. There are rays of light at the outset in the vision of the person [practicing this Târaka-Yoga] [when he is] glancing with fickle vision at the space. [If he] sees that, he is a *yogin*. When he sees rays of light resembling molten gold, [either] at the end of the outer corner [of his sight] or on the ground, that vision [can be said to be] settled. He who sees [thus] twelve thumb breadths beyond his head achieves immortality. If he who is steady [in that vision next has] the vision of the radiance of space in the head, wherever he may be, he surely is a *yogin*. (6)

Now [follows] the perception of the Intermediate Sign. [The *yogin*] sees [phenomena that are] like the entire solar wheel, glittering and so on with morning colors, [or else] like a conflagration of fire, [or] like [the diffusely lit] "mid-region" (*antarîksha*) lacking such [definable radiance]. He abides in the form of their form. Through vision that abounds with these [light phenomena], he becomes the space (*âkâsha*) devoid of qualities. [Then] he becomes the supreme space (*parama-âkâsha*[15]) like deep darkness ablaze with the radiant form of the Deliverer [i.e., Being-Consciousness]. [Then] he becomes the great space (*mahâ-âkâsha*[16]) like the conflagration [at the end] of time. [Then] he becomes the space of Reality (*tattva-âkâsha*[17]) beaming with supreme luminosity superior to everything. [Finally] he becomes the solar space (*sûrya-âkâsha*[18]) resembling the radiant glory of a hundred thousand suns. Thus, the fivefold space, [existing] externally and internally, [constitutes] the Sign of the Deliverer. He who experiences this, released from the fruit [of his actions], becomes like space resembling those [described above]. Hence he becomes the Deliverer, the Sign bestowing the fruit of the transmental (*amanaska*) [Reality]. (7)

That [realization of] the Deliverer is twofold: the former being the Deliverer and the latter the transmental [Condition]. On this there is a stanza: "That [Târaka]-Yoga is to be known as twofold, consisting of a preceding and a succeeding [form], whereby the preceding is to be known as the Deliverer and the transmental [Reality] as that which is succeeding." (8)

In the pupils (*târa*), in the interior of the eyes, there is a replica of the sun and the moon. Through the pupils (*târaka*) [comes about] perception of the solar and the lunar discs, as it were, in the macrocosm, and there is [a corresponding] pair of solar and lunar discs in the space in the middle of the head as the microcosm. Having accepted this, those [internal solar and lunar orbs should be] perceived through the pupils. Here [the *yogin*] should also meditate, mind-yoked, regarding the two as identical, [because if] there was no connection (*yoga*) between these [two levels of reality], there would also be no room for sense activity. Hence the Deliverer should be attended to with introspection only. (9)

*Comments:* This passage introduces a cornerstone of esoteric philosophy, namely the idea that macrocosm and microcosm are mirror images of one another. Here the *yogin* is asked to experience their identity directly through introspection, or inner vision (*antar-drishti*). There also is a pun on the words *târa* ("pupil") and *târaka* ("deliverer").

That Deliverer is twofold: the Deliverer with form and the Deliverer without form. That which "ends" with the senses is "with form." That which transcends the pair of eyebrows is "without form." In every case, in determining the inner import [of a thing] the application of a controlled mind is desirable. [Similarly], by means of Târaka-[Yoga], through vision of that which abides beyond [the senses], with a yoked mind and through introspection (*antar-îkshana*), [the *yogin* discovers] Being-Consciousness-Bliss, the Absolute in its innate form (*sva-rûpa*). Hence [at first] the Absolute formed of white effulgence becomes manifest. That Absolute is known by the eye aided by the mind in introspection. Thus also the "formless" Deliverer [is realized]. Through a yoked mind, through the eye, the *dahara* and other [light phenomena] become known. Owing to the dependence of the process of perception, [both] outwardly and inwardly, on the mind and the eye, it is only through the junction of eye, mind, and Self that perception can take place. Hence mind-yoked inner vision is [instrumental] to the manifestation of the Deliverer. (10)

*Comments:* In ordinary contexts, the term *dahara* mentioned in the above passage refers to a mouse or muskrat. It is derived from the verbal root *dabh* meaning "to injure" or "to deceive." However, in its esoteric application, a more likely derivation is from the root *dah* meaning "to burn." It probably refers to the miniscule space at the heart, which from ancient times has been considered a locus of the effulgent transcendental Self. This *dahara* is also mentioned (verse 10) in the *Kshurikâ-Upanishad*, Source Reading 19.

The sight [should be fixed] in the cavern at the spot between the pair of eyebrows. By this means the radiance abiding above becomes manifest—this is Târaka-Yoga. Having well "conjoined" with careful effort and a yoked mind the Deliverer with [the mind], [the *yogin*] should raise the pair of eyebrows a little upward. This is the former [type] of Târaka-Yoga. The latter, however, is without form and is said to be transmental. There is a great light ray in the area above the root of the palate. That should be contemplated by the *yogins*. Thence comes the power of miniaturization (*animan*), and so on. (11)

*Comments:* The power of "miniaturization" (*animan*), or of becoming as minute as an atom (*anu*), is one of the eight classical paranormal powers (*siddhi*) ascribed to adepts.

When there is the vision of the External Sign and the Internal Sign, [the eyes being] destitute of [the power of] closing and opening—this is the real *shâmbhavî-mudrâ*. Because of being a sojourn to knowers who have "mounted" this seal (*mudrâ*), the earth becomes purified. Through the vision of these [adepts], all spheres (*loka*) become purified. He who is granted [the possibility of paying] homage to such great *yogins* is also delivered [from the cycle of conditioned existence]. (12)

*Comments:* For a description of the *shâmbhavî-mudrâ* see Chapter 18.

The radiant luster of the Internal Sign is the innate form (*sva-rûpa*) [of the nondual Reality]. Through instruction by a superior teacher the Internal Sign becomes the radiant light of the thousand-[petaled lotus at the crown of the head], or the light of Consciousness (*cit*), hidden in the cave of the *buddhi*, or the Fourth Consciousness abiding in the "sixteenth end" (*shodasha-anta*[19]). The sight of that [supreme Reality] depends on a true teacher. (13)

*Comments:* The *buddhi* is the higher mind, the seat of wisdom. The *shodasha-anta*, or "sixteenth end," is a psychic center, or space, that is sixteen digits above the crown of the head. This occult psychoenergetic locus also is referred to in some of the texts of Kashmiri Shaivism.

[A truly competent] teacher is well versed in the *Vedas*, a devotee of Vishnu, free from jealousy, pure, a knower of Yoga, and intent on Yoga, always having the nature of Yoga. (14)

He who is equipped with devotion to [his own] teacher, who is especially a knower of the Self—he who possesses these virtues is designated as a teacher (*guru*). (15)

The syllable *gu* [signifies] darkness. The syllable *ru* [signifies] the destroyer of that [darkness]. By reason of the [ability] to destroy darkness, he is called a *guru*. (16)

The teacher alone is the supreme Absolute. The teacher alone is the supreme way. The teacher alone is supreme knowledge. The teacher alone is the supreme resort. (17)

The teacher alone is the supreme limit. The teacher alone is supreme wealth. Because he is the teacher of that [nondual Reality], he is the teacher greater than [any other] teacher. (18)

He who causes this [scripture] to be recited [even] once becomes released from the cycle [of sorrowful existence]. At that instant the sin committed in all births fades away. He obtains all desires. [For such a *yogin*] there is attainment of the [ultimate] goal of all humanity. He who knows thus, [truly knows] the secret doctrine. (19)

## *Mandala-Brâhmana-Upanishad*

The *Mandala* ("Circle")-*Brâhmana-Upanishad* comprises ninety-two verses distributed over five chapters. The teachings are attributed to Yâjnavalkya, who propounds an eightfold Yoga with some unusual definitions of each limb. Discipline (*yama*), the first limb, is said to encompass the following four practices:

1. Mastery over heat and cold as well as food and sleep at all times

2. Peace (*shânti*)

3. Steadiness (*nishcalatva*) of the mind

4. Restraint of the senses in regard to objects.

Self-restraint (*niyama*), the second limb, consists of the following nine practices:

1. Devotion to the teacher (*guru-bhakti*)

2. Adherence to the path to truth

3. Enjoyment of the Real (*vastu*) as it is glimpsed in pleasurable experiences

4. Contentment

5. Nonattachment (*nihsangatâ*)

6. Living in solitude (*ekânta-vâsa*)

7. Cessation of mental activity

8. Nonattachment toward the fruit of one's actions

9. Dispassion (*vairâgya*), which presumably stands for the renunciation of all desires.

"Postural restraint" (*âsana-niyama*), the third constituent of the eightfold path, is defined as any comfortable posture that can be maintained over a longer period of time. Breath control (*prânâyâma*), again, is divided into inhalation (*pûraka*), retention (*kumbhaka*), and exhalation (*recaka*), which are said to be of a duration of sixteen, sixty-four, and thirty-two "measures" (*mâtrâ*) respectively. In other words, the breathing cycle has the well-known yogic rhythm 1:4:2.

Sensory withdrawal (*pratyâhara*) is explained as restraining the mind from going out toward the sense objects, while concentration, the sixth limb, is defined as stabilizing one's consciousness in the transcendental Consciousness (*caitanya*). Modifying Patanjali's definition, Yâjnavalkya explains meditation (*dhyâna*), the penultimate aspect of the eightfold path, as the "single flow" (*ekatânatâ*) of attention toward the transcendental Consciousness, which is hidden in all beings. Finally, ecstasy (*samâdhi*) is the state of forgetfulness (*vismriti*) in meditation, in which the sense of "I" drops away and there is only the absolute Being-Consciousness-Bliss.

That blissful Reality manifests as different light phenomena, which can be seen within and without. As in the *Advaya-Târaka-Upanishad*, the internal photistic experiences are known as "visions of the inner sign" (*antar-lakshya-darshana*), the external photistic experiences as "visions of the outer sign" (*bâhya-lakshya-darshana*). These phenomena are associated with the idea of

"radiance-space" (*âkâsha*). This is not physical, three-dimensional space, but the expanse of the life force and consciousness itself, as it can be experienced in deep meditation.

Five types of radiance-space are distinguished that appear to be different levels of luminous experience. First, there is the radiance-space (*âkâsha*) existing both within and without, which is said to be "exquisitely dark." Perhaps this corresponds to the experience of the "space of consciousness" at the beginning of meditation. The second level is "superior radiance-space" (*para-âkâsha*), which is as bright as the conflagration at the end of time when the cosmos is destroyed. Next comes the great radiance-space (*mahâ-âkâsha*), which is radiant beyond measure. The fourth is sunlike radiance-space (*sûrya-âkâsha*), while the fifth is supreme radiance-space (*parama-âkâsha*), which is all-pervading and unsurpassably blissful, and whose luminosity is quite indescribable.

We can only guess at the experiential significance of these luminous spaces. They are clearly supraphysical and only vaguely analogous to the ether once thought by physicists to be the medium for the propagation of light. It is easier for meditators than for nonmeditators to appreciate what these potent radiance-spaces might be like.

This *Upanishad*, moreover, makes a distinction between two types of photistic experience. First there is the "deliverer with form" (*mûrti-târaka*), which is within the range of the senses and consists in manifestations of light in the space between the eyebrows. The second type is the "formless deliverer" (*amûrti-târaka*), which is the transcendental Light itself.

The ultimate condition aspired to in this Yoga is called "transmentality" (*amanaskatâ*), or "rapture" (*unmanî*[20]), or "yogic sleep" (*yoga-nidrâ*). The *unmanî* state is the product of prolonged absorption in the formless ecstasy (*nirvikalpa-*

*samâdhi*). This leads to the dissolution of the mind (*mano-nâsha*), whereupon the transcendental Reality shines forth in its solitary majesty.

> The *yogins* immersed in the Ocean of Bliss become that [Absolute]. (2.4.3)

> Compared to that [ultimate bliss], Indra and the other [deities] are only minimally blissful. Thus, he who has attained that bliss is a supreme *yogin*. (2.4.4)

The dissolution of the mind—in fact, the term *nâsha* means "destruction"—must not be misunderstood as a willful obliteration of one's rational faculties. Rather, it stands for the yogic process of transcending the conventional mind, which revolves around the pivot of the ego-sense. The *yogin* who has reached the lofty transmental state is called a supreme swan (*parama-hamsa*) and an *avadhûta*, that is, one who has cast off everything. "Even an ignorant person serving such a one," declares Sage Yâjnavalkya confidently, "is liberated." (5.9)

## V. CUTTING THROUGH THE KNOTS OF ORDINARY AWARENESS

India's famous rope trick is a collective hallucination in which the bystanders witness the following: A fakir throws one end of a rope into the air. Instead of falling back on the ground, it stiffens and stands on its own. Then a boy climbs up the rope, followed by the fakir himself carrying a dagger in his mouth. Both disappear. Suddenly, the boy's severed limbs fall from the sky, seemingly out of nowhere. The fakir reappears and reassembles the youth. When his head is placed back on the neck, the boy comes alive with a broad smile.

The rope trick, though usually performed for public entertainment, has deep symbolic significance, for the dismemberment is a symbolic enactment of the very essence of spiritual life, which is the death of the "old Adam" and the birth of the "new man."

This same motif is present in the *Kshurikâ* ("Dagger")-*Upanishad*.[21] This is a short work with an interesting angle on concentration, which describes well the core of all yogic activity: The *yogin* severs all the bonds that fasten him to conditioned existence, starting with "bioenergetic" blockages, or obstructions in the flow of the life force in the body, and proceeding to faulty attitudes and ideas. Like a sharp blade, the Yoga described in this *Upanishad* cuts through all binding conditions and frees the spirit, which soars like a bird to the Absolute.

Of special interest is the concept of bodily vital points (*marman*), which appear to be places of trapped life energy. By a technique that is the yogic equivalent to contemporary body work, the *yogin* releases the dammed-up life force and then applies it to stimulate the energy flow along the bodily axis (called *sushumnâ*), guiding it gradually to the secret center in the head.

## SOURCE READING 19

# *Kshurikâ-Upanishad*

I will disclose the [doctrine of] the "dagger," the concentration [of attention] for perfection in Yoga, having attained which the Yoga-yoked will not be born again. (1)

That [teaching] is the essence and the goal of the *Vedas*, as has been declared by Svayambhû. Settling in a quiet place, there assume a [suitable] posture, (2)

confining the mind in the heart as a tortoise retracts its limbs—by means of the Yoga of twelve measures (*mâtrâ*) and the *pranava* [i.e., the syllable *om*]—very gradually . . . (3)

. . . one should, all [bodily] openings blocked [by means of the fingers], fill up [with life force] one's whole body (*âtman*) from the chest to the head and from the hips to the nape, with slightly raised chest. (4)

*Comments:* Svayambhû, the "Self-Existent," mentioned in the second stanza is the Creator-God, whether he be called Brahma, Vishnu, or Shiva. The Yoga of twelve measures spoken of in the third stanza presumably refers to the retention of the breath for the duration of twelve repetitions of the syllable *om*.

Therein one should hold fast the [various] life forces (*prâna*) moving through the nostril. Having achieved prolonged breath (*âyata-prâna*), one should gradually exhale ucchvâsa[22]). (5)

*Comments:* Breath (*shvâsa*) and life force are, to the *yogin*, one and the same. Whereas one term emphasizes more the physical aspect, the other reminds us of the metaphysical dimension in which the breath participates. The various life forces are the five types of *prâna* circulating in the human body.

Having made oneself steady and firm, [one should practice breath control] by using the thumb [to close one nostril at a time] [and then draw the life force in] through the ankles and also the calves, "three by three." (6)

*Comments:* The phrase "three by three" (*trayas-trayah*) is not clear. It could refer to the three parts of the process of breath control, namely inhalation, retention, and exhalation, or to the repeated linking of vision, mind, and breath, as one Sanskrit commentator has it.

Then [one should draw the life force in] through the knees and thighs, the penis, and the anus, "three by three." [Lastly], one should cause it to flow and rest in the area of the navel, [having drawn the life force up from] the seat of the anus. (7)

There [at the lowest center of the body] is the *sushumnâ* channel, surrounded by ten [main] channels (*nâdî*): the red, the yellow, and the black, the copper-colored, and the flame-colored ones, . . . (8)

. . . [which are] very fine and tenuous. One should cause the breath to flow to the white channel [of the *sushumnâ*]. Thereupon one should guide the [various] life forces as a spider [ascends] along its thread. (9)

Thence [the *yogin* reaches] that resplendent red lotus, the great seat of the heart, which is called the *dahara* lotus in the Vedânta [scriptures]. (10)

Having broken it open, he proceeds to the throat, and it is said that one should fill that channel [with the life force]. The mind is the supreme mystery, exceedingly spotless wisdom. (11)

The vital place (*marman*) situated on the top of the foot can indeed be contemplated as having that character [of spotless wisdom]. By means of the sharp blade of the mind, constantly devoted to [the practice of] Yoga, . . . (12)

. . . [one should bring about] the cutting of the vital place of the calves, which is said to be "Indra's thunderbolt." He should cut through that [vital point] with the powerful Yoga of meditation, through concentration. (13)

Practicing the four [types of meditation on external and internal as well as coarse and subtle objects], he should, by means of Yoga, unhesitatingly cut through the vital place situated in the middle of the thighs, [thereby] freeing the life force [in that place]. (14)

Thence the *yogin* should gather [the life force and lead it] to the throat, [where] a multitude of channels [exists]. There, one among and above a hundred channels, is the supreme stable . . . (15)

. . . *sushumnâ*, far hidden, pure, embodying the Absolute. *Idâ* stands to the left and *pingalâ* to the right [of the *sushumnâ* channel]. (16)

*Comments:* These three main channels of the life force are explained in Chapter 17.

Between these two is the supreme abode. He who knows it, knows the *Vedas*. Among the seventy-two thousand secondary channels, *taitila* . . . (17)

. . . is cut off by means of the Yoga of meditation, [that is to say,] by the untainted, powerful blade of Yoga with its flaming energy. [However,] the solitary *sushumnâ* is not cut off. (18)

At that moment, the *yogin* can see the *taitila*, which is like a jasmine flower. For the sage should cut, in this very existence, the one hundred channels, because they are the cause [of future births]. (19)

*Comments:* The meaning of the term *taitila* is unclear. It can mean "rhinoceros" and it also is the name of a deity. In his commentary, Upanishad Brahmayogin states that it is "characterized by coming and going," which is not too helpful.

Thus, one should dissociate from auspicious and inauspicious conditions [associated with] these channels. Those who have realized this achieve freedom from rebirth. (20)

With the mind conquered through asceticism, established in a wilderness, unattached, conversant with the limbs of Yoga, desireless, [practicing] step by step—[thus should the *yogin* approach liberation]. (21)

As a swan (*hamsa*) that has cut through its fetters flies straight up into the sky—similarly the psyche (*jîva*), having severed its bonds, always crosses over [the ocean of] existence (*samsâra*). (22)

As a lamp that has burned up [its fuel] at the moment of [the flame's] extinction ceases to function—thus the *yogin*, having burned all karma, ceases to exist [as an individual separate from all other beings]. (23)

> Having cut through the bonds by means of the blade of the measure (*mâtrâ*) [of meditation], well sharpened through breath control and whetted on the stone of renunciation, the Yoga adept is no [longer] fettered. (24)

## VI. BODILY TRANSMUTATION— THE UPANISHADS OF HATHA-YOGA

Sound, light, and breath—these are important tools for the *yogin*. They belong to the oldest and best-tried elements of India's psychotechnology. Their possibilities for psychospiritual transformation have been explored over the centuries by tens of thousands of practitioners. The Sanskrit and vernacular works on Yoga are, therefore, distillates of an immense wealth of factual information, though in many cases we still need to find the right key for unlocking their secrets. The spirit of experimentation on which modern science prides itself is intrinsic to Yoga as well. *Yogins* have always been fearless adventurers in the vast and mostly still unmapped territory of the human body-mind.

At no time has this experimental mood been more prominent than during those centuries that saw the birth and rise of Tantra—in the period between the fifth and the fourteenth centuries C.E. It was during that span of time that India's "athletes of the spirit" intensively explored the hidden potential of the human body. Their curiosity, daring, and persistence led to the creation of what came to be called Hatha-Yoga, which can mean either "Forceful Yoga" or "Yoga of the Force." In the latter case, the "force" is none other than the esoteric "serpent power" (*kundalinî-shakti*) celebrated in the Tantras. This is the universal life energy locked up in the human body, where it is said to be responsible for both bondage and liberation, depending on whether it is functioning unconsciously or consciously. The goal of *hatha-yogins* is to bring the *kundalinî-shakti* under their conscious control, inasmuch as this is possible.

We have encountered that formidable bio-spiritual energy in several of the *Yoga-Upanishads* discussed above, where it is mentioned in passing. The remaining texts of the *Yoga-Upanishads* all focus on Hatha-Yoga and therefore on techniques that are designed to awaken and harness the *kundalinî* energy to the point where it can safely be conducted to the primary bio-spiritual center at the crown of the head, resulting in the blissful state of ecstatic merging with the Divine. The following *Upanishads* are all products of the twelfth to thirteenth centuries C.E. I will outline their contents only briefly here, because I do not want to anticipate too much the contents of Chapters 17 and 18, which discuss the body-positive traditions of Tantra and Hatha-Yoga.

## *Yoga-Kundalî-Upanishad*[23]

The *Yoga-Kundalî-Upanishad*, consisting of three chapters with a total of 171 stanzas, launches straight into an explanation of the serpent power, which it calls *kundalî* and *kundalinî*, both meaning the "coiled one" and referring to the latency of this force. It mentions different types of breath control and the three "locks" (*bandha*)—at the base of the spine, at the abdomen, and at the throat—by which the life force is restrained within the body. Its anonymous author preaches the ideal of disembodied liberation (*videha-mukti*), which is attained when the serpent power reaches the topmost center of the human body where it unites with the transcendental "male" force of Shiva.

The second chapter addresses the highly esoteric practice of the "space-walking seal" (*khecârî-mudrâ*), which, it is emphasized, must be learned from one's teacher. It is performed by using the tongue to block off the cavity behind the palate—a somewhat complicated maneuver that requires the artificial elongation of the tongue. The third chapter consists of speculations about esoteric matters, and it also hints at certain higher yogic processes.

> "The *yogirâj* should not display his abilities to anyone. Rather to keep his abilities concealed from the world, he should live like a fool, an idiot, or a deaf person."
>
> —*Yoga-Tattva-Upanishad* 76b-77

## *Yoga-Tattva-Upanishad*[24]

The *Yoga-Tattva* ("Principles of Yoga")-*Upanishad*, a Vaishnava work of 142 verses, distinguishes and succinctly defines four types of Yoga: Mantra-Yoga, Laya-Yoga, Hatha-Yoga, and Râja-Yoga. This is a fairly systematic text that offers useful definitions of the constituent practices of Hatha-Yoga, as well as the obstacles on the path and also the paranormal attainments that the *yogin* might come to enjoy. It proposes a combination of gnosis (*jnâna*) and yogic technology, with Hatha-Yoga preparing the practitioner for the demands of Râja-Yoga, which calls for both renunciation and discernment. Again the goal is "aloneness" (*kaivalya*), which is explained as disembodied liberation (*videha-mukti*).

## *Yoga-Shikhâ-Upanishad*[25]

With a total of 390 verses, the *Yoga-Shikhâ* ("Crest of Yoga")-*Upanishad* is the most comprehensive of the *Yoga-Upanishads*. It consists of six chapters, of which the concluding chapter appears to have been an independent tract at one time. This Shaiva work, like the *Tantras*, is said to be for spiritual seekers facing the difficulties inherent in the current dark age (*kali-yuga*). Similar to the *Yoga-Tattva-Upanishad*, it propounds a teaching that combines gnosis or wisdom with yogic practice. Again and again the reader is reminded of the importance of transforming the body, so that, as verse 1.168 states, it becomes truly a "temple of Shiva" (*shiva-âlaya*[26]).

By means of the fire [of Yoga], [the *yogin*] should stimulate (*ranjayet*) the body comprised of the seven constituents (*dhâtu*) [i.e., the bodily humors, like wind, bile, gall, blood, etc.]. (1.56a)

All his diseases are cured. How much more so cuts, gashes, and so on. He acquires an embodied shape that is of the form of the supreme radiance-space (*parama-âkâsha*). (1.57)

The Yoga adept is not only Self-realized; his transmuted body is invested with all kinds of paranormal powers (*siddhi*) that are taken to be a sure sign of his spiritual attainment. "One should regard the man lacking powers as bound," declares the anonymous author (1.160). This does not invalidate the generally accepted attitude that the egoic use of these powers is detrimental to the *yogin*'s spiritual welfare. The author, who was obviously an adept himself, also is highly critical of mere book knowledge, speaking of those who are deluded by the little knowledge gleaned from the textbooks (*shastra*).

The *Yoga-Shikhâ-Upanishad* favors an approach that combines wisdom (*jnâna*) and Yoga. Independent of each other, neither wisdom nor Yoga can lead to liberation. Together they can "ripen" a person. The text (1.24–27) distinguishes between "fully cooked" (*paripakva*) and "uncooked" (*apakva*) people. Only the former possess a body that is "not insentient" (*ajada*). In other words, their body is permeated by their disciplined consciousness and therefore yields its full potential, including the paranormal powers. They also are said to be free from suffering (*duhkha*). Indeed, as verses 1.41–42 declare, a *yogin*'s body cannot be seen even by the deities, since it is purer than space (*âkâsha*).

The second chapter deals with Mantra-Yoga, declaring that the subtle inner sound (*nâda*) is the highest *mantra*. In the third chapter, some of the metaphysical aspects of Mantra-Yoga are introduced. Sound is said to have several dimensions of subtlety, starting with the sound-transcending ultimate Reality and its lower or manifest form, the so-called *shabda* ("sound")-*brahman*. Subsequent stages in the progressive manifestation of sound are:

1. *Parâ* ("transcendental"), which is the "seed"-sound or *bindu*.

2. *Pashyantî* ("visible"), which is sound at a level that is inaudible but perceptible through yogic introspection.

3. *Madhyamâ* ("middling"), which can be heard resounding "like a thunderclap" in the heart during deep meditation.

4. *Vaikharî* ("harsh"), which is vocalized sound (*svara*) created by vibrating air.

The fourth chapter of the *Yoga-Shikhâ-Upanishad* is dedicated to expounding the Vedântic doctrine of the unreality of the world and the body, which are nothing apart from the single, all-encompassing Self (*âtman*). In the fifth chapter, we learn about some of the main features of esoteric anatomy, such as the channels (*nâdî*) and the psychospiritual centers (*cakra*) of the body. The concluding chapter covers somewhat similar ground, but focuses on the central channel known as the *sushumnâ-nâdî*, described as the "foremost place of pilgrimage" (6.45). The *yogin* must force the awakened serpent power into this axial channel and then cause it to ascend to the head.

## *Varâha-Upanishad*[27]

The *Varâha* ("Boar")-*Upanishad*, which is a late Vaishnava composition, has 263 verses distributed over five chapters. It begins with an enumeration of the 96 categories (*tattva*) of existence. Vishnu, as the Boar (one of his incarnations), is said to be beyond all categories. Those who take refuge in him become liberated even while alive in the body.

The second and third chapters are a discourse on Vedânta metaphysics, which culminates in the recommendation to contemplate Vishnu in the manner of Bhakti-Yoga. Devotion to the Lord is regarded as the true means of liberation, but Kundalinî-Yoga is also advised.

The fourth chapter explains the seven stages of wisdom, which are also mentioned in the

*Yoga-Vâsishtha* (discussed in Chapter 14). The nature and life of the *yogin* who is embodied yet liberated is described. The *Upanishad* speaks of two approaches—that of the bird, as followed by the sage Shuka, and that of the ant, as followed by the sage Vâmadeva. The former course leads to instant liberation (*sadyo-mukti*), whereas the latter orientation results in gradual liberation (*krama-mukti*).

The fifth chapter, which originally was probably an independent treatise that came to be appended to the *Varâha-Upanishad*, is a longer treatment of Hatha-Yoga. Its author recognizes only three types of Yoga—Laya-Yoga, Hatha-Yoga, and Mantra-Yoga, which should all be mastered. This compound Yoga has eight limbs that match those specified by Patanjali. Its goal is enlightenment in this lifetime.

## Shândilya-Upanishad[28]

The same eightfold Yoga as above is taught in the *Shândilya-Upanishad*, which is a slightly shorter work than the *Varâha-Upanishad* and has a mixture of metric and prose passages. It covers much the same ground as the other texts dealing specifically with Hatha-Yoga concepts and techniques, but again insists on the complementarity of self-knowledge (*jnâna*) and yogic practice. A considerable amount of space is devoted to the channels (*nâdî*) of the life force. Their purification is seen as preparatory for the higher practices of concentration and meditation, by which the vibrations (*spanda*) of the mind are brought under control. The text includes interesting descriptions of methods that the *yogin* is asked to use in order to control and manipulate the life force (*prâna*) in the body. Also a long list of paranormal powers is given.

The last two of the three chapters of this *Upanishad* appear to have been appended. The teachings are ascribed to the sage Shândilya, after whom this work is named.

## Tri-Shikhi-Brâhmana-Upanishad[29]

The *Tri-Shikhi* ("Triple Tuft")-*Brâhmana-Upanishad* is similar to the *Shândilya-Upanishad* both in style and content, though is about half as long. It gets its title from the unnamed brahmin wearing three tufts of hair who received the teachings given in this work directly from God Shiva. The *Upanishad* starts with an exposition of Vedânta metaphysics and then recommends a combination of Jnâna-Yoga and Karma-Yoga (or Kriyâ-Yoga) for the seeker after liberation. It interprets the latter as strict attention to the observances laid down in the scriptures, which presumably means the works of Hatha-Yoga, for the rest of this Vaishnava text covers much the same ground as the above-mentioned works.

## Darshana-Upanishad[30]

The *Darshana* ("Vision/System")-*Upanishad*, which runs over thirty pages in translation, presents itself as the teaching given by Lord Dattâtreya to the sage Samkriti. The title suggests that this is intended as a kind of summary of existing teachings, which probably makes this one of the latest texts of this genre of literature. The *Darshana-Upanishad* expounds Hatha-Yoga on the basis of Patanjali's eightfold path. It defines all the limbs (*anga*) and speaks of ten moral disciplines (*yama*) and ten self-restraints (*niyama*) rather than the five introduced by Patanjali. Under *âsana*, it describes nine postures, which, with the exception of the peacock posture, appear to be primarily meditation *âsanas*. The text mentions, however, that the lotus posture (*padma-âsana*) can conquer all diseases and that the auspicious posture (*bhadra-âsana*) also is capable of removing diseases and the effects of poison.

Under *prânâyâma*, the *Darshana-Upanishad* (section 4) gives a reasonably detailed description of subtle anatomy, which offers no new information. It does, however, relate the circulation of the life force in the body to the course of the sun through the zodiac, and it also speaks of the various somatic loci for yogic concentration as "pilgrimage centers" (*tîrtha*). Thus, Shrî-Parvata is located in the head; Kedâra in the forehead; Varanasi (Benares) at the spot midway between the eyebrows; Kurukshetra (the sacred place of the Bharata war) in the chest; Prayâga (the confluence of the holy rivers Gangâ, Yamunâ, and Sarasvatî) at the heart; Cidambara at the center of the heart; and Kamalâlaya at the base of the spine. These internal pilgrimage centers are said to be superior to any external pilgrimage centers, but the Self (*âtman*) alone is the *tîrtha* that is of ultimate significance.

In addition to the conventional definition of sense-withdrawal (*pratyâhâra*), the *Darshana-Upanishad* (section 7) also offers several other interpretations of this aspect of the yogic path. For instance, it explains it as "seeing the Absolute (*brahman*) in everything" and as the confinement of the life force to certain parts of the body. Concentration (*dhâranâ*) is understood as focusing upon the five material elements as they manifest in the body or, alternatively, as concentration upon the Self. Meditation (*dhyâna*), again, is contemplation of the Self, which is none other than the Absolute. Finally, ecstasy (*samâdhi*) is explained as the realization of the identity of the individual self (*jîva-âtman*) with the supreme Self (*parama-âtman*). This grand recognition is epitomized in the declaration "I am only Shiva." It reveals the world to be mere illusion.

In general the approach of this text is refreshingly systematic. Nevertheless, this late scripture does not add anything significant to our knowledge of Hatha-Yoga.

## Yoga-Cûdâ-Mani-Upanishad [31]

The last work to be examined here is the *Yoga-Cûdâ-Mani* ("Crest-Jewel of Yoga")-*Upanishad*. It teaches a sixfold Yoga but fails to describe the higher stages of yogic practice. The reason for this is that it is a text fragment, namely the earlier portion of the *Goraksha-Paddhati*, which is an important Hatha-Yoga manual (see Source Reading 21).

This concludes our survey of the psychotechnology of the so-called *Yoga-Upanishads*. Their revealed teachings offer a convenient transition to Tantra and Hatha-Yoga discussed in Chapters 17 and 18. But before we turn to these two fascinating interdependent traditions, I would like to conclude Part Four with a short excursion into Yoga in Sikhism.

"O Beloved! You are mind-bedazzling, good looking, life-giving, beautiful, radiant, caring, compassionate, unfathomable, and immeasurable."

—*Âdi-Granth* (5.542)

# *Chapter 16*
# YOGA IN SIKHISM

## *I. OVERVIEW*

Sikhism, which has some thirteen million adherents, is the religio-spiritual tradition founded by Guru Nânak (1469–1538 C.E.), who was born into a family of the *kshatriya* ("warrior") class in a small village near Lahore. The Prakrit word *sikh* is related to the Sanskrit word *shishya* meaning "disciple," and the Sikhs understand themselves as disciples of God. As Guru Râm Dâs (1534–1581 C.E.) affirmed:

My true Guru is eternal and everlasting.
He is free from birth and death.
He is the immortal Spirit,
and is all-pervasive.

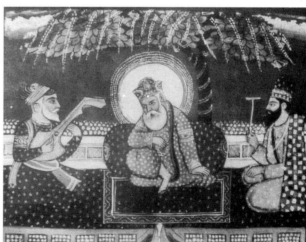

*Guru Nânak*

Discipleship also extends to the great masters of the Sikh tradition, who through their pure lives experienced the full grace of the Divine and were totally surrendered to God, who is typically called Wâhi Guru ("Hail Teacher"). Their teachings, therefore, are regarded as untarnished by ignorance and egotism and consequently can safely guide others on the path to God.

According to tradition, one day during his morning ablutions Guru Nânak disappeared in the water and was considered drowned. He was absent for three days and three nights, and during this time he was removed into the presence of God and was charged with his life's mission to teach humanity to pray. He

443

also was commanded to always praise the divine Name (*nâm*, Sanskrit: *nâma*) and practice charity (*dân*, Sanskrit: *dâna*), service (*sevâ*), prayer (*simran*, Sanskrit: *smarana* or "remembrance"), and ablution (*ishnân*, Sanskrit: *snâna*).

When Nânak, aged thirty, returned, he began his mission with the words, "There is no Hindu; there is no Mussulman [Muslim]." This utterance poignantly characterizes the embracing syncretism of Sikhism, which represents a synthesis of Hindu devotionalism and Islamic Sufism. The Hindu element predominates, and the Muslim aspect of Sikhism manifests primarily in the monotheistic creed and the rejection of idol worship and the caste system.

Guru Nânak lived in an era of great social turmoil when Northern India was governed by Lodhi Afghans, and his gospel of peace and love is one of the most remarkable offshoots of the great *bhakti* movement of medieval India. He was especially influenced by Kabîr, and some scholars have speculated that Kabîr was his teacher. Many Hindus consider Sikhism as part of Hinduism, and many Sikhs do so as well.

His immediate successor, Angad, and the third *guru*, Amar Dâs, were competent teachers but they do not stand out particularly. The fourth lineage *guru*, Râm Dâs, however, achieved fame for laying the foundations of the famous Golden Temple (known as Harimandir or "Temple of Hari") in the middle of a pond in Amritsar ("Lake of Immortality"), which is to this day a popular pilgrimage center for the Sikhs. By the time of the fifth *guru*, Arjun Dev (1581–1606 C.E.), the community had grown considerably in size and influence, so that he was able to organize the Sikhs into a state over which he ruled in royal fashion. Arjun Dev also collected the religious poems of his predecessors and, together with his own compositions, created the *Âdi Granth* ("Original Book"). He was imprisoned by the Muslims and

drowned himself to avoid the ignominy of execution.

His successor, Har Gobind (1606–1645 C.E.), sought revenge by fighting a fierce guerrilla war against the Moghuls. Fighting and internal conflict continued through the reigns of the remaining *gurus*, ending the pacifist phase of Sikhism. In particular, Gobind Singh (1666–1708 C.E.), the last of the original line of ten *gurus*, transformed the Sikh community into an efficient military brotherhood (*khalsa*) trained to defend its faith and cultural/political integrity against the Muslims. He outlawed the caste system and required that his followers adopt the surname Singh (Sanskrit: *simha*, "lion") and, if male, demonstrate their allegiance by wearing the "Five K's" (*panckakâr*, Sanskrit: *panca-kakâra*): long hair (*kesh*, Sanskrit: *kesha*), a comb (*kangha*), a steel bracelet (*kara*), a dagger (*kirpan*), and short pants (*kaccha*). Those who refused to join his sect came to be known as Sahajdhâris, meaning something like "those who take it easy."

Govind Singh composed the *Dasvan Pâdshâh Kâ Granth* ("Book of the Tenth King"), which must be carefully distinguished from the *Âdi-Granth* and which was considered authoritative only by his followers. Only a single poem by this warlike *guru* found its way into the *Âdi-Granth*. With India's independence in 1947, the separation of Bharat (India) from Pakistan drew a brutal line through the middle of the Punjab, the Sikh's homeland, and many members of the community migrated from the new Muslim state of Pakistan to Bharat, where they live an uncertain life.

After Govind Singh's death, the sacred scripture rather than any king-priest was given the role of *guru*, and all Sikhs are expected to venerate and follow the *Âdi-Granth*, also known as the *Guru-Granth-Sahib* ("Teacher Book of the Lord"). Every line of the *Âdi-Granth* is set to music, which affords a parallel to the *Sâma-Veda* of the Hindus. Like the far older Vedic hymns, the Sikh hymns spring from inner illumination and thus represent revealed knowledge.

## II. THE YOGA OF UNITY

The Sikh creed is expressed in the very first hymn of the *Âdi-Granth*, which is known as the *Japji* or *Mûl-Mantra* and is to be recited every morning by the faithful. It begins with the following words:

> There exists only one God, who is called the True, the Creator, free from fear and hate, immortal, not begotten, self-existent, great, and compassionate. The True was at the beginning, the True was in the distant past. O Nânak, the True exists in the present and the True will also exist in the future.

This hymn, which was composed by Guru Nânak, clearly enunciates that God is both transcendent and immanent, pure Being and simultaneously the Creator. The visible and invisible dimensions of existence are all outpourings of the Divine, which is immanent in them. In slight modification of a statement by Nânak we can say that God is writer, tablet, pen, and writing. God also is the sole creator of the three primary qualities (*guna*) of Nature through which illusion (*mâyâ*) and delusion (*moha*) entered the world.

Because God is truly all-comprising, his flawless unity is not fractured by attributing to him such qualities as creatorship, compassion, love, justice, equality. Yet, Sikhism vigorously rejects idolizing the Divine and forbids depicting or worshiping God in any limiting image. God's mystery is inexhaustible and unfathomable.

Under the influence of illusion (*mâyâ*) and the ego (*haumai*, Sanskrit: *ahamkâra*), we fail to realize God's perfect unity and instead experience duality where there is but the one great Being. To discover God's true nature, which is singular, we must cultivate constant remembrance of His name (*nâm*, Sanskrit: *nâma*), which is a form of Bhakti-Yoga. The divine name is of central importance in Sikhism and is said to be the "nectar" (*amrit*, Sanskrit: *amrita*) that is sweeter than honey and more precious than even the wish-fulfilling gem known to mythology. Without remembrance of the divine name (*nâm-simran*), the human body is little more than a corpse, and whatever we do leads only to bondage and suffering. Nânak wrote in *Rag-Sorath*:

> God's name still has all my cravings,
> and the Guru has revealed to me the
> Lord's mansion
> within my own mind, which is completely peaceful.

He also wrote in *Rag-Siri*:

> Your name alone allows people to cross
> the ocean of existence.
> This is my only hope, my only foundation.

And in *Rag-Asa*:

> By repeating God's name I live, and I
> die by forgetting it.

Curiously, the practice of remembrance of the divine name is nowhere defined in the sacred canon, and it must be learned by associating with the community of faithful practitioners. As in Buddhism, the divine Guru is compared to a physician who prescribes the correct remedy for the disease called "ego" and thus lays the foundation for a disciple's ultimate healing. That healing consists in realizing that we are all one and the same Being and in living this realization in the practical details of daily life.

The disciple must walk the path (*panth*, Sanskrit: *patha*) himself or herself by surrendering to the divine will (*hukam*) as manifested in the sacred scripture. This consists, first of all, in diligently practicing the presence of God, that is, feeling the Divine everywhere and aspiring to realize the divine qualities of love, compassion, equality, etc., in one's own life. This inevitably leads one to adopt a lifestyle that has integrity, including proper, honest livelihood (*kirt karni*), as well as sharing the fruit of one's labors generously with others without any expectation of reward—a practice called *vand cakna*. Here Sikhism fully endorses the ideal of Karma-Yoga. An integral part of Sikh morality is the practice of equality, which ignores caste rules and class privileges. Right conduct (*sat acar*, Sanskrit: *sad-âcâra*), wrote Nânak, is even more important than the truth. It is liberating in itself.

Remembrance of the divine name is often practiced as recitation (*japna*, Sanskrit: *japa*) of the various names of God. As Nânak declared in his *Sukhamani-Sahib* (16.5):

> The name of God supports all creatures,
> As well as the universe and its features.
> The name supports nether regions and
> skies,
> The people and the homes they occupy.
> The urge for His name inspired *Smritis*,
> *Vedas* and *Puranas*;
> Those who listen are saved by the
> name, and reach Nirvana.
> The name supports the three worlds and
> fourteen spheres;
> Man will be saved by attending to the
> name with his ears.

Nânak says:
> When by God's mercy a man assimilates the name,
> Spirituality's heights he shall surely gain. [1]

Sikhs are expected to resort daily to the power of *sat-sangat* (Sanskrit: *sat-sanga*), the company of the true or virtuous, which helps them adhere to the principles of the path, especially equality among all people. As Nânak affirms in the *Rag-Wadhans*, "Those who love God love everybody." And Nânak uncompromisingly rejected the caste system and other forms of social disparity, including the inequality between men and women. Nânak especially denounced the ascetical notion of women as evil, pointing out that without women the human race would not exist and that only the Lord himself is independent of the female gender, just as he is independent of the male gender. The egalitarian philosophy of Sikhism is best epitomized in the architectural symbolism of the Golden Temple, which has portals on all four sides suggesting that people from all directions (and walks of life) are welcome to enter.

*Sangat* also entails listening to praiseful chanting (Sanskrit: *samkirtana*) accompanied by music that opens the heart to the great truths of the teaching.

Yoga, for Guru Nânak, consists in meditating on God and remaining detached in the midst of one's daily activities. He strongly criticized sham ascetics, miracle-working *yogins*, and those living in isolation or going about naked. He admonished them in the *Japji* as follows:

> May contentment be their earrings,
> modesty their begging bowl,
> and meditation the ashes smeared on
> their body.

May the thought of death be their
  patched garment,
chastity their way,
and faith in God their walking staff.

May universal brotherhood be their
  order's highest goal,
and may they understand that by controlling the mind
they can subdue the world.

Although the sacred canon favors the lifestyle of the householder rather than the ascetic,
Sikhism also has had its ascetical orders, notably
the Udâsîs, Nirmala-Sâdhus, and Akalîs.

The lovers of God must do everything possible to actualize the ideal of unity in all their
thoughts, words, and actions. In Sikhism this is
exactly what *bhakti* stands for. Yet spiritual discipline is not a sufficient precondition for sainthood. There also must be God's grace (*nadar* or
*prasâd*, Sanskrit: *prasâda*) pouring into the disciple's heart. Then he or she can truly grow in the
stages of the path. There are five such stages or
"realms" (*khând*):

1. *Dharam-khând* (Sanskrit: *dharma-
   khânda*, "realm of virtue"): Here the
   disciple lives in accordance with the
   law of cause and effect, which is seen
   to be valid not only in the material
   world but also in the moral dimension
   of life.

2. *Gyân-khând* (Sanskrit: *jnâna-khânda*,
   "realm of knowledge"): Through increasing insight into the nature of existence and awareness of the vastness of
   the cosmos, the disciple's grip on the
   ego is loosened and a more and more
   benign life is made possible.

3. *Saram-khând* (Sanskrit: *shrama-khân-
   da*, "realm of effort"): In this stage, the
   disciple becomes an adept radiant with
   spiritual illumination.

4. *Karam-khând* (Sanskrit: *karma-khânda*,
   "realm of divine action," that is,
   "grace"): This is the stage of the great
   masters who are united with God and
   who dwell in diverse realms blazing
   with spiritual energy.

5. *Sac-khând* (Sanskrit: *satya-khânda*,
   "realm of truth"): More than a stage on
   the path, this is the ultimate abode of
   the Divine itself, which is absolute
   Truth.

Through deep meditation upon the Divine,
the disciple can hear the "unstruck sound" (*anâhad
shabad*, Sanskrit: *anâhata-shabda*), which liqui-
dates the ego and makes a *gurmukh* ("*guru*-fac-
ing") adept out of the *manmukh* ("self-facing") or
self-cherishing individual. Obviously, for Nânak
this experience represents a very advanced stage of
yogic practice, and thus we must not confuse this
concept with the parallel notion in Hatha-Yoga,
where it represents a lower state of ecstasy.

The various means of Sikh Yoga are all
designed to overcome separation (Sanskrit: *viyoga*) and to cultivate union (Sanskrit: *samyoga*). All
disciplines aim at surpassing the ego, which creates otherness where there is only oneness. The
countless egos are like transparent bubbles arising
from the same ocean and reflecting the same sun-
light. That is to say, we are separated from others
only by a thin skin, which is of no ultimate consequence and can easily be removed by realizing the
divine Being. This realization tears down all barriers between people and does away with conflict.
The person in whom divine unity, or the divine

name, is alive transcends good and evil and becomes a potent transformative spiritual force.

Sikhism subscribes to the ideal of embodied liberation (Sanskrit: *jîvan-mukti*), to which supreme state Nânak also applied the term *sahaj* (Sanskrit: *sahaja*, "spontaneity" or "naturalness"). This state, which is empty of all forms, is not different from God.

## III. YOGA IN CONTEMPORARY SIKHISM

Although Guru Nânak, as we have seen, incorporated certain key yogic practices into his tradition, which can be viewed as a form of Bhakti-Yoga, most Eastern Sikhs do not consider Yoga as part of their faith. This stands in stark contrast to the numerous Western orders of Sikhs established in 1969 by Harbhajan Singh Khalsa—better known as Yogi Bhajan (born 1930).

After emigrating from India in 1968, Yogi Bhajan created the Healthy, Happy and Holy Organization (3HO) in Los Angeles. Three years later, he took eighty-four American students to Amritsar for a pilgrimage to the Golden Temple. His purpose was to expose the students especially to the spiritual heritage of Guru Râm Dâs and to wash away their sins in the pond built by the fourth Guru. Yogi Bhajan had mopped the marble floors of the temple for four-and-a-half years and in the process had purified his own mind.

Yogi Bhajan does not consider himself a *guru*, which would be heretical in the Sikh tradition, although in many ways his role as guide corresponds to what in Hinduism would be considered that of a *guru*. He attributes his own mission in the West to Guru Râm Dâs's blessing and guidance, and points to him as particularly worthy of emulation and veneration.

Yogi Bhajan laid the foundations for the Sikh Dharma in the Western hemisphere and not only brought about a revival of Sikhism but also added a new dimension to it, namely that of Yoga practice. In particular, he teaches "white" Kundalinî-Yoga entailing postures, vigorous breathing exercises, and meditation (mostly combined with chanting). He understands Kundalinî-Yoga as "the yoga of awareness," by means of which the "total potential of the person becomes known to the person."[2]

For Yogi Bhajan, the *kundalinî* is a person's creative potential. He derives the word from *kundala* ("ring"), explaining it as a "lock of the beloved's hair."[3] This potent force must be "uncoiled" through the steady practice of *japa*. By chanting the divine name, a "special heat" is created that completely burns up the practitioner's karma. That heat is not merely figurative but can manifest quite dramatically in the *yogin*'s body. Yogi Bhajan leaves it open which divine name a person should chant, though he recommends *sat nam*, pronounced *sa ta na ma*, which was first given by Guru Nânak and which he explained as "Truth manifested." The individual syllables have the following meaning: *sa* is totality; *ta* is life, *na* is death; and *ma* is resurrection. "The fifth sound," explains Yogi Bhajan, "is the *ah* sound which is common to these four. It is the

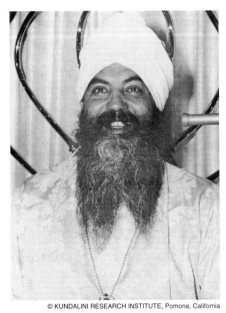

*Yogi Bhajan in his younger years*

creative sound of the universe." The chanting is to be done as follows:

> As you chant, the thumbs are touched to each fingertip in rhythm with the mantra in order to channelize [*sic*] the energy through the nerve endings in the finger which are connected to the brain centers relating to intuition, patience, vitality, and communication. On the sound of Sa touch the thumb to the first finger, with Ta to the second finger, Na to the third, and Ma to the fourth.

> Chant the mantra in three ways: out loud, in the voice of the human being; whispering, in the voice of the lover; and in the silence of your own consciousness, the voice of God. From the depth of your silent meditation, come back to the whisper and then to the full voice. Throughout the meditation, each syllable of the mantra should be projected mentally from the back top of the head, down, and then straight out the third eye point, which is located between the eye-brows at the root of the nose.

> Sit in a comfortable posture with your legs crossed. Keep the spine straight. Chant the mantra out loud for five minutes; whisper for five minutes; and then silently meditate, internally repeating the syllables for ten minutes. Again chant in a whisper for five minutes and then five minutes out loud. Now, inhale and stretch the arms up. Hold the position and exhale. Inhale again, exhale again. Relax. The total time will be thirty-one minutes . . . If you spend two hours per day in meditation, God will meditate on you the rest of the day.[4]

Nânak firmly believed that as long as one surrenders to God, the spiritual process will unfold naturally in one's life. He rejected the fast track promised by certain schools of thought and favored the spontaneous (*sahaj*, Sanskrit: *sahaja*) approach to practice. Everyone, he affirmed, grows according to his or her innate capacity, and forced asceticism or severe self-discipline are ill advised. In all matters, however, he advocated self-initiative. The teacher's role is simply to make the seeker aware that the sought-for treasure lies within.

## Part Five

# POWER AND TRANSCENDENCE IN TANTRA

"I salute you, Goddess, who dispels great fear, averts great difficulties (*durga*), and is of the essence of great compassion."

—*Devî-Upanishad*[1] (25)

"Practice (*prayoga*) is the instrument [of liberation], O Goddess. Bookish scholarship is not [such] an instrument. Scholarship (*shâstra*) is everywhere readily available, but practice is very difficult to accomplish."

—*Vînâ-Shikha-Tantra* (137)

# Chapter 17

# THE ESOTERICISM OF MEDIEVAL TANTRA-YOGA

## I. BODILY PLEASURE AND SPIRITUAL BLISS—THE ADVENT OF TANTRA

The quest for immortality and freedom is fundamental to human civilization. We see it expressed as much in the pyramids of Egypt and in the cathedrals of medieval Europe as in the modern medical search for the fountain of youth and in the race to the stars, as well as in the aspiration to create utopia on Earth. But nowhere has that quest become so obvious a shared cultural motive as in India. Already the Vedic seers were preoccupied with discovering the immortal domain that is the homeland of the Gods, beyond all grief, and even beyond the delightful realms of the ancestral spirits. Later, the Upanishadic sages made the revolutionary discovery that immortality is not part of the topography of the hereafter—even the deities must die—but is an essential characteristic of the ultimate Reality, or Ground of all existence. Consequently, they taught that we only need to realize our inmost nature in order to enjoy the Self, or Identity, of all beings—here and now.

The sages believed that the immortal Self (*âtman*) could never be known, because it is not an object, but that it could be *realized* through direct identification. Such realization consists in a radical shift of our identity-consciousness, of who we experience ourselves to be. Whereas the ordinary mortal thinks of himself or herself as a specific, limited body-mind, the Self-realized being no longer identifies himself or herself as a skin-bound individual but as the timeless quintessence of all beings and things.

The way to that sublime realization, the ancient sages believed, lies in the difficult path of renunciation and asceticism. They maintained that the splendor of the transcendental Reality reveals itself only to those who turn their attention away from the affairs of the world and instead, by exercising conscientious control over body and mind, focus their attention like a laser beam upon the ultimate concern of Self-realization. In the last analysis, in order to *become* the Absolute (*brahman*), one must transcend the human condition and human conditioning. One must desist from investing one's energies in the usual preoccupations through which people reinforce the illusion of being separate entities.

While the Upanishadic ideal of living liberation (*jîvan-mukti*), of enjoying the bliss of the Self while still in the human body, was an important step in the evolution of India's spirituality, it did not entirely overcome the habit of dualistic thinking. This idea raised the following question: If there is only the one Self, why should there be such a struggle involved in realizing it? In other words, why do we have to think of the world, and thus the body-mind, as an enemy that has to be overcome? To put it still more concretely: Why do we have to abandon pleasure in order to realize bliss?

## *The New Approach of Tantra*

A new answer and a new style of spirituality were proposed by the masters of Tantra, or Tantrism, who made their appearance in the opening centuries of the first millennium C.E. Their teachings are embodied in the *Tantras*, which are works similar to the Shaiva *Âgamas* and the Vaishnava *Samhitâs*, but dedicated to the feminine psychocosmic principle, or Shakti.[1] It is sometimes difficult to distinguish between an *Âgama* and a *Tantra* work, because the boundaries between Shaivism and Shaktism are rather fluid.

Goddess worship, which is central to many Tantric schools, existed already in ancient Vedic times. The Tantric masters and practitioners merely drew on the existing sacred lore and ritual practices revolving around the Goddess, as current especially in the rural communities of India. Some scholars have therefore assigned to Tantra an age equaling, if not surpassing, that of the *Vedas*. As a literary phenomenon, however, Tantra does not appear to have emerged much before the middle of the first millennium C.E.

It is widely believed that the Buddhist *Tantras* came first and were closely followed by their Hindu counterparts, though some scholars vehemently contest this. In any case, the Buddhist *Manjushrî-Mûla-Kalpa* ("Fundamental Rules of Manjushrî") and the *Guhya-Samâja-Tantra* ("Tantra of Secret Communion") were probably compiled in the period between 300 and 500 C.E. In the opening chapter of the *Mahâcîna-Âcâra-Krama* ("Process and Conduct of Mahâcîna"),[2] the Goddess advises the sage Vâshishtha to undertake a pilgrimage to Mahâcîna (Tibet, Mongolia, or even China) where he could study with Janârdana in the form of the Buddha.

The earliest Hindu *Tantras* appear to have been lost, and we know of them only from references in later works. Significantly, the seventh-century South Indian saint Tirumûlar refers to a group of twenty-eight *Tantras*. The *Vînâ-Shikha-Tantra* (9), which is the only available left-hand Tantra text dating from around 1200 C.E., mentions the classic set of sixty-four. This suggests that there was considerable literary activity by Tantric masters in the preceding centuries, especially as we know that there were many more *Tantras* even then. One of the oldest extant *Tantras* is the *Sarva-Jnâna-Uttara-Tantra* (written *Sarvajnânottaratantra*), which probably was composed in the ninth century C.E. This work understands itself as containing the essence of many earlier Tantric scriptures.

The original *Tantras* are typically presented in dialogue form and are attributed to the Divine rather than to a particular human author. Their Sanskrit is frequently poor and is grammatically and metrically defective. Later works, especially the summaries, tend to be attributed to human authors and generally are of better grammatical and stylistic quality.

Since Tantrism—whether Buddhist or Hindu—represents a vast, complex, and ill-researched field of study, I am here confining myself to the Hindu *Tantras*, which are more immediately relevant to the Yoga tradition arising out of the Vedic heritage.[3] It should be noted, however, that the Buddhist *Tantras*—as preserved in Tibetan and partly in Sanskrit—are also very important sources for understanding certain yogic processes, especially meditative visualization (*dhyâna, bhâvanâ*) and other higher stages of spiritual practice, as well as the rituals accompanying them.

As indicated above, the Hindu tradition indicates there are sixty-four *Tantras*, but the actual number of these works is much higher. Only a few of the most important texts of this genre of Hindu literature have been translated into European languages. Noteworthy are the *Kula-Arnava-*, the *Mahânirvâna-*, and the *Tantra-Tattva-Tantra*. The scope of topics discussed in the *Tantras* is considerable. They deal with the creation and history of the world; the names and functions of a great variety of male and female deities and other higher beings; the types of ritual worship (especially of Goddesses); magic, sorcery, and divination; esoteric "physiology" (the mapping of the subtle or psychic body); the awakening of the mysterious serpent power (*kundalinî-shakti*); techniques of bodily and mental purification; the nature of enlightenment; and not least, sacred sexuality.

The revolutionary spirituality of Tantra is best captured in the definition of the term *tantra* as given in the old Buddhist *Guhya-Samâja-Tantra*, which explains that "*tantra* is continuity." The word is derived from the root *tan*, meaning "to extend, stretch." It is generally interpreted as "that by which knowledge/understanding is extended, spread out" (*tanyate vistaryate jnânam anena*).

A second meaning of the word *tantra* is simply "book" or "text," as in *Panca-Tantra* ("Five Tracts"), which is a famous Indian collection of fables. Thus a *Tantra* can be defined as a text that broadens understanding to the point where genuine

wisdom arises. All Tantric adepts are agreed that liberation is possible only through the dawning of wisdom (*vidyâ*). Wisdom is liberating because it establishes the Tantric practitioner in the "continuity" of the finite and the infinite dimension, as noted above. The idea of continuity expresses the nature of Tantra well, because this pan-Indian tradition seeks in a variety of ways to overcome the dualism between the ultimate Reality (i.e., the Self) and the conditional reality (i.e., the ego) by insisting on the continuity between the process of the world and the process of liberation or enlightenment.

The great Tantric formula, which is fundamental also to Mahâyâna Buddhism, is "*samsâra equals nirvâna.*" That is to say, the conditional or phenomenal world is coessential with the transcendental Being-Consciousness-Bliss. Therefore, enlightenment is not a matter of leaving the world, or of killing one's natural impulses. Rather, it is a matter of envisioning the lower reality as contained in and coalescing with the higher reality, and of allowing the higher reality to transform the lower reality. Thus, the keynote of Tantra is integration—the integration of the self with the Self, of bodily existence with the spiritual Reality. Orientalist and art historian Ananda Coomaraswamy made this pertinent observation:

> The last achievement of all thought is a recognition of the identity of spirit and matter, subject and object; and this reunion is the marriage of Heaven and Hell, the reaching out of a contracted universe towards its freedom, in response to the love of Eternity for the productions of time. There is then no sacred or profane, spiritual or sensual, but everything that lives is pure and void. This very world of birth and death is also the great Abyss.[4]

It is important to realize that the Tantric revolution was not the product of mere philosophical speculation. Though connected with an immense architecture of old and new concepts and doctrines, Tantrism is intensely practical. It is, above all, a practice of realization or what is called *sâdhana*. Thus Yoga is central to it. Historically, Tantra can be understood as a dialectical response to the often abstract approach of Advaita Vedânta, which was and still is the dominant philosophy of the Hindu elite. Tantra was a grassroots movement, and many, if not most, of its early protagonists hailed from the castes at the bottom of the social pyramid in India—fishermen, weavers, hunters, street vendors, washerwomen. They were responding to a widely felt need for a more practical orientation that would integrate the lofty metaphysical ideals of nondualism with down-to-earth procedures for living a sanctified life without necessarily abandoning one's belief in the local deities and the age-old rituals for worshiping them.

So the teachings of the *Tantras* are marked by an astonishing synthesis between theory and practice based on a vibrant eclecticism with a strong penchant for ritualism. The Tantric teachings were designed to serve the spiritual needs of the "dark age" (*kali-yuga*) that is thought to have commenced with the death of Lord Krishna after the great battle related in the *Mahâbhârata* epic. The psychotechnology described—or, more often than not, only hinted at—in the *Tantras* was invented for those who are barely able to channel their aspirations to the Divine but are easily distracted by their conventional ideas and expectations.

In keeping with the basic nondualist orientation of Tantrism, the adepts of this movement introduced a battery of means that hitherto had been excluded from the spiritual repertoire of mainstream Hindu metaphysics, notably Goddess worship and ritual sexuality. The *tântrikas*, or practitioners of Tantra, rejected the purist attitude of the Hindu and Buddhist orthodoxy and instead sought to ground the spiritual quest in bodily reality. It was the introduction of sexuality that understandably caused the greatest opposition in conventional Hindu and Buddhist circles; the Tantric practitioners were accused of indulging in hedonism under the mantle of spirituality. In some cases, accusations of debauchery were no doubt justified, but such cases were the exception rather than the rule. Today Tantra is held in low esteem in India, and left-hand Tantric gatherings (involving sexual rites) are actively suppressed by the Indian government.

Had it not been for Sir John Woodroffe (alias Arthur Avalon), a British judge of the Calcutta High Court who studied the *Tantras* with native Bengali scholars, we might still share that general prejudice. At the beginning of the twentieth century, Woodroffe boldly disregarded the hostile attitude toward Tantra. In a number of pioneering studies he paved the way for a better understanding and appreciation of this many-faceted movement. In many respects, his writings are still unsurpassed, as is their tolerance.

The so-called sexual revolution of the 1960s and 1970s has, among other things, put Tantra on the map of our contemporary Western culture. Yet Tantra remains widely misunderstood and is often confused by Western neo-Tantrics with the Hindu erotic arts (*kâma-shâstra*). Its sexual practices, which are enacted literally only in the left-hand schools but are understood symbolically by the right-hand *tântrikas*, are merely one aspect of Tantra-Yoga.

It is true that today we are perhaps not as easily shocked by the more controversial features of Tantra, yet the Tantric masters, especially those teaching in the crazy-wisdom mode, can still manage to test even our more enlightened attitudes.

They are spiritual radicals, and notwithstanding our sexual revolution, I believe that most people are still carrying in their heads a rather idealized image of how a spiritual teacher is supposed to behave. We still tend to think of sexuality and spirituality as incompatible, and hence we may be greatly offended by *gurus* who are sexually active.

For instance, how would we relate to the fourteenth-century Bengali adept Candîdâs if he were alive today? He managed to outrage his contemporaries because he, a brahmin, fell in love with a young girl, Ramî, who he had seen washing clothes at the river bank. Their eyes met, and Candîdâs became enchanted by her to the point of neglecting his priestly duties. He was rebuked, and when he continued to openly dedicate love songs to her he was deprived of his offices at the local temple and was "excommunicated." (Since Hinduism has no organized church, however, excommunication is, strictly speaking, not possible.)

Candîdâs's brother finally negotiated an official hearing, during which the adept was given the opportunity to publicly renounce his obsession and be forgiven for his folly. When the maiden heard about this, she went to the hearing. On seeing her, Candîdâs completely forgot the promises he had made to his family and adoringly approached Râmî with folded hands. What Candîdâs's judges and revilers failed to see was that for him that young girl had become an embodiment of the Divine Mother. His love was for the Goddess in human form. It was an emotion of worship triggered by a beautiful maiden.

The liberalism of the Tantric masters, which

> "One day
> while with my sister-in-law,
> I thought of Shyâma,
> and emotion filled my heart.
> I stood transfixed,
> and my body trembled
> uncontrollably.
>
> —*Candîdâs*

has often been confused with hedonism, is of course not unique in the history of religion. Erotic love has been a part of the ritual dimension of many traditions outside India—notably Chinese Taoism—where it has likewise led to occasional excesses and frequent accusations of debauchery. Orgiastic excesses were more likely where ritual practice became separated from lofty metaphysics and associated with magical intentions. A good example of this is found in recent history in the homespun occultism of Aleister Crowley, who encouraged his followers to engage in homosexual activity, premarital and extramarital intercourse, and even bestiality.

## Goddess Worship

The Tantric adepts reclaimed for the spiritual process all those aspects of existence that the mainline traditions excluded by way of renunciation—sexuality, the body, and the physical universe at large. In Jungian terms, we can see this as a concerted attempt at reinstating *anima*, the feminine psychic principle.[5] That this interpretation is correct is borne out by the fact that the unifying element of all schools of Tantra is precisely the attention they pay to the feminine principle, called *shakti* ("power") in Hinduism and depicted in iconography by such Goddesses as Kâlî, Durgâ, Pârvatî, Sîtâ, Râdhâ, and hundreds of other deities.

Often the feminine principle is simply referred to as *devî* ("shining one")—the Goddess.[6] The Goddess is, above all, the Mother of the universe, the spouse of the divine Male, whether he is invoked as Shiva, Vishnu, Brahma, Krishna, or simply Mahâdeva ("Great God").

According to some schools, the Goddess manifests in ten forms. These are known as the "Great Wisdoms" (*mahâ-vidyâ*), which represent an interesting parallel to the Greek gnostic notion of *sophia*. They are as follows:

1. Kâlî—who is the primary form of the Goddess. She is portrayed as dark and unpredictable. She works through the agency of time (*kâla*), which destroys all beings and things. Yet for her devotees she is a loving mother who unfailingly protects and cares for them.

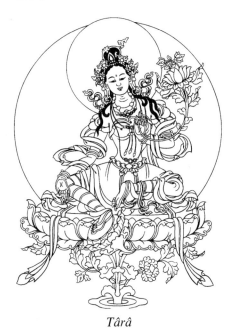

*Târâ*

2. Târâ—who is the saving aspect of the Goddess. Her function is to safely conduct the devotee across the ocean of conditioned existence to the "other shore." Yet, like Kâlî, Târâ is frequently depicted as a terrifying deity who dances on a corpse and holds a severed head in one of her four hands—a reminder that divine grace demands self-sacrifice.

3. Tripurâ Sundarî—who represents the essential beauty of the Goddess. She is called Tripurâ ("Triple City") because she rules over the three states of consciousness—waking, dreaming, and sleeping.

4. Bhuvaneshvarî—who, as the name indicates, is the ruler (*îshvarî*) of the world (*bhuvana*). If Kâlî stands for infinite time, Bhuvaneshvarî represents infinite space and infinite creativity.

5. Bhairavî—who is the fierce, awe-inspiring aspect of the Goddess, demanding the devotee's transformation. She is commonly depicted as a wild woman with bare breasts smeared with blood. Yet her wrath is of the divine variety and is always constructive. Her liberating power is indicated by the fact that two of her hands are in the gesture of bestowing knowledge, while her other two hands are in the gesture of granting protection.

6. Chinnamastâ—who is the mind-shattering aspect of the Goddess. She is portrayed with her own head (*masta*) completely severed (*chinna*) from the body. This gruesome image is a powerful message to her devotees to go beyond the mind and experience Reality directly.

7. Dhûmâvatî—who is that aspect of the Goddess that acts as a divine smoke screen in the form of old age and death, hence her name "Smoky." Only the ardent devotee is able to see beyond the

fear of mortality to the Goddess's promise of immortality.

8. Bagalâmukhî—who, though ravishingly beautiful, carries a cudgel with which she smashes her devotee's misconceptions and delusions.

9. Mâtangî—who in her role as a patron of the arts, especially music, guides her devotee to the uncaused primordial sound.

10. Kamalâtmikâ[7]—who is the Goddess in the fullness of her graceful aspect. She is depicted as seated on a lotus (*kamala*), symbol of purity.

All ten forms of the Goddess, whether gentle or terrifying, are worshiped as the universal Mother. In the *Ânanda-Laharî* ("Wave of Bliss"), a poem ascribed to Shankara, we find this verse, which is characteristic of the Tantric approach:

> He who contemplates You, O Mother, together with Vashinî and the other [attendant female deities] who are lustrous like the moon gem, he becomes a maker of great poems with lovely metaphors, of speech [inspired] by Savitri, and of words that are as sweet as the fragrance of the lotus mouth of that Goddess. (17)

Devî is not only the creatrix and sustainer, whose beauty is beyond imagination; she also is the terrible Force that blots out the universe when the appointed time has come. In the human body-mind, Devî is individuated as the "coiled power" (*kundalinî-shakti*) whose awakening is the very basis of Tantra-Yoga. We will hear more about this shortly.

But Shakti, or Devî, is nothing without the masculine pole of existence. Shiva and his eternal spouse are commonly portrayed in ecstatic embrace—what the Tibetans call *yab-yum*, meaning "Mother-Father." They belong together. On the transcendental plane, they are forever enjoying each other in blissful union. Their transcendental marriage is the archetype for the empirical correlation between body and mind, consciousness and matter, and male and female. "Shiva without Shakti," states a well-known Tantric dictum, "is dead." That is to say, Shiva remains uncreative.

But the same holds true of Shakti on her own, as is emphasized in the Buddhist *Tantras*, which invest the masculine rather than the feminine principle with dynamism. In Hindu Tantra, Shiva represents the primordial Condition in its unqualified aspect, as pure Consciousness or Light. Shakti represents that same Reality in its dynamic motion, its perennial "holomovement," to use David Bohm's quantum-physical phrase. Shakti is the Life Force par excellence, the driving force behind all change and evolution. She is the universal Energy of Consciousness. Thus, Tantric metaphysics conceives of existence as a bipolar process. Creation is simply the effect of the pre-eminence of the feminine or Shakti pole, whereas transcendence is associated with the predominance of the masculine or Shiva pole.

## The Tantric Antiritualist School

Tantra is a comprehensive enough movement to contain its own antithesis. Thus, the pronounced ritualism characteristic of most Tantric schools is, for example, overcome and even criticized in the schools of the Buddhist Sahajayâna, the "Vehicle of Spontaneity." The adepts of this current take the doctrine of the identity between the conditional world and the ultimate Reality as literally as possible. They prescribe neither a path nor a goal, because from the viewpoint of spontaneity (*sahaja*) we are never truly separated from Reality. Our birth, the whole adventure of our life, and also our death occur against the eternal backdrop of Reality. We are like fish who do not know that they are swimming in water and are continuously sustained by it.

The term *sahaja* means literally "born (*ja*) together (*saha*)," which refers to the fact that the empirical reality and the transcendental Reality are coessential. The word has come to connote "spontaneity," the natural approach to existence prior to interfering thought constructs about Reality. The *sahaja-yogin* lives from the point of view of enlightenment, of Reality. When we breathe, it is the Divine that breathes as us. When we think, it is the Divine that thinks as us. When we love and hate, it is the Divine that loves and hates as us. Yet we are forever in search of a "higher" Reality, and this very quest merely reinforces our illusion of being separated from that Reality. The adepts of the Sahaja tradition, therefore, refused to put forward any program of liberation. As the ninth-century adept Lohipâda says in one of his songs (*dohâ*):

> Of what consequence are all the processes of meditation? In spite of them you have to die in weal and woe. Take leave of all the elaborate practices of yogic control (*bandha*) and false hope for the deceptive supernatural gifts, and accept the side of voidness to be your own.[8]

Or as Sarahapâda, a great Buddhist master of the eighth century C.E., declares in his "Royal Song":

> There's nothing to be negated, nothing to be
> Affirmed or grasped; for It can never be conceived.
> By the fragmentations of the intellect are the deluded
> Fettered; undivided and pure remains spontaneity.[9]

The songs of the adept Kanhapâda, who lived in the twelfth century C.E., contain very similar pronouncements. He admonished practitioners to follow the example of the Tantric female consorts who sell their looms and woven baskets to join the Tantric circles. Looms and baskets have been interpreted allegorically as standing for thought constructs and superstitious ideas respectively. The follower of the path of spontaneity must give up the mental habit of experiencing Reality from within the cage of his or her particular "mind-set." This includes the renunciation of magical or wishful thinking, which was as ripe among *tântrikas* as it was and is among most other spiritual traditions.

If the practice-oriented (ritualistic) schools of Tantra were a reaction to the abstractionism of Advaita Vedânta, the Sahajayâna approach can perhaps be regarded as a critique of the extreme ritualism of mainstream Tantra. But the *sâhajîyas*, or *sahaya-yogins*, criticized scholarship as vigorously as they censured religious formalism. With unsurpassed single-mindedness they lived and preached the truth of nondualism.

Strictly speaking, their no-path cannot be characterized as psychotechnology. Rather, Sahajayâna understands itself as the negation of all *techne* (Sanskrit: *upâya*), or "skillful means." It is unquestionably the epitome of the Tantric movement. The principle of *sahaja*, or spontaneity, however, is inherent in all Tantric teachings. After all, the purpose of even the most humble rite is to help the practitioner transcend all the artificial divisions made by the unenlightened mind and to restore the integrity between transcendence and immanence, between bliss and pleasure.

## The Tantric Literature

In addition to the numerous *Tantras*, which form the bedrock of the Tantric corpus, there is a vast number of other works comprising both commentaries and original compositions. The latter consist of monographs (*prakarana*), guides (*paddhati*), digests (*nibandha*, *nirnaya*), dictionaries (*niganthu*), hymns (*stotra*), and magical works (*kavaca*). When viewed broadly, the Tantric tradition also includes aphoristic compositions such as Vasugupta's *Shiva-Sûtra* and Upanishadic texts such as the *Tripurâ-Upanishad* (written *Tripuropanishad*). Tantric scriptures may bear the title *Tantra*, *Âgama*, *Yâmala*, *Rahasya*, *Samhitâ*, *Arnava*, *Shikhâ*, *Purâna*, and so forth.

One of the most significant Tantric works is the erudite Kashmiri adept Abhinava Gupta's monumental *Tantra-Âloka* (written *Tantrâloka*), of which only an Italian rendering is available thus far. Although the author groups this opus with the

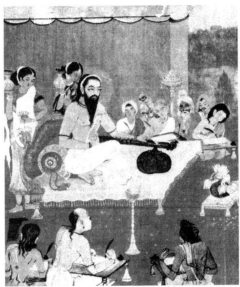

*Reproduced from* Abhinavagupta: An Historical and Philosophical Study
*Abhinava Gupta, adept and scholar*

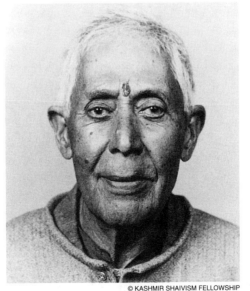

*Swami Lakshmanjoo, who was considered to have been a reincarnation of Abhinava Gupta*

commentarial literature, it is really an original accomplishment that exceeds the traditional criteria for a commentary. Also, according to his disciple Kshemarâja, Abhinava Gupta composed the *Tantra-Âloka* in a state of meditation, which brings it into proximity to the revealed literature. In this work, which comprises nearly six thousand stanzas, we can find references to and quotes from many other Tantric scriptures (nearly two hundred are mentioned by name).[10]

Abhinava Gupta (which appears to be his spiritual rather than his birth name) was born in the mid-tenth century C.E. He created a spate of writings, of which more than forty are known by name. Besides the *Tantra-Âloka*, the most notable are the *Tantra-Sâra* and the *Parâ-Trimshikâ-Vivarana*. He was renowned not only for his erudition, but also for his spiritual accomplishments and miraculous powers. He attained Self-realization through the grace of his teacher Shambhu Nâtha, who initiated him into the secrets of the Kaula school and its literature, but he received teachings in many different subjects and from many other teachers, and he established a thriving school, of which the late Swami Lakshmanjoo was the twentieth century's greatest representative.

The Tantric teachings of Kashmir have become

better known in the West through the scholars who have studied with Swami Lakshmanjoo, especially his disciple Jaideva Singh, the translator of several vitally important works.[11]

The Kashmiri tradition has its counterpart in South India in the widespread Shrî-Vidyâ tradition, whose spiritual treasures also are slowly being brought to light through the diligent labors of scholars like Douglas Renfrew Brooks.[12] As Brooks notes, the Shrî-Vidyâ tradition is among the few branches of Hindu Tantra where we not only have the texts but also living practitioners who are able to expound their esoteric teachings.[13] The most respected text of the Shrî-Vidyâ tradition is the *Vâmaka-Îshvara-Tantra* (written *Vâmakeshvara-tantra*), which has been translated into English.[14] Another work available in English is the *Tripurâ-Upanishad* (written *Tripuropanishad*). Two untranslated but very influential scriptures are the *Tantra-Râja-Tantra* and the *Jnâna-Arnava-Tantra* (written *Jnânârnavatantra*). The sixteenth-century *Shrî-Vidyâ-Arnava-Tantra* must also be mentioned as an authoritative text. Of the later treatises that have been rendered into English, the *Kâma-Kalâ-Vilâsa* must be singled out.[15]

A third stream of

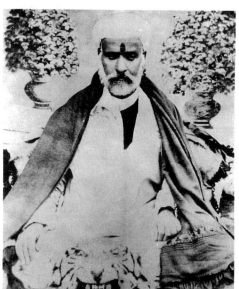

*Swami Mehtabhak, the guru of Swami Lakshmanjoo*

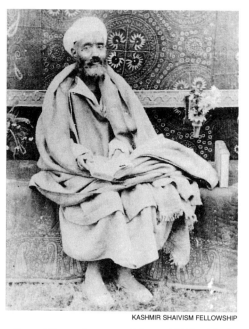

*Swami Ram, the guru of Swami Mehtabhak*

Tantric teachings, called Kaula or Kaulism, is also increasingly being opened up for Western students, especially through the publications by Mark S. G. Dyczkowski and Paul Eduardo Muller-Ortega.[16] Kaulism is one of the oldest branches of Tantra, which achieved fame (or, from a different perspective, notoriety) for its "Five M's" ritual. Some, perhaps even many, Kaula schools understood this ritual metaphorically rather than literally. However, over the centuries critics have always exclusively focused on the left-hand (literalist) variety, as opposed to the conventional (*samâya*) orientation of Tantra, which emphasizes the purely symbolic enactment of the "Five M's" (*panca-makâra*) to be discussed shortly.

The most outstanding (translated) Kaula texts are the *Kula-Arnava-Tantra*, the *Kaula-Jnâna-Nirnaya* attributed to Matsyendra Nâtha, and the *Mahânirvâna-Tantra*.

The closely related Kubjikâ tradition, which may have developed after the original Kaula tradition, produced a large number of texts, most of which seem to have been lost. Of the extant works, the most significant are the *Kubjikâ-Mata-Tantra* and the *Goraksha-Samhitâ* (which is distinct from the Hatha-Yoga manual). Both remain untranslated.

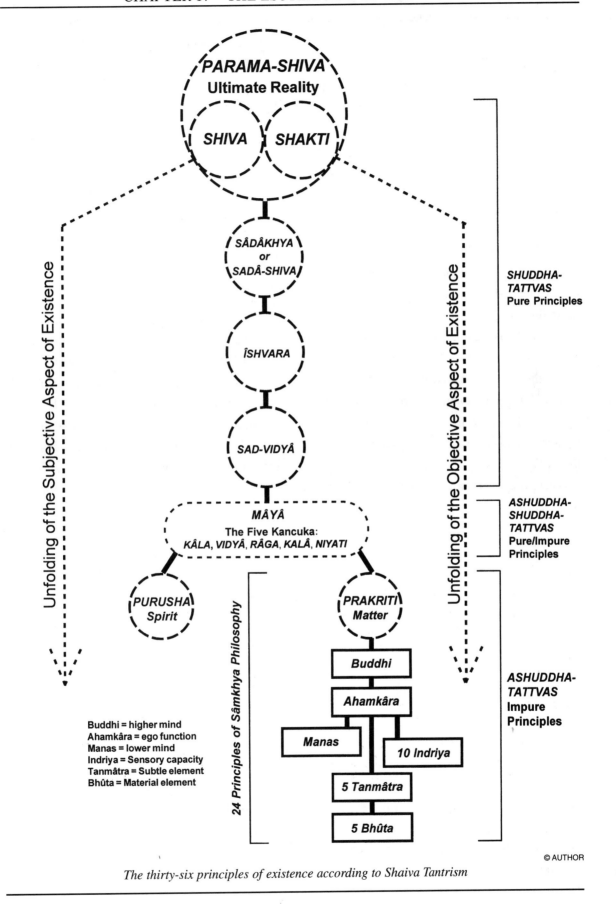

*The thirty-six principles of existence according to Shaiva Tantrism*

For its pervasive influence, Shankara's *Ânanda-Laharî*, noted earlier, deserves further mention. This is a devotional hymn dedicated to the Goddess Tripurâ. Its superlative importance can be gauged from the fact that there are still thirty-six of its commentaries extant today. The *Ânanda-Laharî* has been translated into English together with its complement, the *Saundarya-Laharî*, also attributed to Shankara, the famous Advaita teacher.[17] This attribution is questioned by many scholars, and Shankara (apart from being an epithet of Shiva) is a fairly common name for spiritual preceptors. The same doubt prevails relative to Shankara's authorship of the voluminous *Prapanca-Sâra-Tantra*.

The thousands of Tantric texts composed in Sanskrit, Tamil, and vernacular languages demonstrate the incredible versatility in thought and practice of many generations of adepts. Western students of this ramifying tradition have barely scratched the surface of this literature, never mind the sophisticated psychotechnology described in it. Therefore, it behooves us to be careful in our judgments about this tradition. As the Buddhist scholar Herbert V. Guenther reminds us, "What the *Tantras* say must be lived in order to be understood."[18] And David Gordon White, who wrote a definitive monograph on the medieval Siddha movement, has characterized Tantra as "a wave of genius . . . that has yet to be stilled."[19]

## II. THE HIDDEN REALITY

It is a fundamental premise of all esoteric schools of thought that the world we perceive through our ordinary senses is only a minute slice of a much larger reality and that there are many more subtle planes of existence. Today we can understand this idea in terms of the metaphor of spectral wave bands, or frequencies of vibration.

The distinct levels of existence proposed by traditional esotericism may be viewed as different aspects of the same cosmos vibrating at different rates. Thus, the psyche and mind, which exist on the "subtle" plane, are thought to vibrate many times faster than the material objects of the "gross" plane of space-time. The subtle dimension or dimensions of reality form a fifth axis to the four axes of ordinary space and time, namely length, breadth, height, and duration.

We can perhaps better understand these invisible "higher" dimensions of existence by referring to the new worldview formulated by quantum physicists. Quantum physics operates very comfortably with the notion of electrons and other atomic particles, and yet no one has ever seen any of them directly. The British physicist Harold Schilling proposed that we look upon reality as "a cybernetic network of circuits . . . more like a delicate fabric than an edifice of brick and mortar."[20] But it is a network that has "interior depth." In fact, when we look at the inner hierarchy of reality, we perceive, as Schilling put it, "depth within depth within depth"—an ultimately unfathomable, mysterious well of existence.

As we have seen, Patanjali's philosophy, too, subscribes to the view that there is an "inner" dimension to the universe: The objects we see have an invisible "depth." That depth is progressively disclosed to *yogins* through their sustained effort to internalize their awareness. They experience subtle regions and nonmaterial entities of which modern science knows next to nothing, though thanatologists (death researchers) encounter similar ideas in the reports of subjects who have undergone near-death experiences.

The hidden dimension of macrocosmic existence, of the universe at large, has its precise parallel in the microcosm of the human body-mind. The "deep structures" of the body share in the "deep structures" of its larger environment. All esoteric traditions assume that there is a correspondence between inner and outer reality, and we also encounter the same idea in C. G. Jung's notion of synchronicity, which is really an attempt to explain the fact that there is an occasional surprising coincidence between external events and psychic conditions. For instance, we may recount to a friend a dream we had the previous night about a rare butterfly, and just as we are describing the butterfly, our friend presents us with a gift. When we open the package, we find a book whose cover has a picture of the same type of butterfly.

## The Subtle Body

The earliest explicit model of the inner hierarchy is that of the five "sheaths" (*kosha*)—a doctrine expounded, as we have seen, in the ancient *Taittirîya-Upanishad*. This model is generally accepted by the schools of Vedânta and other nondualist traditions, like Tantra. At any rate, it is widely held in and outside India that the physical body has a subtle counterpart made not of gross matter but of a finer substance, or energy. The "anatomy" and "physiology" of that supra-physical double—the so-called "astral body" or "subtle body" (*sûkshma-sharîra*)— was made the subject of intense yogic investigation particularly in the traditions of Hatha-Yoga and Tantra in general.

The Tantric literature is filled with descriptions of the "centers" (*cakra*) and "currents/pathways" (*nâdî*) that are the basic structures of the subtle body. We will examine this in more detail shortly. Modern physicians typically dismiss these "organs" as entirely fictional, the products of an overheated imagination or an inadequate knowledge of anatomy. Others have suggested that

चक्र । नाडी । कुण्डलिनी ॥

*Cakra, nâdî, kundalinî*

they are merely "maps" for concentration and meditation, or that the *cakras* are created in consciousness through visualization. This point of view is apparently expressed even in some Tantric works, the *Ânanda-Laharî* among them. In general, however, the organs of the subtle vehicle are thought to be as real as the organs of the physical body. Hence they are visible to clairvoyant sight.

But far more than the physical heart, lungs, or liver, the *cakras* and *nâdîs* are subject to great variation. They may be more or less active and

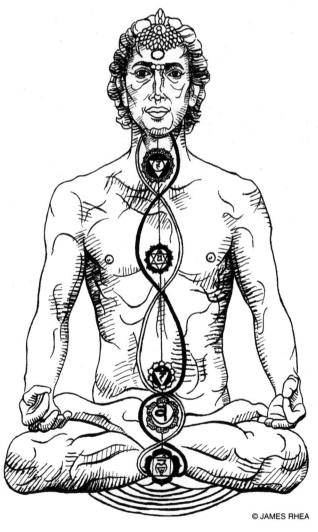

© JAMES RHEA

*The seven psychoenergetic centers (cakra) of the body*

more or less well defined. These differences reflect a person's psychospiritual condition. This explains, in part at least, why the enumerations and descriptions of the *cakras*, as given in various texts, do not always tally. Another reason for these textual variations is that the descriptions are intended to be models for the *yogin*. We can regard them as idealized versions of actual structures of the subtle body which are meant to guide the *yogin*'s visualization and contemplation. Thus, the depiction of the *cakras* as lotuses whose petals are inscribed with Sanskrit letters is clearly an idealization, not an empirical observation, but it is an idealization based on actual perception: The activated *cakras* are, as the Sanskrit word suggests, "wheels" of energy, with radiant spokes that lend themselves to representation as lotus petals.

## The Life Force (Prâna)

The form of "energy" composing the *cakras* and currents in the subtle body is unknown to science. The Hindus call it *prâna*, which means literally "life," that is, "life force." The Chinese call it *chi*, the Polynesians *mana*, the Amerindians *orenda*, and the ancient Germans *od*. It is an all-pervasive "organic" energy. In modern times, it was psychiatrist Wilhelm Reich who attempted to resuscitate this notion in his concept of the orgone, but he only met with hostility from the scientific establishment. More recently, Russian parapsychologists have introduced the notion of bioplasma, which is explained as a radiant energy field interpenetrating physical organisms.

While Western science is still struggling to find explanations for such phenomena as acupuncture meridians, *kundalinî* awakenings, and Kirlian photography, *yogins* continue to explore and enjoy the pyrotechnics of the subtle body, as they have

प्राण । अपान । व्यान । समान । उदान ॥

*Prâna, apâna, vyâna, samâna, udâna*

done for hundreds of generations. Some of their ideas have already fertilized current pioneering research in bioenergy, and I believe it is only a matter of time before the emergent scientific paradigm will generate a comprehensive model of bioenergic fields that can also help us understand and vindicate some of the stranger practices of Hatha-Yoga.

According to the authorities of Yoga, the universal life force is focalized in the individual subtle body, where it branches out into five primary and five secondary energy flows, each with its own specialized function.

1. *Prâna* ("breath" or "in-breath," lit. "breathing forth") — draws the life force into the body (chiefly through the act of inhalation); it is generally thought to be located in the upper half of the trunk, especially in the heart region but also in the head.

2. *Apâna* ("out-breath") — expels the life force (mainly through the act of exhalation); it is associated with the navel and the abdomen but also the anal and genital area.

3. *Vyâna* ("through-breath") — distributes and circulates the life force (chiefly through the action of the heart and lungs); it is always present even when the activity of *prâna* and *apâna* is for some reason suspended; it is widely thought to pervade the entire body.

4. *Samâna* ("mid-breath") — is responsible for the assimilation of nutrients; it is located in the digestive system.

5. *Udâna* ("up-breath") — is primarily responsible for speech but also for belching (which has traditionally been looked upon as a positive sign that the food or drink is being digested properly); it is specifically connected with the throat.

Different scriptures explain these five energies somewhat differently, and also give different locations for them within the body. The above version is the most common.

The five auxiliary bioenergetic functions, or *upa-prânas*, are:

1. *Nâga* ("serpent") — causes vomiting or belching.

2. *Kûrma* ("tortoise") — effects the closing and opening of the eyelids.

3. *Kri-kâra* ("*kri*-maker") — causes hunger.

4. *Deva-datta* ("god-given") — effects yawning or sleep.

5. *Dhanam-jaya* ("conqueror of wealth") — is responsible for the disintegration of the dead organism.

Again, there is no unanimity about the precise functions of these subsidiary energies in the body. The two most important species of the life force are obviously *prâna* and *apâna*, which underlie the breathing process. Their incessant activity is seen as the principal cause for the restlessness of the mind, and their stoppage is the main purpose of breath control (*prânâyâma*). Further details are given in Chapter 18 in connection with the Hatha-Yoga path of realization.

## The Circuitry of the Subtle Body

Rather like electricity, the life force (*prâna*) condensed in the subtle body travels along pathways called *nâdî* in Sanskrit. The word means "duct" or "conduit," but the *nâdîs* must not be mistaken for tubular structures, even though some traditional Yoga texts give this impression. Nor are they identical to the veins and arteries or even the nerves. The *nâdîs* are energy currents, distinguishable flow patterns within the luminous energy field that is the subtle body. The classical drawings of the network of *nâdîs* fail to convey the living, vibrant radiance of the supraphysical vehicle that, to the trained eye, looks like a shimmering, shifting mass of light with foci of different color, and sometimes dark areas suggesting physical weaknesses, perhaps even disease.

Commonly, the Yoga scriptures mention 72,000 *nâdîs* in all. Some speak of as many as 300,000. Several of the *Yoga-Upanishads* name nineteen of them and even give their respective locations, but the names and positions do not always match. The following diagram shows the arrangement of the thirteen principal *nâdîs* based on various Hatha-Yoga texts. The view is from above, looking down into the body.

All the *nâdîs* originate at the "bulb" (*kanda, kânda*), a structure shaped "like a hen's egg," which, according to some texts, is between the anus and the penis (or clitoris), while others locate it in the region of the navel.

## The Three Principal Circuits: Sushumnâ, Idâ, and Pingalâ

There are three chief pathways that are universally recognized in the yogic literature. The central or axial pathway, which runs along the spine, is known as the *sushumnâ-nâdî*, which means "she who is most gracious." It is also called *brahma-nâdî*, because it is the trajectory of the ascending *kundalinî-shakti*, the awakened "serpent power," leading to liberation in the Absolute (*brahman*).

Some works speak of a channel within the *sushumnâ*, which they call *vajrâ* ("thunderbolt")-*nâdî*, and within that channel another still subtler one known as the *citrinî* ("shining")-*nâdî*. This term conveys the idea that within this innermost conduit or flow the *yogin* locates the radiance of Consciousness (*cit*) itself.

To the left of the axial current lies the *idâ-nâdî*, and to the right lies the *pingalâ-nâdî*. The former derives its name from being "pale," the latter from being "reddish." They are respectively symbolized by the cool moon and the hot sun. These pathways wind around the *sushumnâ*, forming a helical stairway. They meet at each of the six lower *cakras* and terminate at the center situated behind and between the eyebrows. Only the *sushumnâ* extends all the way from the bottom *cakra* to the crown center.

The Tantric *yogin*'s principal challenge is to stabilize the flow of bioenergy in the central pathway. So long as the life force oscillates up and down the *idâ* and *pingalâ*, attention is externalized, that is, the *yogin*'s consciousness is dominated by the "lunar" and "solar" forces. By forcing the life energy (*prâna*) along the axial channel, the *yogin* stimulates the dormant *kundalinî* energy until it rushes upward like a volcanic eruption, flooding the crown center and thereby leading to the desired condition of blissful ecstasy (*samâdhi*). According to a widespread esoteric explanation, the word *hatha* signifies the union of "sun" and "moon," that is, the convergence of the life force that ordinarily travels along the *idâ* and the *pingalâ* pathways.

The *kundalinî* has repeatedly been mentioned in these pages, and more will be said about it shortly. Here it is important to point out that the life force, which is responsible for the functioning of the body-mind, and the *kundalinî-shakti* are both an aspect of the Divine Power or Shakti. If we compare the life force to electricity, the *kundalinî* can be likened to a high-voltage electric charge. Or if we regard the life force as a pleasant breeze, the *kundalinî* is comparable to a hurricane.

सुषुम्णा । इडा । पिङ्गला ॥

*Sushumnâ, idâ, pingalâ*

| PÛSHÂ | SARASVATÎ | GÂNDHARÎ |
|---|---|---|
| | PAYASVINÎ | YASHASVINÎ | |
| PINGALÂ | SUSHUMNÂ | IDÂ |
| | SHANKHINÎ | VÂRUNÎ | |
| ALAMBUSÂ | KUHÛ | HASTIJIHVÂ |

© AUTHOR

*Arrangement of the major subtle pathways (nâdî) (viewed from above)*

Once the *kundalinî* power is unleashed in the body, it produces far-reaching changes in one's physical and mental being. If properly managed, this incredible power can, as the adepts of Tantra and Hatha-Yoga promise us, refashion the body-mind into a "divine" vehicle, a transubstantiated form capable of incredible feats.

Knowledge of the functioning of the *idâ-* and *pingalâ-nâdîs* is deemed elementary in Hatha-Yoga. Their activity governs, on the physical level, the responses of the sympathetic and the parasympathetic nervous systems respectively. Thus, through controlled breathing in which the life force is guided along the *pingalâ*, *yogins* can speed up their heart rate and metabolism and improve the functioning of eyes and ears. On the other side, through controlled breathing in which the life force is conducted along the *idâ*, *yogins* can greatly slow down their metabolism. This practice can be pushed to the point where expert *yogins* can, as has been conclusively demonstrated on a number of occasions, remain underground in an airtight container for hours and even days.

But the rationale of breath control (*prânâyâma*) is a different one: Authentic *yogins* do not merely seek to stop their breath and heart and bring about a hibernating condition but to transcend the human condition as such. They want to go beyond the conditioning of the body-mind and break through into the domain of transcendental Being-Consciousness-Bliss. For this, they need to focus the life force like a laser beam and channel it along the spinal axis toward the crown of the head, which is the location of a major esoteric center.

## *The Seven Psychoenergetic Centers (Cakra)*

There are seven major *cakras* in all, which are arranged vertically along the axial channel.

These are pools of life energy, vibrating at different rates. Each *cakra* is associated with specific psychosomatic functions, but these energy whirls must not be confused with the nerve plexuses of the physical body with which they are, however, correlated. From the base up, the sequence of *cakras* is as follows:

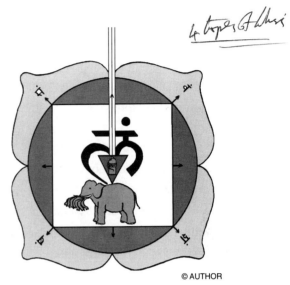
© AUTHOR

*Mûlâdhâra-cakra*

1. *Mûlâdhâra* ("root support," from *mûla* or "root" and *âdhâra* or "support") — Situated at the perineum, this center, which is also called simply *âdhâra*, is associated with the earth element, the sense of smell, the lower limbs, the Sanskrit *mantra lam*, and the elephant (symbol of strength). The presiding deities are Brahma (the creator god) and the Goddess Dâkinî. It is generally depicted as a deep red four-petaled lotus, and it is the seat of the dormant *kundalinî-shakti* and the issue-place of the *sushumnâ*.

2. *Svâdhishthâna* ("own base," from *sva* or "own" and *adhishthâna* or "base") — Located at the genitals, this *cakra* is associated with the water element, the

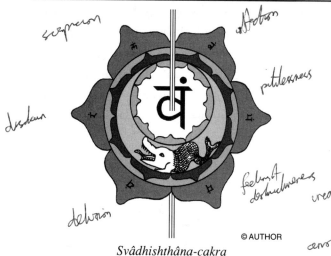

*Svâdhishthâna-cakra*

© AUTHOR

sense of taste, the hands, the *mantra vam*, and an aquatic monster resembling a crocodile (symbol of fertility). The presiding deities are Vishnu and the Goddess Râkinî. This center is depicted as a crimson six-petaled lotus.

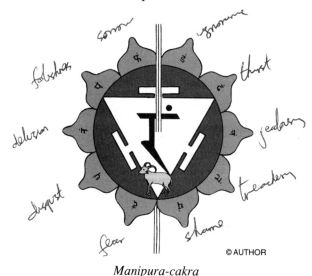

*Manipura-cakra*

© AUTHOR

3. *Manipura* ("jewel city," from *mani* or "jewel" and *pura* or "city/fortress") — Situated at the navel and also called *nâbhi-cakra* ("navel wheel"), this psychoenergetic center is associated with the fire element, the visual sense, the anus, the *mantra ram*, and the ram (symbol of fiery energy). The presiding

deities are Rudra and the Goddess Lâkinî. This center is portrayed as a bright yellow lotus of ten petals.

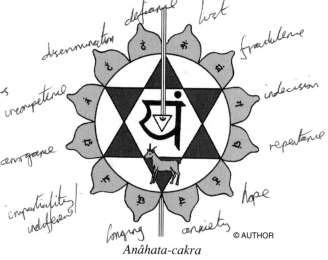

*Anâhata-cakra*

© AUTHOR

4. *Anâhata* ("unstruck") — This center is located at the heart and hence is also widely known as the *hrid-padma* ("heart lotus"), a blue lotus of twelve petals. The designation *anâhata-cakra* derives from the esoteric fact that it is at the heart that the transcendental "sound" (*nâda*) —Pythagoras's "music of the spheres"—which is "unstruck," that is, not produced by mechanical means, can be heard. The heart lotus is associated with the air element, the sense of touch, the penis, the *mantra yam*, and a black antelope (symbol of swiftness). The presiding deities are Îsha and the Goddess Kâkinî.

5. *Vishuddha* ("pure") or *vishuddhi* ("purity") — Situated at the throat, this *cakra*, which is depicted as a smoky violet sixteen-petaled lotus, is associated with the ether element, the auditory sense, the mouth and the skin, the *mantra ham*, and a snow-white elephant (symbol of

470

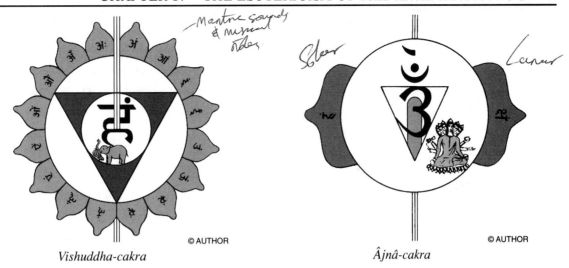

*Vishuddha-cakra* © AUTHOR     *Âjnâ-cakra* © AUTHOR

pure strength). The presiding deities are the androgynous deity Ardhanarîshvara (Shiva/Pârvatî) and the Goddess Shâkinî. It is at this center that the secret *soma* secretion is tasted, which drips from the *lalanâ-cakra*, a minor structure located behind the *vishuddhi-cakra*. The production of this nectar of immortality is stimulated, above all, through the practice of *khecârî-mudrâ* ("space-walking seal"), which is described in Chapter 18.

6. *Âjnâ* ("command") — Located in the brain midway between the eyes, this psychoenergetic center is also known as the "third eye." It is so named because it is through this center that the disciple receives telepathic communications from the teacher. For this reason it is also called *guru-cakra*. This center is associated with the *manas*, or that aspect of the mind which is concerned with the processing of sensory input. The *âjnâ-cakra* is also connected with the sense of individuality (*ahamkâra*) and with the *mantra om*. The presiding deities are Parama-Shiva and the

Goddess Hâkinî. The *âjnâ* center is depicted as a pale gray or white two-petaled lotus. It contains a symbolic representation of the phallus placed within a downward-pointing triangle (the whole signifying the polarity of Shiva and Shakti).

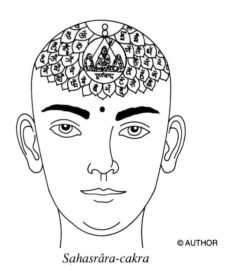

*Sahasrâra-cakra* © AUTHOR

7. *Sahasrâra* ("thousand-petaled," from *sahasra* or "thousand" and *ara* or "petal/spoke") — Situated at the crown of the head, this *cakra* is so called because of the myriad of luminous filaments that compose it. Strictly speaking, it is not part of the *cakra* system at all, but a

body-transcending locus where Consciousness appears to be connected to the human form. This idea is indicated by the luminous *linga*, Shiva's symbol, placed in the middle of this lotus. The symbolic elements connected with each *cakra* serve *yogins* to build up complex visualizations that hold their mind steady and lead to various paranormal powers (*siddhi*), as well as ecstasy.

In modern manuals of Hatha-Yoga, the seven *cakras* are also frequently associated with different psychomental functions. Thus, the lowest *cakra* is said to be connected with fear, the *cakra* in the genital region with sorrow, the navel center with anger, and the heart *cakra* with love. *Kundalinî-yogins* are careful to raise the serpent-power at least to the heart center, because the activation of the lower *cakras* can have undesirable effects on their instinctual life. The center at the throat is sometimes associated with life-positive or life-negative attitudes, the *âjnâ-cakra* or "third eye" with the mood of doubt or basic trust in life, whereas the *sahasrâra-cakra* at the crown of the head may be related to our feeling connected or separated from Reality.

Some schools of thought speak of *cakras* beyond the *sahasrâra*, corresponding to different levels of transcendental realization. Thus, the Shaiva *Âgamas* refer to the so-called *dvâdasha-anta* (written *dvâdashânta*), a locus that is situated, as the name suggests, "twelve digits" above the crown. This idea was undoubtedly conceived as a result of certain advanced yogic experiences and can only really be understood by duplicating those experiences.

The same holds true of the rare concept of the "conduit of immortality" (*amrita-nâdî*) spoken of by Ramana Maharshi, the sage of Tiruvanna-malai in South India, and more recently by the Western adept Da Free John.[21] The latter described this secret channel as the "matrix" of the *sushum-nâ-nâdî*. It manifests only upon full enlightenment, or *sahaja-samâdhi*, at which time it creates a link between the ascending *sushumnâ-nâdî* and the subtle center at the heart. Da Free John writes:

> It is as if a line of Light were plumbed between the deep center of the upper coil (midbrain to crown) and the deep center of the lower coil (below and behind the navel). Not only the sahasrar, but the whole body becomes full of Light or Radiant Bliss. This entire Fullness is the reflection of the Heart [i.e., the transcendental Self]. All of it is Amrita Nâdî.[22]

## The Knots and Vital Places

The classical literature on Hatha-Yoga also knows of "knots" (*granthi*), or bioenergetic constrictions, that effectively prevent the ascent of the life force and then the *kundalinî-shakti* along the spinal axis. The first knot, which is called *brahma-granthi*, is at the base center or the navel; the *vishnu-granthi* is at the throat, and the *rudra-granthi* is at the eyebrow center. These knots must be pierced by the life force so that the *kundalinî* can travel unhindered to the crown center. The texts also speak of the knot or knots in the heart, which consist primarily of doubts (such as doubt about the existence of a nonmaterial reality, or self-doubt).

Some of the later works on Hatha-Yoga recognize the existence of psychosomatic foci of life energy, which are called *marman*. These are the vulnerable places in the body that are particularly critical to a person's well-being. They are supercharged with bioenergy and typically manifest as local blockages that must be removed by means of concentration and guided breath, as taught in the *Kshurikâ-Upanishad*, for instance.

## कुण्डलिणीशक्ति ॥

*Kundalinî-shakti*

### The Serpent-Power (Kundalinî-Shakti)

The most significant aspect of the subtle body is the psychospiritual force known as the *kundalinî-shakti*. What is this mysterious presence in the human body? Metaphysically speaking, the *kundalinî* is a microcosmic manifestation of the primordial Energy, or Shakti. It is the universal Power as it is connected with the finite body-mind. This is sometimes misinterpreted as meaning mere "Force" and is then conveniently contrasted with the principle of love. But, as Sir John Woodroffe noted long ago, Shakti is Power, or cosmic Capacity, and as such is Bliss (*ânanda*), Supraconsciousness (*cit*), and Love (*prema*).[23] Some authorities call it "Divine Intelligence."

So, in some sense, the phrase "*kundalinî* energy" is a misnomer, because we tend to regard energy as a neutral physical force. The term *shakti*, by contrast, connotes something far more positive and creative. Above all, *shakti* is a conscious, intelligent force. Nevertheless, it is convenient to occasionally use such English equivalents as "power" and "energy."

The term *kundalinî* means "she who is coiled" and refers to the fact that the *kundalinî*, or *kundalî*, is envisioned as a sleeping serpent curled three and a half times around a phallus (*linga*) in the lowest bioenergetic center of the human body. That serpent blocks the central pathway with its mouth at the place of the first knot. This symbolism simply suggests that the *kundalinî* is normally in a state of dormancy or latency.

As mentioned before, in the human body the primordial Energy is polarized into potential energy (i.e., the undifferentiated *kundalinî-shakti*) and dynamic energy (i.e., the differentiated *prâna* or *prâna-shakti*). By way of regulating the flow of *prâna*, the potential energy can be mobilized, which results in the well-known phenomenon of *kundalinî* arousal. Thus the *prâna* is used to stir the dormant *kundalinî* energy into action. The situation is analogous to bombarding the atomic nucleus with high-energy particles, which destabilizes the atom and leads to a release of tremendous energy.

Through controlled breathing in which the life energy (*prâna*) is withdrawn from the left and right *nâdîs* and forced into the central pathway, the "sleeping princess" is awakened. Often this process is explained as one of heating the *kundalinî*, and it can be compared to the triggering of a nuclear reaction by means of exploding a conventional bomb. That this comparison is not too far-fetched is evident from Gopi Krishna's description of the moment of *kundalinî* awakening, which, subjectively at least, amounts to a phenomenal burst of energy:

Suddenly, with a roar like that of a waterfall, I felt a stream of liquid light entering my brain through the spinal cord. Entirely unprepared for such a development, I was completely taken by surprise; but regaining self-control instantaneously, I remained sitting in the same posture, keeping my mind on the point of concentration. The illumination grew brighter and brighter, the roaring louder, I experienced a rocking sensation and then felt myself slipping out of my body, entirely enveloped in a halo of light.[24]

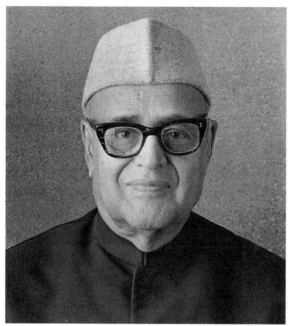

*Gopi Krishna*

In Gopi Krishna's case, this experience was quite unexpected and uncontrolled. The goal of Tantra-Yoga and Hatha-Yoga, however, is to induce this event under controlled conditions so that the practitioner does not have to suffer the kind of disastrous side effects that Gopi Krishna and a good many other meditators as well as nonmeditators have had to endure, often for prolonged periods of time. The symptoms of an unintentionally and wrongly aroused *kundalinî* can be quite severe—from splitting headaches to psychotic episodes.

The traditional model states that when the dormant *kundalinî-shakti* is awakened, it shoots up to the crown center where the blissful meltdown between Shakti and Shiva occurs. Implicit in this is the idea that the *kundalinî* is completely dynamized, and that the body of the *yogin* is now sustained by the "nectar" (*amrita*) that flows from the union of the two poles of Reality. Western students of Kundalinî-Yoga find this model difficult to accept and have proffered other solutions informed by the laws of physics.

A good contender is the model that compares the body to a bipolar magnet. Intense concentration and breath control lead to an "oversaturation," which causes an inductive process in the static pole (i.e., the *mûlâdhâra-cakra*). That is, the life energy begins to stream from that *cakra*. The energy that is released is equivalent to the energy impacting on it, yet of an "opposite" kind, and without depleting itself.

The curious physical phenomena associated with the *kundalinî* awakening, such as the sensation of intense heat, light, sound, pressure, and even pain, must not be confused with the *kundalinî* itself. Hence the American psychiatrist Lee Sannella has dubbed these phenomena collectively as "physio-*kundalinî*."[25] This aspect of the *kundalinî* can be understood in neurophysiological terms, and the model developed by Isaac Bentov and applied by Sannella is thus far the most sophisticated available. Bentov looks at the *kundalinî* process from a mechanical point of view that regards the body as containing, especially in the skull and the heart, standing electromagnetic wave systems. These are thought to trigger the brain into producing the sort of visionary, auditory, and other sensory experiences typical of *kundalinî* awakenings. Undoubtedly, most psychic and mystical phenomena have a physiological basis, but beyond such physiological manifestations of the *kundalinî* lies the mysterious realm of the *kundalinî* as Consciousness-Bliss.

The *kundalinî* experience is presumably as old as humanity's encounter with the spiritual dimension, though the special significance of that experience was not recognized until the dawn of Tantra. Kundalinî-Yoga is the mature product of a long history of psychospiritual experimentation, and it presupposed the discovery of the body as a manifestation or "temple" of the Divine.

More than anyone, it was the Kashmiri pundit Gopi Krishna who has "democratized" the *kundalinî* phenomenon. First, he made it widely known in the modern world and promoted its scientific investigation. Second, he saw in it the engine behind our entire psychospiritual evolution. On one hand, Gopi Krishna was adamant that the *kundalinî* is a spiritual reality, and on the other hand, he passionately advocated it as the biological mechanism that is responsible for sainthood, genius, and insanity alike. As he put it:

> What my own experience has clearly revealed is the amazing fact that though guided by a Super-Intelligence, invisible but at the same time unmistakably seen conducting the whole operation, the phenomenon of Kundalinî is entirely biological in nature.[26]

This states the problem in a nutshell. The *kundalinî* cannot be both a spiritual reality *and* entirely biological, as we would normally understand the term "biological." Of course, from a Tantric point of view, which holds that immanence and transcendence are coessential, any strict distinction between matter and spirit makes little sense, but for this elevated point of view to be relevant, it must be our lived truth. As long as we are not de facto enlightened but experience ourselves as individuated beings, we must concede the usefulness of making practical distinctions. Even though Gopi Krishna's work has contributed greatly toward a phenomenology of the *kundalinî* experience, there is a real need for further research and, not least, conceptual clarification.

Awakening the sleeping princess *kundalinî*, as we have seen, is at the heart of Tantra. We will next turn to the Tantric path itself as codified in Hatha-Yoga, which has as its sole objective arousing the hidden Goddess and inducing her to embrace and melt with the equally hidden God, Shiva, residing at the solitary peak of Mount Meru in the microcosm of the human body.

## III. TANTRIC RITUAL PRACTICE

### The Purification of the Elements (Bhûta-Shuddhi)

Before the prince in the well-known fairy tale could kiss the sleeping princess, he had to combat monsters and cut a path to the castle. Similarly, before the wedding of Shiva and Shakti can occur in the human body-mind, the *yogin* must clear away all kinds of obstructions. The path of realization (*sâdhana*) is, therefore, often couched in terms of purification (*shodhana*). In fact, the very process of *kundalinî* arousal is understood as the progressive purification of the constituent elements (*bhûta*) of the body—earth, water, fire, air, and ether. It is known as *bhûta-shuddhi*.

As the *kundalinî* is conducted upward along the axial channel (*sushumnâ-nâdî*), it gradually "dissolves" the dominant element of each somatic region or *cakra*. Thus, by the time it reaches the sixth or *âjnâ-cakra*, the *kundalinî* has successively dissolved the five elements of earth, water, fire, air, and ether. What this means, in practice, is that the withdrawal of the life force from the body produces a state of coldness and insensitivity in the trunk and the limbs. The *kundalinî's* further progression to the crown, or *sahasrâra-cakra*, signals the temporary dissolution of the mind (*manas*) in the state of "formless" ecstasy or *nirvikalpa-samâdhi*, which completely shuts down *yogins'* individuated awareness of their environment, including their own body. Their awareness-identity now rests in the All-Identity of the transcendental Self, which is indescribably blissful.

On a lower level, *bhûta-shuddhi* is a ritual that is performed as a preliminary practice to the worship of one's chosen deity or deities in the context

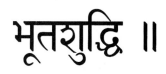
भूतशुद्धि ॥

*Bhûta-shuddhi*

of the Tantric lifestyle. It is the symbolic dissolution of the elements of the body. This procedure, which is described in the *Mahânirvâna-Tantra* (5.93ff.), involves visualizing the process of elemental creation in reverse order. Thus, the *yogin* pictures the lowest element, earth, associated with the center at the base of the spine, as dissolving into the water element at the second *cakra*, and that as dissolving into the fire element at the navel center, and that into the air element at the heart, and that into the ether element at the throat, and that into the infinite space of Consciousness at the crown center. At that point, the practitioner's body-mind is thought to be thoroughly purified.

This ritual is to be followed by a series of other practices by which the body is step by step converted into a temple, or sacred mound, ready to receive the great Being in the form of one's chosen deity (*ishta-devatâ*). Thus, through the practice of "life infusion" (*jîva-nyâsa*), *yogins* assimilate the life force of their chosen (*ishta*) deity. This is done by empowering certain body parts through touch, and infusing them with the life of the God or Goddess of their choice. Another form of "infusion," "installation," or "placement" (*nyâsa*) is *mâtrikâ-nyâsa*, by which the fifty sacred sounds of the Sanskrit alphabet are placed in the *yogin*'s body. The "matrices" or "little mothers" (*mâtrikâ*), as the Sanskrit alphabetic sounds are called, are thought of as the offspring of the primordial sound (*shabda*) of the Absolute. The body parts of the chosen deity are imagined as consisting of the different letters of the alphabet, which are visualized in the respective areas of the *yogin*'s body.

Other similar rites include the "installation of the seers" (*rishi-nyâsa*), the "installation of the six limbs"(*shad-anga-nyâsa*), which is performed by placing the hands on six different bodily parts and empowering them, and the "installation of the hands" (*kara-nyâsa*), which is the same kind of exercise but performed on the fingers and palms

of the hands only. Interspersed between the various rites are complex visualization practices (called *dhyâna*), usually of the deity and his or her celestial abode. All this is a matter of subtle energy experienced by the adept who identifies with the deity of his or her choice. Each deity itself is thought to represent a particular quality of energy. This Tantric practice is combined with a great deal of *mantra* recitation, regulated breathing, and intense concentration. I have already spoken of *mantras* in Chapter 2 in connection with Mantra-Yoga, and they are also the principal tool of the Tantric practitioner.

## Mantra Practice

Under the aegis of Tantra, the age-old practice of *mantra* recitation became a very sophisticated art. The Tantric teachings are also known as *mantra-shâstra*, because their favorite subject matter is the "science of *mantras*" (*mantra-vidyâ*). The Tantric Buddhism of Tibet is known as Mantrayâna. The word *mantra* itself is esoterically explained as being derived from the words *manana* ("thinking") and *trâna* ("liberation")." In other words, a *mantra* is a potent form of thought, an instrument of conscious intention.

> Because the *mantra* is an expression of
> a more evolved consciousness, it offers
> a unique link with that higher level. For
> this reason, it not only makes the path to
> higher consciousness clearer by replacing interfering thoughts, its gradual incorporation pulls consciousness toward
> that state.[27]

Broadly speaking, *mantras* are sounds charged with numinous power. Agehananda Bharati, who was a monk of the Dashanami Order with Tantric leanings, noted that *mantras* can have three possible purposes.[28] They can be used to appease the forces of the universe in order to ward off unpleasant experiences and foster pleasant ones, to acquire things by magical means, and to identify with an aspect of reality (such as a specific deity) or with Reality itself.

As the *Tantras* emphasize, *mantras* are not arbitrary inventions. They are revealed to yogic adepts in heightened states of awareness, and their effectiveness depends entirely on proper initiation (*dikshâ*). According to the esoteric traditions of India, the mere repetition of the archetypal *mantra om*, for instance, will have no spiritualizing effect unless its recitation is empowered by a qualified teacher. As the *Kula-Arnava-Tantra* (chapter 11) declares, there are countless *mantras*

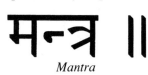

*Mantra*

that only distract the mind. For a *mantra* to bear fruit it must have been received by the teacher's grace. The recitation of a *mantra* that has been overheard or acquired by deceit or accident is considered to lead only to personal misfortune.

The recitation (*japa*) of *mantras* can be done aloud (*vâcika*), whispered (*upâmshu*), or mentally (*mânasa*), which is deemed the best, because it is the most potent. They should be carefully enunciated and never sloppily performed. A fourth way of benefiting from a *mantra* is by writing it out, which is known as "written recitation" (*likhita-japa*).

Whichever form of *japa* is chosen, only conscientious and intensely conscious practice can awaken a *mantra*'s potency and lead to success. Each *mantra* is associated with a specific state of consciousness (*caitanya*), and recitation is thought to be successful when that consciousness is actualized. Without its actualization, a *mantra* is mere sound that has no transformative power. From another point of view, however, a *mantra* is the manifestation of the Absolute as Sound (*shabda-brahman*). The eternal unmanifest sound is the root principle of all manifest sounds—a concept similar to the Greek idea of the *logos*, as found in the opening passage of the gospel of St. John. *Shabda* is the kinetic aspect of the Absolute. In its purely transcendental state, the Absolute is thought of as static and uncreative, and it is through its aspect of sound, or vibration, that it generates the finite realms of existence, such as our space-time universe.

Like the world of forms, sound proceeds from the Absolute in a series of distinct stages. Tantrism proposes a four-phase model of speech (*vâc*, Latin *vox*):

1.  "Supreme speech" (*para-vâc*) — sound as pure potentiality, which is coessential with the Creator's pure cosmic ideation (*shrishti-pratyaya*), or divine will, arising from the union of Shiva and Shakti. This is the level of the subtle inner sound (*nâda*).

2.  "Visible speech" (*pashyantî-vâc*) — sound as mental image prior to thought. This is the level of the seed-point (*bindu*), arising out of the subtle sound.

3.  "Intermediate speech" (*madhyamâ-vâc*) — sound as thought, corresponding to the matrices (*mâtrika*) out of which the distinct audible sounds are created.

4.  "Manifest speech" (*vaikharî-vâc*) — audible sound (*dhvani*), also called "coarse sound" (*sthûla-shabda*), the final step in the process of increasing "densification."

For generations in the East, *mantras* have been employed not only in sacred contexts, but have widely served as magical spells for profane ends, including healing and occasional black magic. However, their nuclear significance is as a means of internalizing and intensifying awareness to the point of transcendence of all contents of consciousness. It is impossible to do justice to this far-ranging and recondite subject here, and I refer the reader to the works of Sir John Woodroffe for an abundance of technical details, notably his *The Garland of Letters*.[29]

In addition to *mantras*, there are two other important elements of Tantric practice, namely hand gestures (*mudrâ*) and geometric representations of the levels and energies of the psychocosmos, which are known as "devices" (*yantra*).

## Symbolic Gestures (Mudrâ)

The word *mudrâ* is derived from the root *mud*, "to be glad, delight in," because *mudrâs* bring delight (*mudâ*) to the deities and cause the dissolution (*drava*) of the mind. But the term *mudrâ* also denotes "seal," and it is employed in Tantric contexts in this sense, because the hand gestures (or, in Hatha-Yoga, the bodily postures), "seal" the body, thus bringing joy. They are means of controlling the energy in the body. They are also symbolic

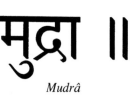
*Mudrâ*

representations of inner states. People who are even a little bit sensitive to the body's energies can easily verify that by folding one's hands a change of mood is effected: We begin to feel more mentally collected. With a little experience, the different inner states associated with the *mudrâs* become clearly discernible.

There are said to be 108 hand gestures—108 being a favorite sacred number among Hindus. In

reality, there are many more, though according to the *Nirvâna-Tantra* (11) fifty-five are most commonly used. The origin of the hand gestures used in the Tantric rituals is obscure. They probably go back to Vedic times, when the sacrificial cere-

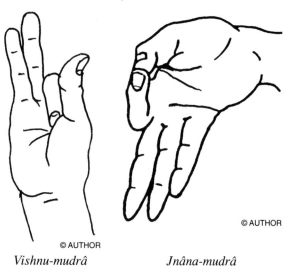
*Vishnu-mudrâ*          *Jnâna-mudrâ*

monies involved the meticulous handling of implements such as the ladle during the pouring of the soma libations. The Japanese tea ceremony is a good example of the intensely conscious conduct called for in such rituals. Another, later source of inspiration was Indian dance, which knows a great repertoire of *mudrâs*, though the possibility that the Tantric *mudrâs* cross-fertilized Indian dance cannot be ruled out. The *Natya-Shâstra* ("Textbook of Dance"), created around 200 C.E. but attributed to the ancient sage Bharata, mentions thirty-seven positions of the hands but also thirty-six specific ways of gazing, closing the eyes, or raising the eyebrows.

The most commonly used Tantric hand gesture, which is also widely employed as a meditation gesture in Yoga, is the *jnâna-mudrâ* ("wisdom seal") or the *cin-mudrâ* ("consciousness seal") depicted above.

In the various Tantric rituals, many other *mudrâs* are used, often specific to the deity invoked. Thus, according to the *Mantra-Yoga-Samhitâ* (53), nineteen seals are necessary in the worship of Vishnu, ten for Shiva and the Goddess Tripurâ Sundarî, nine for Durgâ, seven for Ganesha, five for Târâ, four for Sarasvatî, two for Râma and Parashu-Râma, and only one for Lakshmî. In the Shrî-Vidyâ tradition, the Goddess Tripurâ Sundarî is invoked by means of ten hand gestures, which are symbolically related to the nine sets (called *cakra*) of subsidiary triangles composing the famous *shrî-yantra* (or *shrî-cakra*), with the tenth *mudrâ* representing the *yantra* and Goddess as a whole.

## Common ritual hand gestures

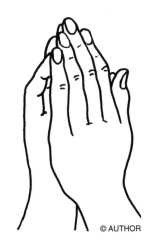

© AUTHOR

1. *Anjali-mudrâ* ("seal of honoring"): Bring the palms of your hands together in front of the heart, with the extended fingers pointing upward. Particularly when done at the level of the forehead, this prayerful gesture is used to welcome the deity.

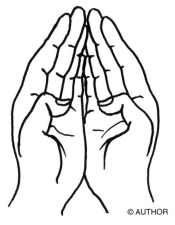

© AUTHOR

2. *Âvâhani-mudrâ* ("seal of invitation"): Bring your hands together, palms up and forming an offering bowl, with thumbs curled and the other fingers fully extended. This gesture is used, for instance, when offering a flower to the deity.

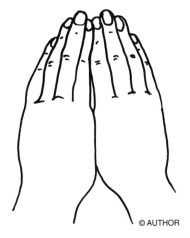

© AUTHOR

3. *Sthâpana-karmanî-mudrâ* ("seal of fixing action"): Bring your hands together, palms down, with thumbs tucked underneath. This is essentially the same gesture as the one above, but in reverse.

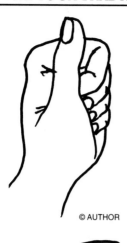

© AUTHOR

4.  *Samnidhâpanî-mudrâ* ("seal of bringing close"): Bring your closed fists together, with thumbs placed on top.

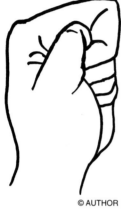

© AUTHOR

5.  *Samnirodhanî-mudrâ* ("seal of full control"): Same as the preceding gesture but with thumbs tucked into the fists.

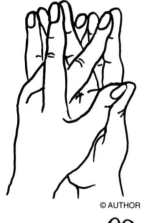

© AUTHOR

6.  *Dhenu-mudrâ* ("cow seal"), also called *amritî-karana-mudrâ* ("seal creating the nectar of immortality"): Place the tip of the right index finger on the tip of the left middle finger, the tip of the right middle finger on the tip of the left index finger, the tip of the right ring finger on the tip of the left little finger, and the tip of the right little finger on the tip of the left ring finger.

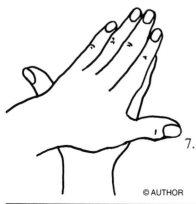

© AUTHOR

7.  *Matsya-mudrâ* ("fish seal"): Place the palm of the left hand on top of the right hand with the fingers fully extended and the thumbs pointing outward at right angles.

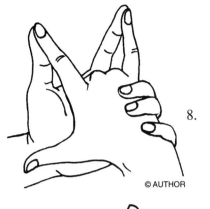
© AUTHOR

8. *Kûrma-mudrâ* ("tortoise seal"): Place the palms together in such a way that the right thumb rests on the left wrist, the right index finger touches the tip of the left thumb, and the tips of the right little finger and left index finger touch.

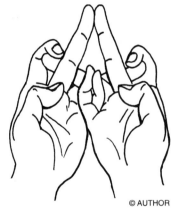
© AUTHOR

9. *Padma-mudrâ* ("lotus seal"): Bring the wrists together, with the fingers forming the petals of a lotus blossom. The fingertips do not touch.

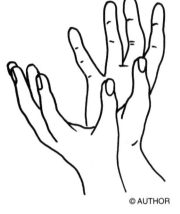
© AUTHOR

10. *Yoni-mudrâ* ("seal of the womb/vulva"): Bring your hands together, palms up. Interlace the little fingers, and cross the ring fingers behind the fully extended middle fingers, which touch at the tips. The ring fingers are held down by the index fingers. This is the classic symbol of the Goddess.

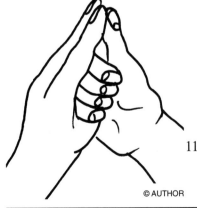
© AUTHOR

11. *Shanka-mudrâ* ("conch seal"): Hold the thumb of your left hand with four fingers other than the thumb of your right and bring the right thumb to the extended fingers of the left hand.

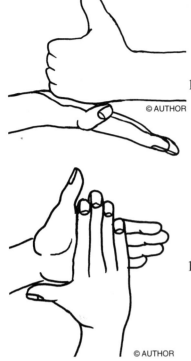

© AUTHOR

12.  *Shiva-linga-mudrâ* ("seal of Shiva's mark"): Place the left hand palm up near the chest; make the right hand into a fist and place it on the left palm. The right thumb is extended upward. (This illustration is shown from the viewpoint of an observer.)

13.  *Cakra-mudrâ* ("wheel seal"): Place the left hand with extended fingers in front of the chest, with the palm facing the chest and the thumb extended. Then place the extended right hand, facing downward, on top of the left palm, again with the right thumb extended and at the left wrist.

© AUTHOR

Tantrism also knows of therapeutic *mudrâs*, which operate on the principle that the body mirrors macrocosmic realities and that disease is caused by an imbalance of the five material elements (earth, water, air, fire, and ether/space).[30] The above-mentioned *jnâna-mudrâ* is thought to be excellent for combating insomnia, nervous tension, and weak memory. *Prâna-mudrâ* is recommended in the case of a heart attack. It is performed by pressing the index finger down on the mound of the thumb, with the other fingers pushing the index finger. *Shûnya-mudrâ* ("seal of emptiness"), which is said to be good for curing deafness, is executed by placing the middle finger against the root of the thumb. *Sûrya-mudrâ* ("solar seal"), which is recommended when feeling a sense of heaviness, is done by placing the ring finger against the root of the thumb. In all cases, the seal is to be practiced with both hands simultaneously.

## Geometric Meditation Devices (Yantra)

A *yantra* is a thumbnail sketch of the levels and energies of the universe—personalized in the shape of a given deity (*devatâ*)—and thus the human body (as a microcosmic replica of the macrocosm). A *yantra* may be drawn on paper, wood, cloth, or any other material, or into sand if nothing else is available. Three-dimensional models made of clay or metal are also known. A *yantra* has a similar function to the *mandala* ("circle") used in Tibetan Tantrism. The difference between them is that *mandalas* tend to be more pictorial and are based on a circular arrangement of their constituent elements. A *yantra* typically consists of a square surround, circles, lotus petals, triangles, and at the center the "seed-point" (*bindu*). Each component has a more or less elaborate symbolism attached to it. Thus, the upward-pointing triangle denotes the masculine or Shiva pole of reality, while the downward-pointing triangle represents the feminine or Shakti pole. The point in the middle is the creative matrix of the universe, the gateway to the transcendental Reality itself.

In the higher stages of Tantric practice, the *yantra* must be completely internalized, that is, *yogins* must construct its complex geometrical pattern mentally through visualization. The *yantra* is erected either from the innermost point outward—in accordance with the process of macrocosmic evolution—or from the outermost

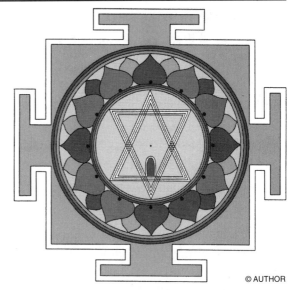

*Tripurâ-sundarî-yantra*

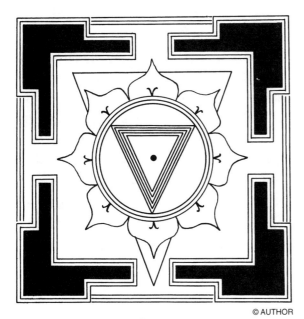

*Kâlî-yantra*

circumference toward the center—in alignment with the microcosmic process of meditative involution. After having elaborately constructed the *yantra* internally, *yogins* proceed to dissolve it again. Since they are, in consciousness, identical with the structure of the *yantra*, its dissolution necessarily implies their own extinction as an experiencing subject. In other words, *yogins*, if successful at this advanced practice, transcend their conditioned mind and are catapulted into pure Being-Consciousness-Bliss, where the distinction between subject and object does not exist.

Tantrism employs a large number of *yantras*. In Chapter 20 of the *Mantra-Mahodadhi* ("Great Ocean of *Mantras*") twenty-nine *yantras* are described. The most celebrated of all is undoubtedly the *shrî-yantra* depicted below. The name *shrî* refers to Lakshmî, the goddess of fortune. This *yantra* is composed of nine juxtaposed triangles that are arranged in such a way that together they produce a total of forty-three smaller triangles. Four of the nine primary triangles point

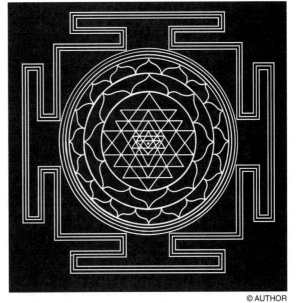

*Shrî-yantra*

upward, representing the male cosmic energy (Shiva); five of them point downward, symbolizing the female power (Shakti). These triangles are surrounded by an eight-petaled lotus symbolizing the deity Vishnu, who stands for the all-pervading ascending tendency in the universe. The next lotus, with sixteen petals, represents the attainment of the desired object, particularly *yogins'* power over their mind and senses. Enclosing this lotus are four concentric lines that are symbolically connected with the two lotuses. The triple line surround is called "earth-city" (*bhû-pura*), which designates the consecrated place that may be the entire universe or, by way of analogy, the human body.

Some ritual *yantras* are also employed for therapeutic purposes. In addition, *yantras* specific to an illness or a person can be created as amulets to effect magical cures. In every case, the effectiveness of a *yantra* depends on the adept's quality of concentration and visualization, as well as on his or her mastery of the subtle energies.

## The Ritual of the "Five M's"

The term *mudrâ*, mentioned above, is applied to another practice of Tantrism. It refers to one of the elements of the central Tantric ritual of the "Five M's" (*panca-makâra*). These five practices, which in Sanskrit all have names beginning with the letter *m*, are the following: (1) *madya* or wine; (2) *matsya* or fish; (3) *mâmsa* or meat; (4) *mudrâ* or parched grain; (5) *maithunâ* or sexual intercourse. These five are understood metaphorically (in right-hand schools) and performed literally (in left-hand schools).

According to the *Kula-Arnava-Tantra* (chapter 4), wine is used in the left-hand ritual as a cathartic agent, cleansing the mind from the worries and concerns of everyday life. The object,

however, is not drunkenness, which induces stupor rather than clarity. Similarly, the consumption of fish and meat, which are as strictly forbidden to the ordinary Hindu as is wine, has the sole purpose of achieving a higher state of awareness. Parched grain, like wine, fish, and meat, is supposed to act as an aphrodisiac—again an awareness-altering substance. Why parched grain should have this property is nowhere explained in the classical or exegetical literature, though it is possible that ergot might be involved, which was apparently also used in the ancient Greek cult of Demeter.

Not mentioned among the "Five M's" but also prominent in Tantric rites are narcotic drugs (*aushadhi*). Commenting on the widespread use of awareness- or mood-altering drugs, Swami Satyananda Saraswati of Bihar made the observation that, to this day, India's holy men take drugs such as *ganja* (marijuana) and datura (jimsonweed), while *bhang* (a preparation made from marijuana) is universally used during the Shivaratri festival, in which the marriage of Shiva and Parvati is celebrated. However, the Swami did not fail to remind us that drugs "allow us to taste the beyond but do not make us masters of the transcendental."[31]

Practitioners of the left-hand path (*vâma-mârga*)—*vâma* means both "left" and "woman"—know they are breaking profound social taboos, and their only justification for their conduct is that their goal is not sensual gratification but self-transcendence in the context of bodily existence. The philosophy of Tantrism is summarized in the following words from the *Mahâcîna-Âcâra-Krama-Tantra*:

> The *yogin* cannot be a sensualist (*bhogin*), and the sensualist is not one endowed with Yoga. Hence the *kaula* whose essence is Yoga and sensuality is held to be superior to everyone.[32]

## Ritual Sex (Maithunâ)

The *Tantras* make it clear that to be successful in this dangerous approach, the (male) practitioner must not suffer from doubt, fear, or lust. He must be a "hero" (*vîra*). This is especially important in the execution of the fifth practice, which is sexual congress—a practice that the *Tantras* generally direct to male practitioners. The female partner in this rite must be duly consecrated through ritual bathing and other ceremonies of purification, and ideally she should be a spiritual practitioner herself. The *yogin* must see in her not a person of the opposite sex, but the Goddess, Shakti, just as he must experience himself as Shiva. The ideal female partner should be lovely and quite uninhibited. Any woman qualifies, except one's mother. However, in an appendix to the *Yoga-Karnikâ* ("Ear-Ornament of Yoga"), a work of the eighteenth century, we find Shiva himself give the following instruction:

> One should place one's penis into the vagina of one's mother and one's sandals on one's father's head, while fondling [or licking] one's sister's breasts and kissing her fair seat. He who does this, O great Goddess, reaches the Abode of Extinction. He who worships day and night an actress, a female skull-bearer, a prostitute, a low-caste woman, a washerman's wife—he verily [becomes identical with] the blessed Sadâ-Shiva.

More likely than not, even extreme left-hand *tântrikas* would interpret the opening sentence metaphorically. Tantrism has a fully developed "twilight language" (*sandha-bhâsha*), or secret symbolic language, which can be very misleading to the uninitiated. Initiates must learn from a knowledgeable teacher how to navigate the symbolism of their respective tradition lest they become shipwrecked on the rock of literalism.

In left-hand Tantrism, the term *mudrâ* also refers to the female partner in the metasexual ritual. She also is called *vâma*, simply meaning "lovely woman." The *maithunâ* rite, which

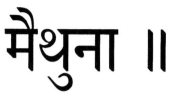

*Maithunâ*

incidentally has Vedic antecedents, often bears the technical designation *yoni-pûjâ* or "worship of the vulva." This is meant to suggest that the rite is a sacred procedure. In fact, it can be an exceedingly complex affair, consisting of hours of painstaking ceremonial preparation and then an equally formal period of actual intercourse. Ordinarily, this ritual is performed among a circle (*cakra*) of initiates with the teacher present. The partners embrace as male and female deities, not ordinary mortals. There is of course delight, since the whole point of the ritual is to generate bliss (*ânanda*) through bodily means, but there should be no self-indulgence, no egoic exploitation of the experience.

It is incumbent on the *yogin* to prevent the discharge of his semen at all cost. Semen (*bindu*, *retas*) is considered a most precious product of the life force and must be conserved. The significance of *coitus reservatus* is that the semen is transmuted into a finer substance, called *ojas*, that nourishes the higher centers of the body, thereby facilitating the difficult ordeal of psychosomatic transformation attempted in Tantrism. From ancient times a spiritual practitioner who is adept at this inner alchemy has been known as *ûrdhva-retas* or "one whose semen flows upward." This can be experienced as a literal event, as is clear from Gopi Krishna's description:

There was no doubt an extraordinary change in my nervous equipment, and a new type of force was now racing through my system connected unmistakably with the sexual parts, which also seemed to have developed a new kind of activity not perceptible before. The nerves lining the parts and the surrounding region were all in a state of intense ferment, as if forced by an invisible mechanism to produce the vital seed in abnormal abundance to be sucked up by the network of nerves at the base of the spine for transmission into the brain through the spinal cord. The sublimated seed formed an integral part of the radiant energy which was causing me such bewilderment and about which I was as yet unable to speculate with any degree of assurance.[33]

The climax of Tantric Yoga is not orgasm but ecstasy—the practitioner's abiding in and as the transcendental Self beyond the ego-self-personality. The female partner, however, may come to orgasm during the *maithunâ* ritual. Her sexual excitement produces a much-desired vaginal secretion that the competent *tântrika* knows how to suck up through his penis. The female ejaculate is thought to enrich the *yogin*'s hormonal system. This practice is called *vajrolî-mudrâ* and belongs to the repertoire of Hatha-Yoga. But primarily the interaction between *yogin* and *yoginî* is one of energy exchange that goes far beyond what occurs in ordinary intercourse.

More than any other feature of Tantrism, the "Five M's" embody its antinomian spirit: Tantric practitioners deliberately break with conventional life. Their behavior is based on the principle of reversal (*viparîta*). They seem to indulge in sensual pleasure (*bhoga*), whereas in reality they cultivate transcendental bliss (*ânanda*). In this way they lend a new, esoteric significance to all their seemingly mundane actions. In Hatha-Yoga, it is the headstand that best symbolizes this principle of reversal. The Tantric procedures are all intended to construct a new reality for the *yogin* or *yoginî*—a sacred reality that is analogous to the transcendental Reality: The practitioner's body becomes the body of the chosen deity (*ishta-devatâ*). That is to say, it is as that deity that the *yogin* or *yoginî* approaches the transcendence of all forms, until he or she is one with the supreme Deity, or Godhead, which is sheer Being.[34]

## IV. THE MAGIC OF POWERS

Tantrism, or Tantra, is concerned with *siddhi* ("attainment, realization"), both in the sense of ultimate liberation and magical power. Since the Tantric viewpoint affirms the phenomenal world, it also has a positive relationship to the cultivation of the body-mind's innate psychophysical potential. Unlike certain schools of Vedânta, which anxiously avoid paranormal abilities (*siddhi, vibhûti*),

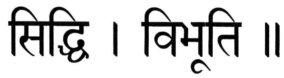

*Siddhi, vibhûti*

Tantrism regards them as an advantage, allowing practitioners to accomplish their spiritual goals in the world more readily and fully. As can be expected, however, *tântrikas* have also cultivated such powers for less noble goals, and entire *Tantras* have been composed dealing with unsavory practices with the explicit purpose of controlling or harming others. This orientation is sometimes referred to as "lower Tantrism," as opposed to the "higher Tantrism" motivated by liberation and the spiritual upliftment of other human and nonhuman beings.

The Yoga and Tantra scriptures mention numerous paranormal abilities, which are presented as being part of the accomplished adept's arsenal of skillful means. The *Yoga-Bîja* (54) states:

> The *yogin* is endowed with unthinkable powers. He who has conquered the senses can, by his own will, assume various shapes and make them vanish again.

According to the *Yoga-Shikhâ-Upanishad* (1.156), these abilities are the mark of a true Yoga adept and are encountered in the course of one's spiritual practice, just as a pilgrim on the way to the sacred city of Kâshî (modern Benares/ Varanasi) passes by a number of sacred spots (*tîrtha*). Conversely (1.160), in the absence of such abilities, a person can be said to be bound.

This text (1.151–155) distinguishes two fundamental types of paranormal abilities, namely those that are artificial (*kalpita*) and those that are nonartificial (*akalpita*), or spontaneously arising. The former are produced by means of herbal concoctions (*aushadhi*), ritual (*kriyâ*), magic (*jâla*), *mantra* recitation, and alchemical elixirs (*rasa*). In an aphorism that was probably interpolated, the *Yoga-Sûtra* (4.1) similarly explains that *siddhis* can arise from birth (*janman*), herbal concoctions (*aushadhi*), *mantra* recitation, asceticism (*tapas*), and ecstasy (*samâdhi*). The nonartificial or spontaneous abilities are said in the *Yoga-Shikhâ-Upanishad* to spring from self-reliance (*svatantrya*), and to be permanent, greatly efficacious, and pleasing to the Lord (*îshvara*). They manifest naturally in those who are free from desire.

The third chapter of Patanjali's *Yoga-Sûtra* contains a long list of *siddhis* and therefore bears the title *vibhûti-pâda*. The term *vibhûti* means

"manifestation" and probably stems from the *Bhagavad-Gîtâ* (10.16), which speaks of the far-flung powers of Lord Krishna. The fully realized adept, who is one with the Divine, has access to all the divine powers. He or she is a *mahâ-siddha* ("great adept") who enjoys the *mahâ-siddhis*, or great powers.

Usually eight great powers are mentioned, and according to the *Yoga-Bhâshya* (3.45) they are the following:

1.  *Animan* ("miniaturization")[35] — the ability to shrink oneself to the size of an atom (*anu*). According to the *Yoga-Sûtra* (3.44), this results from mastery over the material elements. The *Yoga-Bhâshya-Vivarana* (3.45) states that by means of *animan* one becomes more subtle than the subtle and thus can no longer be seen.

2.  *Mahiman* ("magnification") — the ability to expand to a vast size. In his *Tattva-Vaishâradî* (3.45), Vâcaspati Mishra explains this as the ability to become as large as an elephant, a mountain, or a whole town, and so on. However, the *Mani-Prabhâ* (3.45) defines *mahiman* as "pervasiveness" (*vibhûtva*), which suggests that it is not the physical body that expands but the subtle body, or mind.

3.  *Laghiman* ("levitation") — the ability to become weightless "like the tuft of a reed" (*Tattva-Vaishâradî* 3.45).

4.  *Prâpti* ("extension") — the ability to bridge great distances instantly. The *Yoga-Bhâshya* (3.45) seriously suggests that by means of this power the

*yogin* can touch the moon with his fingertips.

5. *Prâkâmya* ("[irresistible] will") — the ability to realize one's will. The *Yoga-Bhâshya* (3.45) gives the example of diving into solid earth as if it were liquid.

6. *Vâshitva* ("mastery") — complete mastery over the material elements (*bhûta*) and their products or, as the *Yoga-Bhâshya-Vivarana* (3.45) puts it, over all the worlds.

7. *Îshitritva* ("lordship") — perfect mastery over the subtle causes of the material world, bringing the *yogin* on a par with the Creator (Brahma) himself.

8. *Kâma-avasâyitva* ("fulfillment of [all] desires," written *kâmâvasâyitva*) — the unobstructed ability to will into being whatever one sees fit. The *Yoga-Bhâshya* (3.45), however, makes it clear that the adept's will does not go against the will of the Lord (*îshvara*). Thus, as the *Yoga-Bhâshya-Vivarana* (3.45) explains, he does not make fire cold because he respects the preestablished order of things.

In addition to the eight classic *siddhis*, which vary somewhat from school to school, Tantrism also recognizes a set of six magical actions (*shat-karman*), which are treated in many short *Tantras*. One of the most widely disseminated (and medium-size) scriptures dealing with the *shat-karmans* is the *Dattâtreya-Tantra* comprising seven hundred stanzas. Even more popular is the *Shat-Karma-Dîpikâ* ("Light on the Six Actions")

authored by the renowned sixteenth-century Bengali adept Krishnânanda Vidyâvâgîshvara, who also composed the *Tantra-Sâra* (to be distinguished from Abhinava Gupta's earlier work of the same title). The six magical actions are standardized as follows:

1. *Shânti* ("peace") — the ability to pacify another being by magical means, such as *mantra*, *yantra*, and visualization. As the *Kalpa-Cintâmani*, an abridgment of the *Mahâkalpa-Cintâmani*, states in the section on *shânti*, this practice can be used to eradicate fever.

2. *Vashîkarana* ("subjugation") — the ability to bring others under one's complete control and make them subservient like slaves.

3. *Stambhana* ("stoppage") — the ability to completely immobilize another being or render a situation ineffective.

4. *Uccâtana* ("eradication") — the ability to destroy someone at a distance and without visible means.

5. *Vidveshana* ("causing dissension") — the ability to create discord among people.

6. *Mârana* ("death-ing") — the ability to kill someone at a distance.

The above practices amount to black magic and seem to fall short of the high Tantric ideal of liberation through gnosis and spiritual upliftment. They have, no doubt, been deployed for millennia, however, and even today it is not difficult to find *tântrikas* who, for a few rupees, will use their magical skills to harm others. In this respect, India is not different from other countries with a strong premodern cultural base. Such degenerate practices, however, do not characterize higher Tantrism, which is first and foremost a path to liberation that entails elevated moral values.

What are we to make of these abilities? Are they merely the product of a lively imagination triggered by too much solitary introspection? Or are they manifestations of a psychic dimension of reality that science still needs to discover? Over the centuries, all kinds of anecdotal reports have come down to us of the uncommon powers of *yogins* and strange phenomena witnessed in their company. While there is today ample evidence of *yogins'* incredible control over bodily and mental functions that had long been thought to be outside the reach of our personal will, their claims to paranormal abilities have so far been only scantily researched. The cumulative weight of the findings of parapsychological research on nonyogic subjects, however, increasingly lends credence to at least some of the claims made in yogic circles.

Rather than offhandedly dismissing the *siddhis* as mere fantasy, it would be more prudent to appreciate them as an integral aspect of the experiential world of *yogins* and as worthy of unbiased investigation. As is evident from the massive evidence accumulated by parapsychology, the human potential is extraordinary. Anyone who reads, for instance, Michael Murphy's *The Future of the Body* with an open mind cannot fail to be struck by the scope of the available scientific and anecdotal evidence for paranormal abilities.[36]

---

**SOURCE READING 20**

## *Kula-Arnava-Tantra (Selection)*

The *Kula-Arnava-Tantra* (written *Kulârnavatantra*), one of the most important scriptures of the Kaula tradition, was probably composed between 1000 and 1400 C.E. According to its own testimony, the extant version of a little over 2,000 stanzas constitutes only the fifth chapter of a text that originally comprised 125,000 stanzas but is no longer available (if it ever existed in such a comprehensive form). Following is a rendering of the ninth chapter, which contains many valuable definitions of the Kaula approach.

Shrî Devî said:
Kula Lord! I desire to hear about Yoga, the characteristics of the foremost of *yogins*, and the fruit of adoration for the *kula* worshiper. Tell me that, O embodiment (*nidhi*) of compassion! (1)

The Lord (*îshvara*) said:
Listen Goddess! I will tell you what you ask of me. Merely by listening to this, Yoga is revealed directly. (2)

Meditation is said to be twofold, due to the difference between coarse (*sthûla*) and subtle (*sûkshma*) [objects]. They call the coarse [meditation] "with form" and the subtle [meditation] "formless." (3)

*Comments:* This distinction is also found in the scriptures of Hatha-Yoga, where coarse meditation is meditation having an internalized image of a deity, one's teacher, and so forth. Subtle meditation is equated in the *Gheranda-Samhitâ* (6.9) with the *shâmbhavî-mudrâ* ("Shambhu's seal"), which consists in the direct experience of the union of Shambhu (i.e., Shiva) and Shakti.

When the mind has a stable object [to concentrate on], this is styled "coarse meditation" by some. The mind must be immobile in the coarse [meditation] and likewise immobile in the subtle [meditation]. (4)

One should contemplate the supreme Lord [who is] impartite Being-Consciousness-Bliss lacking hands, feet, belly, face, and so forth and consisting entirely of [unmanifest] light. (5)

He does not rise; he does not sink; he does not undergo growth; he does not undergo diminution. Himself being resplendent, he illumines others, without performing [any actions whatsoever]. (6)

When the infinite, luminous, pure, transcendental (*agocara*) Being is experienced purely by the mind, then the [arising] wisdom is designated as the Absolute (*brahman*). (7)

*Comments:* From the vantage point of enlightenment, there is no distinction between the Absolute, or Self, and the enlightened being's knowledge thereof.

The *yogin* who knows the singular splendor (*dhâman*) of the supreme entity (*jîva*), [which is] immovable like stone [or like] the discontinued motion of the wind [i.e., windstillness], is called a knower of Yoga. (8)

That meditation that is devoid of its essence but illuminating and steady like the unruffled ocean is styled "ecstasy" (*samâdhi*). (9)

*Comments:* This stanza echoes the *Yoga-Sûtra* (3.2–3). The "essence" (*sva-rupa*) of meditation is the contemplation of a chosen object, implying a division between subject and object. In the ecstatic state, this schism is overcome, and instead the *yogin* becomes identified with the object of contemplation, in the present case the Divine itself.

The [ultimate] Reality shines forth of itself, not by any mental effort (*cintana*) whatsoever. When Reality shines forth of itself, one should immediately assume its form. (10)

He who abides sleeplike in the dream and waking state, without inhaling or exhaling, is certainly liberated. (11)

*Comments:* Here liberation is equated with the state of trancelike ecstasy. A higher realization is the open-eyed state of *sahaja-samâdhi*, which includes the external world in the blissful condition of enlightenment.

He who is like a corpse, having the "wind" [i.e., the breath and subtle life energy] and the mind merged in his Self, with the host of senses motionless, he is clearly called "liberated while alive." (12)

*Comments:* The supreme realization of living liberation (*jîvan-mukti*) is here identified with the state of trancelike ecstasy corresponding to *asamprajnâta-samâdhi* in Patanjali's Classical Yoga. In other schools, living liberation is based on *sahaja-samâdhi*.

[The *yogin* in the ecstatic state] does not hear, smell, touch, see, or experience pleasure and pain, and his mind does not conceptualize. (13)

He experiences nothing and, like a log, does not comprehend [anything]. Thus, with the [individual] self merged into Shiva, [the *yogin*] is here called "ecstasy abiding" (*samâdhi-stha*). (14)

As water poured into water, milk into milk, and ghee into ghee becomes indistinguishable, so [also is the merging of] the individual self with the supreme Self. (15)

*Comments:* This definition of ecstasy, or of the goal of Yoga, is widely found in the *Tantras* and *Purânas*, as well as in the textbooks of Vedânta.

Just as through the capacity for meditation a worm comes to be a bee, so a man, through the capacity for ecstasy, will assume the nature of the Absolute (*brahman*). (16)

*Comments:* The ancient Hindus believed that a worm becomes a bee because of its mental focus.

Like ghee extracted from milk when poured back into it is not as before, so is said to be the [individual] self here [in this world], which is rendered distinct [from the transcendental Self] by the qualities (*guna*) [of Nature]. (17)

*Comments:* The three qualities are *sattva* (principle of lucidity), *rajas* (principle of dynamism), and *tamas* (principle of inertia). These define a person's body-mind and create the illusion of the individual being separate from every other individual and from the divine Source itself. Upon enlightenment, this misapprehension falls away, and the *yogin* realizes the supreme Self, which is said to be *nirguna*, that is, beyond the qualities of Nature.

Just as one afflicted with total blindness perceives nothing here, similarly the *yogin* does not perceive the manifest world (*prapanca*), [which is] invisible [to him]. (18)

Just as upon closing (*nimîlana*) [one's eyelids] one does not perceive the manifest world, so will be [the *yogin*'s consciousness] upon opening (*unmîlana*) [the eyelids]; this is a sign of meditation. (19)

*Comments:* In the state of deep meditation, or ecstasy, *yogins* do not perceive the ordinary world, regardless of whether their eyes are open or shut. Their field of vision is the infinite Self itself.

Just as a person experiences an itch in the body, similarly he who is coessential (*svarûpin*) with the supreme Absolute knows the motion of the world. (20)

*Comments:* For the *yogin* who has realized the Divine, that is, become identical with Shiva, the world is like the body is to the mind.

When the unchanging supreme Reality (*tattva*) transcending [all] letters (*varna*) is known, the *mantras* go into servitude together with the *mantra* rulers [i.e., the deities]. (21)

Whatever activity [is engaged] by him who abides in the condition of the singular Self, that is adoration (*arcana*). Whatever conversation [he makes], that is true *mantra*. That which is called "meditation" is introspection (*nirîkshana*). (22)

When identification with the body has ceased and the supreme Self is known, then wherever the mind roams it [experiences] ecstasy (*samâdhi*). (23)

Upon seeing this supreme Self, the knot at the heart is pierced, all doubts are removed, and his karmas disappear. (24)

If the chief of *yogins* attains the pure supreme State, he is not captivated even if he attains the state of the deities and *asuras*.[37] (25)

He who sees the omnipresent, tranquil, blissful, immutable Self (*âtmaka*), for him nothing is unattainable and nothing remains to be known. (26)

Upon attaining wisdom and knowledge as well as the Object (*jneya*) residing at the heart, upon ascertaining the tranquil state, O Goddess, [there is] no Yoga, no concentration. (27)

*Comments:* When the Self, which can be contacted at the heart, is fully realized, the work of Yoga is accomplished, and then all yogic means, including concentration and meditation, are transcended.

When the supreme Absolute is known, [then the *yogin*] is through with all rules, measures, and regulations. What use is a palmyra fan when the wind blows from [Mount] Malaya? (28)

For him who sees himself as *om* [i.e., the Self], there is no binding of the life force (*âsikâ*) and no binding of the nostrils (*nâsikâ*); there is no discipline (*yama*) and no self-restraint (*niyama*). (29)

Yoga is not [attained] through the lotus posture and not by gazing at the tip of the nose. Yoga, say the experts of Yoga, is the identity (*aikya*) of the psyche (*jîva*) with the [transcendental] Self. (30)

When the Supreme is contemplated here [on Earth] with faith even for an instant, the great merit that is gained thereby is incalculable. (31)

He who practices even for an instant the self-reflection "I am the Absolute" wipes out all sin, just as sunrise [dispels] darkness. (32)

The knower of Reality (*tattva*) obtains a crore[38] of virtues, which are the fruit of vows, rites, austerities, pilgrimages, gifts, worship of the deities, and so forth. (33)

The natural state (*sahaja-avasthâ*) is highest; meditation and concentration are middling; recitation and praising are low; sacrificial worship is lowest. (34)

Thinking (*cintâ*) about Reality is highest; thinking about recitation is middling; thinking about the textbooks (*shâstra*) is low; thinking about the world is lowest. (35)

A crore of ritual worships (*pûjâ*) is equal to one hymn of praise (*stotra*); a crore of hymns of praise is equal to one recitation (*japa*); a crore of recitations is equal to one meditation; a crore of meditations is equal to one [moment of complete] dissolution (*laya*) [into the transcendental Self]. (36)

*Mantra* is not superior to meditation; a deity is not superior to the Self; worship is not superior to application [of the limbs of Yoga]; reward is not superior to contentment. (37)

Inaction is supreme worship; silence is supreme recitation; nonthinking is supreme meditation; desirelessness (*anicchâ*) is the supreme fruit. (38)

The *yogin* should daily practice the worship at twilight without ablutions and *mantras*, [and he should practice] asceticism (*tapas*) without sacrifices (*homa*) and rituals of worship (*pûjâ*), and worship without garlands. (39)

[He who is] indifferent, unattached, free from desire (*vâsana*) and superimposition (*upâdhi*), absorbed in the essence of his innate [power] is a *yogin*, a knower of the supreme Reality. (40)

*Comments:* The term *upâdhi* stems from Vedânta and signifies the mind's habit of attributing finite aspects to the Infinite.

The body is the abode (*âlaya*) of God (*deva*), O Goddess! The psyche is God Sadâ-Shiva. One should abandon the offering-remains of ignorance; one should worship with the thought "I am He." (41)

*Comments:* The psyche (*jîva*) is the individuated consciousness deeming itself other than the omnipresent Divine. It is powered by the life force (*prâna*), which in turn is driven by the individual's karmic stock. In truth, however, the psyche is not a limited consciousness trapped in a material body but the all-comprising Being-Consciousness, the eternal Shiva. This and the next stanza are built on the word play *jîva*/Shiva.

The psyche is Shiva; Shiva is the psyche. The psyche is Shiva alone. The [unliberated] psyche is known as the fettered beast (*pâshu*). Sadâ-Shiva is one who is released from [all] bonds (*pâsha*). (42)

Rice is imprisoned in the husk; when the husk is gone, the grain [becomes visible]. [Similarly,] the psyche is known as imprisoned by karma; Sadâ-Shiva is [that Reality which is eternally] free from [the "husk" of] karma. (43)

God abides in fire in the heart of devout worshipers (*vipra*)[39] who have themselves awakened to the likeness (*pratimâ*) [within], who know the Self everywhere. (44)

*Comments:* The inner likeness is none other than the Self.

He who is the same in praise and abuse, cold and heat, joy and sorrow, and [who is always the same] toward friend and foe is chief among *yogins*, beyond excitement and nonexcitement. (45)

The *yogin* who is desireless and always content, seeing the same [in all], with his senses controlled and sojourning as it were in the body knows the supreme Reality. (46)

He who is free from thought, free from doubt, unsullied by desire and superimposition (*upâdhi*), and immersed in his innate essence is a *yogin* who knows the supreme Reality. (47)

As the lame, blind, deaf, timid, mad, dull-witted, etc., live, O Mistress of Kula, so [lives] the *yogin* who knows the [ultimate] Reality. (48)

He who is keen on the supreme bliss produced by the five seals (*mudrâ*) is chief amongst *yogins*; he perceives the Self within himself. (49)

*Comments:* Sanskrit does not have upper- and lowercase letters. Therefore the phrase *pashyaty âtmânam âtmani* could also be translated as "he perceives the self within the Self," "he perceives the self within the self." But *âtman* also can simply mean "oneself." The five seals referred to here are better known as the "Five M's," which comprise the core of the Kaula ritual: wine, meat, fish, parched grain (thought to have aphrodisiacal properties), and sexual intercourse.

O Beloved, the joy that comes about from wine (*ali*), meat, and intercourse [causes] liberation for the wise but sin (*pâtaka*) for the ignorant. (50)

He who ever enjoys liquor and meat, ever cares for [ritual] practice, and is ever free from doubt is called a *kula-yogin*. (51)

Drinking liquor, eating meat, intent on behaving according to his will, contemplating the identity of "I" and "That," he should live happily. (52)

He who does not have the smell of flesh or liquor [coming from] his mouth is undoubtedly merely a "beast" who must make atonement and must be shunned. (53)

So long as there is the smell of liquor [on his breath], the "beast" is Pashupati [i.e., Shiva] himself. Without the smell of wine and flesh even Pashupati is obviously a "beast." (54)

In the world the lowly are elevated and the elevated are lowered: This has been declared to be the path of Kula by Bhairava, the great Self. (55)

Bad behavior is good behavior; what should not be done is the best of what should be done. O Mistress of Kula, for the *kaulikas* untruth is truth. (56)

O Mistress of Kula, the *kaulikas* should drink forbidden drinks, eat forbidden food, and enjoy forbidden intercourse. (57)

O Mistress of Kula, for the *kaulikas* there is no rule, no prohibition, no virtue, no sin, no heaven, and no hell. (58)

O Lady of Kula, even if they are ignorant the *kaulikas* know, even if poor they are rich, even if ruined they flourish. (59)

O Mistress of Kula, even enemies are friendly to the *kaulikas*, kings serve them, and all the people are loyal to them. (60)

O Mistress of Kula, the indifferent become partial toward the *kaulikas*, all those who are haughty pay tribute to them, and harassers become helpful. (61)

O Mistress of Kula, for the *kaulikas* worthless [things] are endowed with [excellent] qualities (*guna*), what is *akula* is fit for the *kula*, and nonvirtuous [qualities] are virtuous. (62)

*Comments:* As a branch of Tantrism, the Kaula school adheres to the principle of reversal (*parâvritti*) by which seemingly unspiritual actualities are viewed as spiritual. In Buddhist parlance, the world of change is the changeless Reality, or *samsâra* equals *nirvâna*.

O Goddess, for the *kaulikas* death is actually a physician, one's home is heaven, and, O Mistress of Kula, intercourse with a woman is meritorious. (63)

O Beloved, why say more? The adept *kula-yogins* have all their desires fulfilled. One should not doubt this. (64)

O Mistress of Kula, in whatever stage of life (*âshrama*) the *kula-yogin* may be, he is unsullied by whatever disguise (*vesha*) [he may adopt]. (65)

Desiring the welfare of human beings, *yogins* roam the earth in various guises, with their true nature unrecognized. (66)

O Mistress of Kula, they do not easily divulge their Self-knowledge but live among people as if intoxicated, dumb, and stupid. (67)

*Comments: Kula-yogins* conceal their spiritual attainment and do not mind looking foolish in the eyes of others. This shows the level of their realization, contentment, and inner certainty.

Just as the constellations and planets become invisible in the world through a conjunction of sun and moon [i.e., at the time of an eclipse], so the behavior of *yogins* [is too subtle to be understood]. (68)

Just as one cannot see the trail of water creatures in water or of birds in the sky, so the behavior of *yogins* [is invisible, or unintelligible, to the ordinary person]. (69)

The experts of *kula-yoga*, O Beloved, speak like liars, behave like fools, and look like rogues. (70)

They behave in this way so that people despise them, do not seek out their company, and say nothing [to them]. Thus does a *yogin* live. (71)

O Great Goddess, the knowing *kula-yogin*, even though liberated and a master of Kula, plays like a child, behaves like a simpleton, and speaks like a madman. (72)

Just as people laugh at, despise, and ridicule what comes from afar [i.e., what is strange and foreign], so fares the *yogin*. (73)

The *yogin*, wearing various garments (*vesha*), moves on the surface of the earth at times [like someone who is] honored and at times [like someone who is] downtrodden, or like a demon or ghost. (74)

The *yogin* enjoys enjoyments not out of desire but for the benefit of the world. Favoring all people, he plays [freely] upon the surface of the earth. (75)

Just as the sun dries out everything, just as fire is all-consuming, so the *yogin* enjoys all enjoyments but is not tainted by sin. (76)

Just as the wind touches everything, just as space (*âkâsha*) is omnipresent, just as all who bathe in rivers [for the daily ablutions are pure], so the *yogin* is ever pure. (77)

Just as the water of a village becomes purified when entering a river, so too what has been touched by a barbarian (*mleccha*), and so forth, becomes pure in the hands of a *yogin*. (78)

O foremost Goddess, just as the experts of the *kula* wisdom do not stir, so the sages desiring the [highest] good (*hita*) honor the Self. (79)

That on which the master *yogins* move is deemed the supreme path, just as where the sun rises is called the eastern quarter. (80)

Wherever an elephant walks there is a [new] path. Similarly, O Mistress of Kula, wherever the *kula-yogin* moves there is the path [to liberation]. (81)

Who is capable of making a winding river straight or stopping its flow? Similarly, who can deter [the *yogin*] roaming peacefully and at will? (82)

Just as [a snake charmer] fortified by *mantras* is not bitten by his playthings, so also the knower (*jnânin*) playing with the serpents of the senses is not bitten. (83)

Beyond suffering, contented, beyond the opposites, and free from envy, the peaceful *kaulikas* are dedicated to the *kula* wisdom and devoted to you. (84)

Free from pride, anger, arrogance, hopefulness, egotism (*ahamkâra*), truthful in speech, the foremost *kaulikas* are not controlled by the senses and are stable. (85)

O Goddess, those whose hair stands on end, whose voice shakes [with emotion], and who shed tears of bliss when the *kula* [way of life] is praised are called the foremost of *kaulikas*. (86)

Those who consider the *kula* teaching (*dharma*) arising from Shiva as the best of all teachings in the world are the foremost of *kaulikas*. (87)

O Beloved, he who knows the truth of the *kula*, is an expert of the *kula* doctrine, and fond of *kula* worship is a *kaulika*, and none other. (88)

He who delights in encountering *kula* devotees [endowed] with *kula* wisdom, *kula* behavior, and *kula* vows is a *kaulika* dear to Me [i.e., Shiva]. (89)

He who is devoted to *guru* and deity and who knows the reality of the three principles (*tattva*), the sacred path (*carana*), and the meaning of the root *mantra* is a *kaulika* through initiation. (90)

O Beloved, the sight (*darshana*) of a *kula* teacher is difficult to obtain in all the worlds. It can be obtained only through the ripening of [previously accumulated karmic] merit, not otherwise. (91)

If he is merely remembered, lauded, seen, saluted, or spoken to, the adherent of the *kula* teaching instantly purifies even a *cândâla*.[40] (92)

O Goddess, wherever there is a *kula* knower, be he omniscient or a fool, the lowest or the most exalted, there I [Shiva] am with you. (93)

I do not dwell on Kailâsa, Meru, or Mandara. O Bhâvini, I am wherever the knowers of *kula* dwell. (94)

Even if such people of the Great Lord be very far, one must go to them and [make every] effort to see them, for I am close [to them]. (95)

A *kula* teacher should be seen even when he dwells very far away. But, O Beloved, a beast [i.e., an uninitiated individual] should be ignored even when he is nearby. (96)

Wherever a *kula* knower lives, that place is blessed. By gazing upon and venerating him twenty-one generations (*kula*) are uplifted. (97)

When the ancestors behold a *kula* knower abiding in the family home, they praise him [saying,] "We shall go to the supreme State." (98)

As farmers [appreciate] abundant rain, so the ancestors welcome into their families a son or grandson who is a *kaulika*. (99)

O Beloved, the sinless person whom the teachers of *kula* approach with delight (*mudrâ*) is indeed rich in this world. (100)

O Goddess, when a foremost *kaulika* is present, *yogins* together with *yoginîs* approach the *kaulika's* dwelling with delight. (101)

The ancestors and deities worship him who has joined the foremost of *kula-yogins*. Therefore those fond of *kula* wisdom should be worshiped with devotion [by everyone]. (102)

The sinners who do worship those of your devotees who have adored you, O Goddess, should not become receptacles of your grace. (103)

O Lotus-eyed [Goddess], you accept the offerings placed before you while I eat their essence from the tongue of devotees [who chant the sacred *mantras*]. (104)

O Goddess, I am the one who is undoubtedly worshiped by the worship of your devotees. Therefore he who seeks my favor should indeed worship your devotees. (105)

What is done for those who rely on *kula* is done for the deities. All the deities are fond of *kula*. Therefore one should adore the *kaulika*. (106)

Just as I am not pleased unless I am properly worshiped with devotion, so I am completely pleased, O Pârvatî, when one adores the foremost of *kaulikas*. (107)

The fruit that is obtained by the worship of the foremost *kaulikas*, that fruit, O Beloved, one cannot acquire by means of pilgrimages, austerities, charity, sacrifices, or vows. (108)

O Ambikâ, by disregarding a *kula* knower, [whatever one] gives, offers, sacrifices, does penance for, worships, or recites becomes useless for a *kaulika*. (109)

O Goddess, he who enters the *kula* teachings but does not know the way of *kula* is a sinner, a lowest dog-cooker, and his house is a cemetery. (110)

O Goddess, he who has abandoned the adherents of the *kula* [teachings] and gives to others, his charity is fruitless, and the donor himself goes to hell. (111)

The gift made to someone who is not a *kaulika* is like water in a broken vessel, seed sown on rock, or ghee poured into ashes [rather than the sacrificial fire]. (112)

Whatever is given to a *kula-yogin* according to one's ability and with love on specific days [bears] fruit that is not tainted. (113)

O Goddess, he who calls upon the *kula* wisdoms on auspicious days, worships—mindful of the deities—by means of fragrant flowers or grain, and so forth, . . . (114)

. . . with devotion fully satisfies [the deities] by means of the five seals beginning with [the letter] "m." All the deities become satisfied with these, and I become satisfied as well. (115)

O foremost Goddess, the merit of someone who offers his sister, daughter, or wife to an intoxicated *kula-yogin* is incalculable. (116)

The "honey" (*madhu*) [i.e., wine] given freely in the heroic circle (*vîra-cakra*) facilitates the pathway to the other world. (117)

"Honey" associated with evil conduct and rejected by the whole world yields, when offered to a *kula-yogin*, the [precious] *kula* substance. (118)

O Goddess, a country in which a hero (*vira*) fond of *kula* worship dwells is a pure country. Where better to reside? (119)

By once eating [from the food of] a foremost *kaulika*, one acquires a crore of merit. How can one calculate the merit of someone who eats [from the food of a foremost *kaulika*] repeatedly? (120)

Therefore with every effort, in all conditions, and at all times, one who is fond of the *kula* teachings should venerate a *kula* knower. (121)

Whether knowledgeable or ignorant, as long as one retains a [physical] body one must observe the conduct [proper to one's] class (*varna*) and stage of life (*âshrama*) in order to free oneself from karma. (122)

When ignorance is uprooted through [appropriate] action, one attains Shivahood (*shi-vatâ*) by means of wisdom. In Shiva there is liberation. Hence one should cultivate [appropriate] action. (123)

One should engage in blameless actions and perform the [prescribed] daily actions. Dedicated to [appropriate] action, desiring joy, and being free [in the midst of] action, one finds joy. (124)

It is not possible for an embodied person (*deha-dhârana*) to abandon all actions. He who gives up the fruit of his actions is called a [true] renouncer (*tyâgin*). (125)

Casting off the I-sense (*aham-bhâva*), one should think that [merely] one's organs are engaged in their respective functions. He who does this is not tainted. (126)

Actions done after the attainment of wisdom do not touch the knower of Reality, just like [muddy] water [does not stain] the leaves of the lotus. (127)

Meritorious and demeritorious actions cease for one who is established in this [ego-transcending attitude]. They move on but do not taint him; neither do further actions. (128)

502

O Beloved, the sage who has abandoned all thoughts (*samkalpa*) and who delights in the knowledge of spontaneously arising bliss should also renounce [all] actions. (129)

O Beloved, the ignorant who, pretending to learning, abandon the action part [of the Vedic revelation] as useless are impostors who go to hell. (130)

*Comments:* The Vedic revelation is thought to consist of two parts (*kânda*). The *karma-kânda* is concerned with the ritual actions that maintain the social order, and the *jnâna-kânda* is concerned with liberating wisdom.

Just as a tree indifferently sheds its blossoms when carrying fruit, similarly the *yogin* who has attained Reality (*tattva*) abandons his fondness for rituals. (131)

Those in whose heart the Absolute (*brahman*) is [firmly] stationed are not affected by the merit arising from [participation in the greatly meritorious] horse sacrifice or by the demerit caused by slaying a brahmin. (132)

On Earth, actions proceed by means of tongue, genitals, [and so forth]. He who has renounced tongue and genitals, what can he [possibly] have to do with actions? (133)

*Comments:* This stanza expresses the grand ideal of inaction-in-action (*naishkarmya-karman*), first propounded in the *Bhagavad-Gîtâ*. It is the key concept of Karma-Yoga, according to which we do not avoid becoming embroiled in the nexus of karma if we avoid charging our actions with selfish intent and instead stand aloof while simply carrying out what is necessary and appropriate.

Thus I have told you briefly some of the characteristics of Yoga and the foremost of *yogins*. O Mistress of Kula, what more do you desire to hear? (134)

"When the mind is held stable, then breath (*vâyu*) and semen (*bindu*) are also stable. Through stability of the semen, stability of the body is truly always generated."

—*Goraksha-Vacana-Samgraha* (132)

# Chapter 18
# YOGA AS SPIRITUAL ALCHEMY: THE PHILOSOPHY AND PRACTICE OF HATHA-YOGA

## I. THE ENLIGHTENMENT OF THE BODY—THE ORIGINS OF HATHA-YOGA

The human body-mind is not what it appears to be: a limited, mobile digestive tube. We only need to relax or meditate to discover that this popular materialistic stereotype is untrue, for it is then that we begin to discover the energy dimension of the body and the "deep space" of consciousness. As the hard boundaries that we normally draw around ourselves dissolve, we feel more alive and enter a world of greater experiential intensity. Relaxation and meditation replace our ordinary body image with an experience of ourselves as a fluid process that is connected with the larger, vibrant whole. In this experience, the boundaries of the ego lose their rigidity. Quantum physics tells us that everything is interconnected and that the idea that "I" am a separate physical entity is an illusion. It tells us, moreover, that the so-called objective world is a "hallucination," a projection of that imaginary point of subjectivity within us. We are slow in acknowledging the profound practical implications of the quantum-physical view, obviously because it requires us to make far-reaching and demanding changes in the way we think of ourselves and our universe. The quantum-physical perspective is not as new as we would like to believe. It underlies the entire Tantric tradition, notably the schools of Hatha-Yoga, which are an offshoot of Tantrism.

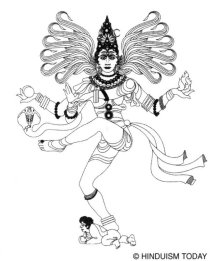

© HINDUISM TODAY

*Shiva Nata-Râja*

The image of the "dance of Shiva" best captures this orientation: Shiva, as Nata-Râja or "Lord of Dance," is forever dancing out the rhythms of the universe—the cycles of creation (*sarga*) and destruction (*pralaya*). He is the master weaver of space and time. This classical Hindu image has fascinated a number of quantum physicists. The first to draw attention to it was Fritjof Capra in his widely read book *The Tao of Physics*:

> The ideas of rhythm and dance naturally come to mind when one tries to imagine the flow of energy going through the patterns that make up the particle world. Modern physics has shown us that movement and rhythm are essential properties of matter; that all matter, whether here on earth or in outer space, is involved in a continual cosmic dance. The Eastern mystics have a dynamic view of the universe similar to that of modern physics, and consequently it is not surprising that they, too, have used the image of the dance to convey their intuition of nature.[1]

It was the adepts of Tantrism who pioneered this dynamic view of the universe, and it was also they who inaugurated a new attitude toward the human body and bodily existence in general. In pre-Tantric times, the body was often looked upon, in Gnostic fashion, as a source of defilement, as the enemy of the spirit. This attitude prompted the anonymous author of the *Maitrâyanîya-Upanishad* to compose the following litany:

> Venerable, in this ill-smelling, unsubstantial body [which is nothing but] a conglomerate of bone, skin, sinew, muscle, marrow, flesh, semen, blood, mucus, tears, rheum, feces, urine, wind, bile, and phlegm—what good is the enjoyment of desires? In this body, which is afflicted with desire, anger, greed, delusion, fear, despondency, envy, separation from the desirable, union with the undesirable, hunger, thirst, senility, death, disease, sorrow, and the like—what good is the enjoyment of desires? (1.3)

We may find the pessimistic tone of this passage strange and exaggerated, and yet it expresses our own culture's materialistic point of view very well. As long as we consider the body to be a walking alimentary canal, there is little solace in the pursuit of pleasure, since any pleasure the body can afford us is inevitably limited in intensity and duration and usually purchased at great cost. Besides, the pursuit of pleasure certainly cannot save us from death. The Tantric revolution led away from the model of the body as an "inflated bladder of skin."[2] "In tantrism," observed historian of religion Mircea Eliade, "the human body acquires an importance it had never before attained in the spiritual history of India."[3] This new attitude is pithily expressed in the *Kula-Arnava-Tantra*, an important Hindu Tantric work, thus:

> Without the body, how can the [highest] human goal be realized? Therefore, having acquired a bodily abode, one should perform meritorious (*punya*) actions. (1.18)

> Among the 840,000 types of embodied beings, the knowledge of Reality cannot be acquired except through a human [body]. (1.14)

What the Tantric masters aspired to was to create a transubstantiated body, which they called "adamantine" (*vajra*) or "divine" (*daiva*)—a body not made of flesh but of immortal substance, of Light. Instead of regarding the body as a meat tube doomed to fall prey to sickness and death, they viewed it as a dwelling place of the Divine, and as the cauldron for accomplishing spiritual perfection. For them, enlightenment was a whole-body event. As the *Yoga-Shikhâ-Upanishad* puts it:

> He whose body (*pinda*) is unborn and deathless is liberated in life (*jîvan-mukta*). Cattle, cocks, worms, and the like verily meet with their death.

> How can they attain liberation by shedding the body, O Padmaja? The life force [of the *yogin*] does not extend outward [but is focused in the axial channel]. How then can the shedding of the body [occur]?

> The liberation that is attainable by the shedding of the body—is that liberation not worthless? Just as rock-salt [is dissolved] in water, so the Absolute (*brahmatva*) extends to the body [of the enlightened *yogin*].

> When he reaches the [condition of] non-otherness (*ananyatâ*), he is said to be liberated. [But others continue to] distinguish different bodies and organs.

> The Absolute has attained embodiment (*dehatva*), even as water becomes a bubble. (1.161–165a)

The embodiment of enlightened masters is not limited to the physical organism with which they appear to be specifically associated. Their body is really the Body of all, and therefore they can assume any form at will—a feat that is attributed to many ancient and contemporary adepts. This transubstantiated body is also styled *ativâhika-deha* or "superconductive body." This omnipresent, luminous vehicle is endowed with the great paranormal powers (*siddhi*) acknowledged in all the scriptures of Yoga and Tantra. In the *Yoga-Bîja*, we find the following stanzas:

> The fire of Yoga gradually bakes the body composed of the seven constituents [such as bone, marrow, blood, etc.].

> Even the deities cannot acquire the exceedingly powerful yogic body. [The *yogin*] is freed from bodily bonds, endowed with various powers (*shakti*), and is supreme.

> The [*yogin*'s] body is like the ether, even purer than the ether. His body is more subtle than the subtlest [objects], coarser than any coarse [objects], more insensitive [to pain, etc.,] than the [most] insensitive (*jada*).

> The [body of] the lord of *yogins* conforms to his will. It is self-sufficient, autonomous, and immortal. He entertains himself with play wherever in the three realms [i.e., on Earth, in the mid-region, and in the celestial worlds].

> The *yogin* is possessed of unthinkable powers. He who has conquered the senses can, by his own will, assume various shapes and make them vanish again. (50b-54)

Thus, the adept is not merely an enlightened being but a magical theurgist, who is on a par with the Creator-God. There are few Yoga and Tantra scriptures that do not make reference to this occult aspect of the yogic way of life, and the texts of Hatha-Yoga are no exception.

## The Siddha Movement

The ideal of the adamantine body was at the core of a ramifying cultural movement comparable perhaps to the body-awareness movement of the 1970s and 1980s. This was the so-called Siddha cult, which flourished between the eighth and the twelfth centuries and which was a vital factor in completing the great pan-Indian synthesis of the spiritual teachings of Hinduism, Buddhism, and Jainism, as well as alchemy and popular magic.

The designation *siddha* means "accomplished" or "perfected" and refers to the Tantric adept who has attained enlightenment as the ultimate perfection (*siddhi*) and also possesses all kinds of paranormal powers (*siddhi*). The South Indian adept Tirumûlar defined a *siddha*, or *cittar* in the Tamil language, as someone who has realized, through yogic ecstasy, the transcendental Light and Power (*shakti*).

The *siddha* is a spiritual alchemist who works on and transmutes impure matter, the human body-mind, into pure gold, the immortal spiritual essence. However, he is also said to be capable of the literal transmutation of matter, and the renowned Czech Indologist Kamil V. Zvelebil recalled a baffling demonstration of this power by one of his *siddha* teachers.[4] The yogic process peculiar to this Tantric tradition, which straddled Hinduism and Buddhism, is known as *kâya-sâdhana* or "body cultivation." It was the cradle of Hatha-Yoga.

The most important schools of the Siddha movement were those of the Nâthas and the Maheshvaras. The former had their home in the north of the subcontinent, especially Bengal. The latter had their provenance in the South. The Buddhist *Tantras* speak of a pantheon of eighty-four great adepts, or *mahâ-siddhas*, many of whom are even today revered as demi-gods. They were "mostly rustic folk without much liking for and no pretense to learning,"[5] but among them we also find royal personages and great scholars. The Tibetan sources, relying on no longer available Sanskrit works, furnish us with biographical sketches of these adepts. While the bulk of the material is entirely legendary, there is good reason to assume that the individuals behind these wonderfully imaginative stories were historical. For some of them, we even have extant literary works and mystical songs.

According to the Tibetan tradition, the first and foremost adept of the eighty-four *siddhas* was Luipâ, whom some scholars identify with Matsyendra Nâtha, the famous teacher of the still more famous Goraksha Nâtha. Innumerable legends and songs tell of the magical and spiritual accomplishments of these two great masters (see below). Another remarkable *siddha* was the Buddhist Nâgârjuna, the teacher of Tilopa, who initiated Nâropa, the *guru* of Marpa, who, in turn, instructed the illustrious *yogin*-poet Milarepa. The Tibetan list of *mahâ-siddhas* includes several names that are also recognized by the Hindus.

The Tamil tradition of South India remembers eighteen *siddhas,* some of whom were of Chinese and Singhalese origin, and one is said to have hailed from Egypt. The number eighteen is as symbolic as the number eighty-four is for the *siddhas* of the North, both suggesting completeness. Among the *siddhas* of the South, it is particularly Akkattiyar (Sanskrit: Agastya), Tirumûlar,

Civavakkiyar, and Bhogar whose teachings and magical feats have captivated the imagination of the people.

Bhogar, a seventeenth-century adept, alchemist and poet who belonged to the potter caste, is said to have immigrated from China together with his teacher Kalangi Nâthar. Bhogar composed an important work on Kundalinî-Yoga in 7,000 verses. Layne Little, an American scholar of Tamil, has begun to translate this comprehensive and difficult text. In verse 20 of his mystical poem, Bhogar declares:

> Time was when I despised the body;
> but then I saw the God within.
> The body, I realized, is the Lord's
> temple;
> And so I began preserving it with care
> infinite.

This sentiment expresses perfectly the Tantric view of embodiment. In the nineteenth century, it was Râmalingar who reiterated and also demonstrated the tradition of bodily transmutation. Because of his profound spiritual realization, Râmalingar was able to describe the path to freedom with overwhelming immediacy, and in his *Tamil Literature*, Kamil V. Zvelebil rightly calls him "the great Tamil poet of the 19th century." He started composing mystical and devotional poems at the age of nine, and inspired words continued to pour from him until his mysterious

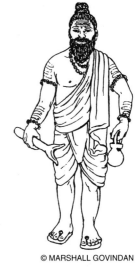

© MARSHALL GOVINDAN
*Agastya*

disappearance in 1874. It is said that he had reached such a high level of spiritual accomplishment that he was able to dissolve his physical body into light without leaving a trace behind.

It appears that the southern branch of the diffuse Siddha movement tended to be more radical in its rejection of ritualism and other establishment values than its northern counterpart.[6] One of Civavakkiyar's poems reads:

Why, you fool, do you utter mantras, murmuring them, whispering, going around the fixed stone as if it were god, putting garlands of flowers around it? Will the fixed stone speak—as if the Lord were within? Will the cooking vessel, or the wooden ladle, know the taste of curry?[7]

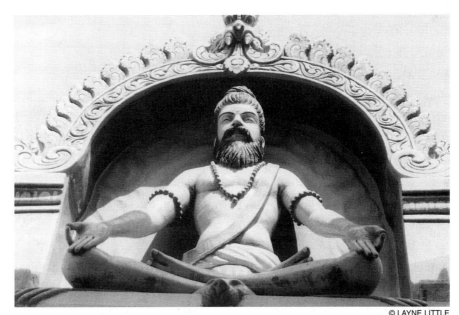

© LAYNE LITTLE
*Bhogar*

But this rejection of popular forms of worship often amounting to idolatry can be met with also among the *siddhas* of the North, notably the followers of the Buddhist Sahajîyâ tradition of spontaneity, as well as the Bauls of Bengal who, to this day, roam the countryside, singing their initiatory songs. Of course, the *siddhas* did not dismiss devotional feelings as such. Rather, their criticism typically targeted automatic behavior, whether secular or religious. Even sentiments of devotion can be made into a soul-destroying "ism" that obscures rather than reveals the mind-transcending Reality.

The trenchant criticism of the *siddhas* notwithstanding, we can detect a certain trend toward "technologism" among members of the Nâtha sect, who place magical rituals and Hatha-Yoga practices above ego-transcendence, leaving little room for the cultivation of authentic spiritual values and attitudes. Where the acquisition of power is given priority over self-transcendence, it is easy enough to succumb to ego-inflation and a stony heart. Or, to put it differently, when the *kundalinî* produces its characteristic kaleidoscope of fascinating inner phenomena, we are apt to forget that the *kundalinî* is, ultimately, the Goddess, and that the inner display is only her play. Like modern scientific technology, Indian psychotechnology is not without its perils. When the supreme value of self-transcendence is lost from sight, any technology is in danger of becoming the servant of merely egoic purposes.

It was none other than Jnânadeva, the great thirteenth-century adept of Maharashtra, who criticized those *hatha-yogins* that "day and night measure the wind with upstretched arms" but sadly lack the slightest degree of devotion. They should, he predicted, only expect sorrow and tribulations in their path. Jnânadeva was initiated into Hatha-Yoga by his elder brother Nivritti Nâtha, who is said to have been a disciple of Goraksha. Jnânadeva's *Jnâneshvarî*, composed in melodious Marathi, is one of the most illumined independent commentaries on the *Bhagavad-Gîtâ*. It represents a successful attempt to combine the Hatha-Yoga teachings Jnânadeva received from his family with the way of the heart taught by Lord Krishna of yore. It is difficult to read this work without being deeply touched by its wisdom and lyrical beauty.

## Matsyendra and Goraksha

Hindu tradition associates the creation of Hatha-Yoga with Goraksha Nâtha (Hindi: Gorakhnâth) and his teacher Matsyendra Nâtha, both of whom were born in Bengal. In his *Tantra-Âloka*, Abhinava Gupta salutes Matsyendra as his *guru*, which means that the latter must have lived before the middle of the tenth century C.E.[8] Matsyendra was a chief representative, if not the originator, of what is known as Nâthism. But Shiva himself is considered as the source of the Nâtha lineage and is invoked as Âdinâtha or "Primordial Lord." The term *nâtha* simply means "lord" or "master" and refers to a yogic adept who

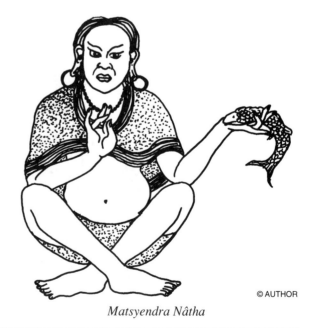

© AUTHOR

*Matsyendra Nâtha*

enjoys both liberation (*mukti*) and paranormal powers. Such *nâthas* are thought of as immortal beings who roam the Himalayan region. Matsyendra himself is venerated as the guardian deity of Kathmandu, in the form of Shveta Matsyendra ("White Matsyendra"), whose transcendental essence is the *bodhisattva* Avalokiteshvara. The followers of these masters—specifically Goraksha—are also known as *nâthas*, and Nâthism is recognized as one of the strands of the tapestry of contemporary Tantrism.

Matsyendra ("Lord of Fish," from *matsya* "fish" and *indra* "lord") is also known as Mîna, which has the same connotation. The name also may contain a reference to his occupation: fisherman. According to the legendary account given in the *Kaula-Jnâna-Nirnaya* ("Ascertainment of Kaula Knowledge"), which belongs to the eleventh century and is the oldest available source of information about Kaulism, Matsyendra recovered the canon of the Kaulas (called *kula-âgama*, written *kulâgama*) from a large fish that had swallowed it. Some scholars understand Matsyendra's name symbolically and argue that it suggests a level of spiritual attainment, which is possible and need not conflict with the conclusion that he earned his living from the sea. Some traditions state that a person who carries the title *matsyendra* has mastered the practice of suspending breath and mind by means of the space-walking seal (*khecârî-mudrâ*), one of the most important bodily seals of Hatha-Yoga.

Matsyendra is known to the Tibetans as Jowo Dzamling Karmo ("White Lord of the World"), one of the four exalted brothers, who are said by some to have lived in the seventh century. He is specifically associated with the Kaula sect of the Siddha movement, within which he may have founded the Yoginî-Kaula branch. This Tantric sect derives its name from its primary doctrinal tenet, the *kula*. This *kula* is the ultimate Reality in its dynamic or feminine aspect, as Shakti, specifically *kundalinî-shakti*. The literal meaning of *kula* is "flock" or "multitude" but also, more significantly, "family" and "home." Thus, the term evokes both the sense of differentiation and protectedness, which is pertinent in regard to the serpent power, since the *kundalinî* is both the source of the multitudinous universe and the ultimate security for the *yogin* who knows the *kula* secret. In this school, Shiva is often referred to as *akula*—the principle that transcends differentiation. The related concept of *kaula* stands for the condition of enlightenment or liberation, gained through the union of Shiva and Shakti. The word, however, also refers to the practitioner of this esoteric path. Some lists of teachers name Matsyendra and Mîna as separate individuals, which is possible but not highly likely. Other sources equate him with Luipâ, whom the Tibetans, however, regard as a distinct adept. Lore about Luipâ—the Tibetan name means something like "fish gut eater"—can be found throughout Northern India. The stories portray him as a *yogin* fond of eating the innards of fish. In Bengali, a *lui* is a small fish-catching device made of cane. Some authorities derive the name from *lohi-pâda*, meaning someone hailing from Lohit (the Assamese name for the Brahmaputra River, which is reddish in color). Luipâ is thought to have coauthored a book with the Buddhist adept-scholar Dîpamkara Shrîjnâna (=Atîsha), who was born in 980 C.E.

In the Tibetan hagiography of the eighty-four *mahâ-siddhas*, the following story is told of Mîna Nâtha (who probably is identical with Matsyendra). The fisherman spent most of his time in his small boat in the Bay of Bengal. One day, he hooked a huge fish that pulled so hard on his fishing line that he was thrown overboard. Like Jonah in the biblical story, Mîna ended up in the fish's enormous stomach, protected by his good karma.

It so happened that at that time Lord Shiva was instructing his divine spouse Umâ in secret teachings he had thus far been keeping to himself. She had created a special environment at the bottom of the ocean where no one could overhear the discourse. Many fish were drawn to the luminous undersea structure, including the leviathan that had gulped down Mîna. So it came to pass that the fisherman was able to listen to Shiva's secret instructions without being noticed. At one point, the Goddess fell asleep. When Shiva asked, "Are you listening?" a prompt "Yes!" came from the belly of the fish. Using his third eye, Shiva gazed straight through the mountain of flesh into the fish's stomach, where he saw Mîna. He was thrilled at the discovery, saying, "Now I see who my real disciple is." Turning to his sleepy spouse, he said: "I will initiate him rather than you."

Mîna gratefully took the initiation and then for the next twelve years—all the while remaining in the fish's belly—dedicated himself exclusively to the esoteric practices given to him by the great God himself. At the end of this period, another fisherman caught the monster and hacked it open, with Mîna emerging as a fully realized master.

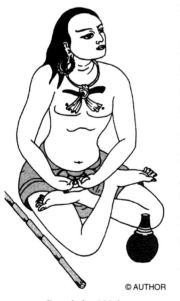
*Goraksha Nâtha*

Mîna's, or Matsyendra's, chief disciple was Goraksha. Legend has it that a peasant woman once implored Shiva to grant her a son. Touched by her fervent prayers, the great God gave her magical ash to eat, which would ensure her pregnancy. In her ignorance, the woman discarded the priceless gift on a dung heap. Twelve years later, Matsyendra happened to overhear a conversation between Shiva and his divine spouse Pârvatî. Wishing to see the child granted to the peasant woman, Matsyendra went to visit her. She sheepishly confessed what had happened to Shiva's graceful gift. Unperturbed, the *siddha* asked her to search the dung heap again, and—lo and behold!—she found a twelve-year-old boy who she named Goraksha ("Cow Protector").

Matsyendra adopted Goraksha as his disciple, and soon the student's fame exceeded that of his teacher. In some stories, Goraksha is portrayed as using his considerable magical powers for the benefit of his *guru*. Thus, according to one legend, Matsyendra went to visit Ceylon, where he fell in love with the queen. She invited him to stay with her in the palace, and before long Matsyendra was thoroughly ensnared in courtly life. When Goraksha heard about his teacher's fate, he at once went to rescue him. Goraksha assumed a female form so that he could enter the king's harem and confront him. Thanks to his disciple's timely intervention, Matsyendra came to his senses and returned to India, accompanied by his two sons Parasnâth and Nimnâth (two Hindi names).

Later, another story relates, Goraksha killed Matsyendra's sons, only to restore them to life. All these legends have, of course, deep symbolic significance. For instance, the murder of the two boys can be interpreted as the yogic act of withdrawing the life force (*prâna*) from the *idâ*- and the *pingalâ-nâdî*, the currents to the left and right of the axial current (*sushumnâ-nâdî*), and gathering it in the esoteric energy center at the base of the spine, from where the awakened *kundalinî* ascends to the crown center.

Goraksha, who lived in the late tenth and early eleventh century C.E., is remembered as a miracle worker second to none. He was obviously a realized adept and a charismatic personality of considerable social influence. Yet, according to most traditional accounts, he hailed from a lower, if not the lowest, social class. They are also agreed that he embraced the ascetic life at an early age and practiced lifelong celibacy. He was apparently a very handsome and charismatic individual who traveled widely throughout India. Kabîr, who had few good words for the *yogins* of his day, praised Goraksha, Bhartrihari, and Gopîcanda as masters who had found union with the Divine. He also acknowledged his indebtedness to them for their teachings about the six psychospiritual centers (*cakra*) of the body and the Yoga of sound (*shabda-yoga*).

The invention of Hatha-Yoga is often attributed to Goraksha alone, though many of the tenets and practices of this school were in existence long before his time.[9] Goraksha is also said to have founded the Kânphata ("Split-ear") order of the Nâthas, which gets its curious name from one of the distinguishing marks of its members, namely their split earlobes into which large rings (called *mudrâ* or *darshana*) are inserted. Some members

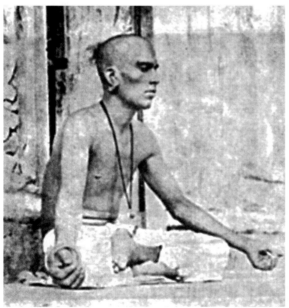

*Reproduced from* Gorakhnath and the Kanphata Yogis
*A kânphata yogin in meditation,
with uncharacteristically slumped posture*

claim that this custom affects an important current (*nâdî*) of life force at the ear that facilitates the acquisition of certain magical powers.

The Kânphata order, whose members are also called *jogîs*, is scattered throughout India and includes hermits and monastic groups, as well as a small number of married men and women. The 1901 census of India reported 45,463 Nâthas, almost half of whom were women. They generally have a low social status, and, as George Weston Briggs reported, they

> make charms for themselves, and some sell them to others; they pronounce spells and practice palmistry and juggling, tell fortunes, and interpret dreams; they sell a woolen amulet to protect children from the evil eye; and they pretend [?] to cure disease, muttering texts over the sick and practising medicine and exorcism, and vending drugs.[10]

The picture painted by Briggs and others suggests that the order founded by Goraksha is in a state of decline, and many of its members are both despised and feared for their actual or putative magical powers and ever ready curses. But there are also those who continue to instruct the villagers in spiritual and worldly matters and who, like those in the lineage of Bhartri Nâtha, entertain and edify through their music and songs. While it is true that the danger of narcissism lurks in all body-centered paths, it is also true that self-transcending love is not absent from any genuine spiritual approach, including Hatha-Yoga.

## Other Masters of Nâthism

After Goraksha, the most prominent adepts of Nâthism are Jâlandhari (disciple of

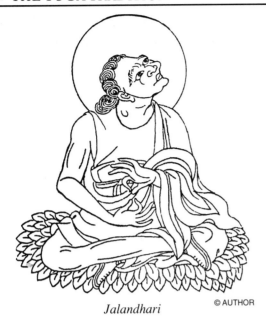

*Jalandhari*                © AUTHOR

Matsyendra), Bhartrihari (disciple of Jâlandhari), Gopîcandra (disciple of Jâlandhari or Kanhu), and Caurangî (whose stepmother abandoned him in the forest after cutting off his hands and feet, and who became a disciple of Matsyendra), as well as Carpata (or Carpati) and Gahini (both of whom were disciples of Goraksha).

Before renouncing the world, Jâlandhari ruled over the thriving city of Hastinâpura in North-Western India. In the east, in Bengal, he is also known as Hâdipâ, which indicates his occupation as a lowly menial laborer. Legend has it that because he, the great *siddha*, coveted Shiva's spouse herself, she cursed him to live out his life as a *hâdi* in service to the beautiful queen May-nâmati of Comilla (in what is now Bangladesh). He is remembered as a great miracle worker, who is said to have been able to bring back the dead— a feat he performed on his most famous disciple, King Gopîcandra (see below).

Bhartrihari was the king of Ujjain, and, according to some legends, the brother of Queen Maynâmati, the mother of Gopîcandra. He was initiated by Jâlandhari and also is considered to have been a disciple of Goraksha. After his abdication, his brother Vikramâditya (Candragupta II)

ascended the throne and ruled from 1079 to 1126 C.E. One of the subsects of the Kânphatas is named after Bhartrihari, whose renunciation, prompted by his beloved wife Pingalâ's death, is still celebrated in popular songs, especially in Western India.

Another of Goraksha's twelve main disciples was Baba Ratan Haji, a Muslim, who still has followers in Kabul and may have authored the *Kafir-Bodha* (which is also ascribed to Goraksha). He appears to have died at the end of the twelfth century, however, which would rule out a direct contact with Goraksha, unless we assume that the latter was extremely long lived.

Caurangî, who was the son of King Devapâla of the Pâla dynasty of Bengal, is credited with the authorship of the *Prâna-Sankali* (composed in medieval Hindi). The Tibetan hagiography of the eighty-four great adepts relates the story of his stepmother's amorous advances toward him, which he rejected. Feeling humiliated, she plotted revenge. One day she inflicted scratches over her entire body and blamed Caurangî for them. King Devapâla, who had no reason to disbelieve his new wife, ordered the executioners to abandon the prince in the forest after cutting off his arms and legs. Before Caurangî could bleed to death, Mîna Nâtha appeared before him. He initiated the dying prince into Yoga and promised that, after successful completion of the practices he had given him, his limbs would grow back.

One night, after twelve long years, a caravan laden with gold and precious stones camped nearby. Caurangî called out to them from the dark. Fearfully, they identified themselves as merchants carrying simple charcoal. "So be it," he replied. On sunrise, they discovered to their horror that all their chests and sacks were filled with charcoal. The merchants remembered the disembodied voice of the previous night and looked for

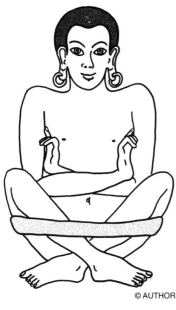

© AUTHOR

*Caurangî*

Caurangî. They were shocked to find his limbless body propped up against a tree. But they also sensed that he was a man of great power, and so they confessed their little lie and asked for his help. Caurangî explained that he probably had nothing to do with the incident, but if his words were responsible for their fiasco then the charcoal should be transformed back into gold and precious stones that instant. When they checked their chests and sacks, the merchants were overjoyed to discover that their property had been restored to its right form. Caurangî, however, was as surprised as they were. He remembered Mîna Nâtha's promise, and then purely through visualization he grew his missing limbs back that same day.

Carpata, or Carpati, had King Sahila Varma of Chamba as his disciple, who flourished in the early tenth century C.E. Carpata is credited with the authorship of a work entitled *Carpata-Shataka* (or *Carpata-Paddhati*), which shows a strong Jaina influence. According to some scholars, however, he was an alchemist who had followed Buddhism but later became a disciple of Goraksha. It is clear from this work and other teachings of Nâthism that this movement unfolded at the confluence of Hinduism, Buddhism, and Jainism. There also is a *Carpata-Panjarikâ-Stotra*, wrongly attributed to Shankara, which appears to be modeled on the *Shataka*.[11] Tibetan

sources, who list Carpati among the eighty-four great adepts, know him as Carbaripâ. He is said to have had the peculiar ability of turning people into Buddha sculpture made from stone. Legend has it that the sculptures come back to life in order to manhandle faltering practitioners until their clarity and motivation are restored.

Gahini (Marathi: Gaini), of Maharashtra, is said to have been a disciple of Goraksha. His date of birth is traditionally given as 1175 C.E., which is too late for Goraksha. Goraksha could, however, have been his *parama-guru*, or teacher's teacher. Gahini Nâtha initiated Nivritti (see below).

Gopîcandra, erstwhile king of East Bengal (now Pakistan), is the subject of numerous popular legends and ballads that are still recited in Northern India today. Some scholars associate him with Pattikânâgara in Tripura (Chittagong district on the Bay of Bengal) rather than with the Pâla dynasty of Bengal. It appears his family may have leased a portion of Bengal. He married the two daughters of King Harishcandra, who may have ruled over Savar in the Dacca district, Bengal.

According to one account, Gopîcandra was born as a direct result of Shiva's grace, for there was no son written in his royal mother's destiny. Queen Maynâmati, wife of King Manikcandra, was told that her newborn son was a disciple of the adept Jâlandhari and would have to be returned to that teacher after Gopîcandra had ruled over his kingdom for twelve years. She was also told that if Gopîcandra were to submit to his *guru* at that point in time, he would acquire immortality. If, however, he were to reject his teacher and fail to renounce the world, his fate would be to die instantly.

Gopîcandra was brought up in luxury, free from worldly cares, and became a successful ruler. In the twelfth year of Gopîcandra's reign,

Jâlandhari (disguised as a low-caste sweeper bearing the name Hâdi) arrived at the palace gardens and demanded what was rightfully his. The queen mother, who was a disciple of Jâlandhari, broke the news to Gopîcandra. After questioning her closely, he arrived at a decision. He went straight to Jâlandhari/Hâdi and, to everyone's horror, threw the adept into a deep well. He blocked the well with a huge rock, and then had seven hundred cartloads of horse manure dumped on top of the rock.

As prophesied by Jâlandhari many years ago, Gopîcandra instantly found himself in the throes of death. Suddenly Jâlandhari, who had been quite unperturbed by his disciple's cruel treatment, materialized in front of him. His superior power quickly restored Gopîcandra's departing psyche to the body. Although he was glad to be alive, the king only reluctantly accepted the life of a renouncer. In fact, Jâlandhari had to intervene many more times in his disciple's life, because Gopîcandra was strongly attached to his eleven hundred wives, his sixteen hundred slave girls, and their children, as well as the luxurious life, power, and glory of a regent. He is probably the most insubordinate disciple on record in the history of Yoga and suffered greatly in the course of his discipleship. But he also won the supreme prize of liberation in this life because of his *guru*'s grace, his good karma, and not least his persistence.

In addition to the above masters, the *Hatha-Yoga-Pradîpikâ* (1.5–9) mentions Shâbara, Ânanda Bhairava, Mîna (as distinct from Matsyendra), Virûpâksha, Bileshaya, Manthâna Bhairava Yogin, Siddhi, Buddha, Kanthadi, Korantaka, Surânanda, Siddhipâda, Kânerin, Pûjyapâda, Nitya Nâtha, Niranjana, Kapâlin, Bindu Nâtha, Kâkacandîshvara, Allâma Prabhudeva, Ghodâcolin, Tintini, Bhânukin, Nâradeva, Khanda, Kâpâlika. We know next to nothing about many of these personages, but numerous legends are told about the most important of these adepts.

If Ânanda Bhairava is the same as the Bhairava Ânanda mentioned in King Shekhara's *Karpura-Manjari*, we can place him in the early tenth century.

Virûpâksha may be the same as the adept Virûpa whom Tibetan sources regard as one of the eighty-four *mahâ-siddhas*. He was born in Bengal during the reign of King Devapâla and entered the Buddhist monastic university of Somapuri at a young age. When after twelve years of dedicated practice no spiritual breakthrough occurred, he discarded his rosary in utter frustration. That evening, his chosen deity, Goddess Vajra Varahi, appeared to him with the gift of a new rosary. His motivation greatly strengthened by this extraordinary event, he spent another twelve years pursuing his particular meditation practice and gained the longed-for realization. Shortly after his enlightenment, Virûpa was discovered in his cell feasting on pigeon meat and wine. He was defrocked and asked to leave the monastery. Outside the monastery gates, he happily walked across the lake, stepping light-footedly from lotus leaf to lotus leaf until he reached the other shore.

Dumbfounded and remorseful, the monks begged him to return, which he did. When asked why he killed the pigeons for a meal, he explained that it had all been an illusion, like everything else. He snapped his fingers, and the pigeons came back to life. After this demonstration he left the monastery for good to roam the countryside at his leisure.

Kanthadi may be the same *siddha* whom the Chalukya king Mûlrâj I (941–996 C.E.) found living on the banks of the Sarasvatî River.

Pûjyapâda may be the great philosopher-physician who was a Jaina by birth and lived in Karnataka perhaps around 600 C.E. His original name was Devanandi, and he wrote a medical

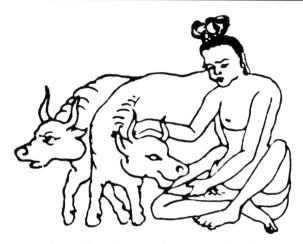

*Goraksha with cows (from a woodblock)*

work entitled *Kalyana-Kâraka*. It is not clear whether he is the same as the Pûjyapâda to whom several medical works, including the *Samâdhi-Shataka*, in the Telugu script are attributed.

Nitya Nâtha was the name of a great fifteenth-century adept who authored the *Rasa-Ratna-Âkâra* (written *Rasaratnâkâra*), which is a thousand pages long and purports to be a digest of all earlier Âyurvedic works. He is also sometimes credited with the authorship of the *Kaksha-Pûta-Samhitâ* (a manual of sorcery) and the *Siddha-Siddhânta-Paddhati*.

Kapâlin could be identical with Kapâlapâ mentioned in the hagiography of the eighty-four *mahâ-siddhas*. He is said to have been a laborer in Râjapuri, where an epidemic claimed the life of his beloved wife and five children. He was initiated into the Buddhist tradition by Krishnâcârya, who converted the decapitated head of Kapâlapâ's wife into a skull bowl and carved ritual ornaments from the bones of the five children. He instructed the grieving man to meditate on the emptiness of the skull bowl. After nine years, Kapâlapâ met with success and in due course became a renowned teacher with six hundred disciples.

Bindu Nâtha may be the same as the author of the *Rasa-Paddhati*, a medical work.

Kâkacandîshvara authored several works on Yoga and the medical text *Kâkacandîshvara-Kalpa*.

Allâma Prabhudeva was a contemporary of Basava (1120–1168 C.E.) and the head of an order that included three hundred realized practitioners, sixty of whom are said to have been women. His life story is related in the *Prabhulinga-Lîlâ*, a mid-sixteenth-century work, according to which Goraksha took initiation from Allâma. As a result of the practices given to him, Goraksha acquired immunity from all weapons. He proudly demonstrated his newly won paranormal ability to his teacher. To teach Goraksha a lesson in humility, Allâma asked his disciple to strike him with a sword. To his astonishment, Goraksha found that the sword passed through the great *siddha* as if he were made of empty space. Allâma explained that all forms are but frozen shadows produced by illusion (*mâyâ*). When the knot at the heart is untied and the spell of *mâyâ* is lifted, then the body is realized to be nothing but the singular Reality, which is omnipresent. Allâma dropped his shadow-body in 1196 C.E.

## II. WALKING THE RAZOR'S EDGE— THE HATHA-YOGIC PATH

The body is the abode of God, O Goddess. The psyche (*jîva*) is God Sadâ-Shiva. One should abandon the offering-remains of ignorance; one should worship with the thought "I am He."

This quote from the *Kula-Arnava-Tantra* (9.41) states the ultimate purpose of Hatha-Yoga, which is God-realization, or enlightenment, here and now, in a divinized or immortal body. This is often expressed as the state of balance or harmony (*samarasa*) in the body, when the ordinarily diffuse life energy is stabilized in the central channel.

This idea is present in the term *hatha-yoga* itself, which is esoterically explained as the union (*yoga*) between "sun" and "moon," the conjunction of the two great dynamic principles or aspects of the body-mind.

The life force (*prâna*) is polarized along the spinal axis, where the dynamic pole (represented by Shakti) is said to be at the base of the spine and the static pole (represented by Shiva) at the crown of the head. The *hatha-yogin*'s work consists in uniting Shakti with Shiva. For this marriage to come about, however, he must first stabilize the alternating life current animating the body. This dynamic flow (often referred to as *hamsa*) is polarized positively and negatively, rushing up and down on the left and the right side of the body 21,600 times in the span of a day.[12] The positive current is experienced as heating, the negative as cooling. On the material level, they correspond to the sympathetic and the parasympathetic nervous system respectively.

According to the Tantric model of the human body, the axial channel (called *sushumnâ*) is entwined by the helical *idâ-* and *pingalâ-nâdîs*. The *idâ* is the carrier or flow of the lunar force on the left of the bodily axis, and the *pingalâ* is the conduit or flow of the solar force on the right. The syllable *ha* in the word *hatha* also represents the solar force of the body, and the syllable *tha* represents the lunar force.[13] The term *yoga* stands for their conjunction, which is the ecstatic state of identity between subject and object.

The *hatha-yogin*'s primary objective is to intercept the left and right current and draw the bipolar energy into the central channel, which commences at the anal center or *mûlâdhâra-cakra*, where the *kundalinî* is thought to be asleep. This persistent effort to redirect the life force acts upon the *kundalinî*, which is mobilized. This action can be compared to a hammer striking an anvil; hence, the regular exoteric meaning of the word hatha is "force." Hatha-Yoga is a forceful enterprise in which the body's innate life force is utilized for the transcendence of the self.

## Purificatory Techniques

Breath control (*prânâyâma*), which is the most immediate way of effecting the life force, is at the heart of Hatha-Yoga practice. In their long experimentation with the breath, however, early *yogins* found that most aspirants should undergo more or less extensive purification prior to embarking on breath control. They thus invented a large array of cleansing techniques to prepare the body for the demands of the higher stages of practice. The *Gheranda-Samhitâ* has the following pertinent stanzas:

> Purification, strengthening, stabilizing, calmness, lightness, perception [of the Self], and the untainted [condition of liberation] are the seven means of [the Yoga of] the pot (*gatha*) [i.e., the body]. (1.9)

> Purification [is accomplished] by the six acts; [the *yogin*] becomes strong through postures (*âsana*); stability [is acquired] through the seals (*mudrâ*) and calmness through sense-withdrawal (*pratyâhâra*). (1.10)

> Lightness [results] from breath control (*prânâyâma*), perception of the Self from meditation (*dhyâna*), and the untainted [state] from ecstasy (*samâdhi*); [this last state] is undoubtedly liberation (*mukti*). (1.11)

Sage Gheranda continues to describe the "six acts" (*shat-karman*), which comprise the following six purificatory practices:

1.  *Dhauti* ("cleansing") consists of the following four techniques:

    (i)   *Antar-dhauti* ("inner cleansing") is of four types: The first technique is performed by means of swallowing the breath and expelling it through the anus; the second by means of completely filling the stomach with water; the third by stimulating the "fire" in the abdomen through repeatedly pushing the navel back toward the spine; the fourth is executed by washing the prolapsed intestines (a risky undertaking). These are respectively known as *vâta-sâra-* ("relating to air"), *vâri-sâra-* ("relating to water"), *vahni-sâra-* ("relating to fire"), and *bahish-krita-* ("externally performed") *antar-dhauti*.

    (ii)  *Danta-dhauti* ("dental cleansing") includes cleaning teeth, tongue, ears, and frontal sinus. The cleansing of the tongue involves rubbing butter on it and then milking and pulling it in preparation for the *khecârî-mudrâ*, which requires that one insert the tip of the tongue into the nasal opening at the palate. Some *yogins* even use metal instruments to elongate the tongue.

    (iii) *Hrid-dhauti* ("heart cleansing") consists in the cleansing of the throat by means of a plantain stalk, turmeric, a cane, or a piece of cloth, or by self-induced vomiting, which is beneficial for those suffering from diseases of the chest ("heart"). Cleansing the throat and stomach by means of a long four-finger-wide cloth is called *vâso-dhauti*, which is said to cure tumors, an enlarged spleen, skin diseases, and various disorders of phlegm and bile.

    (iv)  *Mûla-shodhana* ("root purification") is the cleansing of the anus (*mûla*) manually, with water, or with a turmeric stalk, which heals gastrointestinal diseases and increases bodily vigor.

2.  *Vasti* or *basti* ("bladder") consists in the contraction and dilation of the sphincter muscle to cure constipation, flatulence, and urinary ailments and can also be performed while standing in water. Sometimes a tube is inserted into the rectum while seated in the *utkata-âsana*, which is the yogic version of an enema.

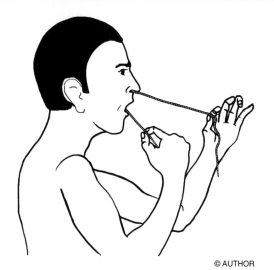

© AUTHOR

*Sûtra-neti, nasal cleansing by means of a thread*

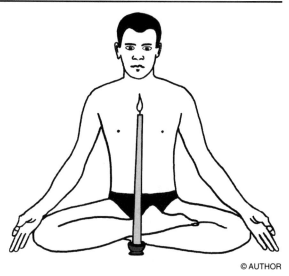

© AUTHOR

*Trâtaka*

3. *Neti* (untranslatable) refers to a thin thread of around nine inches that is inserted into one nostril at a time and passed through the mouth to remove phlegm and, because of its action upon the *âjnâ-cakra*, induce clairvoyance (*divya-drishti*).

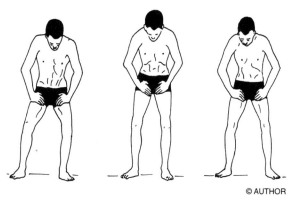

© AUTHOR

*Naulî-kriyâ*

4. *Lauli* or *laulikî* ("to-and-fro move-ment"), also called *naulî* or *naulî-kriyâ*, consists in rolling the abdominal mus-cles sideways to massage the inner organs, which is thought to cure a vari-ety of diseases.

5. *Trâtaka* (untranslatable) refers to the

steady, relaxed gazing at a small object until tears begin to flow, which is said to cure diseases of the eye and also induce clairvoyance.

6. *Kapâla-bhâti* ("skull-luster") comprises three practices that are held to remove phlegm, and the last is additionally said to make the *yogin* as attractive as the God of love, Kâmadeva:

(i) The "left process" (*vâma-krama*) consists in breathing through the left nostril and expelling the air through the right, and vice versa.

(ii) The "inverted process" (*vyut-krama*) consists in drawing water up through the nostrils and expelling it through the mouth.

(iii) The *"shît* process" (*shît-krama*) consists in sucking water up through the mouth and expelling it through the nose. The phrase *shît* is ono-matopoeic for the sound produced by this practice.

Other texts occasionally give different definitions of the above practices, and some scriptures mention further techniques for purifying the body and preparing it for the advanced art of breath control. Noteworthy is the work *Sat-Karma-Samgraha* (also titled *Karma-Paddhati*) of Cidghanânanda, which is a manual perhaps dating back to the eighteenth century and comprising 149 stanzas. It deals extensively with purificatory techniques and ailments resulting from faulty Yoga practice. According to the *Hatha-Yoga-Pradîpikâ* (2.21), only those who are flabby and phlegmatic need to resort to the "six actions" to purify the body.

## Postures

Sage Gheranda treats Hatha-Yoga as having seven rather than eight limbs, whereby the postures (*âsana*) and the seals (*mudrâ*) are respectively the second limb and the third limb, while the moral rules (that is, *yama* and *niyama*) are not regarded as independent aspects. The *Gheranda-Samhitâ* (2.1) makes the point that there are as many *âsanas* as there are animal species. Gheranda claims that Shiva taught as many as 840,000 postures, of which eighty-four are considered important by *yogins*. According to the *Hatha-Yoga-Pradîpikâ* (1.33), however, Shiva taught only eighty-four postures. Of these postures, the following thirty-two are described in the *Gheranda-Samhitâ*: (1) *Siddha-âsana* ("adept posture"), (2) *padma-âsana* ("lotus posture"), (3) *bhadra-*

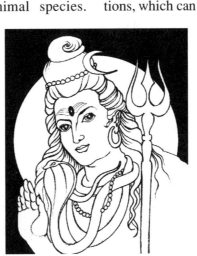
© HINDUISM TODAY
*Shiva, primordial teacher of Yoga*

*âsana* ("auspicious posture"), (4) *mukta-âsana* ("liberated posture"), (5) *vajra-âsana* ("diamond posture"), (6) *svastika-âsana* ("*svastika* posture"), (7) *simha-âsana* ("lion posture"), (8) *go-mukha-âsana* ("cow-face posture"), (9) *vîra-âsana* ("hero posture"), (10) *dhanur-âsana* ("bow posture"), (11) *mrita-âsana* ("corpse posture"), (12) *gupta-âsana* ("hidden posture"), (13) *matsya-âsana* ("fish posture"), (14) *matsyendra-âsana* ("Matsyendra's posture"), (15) *goraksha-âsana* ("Goraksha's posture"), (16) *pashcimot-tana-âsana* ("back-stretch posture"), (17) *utkata-âsana* ("extraordinary posture"), (18) *samkata-âsana* ("dangerous posture"), (19) *mayûra-âsana* ("peacock posture"), (20) *kukkuta-âsana* ("cock posture"), (21) *kûrma-âsana* ("tortoise posture"), (22) *uttâna-kûrmaka-âsana* ("extended tortoise posture"), (23) *uttâna-manduka-âsana* ("extended frog posture"), (24) *vriksha-âsana* ("tree posture"), (25) *manduka-âsana* ("frog posture"), (26) *garuda-âsana* ("eagle posture"), (27) *vrisha-âsana* ("bull posture"), (28) *shalabha-âsana* ("locust posture"), (29) *makara-âsana* ("shark posture"), (30) *ushtra-âsana* ("camel posture"), (31) *bhujanga-âsana* ("serpent posture," often called "cobra"), and (32) *yoga-âsana* ("Yoga posture"). In place of lengthy descriptions, which can be found in numerous books, the following illustrations depict each posture.

Contemporary manuals describe over a thousand postures. Some of these postures—like the adept and the lotus posture—are clearly intended for prolonged sitting in meditation. Most of them, however, are designed to regulate the life force in the body in order to balance, strengthen, and heal it. It appears from the outset that Hatha-Yoga has

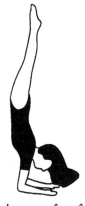

*piccha-mayûra-âsana*
("feathered peacock posture")

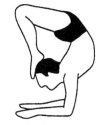

*vrishcika-âsana*
("scorpion posture")

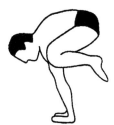

*baka-âsana*
("crane posture")

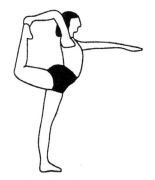

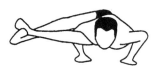

*ashtâvakra-âsana*
("Ashtâvakra's posture")

*nata-râja-âsana*
("King of Dance posture")

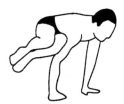

*pârshva-baka-âsana*
("lateral crane posture")

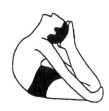

*râja-kapota-âsana*
("king pigeon posture")

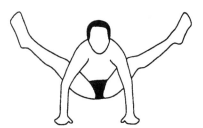

*tittibha-âsana*
("fire-fly posture")

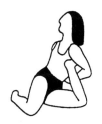

*yoga-danda-âsana*
(yogic staff posture)

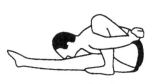

*marîci-âsana*
("Marîci's posture")

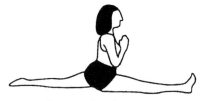

*hanumân-âsana*
("Hanumat's posture")

© AUTHOR

*Various advanced Hatha-Yoga postures*

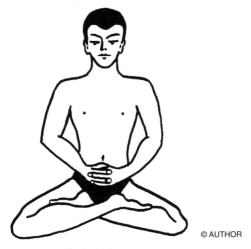

*Padma-âsana*

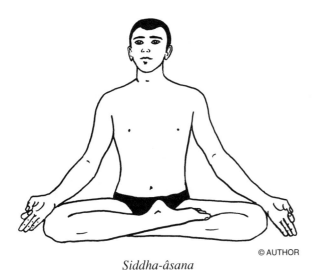

*Siddha-âsana*

*Svastika-âsana*

included a therapeutic dimension, which today is being professionalized as "Yoga therapy."[14]

Even the meditation postures are said to have therapeutic value, and in some instances rather exaggerated claims are made in the Sanskrit texts. In both Eastern and Western Yoga circles, postural practice is often overemphasized, and the following observation found in the *Kula-Arnava-Tantra* is pertinent:

> Yoga is not [attained] through the lotus posture and not by gazing at the tip of the nose. Yoga, say the experts of Yoga, is the identity of the psyche (*jîva*) with the [transcendental] Self. (9.30)

## Seals and Locks

Related to the postures are the seals (*mudrâ*) and locks (*bandha*), which form the third limb of Hatha-Yoga. The seals represent more advanced techniques, which, as is clear from the last five techniques, even merge with meditative practices. "They are divine," declares Svâtmârâma, the author of the *Hatha-Yoga-Pradîpikâ* (3.8), "and they bestow the eight [great paranormal] powers. They are favored by all the adepts and are difficult to obtain even by the deities." Svâtmârâma further states that they should be kept secret, just as, in his words, one would not divulge one's sexual intimacies with a well-bred woman. The locks (*bandha*) are special bodily maneuvers that are designed to confine the life force within the trunk and thereby stimulate it. In the *Gheranda-Samhitâ* (chapter 3), the following twenty-five *mudrâs*, including the *bandhas*, are described in the order given:

1. *mahâ-mudrâ* ("great seal"), performed by pressing the left heel against the perineum and grasping the toes of the right

outstretched leg while contracting the throat;

2.   *nabho-mudrâ* ("sky seal"), which is executed by turning the tongue upward against the palate, and which can be done during any activity;

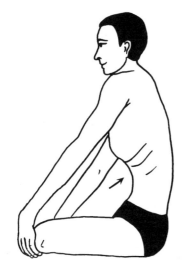

*Uddiyâna-bandha*

3.   *uddîyâna-bandha* ("upward-going lock"), performed by drawing back the abdomen;

4.   *jalandhara-bandha* ("Jalandhara's lock"), done by contracting the throat;

5.   *mûla-bandha* ("root lock"), executed by contracting the anal sphincter muscle;

6.   *mahâ-bandha* ("great lock"), performed by pressing the left ankle against the perineum while placing the right foot on top of the other foot and contracting the anal sphincter muscle;

7.   *mahâ-vedha* ("great penetrator"), executed by engaging the *uddîyâna-bandha* during the application of the great seal;

8.   *khecârî-mudrâ* ("space-walking seal"), a very important technique, which is performed by inserting the elongated tongue into the passage above the upper palate and by fixing the gaze on the spot between the eyebrows; this is said to release the "nectar of immortality" (*amrita*), which leads to health, longevity, and a host of paranormal powers; the *amrita* is sweet-tasting saliva;

9.   *viparîta-karî-* or *viparîta-karanî-mudrâ* ("inverted action seal"), also known as the headstand or shoulderstand, which prevents the ambrosia (*amrita*, *soma*) from dripping into the "fire" at the navel;

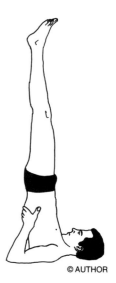

*Viparîta-karanî-mudrâ, also called sarva-anga-âsana*

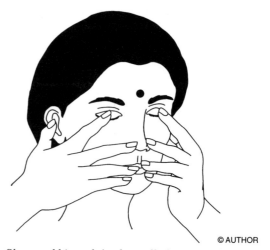

*Shan-mukhi-mudrâ, also called yoni-mudrâ*

10.   *yoni-mudrâ* ("womb seal"), performed by sitting in the adept posture and closing the eyes, ears, nostrils, and the mouth with the fingers, followed by breath retention and simultaneous

contemplation of the six centers (*cakra*); this practice is also called *shan-mukhi-mudrâ;*

11. *vajrolî-mudrâ* ("thunderbolt seal"), executed by raising oneself off the ground while winding the legs around the neck; other texts, however, provide a completely different explanation of this practice, which involves drawing up liquids through the penis;

12. *shakti-câlanî-mudrâ* ("power-stirring seal"), performed by forcibly joining the life force in the chest with that in the abdomen while contracting the anal sphincter muscle by means of *ashvinî-mudrâ* and while sitting in the adept's posture;

13. *tâdâgî-mudrâ* ("pond seal"), performed by pulling back the abdomen while lying prone;

14. *mândukî-mudrâ* ("frog seal"), done by moving the tongue until the "nectar" flows profusely, which is then swallowed;

15. *shâmbhavî-mudrâ* ("Shambhu's seal"), a most important technique that consists in gazing at the spot between the eyebrows while inwardly contemplating the transcendental Self; Shambhu is another name for God Shiva, and the *yogin* who has mastered this technique is said to resemble the great God himself;

16. *ashvinî-mudrâ* ("dawn-horse seal"), performed by repeatedly contracting the anal sphincter muscle;

17. *pâshinî-mudrâ* ("bird-catcher seal"), executed by crossing the legs behind the neck, though not raising the body off the ground, as in the *vajrolî-mudrâ;*

18. *kâkî-mudrâ* ("crow seal"), done by slowly inhaling through the mouth which is formed into a crow's beak;

19. *mâtangî-mudrâ* ("elephant seal"), performed by standing neck-deep in water and sucking up water through the nose and expelling it through the mouth;

20. *bhujanginî-* or *bhujangî-mudrâ* ("serpent seal"), executed by drawing in air through the mouth while making a slight rasping noise with the throat;

21–25. the five concentrations (*dhâranâ*) upon the material elements, which involve focusing the life force and the mind on each respective element for two hours while imaging the various symbolic forms associated with each (such as the presiding deity of each element, its seed mantra, and so on). The five elements are earth, water, fire, air, and space/ether (*âkâsha, kha*). The inclusion of these concentration practices under the heading of *mudrâs* is curious, but illustrates the close relationship that exists in Yoga between physical practice and mental focus.

## Sense-Withdrawal

According to Gheranda's path, the fourth limb of Hatha-Yoga is sense-withdrawal (*pratyâhâra*), which he deals with only very cursorily.

It simply consists in withdrawing attention from external, sensory objects. The fact that this practice is placed before breath control, the fifth limb, indicates that yogic breathing presupposes a great measure of mental discipline.

## Breath Control

Breath control (*prânâyâma*) is the careful regulation of the life force (*prâna*) in its different forms. From the point of view of the *hatha-yogin*, the work of Yoga is impossible to accomplish without mastery of the breath/life force. As the *Yoga-Bîja* puts it:

> He who desires union (*yoga*) without controlling the breath (*pavana*) is, to *yogins*, like someone who wants to cross the ocean in an unbaked [earthen] vessel. (77)

In the words of the *Hatha-Yoga-Pradîpikâ*:

> When the breath moves, consciousness (*citta*) [also] moves. When it is immobile, [consciousness is also] immobile, and the *yogin* attains stability. Therefore, one should restrain the breath.

> It is said that as long as there is breath in the body, as long there is life. Its departure is death. Therefore, one should restrain the breath. (2.2–3)

Before describing the various techniques of breath control, Sage Gheranda stresses the importance of proper diet and environment. Among other things, he states that the *yogin* should commence *prânâyâma* during the spring or autumn season, when the weather is neither extremely hot nor excessively cold. He also emphasizes the importance of purifying the "conduits" (*nâdî*), the channels along which the life force flows. This purification process is said to be of two kinds, which are technically (and untranslatably) known as *samanu* and *nirmanu* respectively. The former is a meditative exercise by means of which the presiding deities of the various occult bodily centers (*cakra*) are invoked and "installed" in the body. This is combined with the recitation of their respective *bîja*- or "seed" *mantras*. The *nirmanu* type of purification is the practice of cleansing (*dhauti*), as described above under the "six actions" (*shat-karman*).

Gheranda distinguishes the following eight types of breath control, which he calls "retentions" (*kumbhaka*, lit. "pot"):

1. *Sahita-kumbhaka* ("joined retention"), which is a complex breathing technique involving visualization of different deities in conjunction with inhalation, retention, and exhalation; the rhythm is 1:4:2. Thus, if inhalation lasts five seconds, the breath has to be held for twenty seconds, while exhalation extends over ten seconds. The rhythm is measured in so-called *mâtrâs*, a *mâtrâ* being several seconds long. The maximum duration is given as 20:80:40 *mâtrâs*, which, depending on the system used, can total as much as seven minutes or more. The breathing is done alternately through the left and the right nostril, and after inhalation and prior to retention the *yogin* performs the abdominal lock (*uddîyâna-bandha*).

Svâtmârâma, the author of the *Hatha-Yoga-Pradîpikâ*, understands *sahita-kumbhaka* differently. He uses it as a generic term for all forms of *prânâyâma* that entail inhalation and exhalation, contrasting them with *ke-vala-kumbhaka* or full-blown retention of the breath, which skilled *yogins* can perform for several hours at a time. According to the *Gheranda-Samhitâ*, however, *sahita-kumbhaka* is of two kinds:

(i) *Sagarbha* ("with seed"), which is performed while mentally repeating a "seed" or *bîja-mantra*, such as *om*, *ram*, or *yam*.

(ii) *Nigarbha* ("without seed"), which is performed without the aid of a *bîja-mantra*.

2. *Sûrya-bheda-kumbhaka* ("sun-piercing retention"), which gets its name from the fact that in this technique *yogins* inhale exclusively through the right (solar) nostril and exhale only through the left (lunar) nostril; in between they practice the throat lock (*jalandhara-bandha*) while forcibly retaining the air in their lungs until they experience heat in the roots of their hair and fingertips.

3. *Ujjâyî-kumbhaka* ("victorious retention"), which is executed by inhaling through both nostrils, retaining the air (or life force) in the nose, then drawing it further into the mouth and holding it there for as long as it is comfortable by means of the throat lock (*jalandhara-bandha*); according to the *Hatha-Yoga-Pradîpikâ* (2.51), this practice is performed in such a way that during inhalation a sonorous sound is produced in the throat.

4. *Shîtalî-kumbhaka* ("cooling retention"), which is executed by drawing in the air through the mouth and exhaling it through both nostrils after a short period of breath retention. In the *Hatha-Yoga-Pradîpikâ* (2.54), this technique is to be done by curling the tongue. A related technique, also described in the *Pradîpikâ* (2.54), is *sîtkarî* ("sît-maker"), which is executed by making a hissing sound (i.e., *sît*) during inhalation through the mouth, while exhalation should be done through the nostrils.

5. *Bhastrikâ-kumbhaka* ("bellows retention"), which is performed by rapid inhalation and exhalation through both nostrils simultaneously; the cycle should be repeated three times in all; this practice is said to awaken the *kundalinî* force very quickly.

6. *Bhrâmarî-kumbhaka* ("bee-like retention"), which is performed by inhalation and prolonged retention of the breath, while blocking the ears and intently listening to the various inner sounds generated in the right ear; according to the *Hatha-Yoga-Pradîpikâ* (2.68), a bee-like sound is produced during inhalation and exhalation.

7. *Mûrcchâ-kumbhaka* ("swooning retention"), which consists in gentle retention effected by the neck lock (*jaland-hara-bandha*) while fixing attention on the spot between the eyebrows and detaching oneself from all objects; this

is followed by slow exhalation. This technique produces a euphoric state.

8. *Kevalî-kumbhaka* ("absolute retention"), which is simply retention of the breath for as long as possible. It should be performed five to eight times a day, with one to sixty-four repetitions per session.

Breath control has a range of physiological and psychological effects, and Gheranda differentiates between three levels of mastery: At the lowest level, *prânâyâma* generates heat in the body. At a higher level, it causes tremor in the limbs, especially in the spinal column. At the highest level, it leads to actual levitation ("leaving the ground").

*Prânâyâma* is also held to cure a great variety of diseases, awaken the serpent power, and create blissful states of consciousness.

## Meditation

In Hatha-Yoga and Tantrism in general, *dhyâna* is characteristically understood as visualization. The *Gheranda-Samhitâ* (6.1) speaks of three types of *dhyâna*: (1) visualization having a "coarse" (*sthûla*) object, such as a carefully visualized deity; (2) visualization having a "subtle" (*sûkshma*) object, namely the Absolute in the form of the transcendental point-origin (*bindu*) of the universe, as explained in connection with Tantrism; and (3) contemplation of the Absolute as light (*jyotis*). The *Gheranda-Samhitâ* states:

The contemplation of light (*tejo-dhyâna*) is understood to be a hundred times better than coarse visualization (*sthûladhyâna*). Subtle visualization (*sûkshma-dhyâna*), the greatest of all, is a

hundred thousand times better than the contemplation of light. (6.21)

In subtle visualization or contemplation, attention is simply introverted upon the inner essence, the Self (*âtman*), and a degree of unitive consciousness is achieved. Sage Gheranda explains this process in terms of the awakened *kundalinî* uniting with the Self and rising to the center at the crown of the head, which brings us to the crowning accomplishment of the *hatha-yogin*.

## Ecstasy

The ascent of the *kundalinî* to the top center signals the *yogin*'s transcendence of the ego-consciousness in ecstatic unity or *samâdhi*, which is the seventh and final limb of Hatha-Yoga. The *Gheranda-Samhitâ* features these pertinent definitional stanzas:

Separating the mind from the "pot" [i.e., the body], one should identify it with the transcendental Self (*paramaâtman*)[15]: This is to be known as ecstasy (*samâdhi*), which means liberation from the states [of consciousness], and so on.[16]

I am the Absolute (*brahman*). I am no other. Verily, I am the Absolute, not an experiencer of grief. I am of the form of Being-Consciousness-Bliss, ever free, self-existent (*svabhâvavat*). (7.3–4)

The *Hatha-Yoga-Pradîpikâ* offers the following helpful explanations:

Just as salt becomes identical with water through union [with it], so the

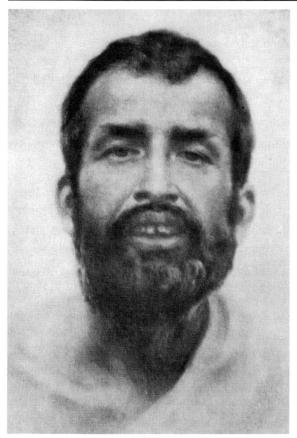

*Sri Ramakrishna, a virtuoso of both savikalpa- and nirvikalpa-samâdhi*

identity (*aikya*) of mind and Self is named "ecstasy" (*samâdhi*).

> When the mind and the life force merge and dissolve, the [resulting state of] balance (*samarasatva*) is named "ecstasy."
>
> That [state of] balance (*sama*), which is the identity of the individuated self (*jîva-âtman*) and the transcendental Self (*parama-âtman*), in which all conceptualization (*samkalpa*) is vanished, that is named "ecstasy." (4.5–7)

It is clear that ecstasy refers here not to one of the lower types of *samâdhi*, which are associated with spontaneously arising thought forms and imagery, but to the ultimate realization of perfect identity with the transcendental Reality. That is to say, the *samâdhi* intended is *nirvikalpa-samâdhi* or "formless ecstasy," which is thought to be synonymous with liberation or enlightenment itself.

Thus, at the end of the long and arduous journey the *hatha-yogin* enjoys the same condition of utter simplicity to which the *râja-yogin* also aspires. The apparent detour of Kundalinî-Yoga, however, which seeks to realize the psychospiritual potential of the body, was not futile, for the *yogin* does not view Self-realization as an event that is separate from life in the physical realm. The realization of the *hatha-yogin* is portrayed as being more complete than that of the *râja-yogin*, simply because it includes the body. The high risks and difficulties of Kundalini-Yoga are compensated by the advantage of extending enlightenment to the body and to physical existence in general, which is expressed in the Tantric formula that liberation (*mukti*) and enjoyment (*bhukti*) are one and the same. For the Tantric *yogin*, the body is indeed a manifestation of the ultimate Reality. As Sir John Woodroffe, the pioneer of Tantric studies, put it:

> He [the *yogin*] realises in the pulsing beat of his heart the rhythm which throbs through, and is the sign of, the universal life. To neglect or to deny the needs of the body, to think of it as something not divine, is to neglect and deny that greater life of which it is a part, and to falsify the great doctrine of the unity of all and of the ultimate identity of Matter and Spirit. Governed by such a concept, even the lowliest physical needs take on a cosmic significance. The body is Shakti. Its needs are Shakti's needs; when man enjoys, it is Shakti who enjoys through him. In all

he sees and does it is the Mother who looks and acts. His eyes and hands are Hers. The whole body and all its functions are Her manifestation. To fully realise Her as such is to perfect this particular manifestation of Hers which is himself.[17]

In Hatha-Yoga, humanity's hope for physical immortality merges with the spiritual impulse toward liberation from the shackles of the ego-ensconced mind. While the dream of an incorruptible earthly body is only a dream, the tradition of Hatha-Yoga has an immense wealth of hard-won information about the hidden potential of the human body-mind from which we can greatly benefit in our own quest for ultimate meaning and happiness. Gradually, modern medicine and psychology, aided by advanced scientific concepts, methods, and instrumentation, are rediscovering some of the amazing facts that *yogins* have talked about and demonstrated for centuries.

It is also obvious that, once the materialistic bias of mainstream science is overcome, we will not only be able to confirm many yogic theories and validate their associated practices but also improve on them and move beyond them. A careful study of Hatha-Yoga, in particular the *kundalinî* phenomenon, could greatly extend our understanding of the human body-mind and its surprising abilities. We must, of course, be willing to step into the *yogin*'s laboratory, and to replicate these experiments in our own person. Subjective testing is, in this case, a reasonable approach; it also happens to be the only logical way of meeting the current scientific ideal of "objectivity."

## III. THE LITERATURE OF HATHA-YOGA

*Yogins* have always been wary of the written word, and those who have written down their insights and experiences have been the exception rather than the rule. As I have tried to show in this volume, however, there is nonetheless a considerable Yoga literature. It primarily exists in manuscript form only, and published editions and translations represent a mere fraction of what is available in the libraries and learned homes of India. Not a few of these works concern Hatha-Yoga. The *Yoga-Upanishads* were discussed in Chapter 15, and several of these texts address Kundalinî-Yoga, which overlaps with Hatha-Yoga insofar as the serpent power (*kundalinî-shakti*) is at the core of higher Hatha-Yoga practice. In the following sections I will briefly describe the most important Hatha-Yoga scriptures that exist in addition to the so-called *Yoga-Upanishads*.

### Goraksha's Writings

Perhaps the earliest work of this branch of the Yoga tradition is the text entitled *Hatha-Yoga*, which is attributed to Goraksha himself. Unfortunately, it is no longer available, though some of its stanzas may well have survived in other works. In fact, the extant texts of Hatha-Yoga share many stanzas between them. Goraksha is also credited with the authorship of a number of other texts, including the *Goraksha-Paddhati* ("Track of Goraksha"), which consists of 200 stanzas outlining the Hatha-Yoga path and which is translated below; the *Goraksha-Shataka* ("Goraksha's Century [of Stanzas]"), which is a fragment of the former work; the *Goraksha-Samhitâ* ("Goraksha's Collection"), which appears to be identical with the *Paddhati* and is different from the alchemical work by this title; the *Hatha-Dîpikâ* ("Lamp of Hatha"), about which nothing is known; the *Jnâna-Amrita* ("Nectar of Wisdom"), a work dealing with the sacred duties of a *hatha-yogin*; the *Amanaska-Yoga* ("Transmental Yoga"), which has 211 stanzas; the *Amaraugha-Prabodha* ("Understanding the Immortal Flood"), a work of 74 stanzas that defines Mantra-, Laya-, Râja-, and Hatha-Yoga and speaks of the *bindu* and the *nâda* as the two great remedies present in every human body that alone can save the *yogin* from death; and the *Yoga-Mârtanda* ("Sun of Yoga"), which has 176 stanzas, many of which are similar to those found in the *Hatha-Yoga-Pradîpikâ*.

## SOURCE READING 21

# *Goraksha-Paddhati*

The importance of the *Goraksha-Paddhati* ("Tracks of Goraksha") can be gauged by the fact that many of its verses are found scattered throughout the later literature of Hatha-Yoga. It is unlikely to have been authored by Goraksha, however, because its concepts and terminology belong to the twelfth or thirteenth rather than the tenth century. This text is here translated in full for the first time, based on the Sanskrit edition by Khemarâja Shrîkrishnadâsa (Bombay).

## Part I

Bowing to the Blessed Âdinâtha—his own teacher, Hari, the sage and *yogin*—Mahîdhara has undertaken to present a commentary on Goraksha's teaching (*shâstra*) that provides a proper understanding of Yoga. (1.1)

*Comments:* This opening stanza is presumably an interpolation, because in the third stanza the author is identified as Goraksha. The name Mahîdhara, which means "Supporter of the Earth," could refer to the well-known sixteenth-century Yoga master who authored the *Mantra-Mahodadhi* together with the auto-commentary *Naukâ*. The Hatha-Yoga literature is full of incongruities, and many texts contain fragments of other scriptures.

I venerate the blessed teacher, the supreme bliss (*parama-ânanda*[18]) who is an embodiment of the innate bliss (*sva-ânanda*[19]) and in whose mere proximity [my] body becomes blissful and conscious. (1.2)

*Comments:* Tradition unanimously names Matsyendra as Goraksha's teacher. In this stanza, he is identified with the unalloyed bliss of the ultimate Reality, unless we interpret *parama-ânanda* as the name of an individual other than Matsyendra.

Devotedly saluting his teacher as supreme wisdom, Goraksha expounds what is desired to bring about the ultimate bliss in *yogins*. (1.3)

With the desire to benefit *yogins*, he declares the *Goraksha-Samhitâ*. By comprehending it, the supreme State is surely attained. (1.4)

It is a ladder to liberation, a [means of] cheating death, by which the mind is turned away from pleasure (*bhoga*) and attached to the transcendental Self (*parama-âtman*[20]). (1.5)

The most excellent ones resort to Yoga, which is the fruit of the wish-fulfilling tree of revelation (*shruti*), whose branches are frequented by the twice-born, and which pacifies the tribulations of existence. (1.6).

*Comments:* This stanza contains a pun on the word *dvija*, which means both "twice-born" and "bird." The twice-born are those who have been duly invested with the sacred thread and are entitled to study the revealed scriptures. Like birds, they are seated on the branches of Vedic learning, feasting on the delicious fruit of perennial wisdom.

They name posture, breath restraint (*prâna-samrodha*), sense-withdrawal, concentration, meditation, and ecstasy as the six limbs of Yoga. (1.7)

There are as many postures as there are species of beings. [Only] Maheshvara[21] [i.e., Shiva] knows all their varieties. (1.8)

Of the 840,000, one for each [100,000] has been mentioned. Thus Shiva created eighty-four seats (*pîtha*) [for *yogins*]. (1.9)

Of all the postures, two are special. The first is said to be the hero's posture (*siddha-âsana*[22]); the second is the lotus posture (*kamala-âsana*). (1.10)

[The *yogin*] should firmly place one [i.e., the left] heel against the perineum (*yoni-sthâna*), while placing the other heel above the penis and pressing the chin against the chest (*hridaya*). With the senses restrained like a log, he should direct his gaze steadily at the [third eye] between the eyebrows. This is said to be the hero's posture, which bursts open the door to liberation. (1.11)

Placing the right [lower] leg on top of the left [thigh] and the left [lower leg] on top of the right [thigh], firmly grasping the big toes with the hands crossed behind the back, while placing the chin on the chest, he should look at the tip of the nose. This is said to be the [*baddha* or "bound"] lotus posture, which removes various kinds of diseases. (1.12)

How can those *yogins* succeed who do not know the six centers, the sixteen props, the 300,000 [channels],[23] and the five ethers/spaces in their own body? (1.13)

*Comments:* The six psychoenergetic centers (*shat-cakra*) are the well-known *mûlâd-hâra* (at the base of the spine), *svâdhishthâna* (at the genitals), *manipûra* (at the navel), *anâhata* (at the heart), *vishuddha* (at the throat), and *âjnâ* (in the middle of the head). The *Siddha-Siddhânta-Paddhati* (2.10) mentions the following sixteen props (*shodasha-âdhâra*, written *shodashâdhâra*): the two big toes, perineum (*mûla*), anus, penis, lower abdomen (*udyâna*), navel, heart, throat, "bell" (*ghantikâ*, corresponding to the uvula), palate, tongue, point midway between the eyebrows, nose, root of the nose, and forehead. The 300,000 channels (*nâdî*) that crisscross the subtle body are the carriers of the life force. Of these, the central channel (*sushumnâ*), the lunar channel (*idâ*), and the solar channel (*pingalâ*) are the most important. The five ethers/spaces (*vyoman*) are distinct yogic experiences of the space of consciousness.

How can those *yogins* who do not know their own body as a single-columned dwelling with nine openings and five divinities (*adhidaivata*) be successful? (1.14)

*Comments:* The single column is the trunk, and the nine openings are the eyes, ears, nostrils, mouth, anus, and urethra. The five divinities are the five senses.

The "prop" [i.e., the *mûlâdhâra* lotus at the base of the spine] has four petals. The *svâdhishtâna* has six petals. At the navel is a ten-petaled lotus, and at the heart [is a lotus having as many] petals as the number of solar [months, i.e., twelve]. (1.15)

At the throat is a sixteen-petaled [lotus] and between the eyebrows is a two-petaled [lotus]. At the brahmic fissure (*brahma-randhra*), at the great path, [there is a lotus] called "thousand-petaled." (1.16)

The "prop" (*âdhâra*) is the first center; *svâdhishthâna* is the second. Between them is the perineum named *kâma-rûpa*. (1.17)

*Comments:* The name *kâma-rûpa* means literally "desire-formed." This is also the name of a sacred geographical area famous for Tantric study and practice, which has been identified as Assam. In the human body, this too designates a sacred spot, a place of power, which harbors the potential for liberation as well as self-destruction.

The four-petaled lotus called "prop" is at the place of the anus (*guda-sthâna*). In the middle of it is said to be the "womb" (*yoni*) praised by adepts under the name of desire (*kâma*). (1.18)

*Comments:* The technical term *yoni* can stand for either the perineum or an esoteric energy structure associated with the *kundalinî*. In the latter case, it is the "womb" for Shiva's phallus/symbol (*linga*), as mentioned in the next stanza.

In the middle of the "womb" stands the great phallus/symbol [of Shiva] facing backward. He who knows the disk, which is like a [brightly shining] jewel, in [its] head is a knower of Yoga. (1.19)

*Comments: Yoni* and *linga* represent Shakti and Shiva respectively. The sexual symbolism conceals a sweeping cosmic reality: the eternal play between feminine power and masculine consciousness, which are always united on the transcendental level but are experienced as separate on the empirical level. The luminous disk/mirror (*bimba*) mentioned in this stanza is pictured as being fastened to the "head" (*mastaka*) of Shiva's symbolic phallus. Presumably it stands for the *linga's* native luminosity, which is reflected back upon itself—in evidence of Shiva's perfect autonomy.

Situated below the penis is the triangular city of fire,[24] flashing forth like lightning bolts and resembling molten gold. (1.20)

When in the great Yoga, in ecstasy, [the *yogin*] sees the supreme, infinite, omnipresent Light, he does not experience [any further] coming and going [i.e., births and deaths in the finite world]. (1.21)

The life force arises with the sound *sva*. The resting place of this [life force] is the *svâdhishthâna*[*-cakra*]. Thus the penis is named after this place as *svâdhishthâna*. (1.22)

Where the "bulb" (*kanda*) is strung on the *sushumnâ* [i.e., the central channel] like a jewel on a thread, that region is called the *manipûraka-cakra*.[25] (1.23)

So long as the psyche (*jîva*) roams at the great twelve-spoked center [at the heart], which is free from merit (*punya*) and demerit (*pâpa*), it cannot find Reality. (1.24)

*Comments:* The psyche, or individuated consciousness, is thought to restlessly move in the petals of the heart lotus, driven by its own karma and trapped by its own ignorance (*avidyâ*). That nescience is the psyche's ignorance of its true nature as the Self. When wisdom dawns, the *jîva*'s centrifugal movement ceases, and consciousness finds its real source at the center of the heart, which is the free and blissful consciousness of the Self. For the liberated individual, there is neither merit nor demerit, which are karmic realities that pertain only to the condition of unenlightenment.

Below the navel and above the penis is the "bulb" (*kanda*), the "womb" (*yoni*), which is like a bird's egg. In it the 72,000 channels originate. (1.25)

Among these thousands of channels, seventy-two are described. Again, of these carriers of life force ten are mentioned as primary. (1.26)

*Idâ* and *pingalâ*, and *sushumnâ* as the third, as well as *gândhârî, hasti-jihvâ, pûshâ, yashasvinî,* . . . (1.27)

. . . *alambushâ, kuhû¸* and *shankhinî* as the tenth are mentioned. *Yogins* should always understand this network (*cakra*) composed of channels. (1.28)

*Idâ* is located on the left side; *pingalâ* is located on the right. *Sushumnâ* is in the central place, while the *gândhârî* is in the left eye. (1.29)

*Hasti-jihvâ* is on the right, and *pûshâ* is in the right ear, while *yashasvinî* is in the left ear and *alambhushâ* is in the mouth. (1.30)

*Kuhû* is at the place of the penis (*linga*) and the *shankhinî* at the place of the anus. Thus there are ten channels, [each of which is] connected with an opening. (1.31)

*Idâ, pingalâ,* and *sushumnâ* are connected to the path of the life force. The [ten] are always carriers of the life force, [and they are respectively associated with] the deities of moon (*soma*), sun, and fire. (1.32)

*Prâna, apâna, samâna, udâna,* as well as *vyâna* are the [principal] "winds." *Nâga, kûrma, kri-kala, deva-datta,* and *dhanam-jaya* [are the secondary types of life force in the body]. (1.33)

*Comments:* These ten names are technical terms in Yoga and are not readily translatable. They stand for various aspects or functions of the life force as it manifests in the human body.

*Prâna* dwells at the heart; *apâna* is always in the region of the anus; *samâna* is at the location of the navel; *udâna* is in the middle of the throat; . . . (1.34)

. . . *vyâna* pervades the [whole] body. [These are] the five principal "winds." The five beginning with *prâna* and the [other] five "winds" beginning with *nâga* are well known. (1.35)

*Nâga* is said to be [present in] eructation; *kûrma* is said [to manifest in] the opening [of the eyes]; *kri-kâra* [or *kri-kala*] is known as causing sneezing; *deva-datta* [is present in] yawning. (1.36)

*Dhanam-jaya* is all-pervasive and does not even quit a corpse. These [ten forms of the life force] roam in all the channels in the form of the psyche (*jîva*). (1.37)

As a ball struck with a curved staff flies up, so the psyche, when struck by *prâna* and *apâna* [in the form of the in-breath and out-breath], does not stand still. (1.38)

Under the force of *prâna* and *apâna* the psyche moves up and down along the left and right pathways, [even though] it cannot be seen because of its mobility. (1.39)

Like a falcon tied with a string can be pulled back when it has taken off, so the psyche, tied by the qualities (*guna*) [of Nature] can be pulled back by means of [controlled] *prâna* and *apâna*. (1.40)

*Apâna* pulls *prâna*, and *prâna* pulls *apâna*. [These two forms of the life force are respectively] situated above and below [the navel]. The knower of Yoga joins both [to awaken the serpent power]. (1.41)

[The psyche] exits [the body] with the sound *ha* and reenters it with the sound *sa*. The psyche continually recites the *mantra* "*hamsa hamsa*." (1.42)

*Comments:* This natural, spontaneous recitation, caused by inhalation and exhalation, is known as the *ajapa-gâyatrî*. When the *yogin* engages this recitation consciously, *hamsa hamsa hamsa* is converted into the *mantra* "*so' ham so' ham so' ham*," meaning "I am He; I am He; I am He."

The psyche continually recites this *mantra* 21,600 times day and night. (1.43)

The *gâyatrî*[-*mantra*] named *ajapa* bestows liberation upon *yogins*, and merely by the desire [to recite] it one is released from all sin. (1.44)

Knowledge like this, recitation (*japa*) like this, and wisdom like this did not exist [before now] nor will exist [ever again]. (1.45)

The life-sustaining *gâyatrî* is born from the *kundalinî*. He who knows this knowledge of the life force, the great science, is a knower of the *Vedas*. (1.46)

*Comments:* Here the yogic science of the breath, or life force, is presented as the quintessence of the Vedic revelation. This is not far from the truth, because breath control together with curbing the mind was the earliest form of Yoga, practiced already in Vedic times. It was fundamental to the Vedic ritual, especially in connection with the disciplined chanting of the sacred hymns.

The *kundalinî* power folded into eight coils always resides above the "bulb," closing the opening of the "brahmic gate" (*brahma-dvâra*) with its face. (1.47)

*Comments:* The eight coils of the serpent power are named in the *Yoga-Vishaya* (22) as follows: *pranavâ, guda-nâlâ, nalinî, sarpinî, vanka-nâli, kshayâ, shaurî,* and *kundalî.*

Through that gate one should go to the state of the Absolute[26] beyond ill, [but] Parameshvarî is asleep covering that gate with her face. (1.48)

[When the *kundalinî*] is awakened through *buddhi-yoga* together with the mind and the breath (*marut*), it moves upward through the *sushumnâ* like a needle drawing a thread. (1.49)

*Comments:* The term *buddhi-yoga* stands for the disciplined application of the higher mind (*buddhi*) through which the lower mind (*manas*) becomes pliable enough for attention to become linked with the movement of the life force, or breath. By their combined action, the dormant *kundalinî* is aroused and gradually guided along the spinal axis toward the crown center.

[When the *kundalinî*], having the form of a sleeping serpent and being splendid like a lotus fiber, is awakened through *vahni-yoga*, it moves upward through the *sushumnâ*. (1.50)

*Comments:* The compound *vahni-yoga*, or "Yoga of fire," refers to the combustion created by uniting the mind (attention) with the life force (breath). It is the physiological counterpart to *buddhi-yoga*.

Just as one forcibly opens a door with a key, so the *yogin* should break open the door to liberation by means of the *kundalinî*. (1.51)

*Comments:* There is a pun here on the word *hatha* ("force"), which in the ablative *hathât* means "by force" or "forcibly." The *kundalinî* process is quintessential in Hatha-Yoga, the forceful Yoga.

Cupping the hands firmly and assuming the lotus posture while placing the chin tightly against the chest and [practicing] meditation in the mind (*cetas*), he should expel again and again the *apâna* air above, after having filled [the chest with it]. [Thus] upon releasing the life force, he acquires unequaled understanding (*bodha*) through the awakening of the power (*shakti*). (1.52)

He should rub his limbs with the liquid [i.e., the perspiration] produced by the effort. He should consume milk and abstain from bitter, sour, and salty [food]. (1.53)

He who practices [this kind of] Yoga should be a celibate (*brahmacârin*) and a renouncer (*tyâgin*), living on a modest diet (*mita-âhârin*[27]). He will become an adept after a year. There should be no doubt about this. (1.54)

*Comments:* While engaging the difficult *kundalinî* process, *yogins* must take great care about their diet. Neither fasting nor overeating is recommended.

He who consumes[28] oil-rich and sweet food, delighting in its taste and leaving a fourth part, is called a modest eater (*mita-âhârin*). (1.55)

*Comments:* The traditional recommendation is to fill two parts of the stomach with food and one part with water, leaving the fourth part empty. A quarter portion of the food itself should be offered to the deities and ancestors before eating.

He who knows the *kundalinî-shakti* [situated] above the "bulb" and bestowing splendid liberation, but [causing greater] bondage for fools, is a knower of the *Vedas*. (1.56)

*Comments:* The serpent power is a two-edged sword. For wise practitioners it brings the fruit of liberation, but for others it merely deepens their ignorant involvement in the painful cycle of existence (*samsâra*).

The *yogin* who knows the *mahâ-mudrâ*, *nabho-mudrâ*, *uddîyâna*[*-bandha*], *jalandhara*[*-bandha*], and *mûla-bandha* partakes of liberation. (1.57)

Placing the chin on the chest, pressing continually the left heel against the perineum (*yoni*), and holding the extended right foot with the hands, [the *yogin*] should, after inhaling the air and holding it on both sides of the chest, expel it gradually. This great seal [i.e., mahâ-mudrâ] is said to remove people's diseases. (1.58)

*Comments:* The expression *kakshi-yugalam*, here translated as "on both sides of the chest," corresponds to the sensation of filling the lungs to capacity so that the rib cage expands.

After practicing [the *mahâ-mudrâ* first] with the lunar part [i.e., the left nostril], he should practice it with the solar part [i.e., the right nostril]. He should discontinue this seal after achieving an equal number [of repetitions]. (1.59)

[For the adept who is successful in the practice of the *mahâ-mudrâ*] there is no proper or improper [food]. All tastes are indeed without taste. Even virulent poison when swallowed is digested as if it were nectar (*pîyûsha*). (1.60)

For him who practices the *mahâ-mudrâ*, [all] diseases are eliminated, notably consumption, leprosy, constipation,[29] abdominal swelling, and decrepitude. (1.61)

This *mahâ-mudrâ* that has been described brings great accomplishments for people. It should be diligently guarded and not given to anyone. (1.62)

*Comments:* The phrase *mahâ-siddhi*, here rendered as "great accomplishments," can also be understood in the singular as the great accomplishment of liberation. Alternatively, it could refer to the eight great paranormal powers traditionally associated with fully realized adepts.

The *khecârî-mudrâ* consists in turning the tongue backward into the hollow of the skull while fixing the gaze between the eyebrows. (1.63)

He who knows the *khecârî-mudrâ* does not experience sleep, hunger, thirst, fainting, or death from disease. (1.64)

He who knows the *khecârî-mudrâ* is not troubled by grief, tainted by actions [or karma], or bound by anything. (1.65)

The mind (*citta*) does not move because the tongue assumes the *khecârî*. Because of this, the perfected *khecârî* is adored by all the adepts. (1.66)

The semen (*bindu*) is the root of [all] bodies in which the veins [i.e., the channels of the life force] are established. They constitute [all] bodies from the head to the soles of the feet. (1.67)

For him who [enters] the cavity above the uvula by means of the *khecârî-mudrâ*, the semen is not wasted, [even if he is] embraced by a woman. (1.68)

*Comments:* Through mastery of the *khecârî-mudrâ*, the *yogin* can engage in sexual activity without the risk of seminal discharge, which is traditionally avoided because of the depletion of vital energy (*ojas*) entailed.

So long as the semen remains in the body, how can there be fear of death? So long as the *nabho-mudrâ* is maintained, the semen does not stir. (1.69)

*Comments:* The term *nabho-mudrâ* is similar to *khecârî-mudrâ*, and *nabhas*[30] is another word for *kha* (in *khecarî*); both mean "ether/space."

Even if the semen has dropped into the "sacrifice consuming" (*huta-âshana*) [female womb], it moves back up again, having been stolen, when it is restrained by the power of the *yoni-mudrâ*. (1.70)

*Comments:* The *yoni-mudrâ* consists in the skillful contraction of the perineum.

Moreover, the semen is twofold: white and red. They call the white one *shukra*, while the red one is named *mahâ-rajas*. (1.71)

*Comments:* The white *shukra* is the male semen, and the red *mahâ-rajas* refers to the female vaginal secretion, which is sometimes (mis-)understood as menstrual blood or ovâ.

The *rajas* is located at the place of the navel and resembles a red liquid. The *bindu* is located at the place of the moon [i.e., at the palate]. Their union is difficult to achieve. (1.72)

*Comments:* It is clear from this stanza that, from a yogic perspective, the *bindu* represents more than the sperm produced in the testicles, just as the *rajas* stands for more than female genital secretion. Both have their energetic aspects as well. Thus, the *rajas* is associated with the solar element in the abdomen and the *bindu* with the lunar element in the head.

The *bindu* is Shiva; the *rajas* is Shakti. The *bindu* is the moon; the *rajas* is the sun. Only through the union of both does [the *yogin*] attain the supreme State. (1.73)

When the *rajas* is activated by stirring the [*kundalinî-*]power through the breath (*vâyu*), then it achieves union with the *bindu*, whereupon the body becomes divine. (1.74)

*Comments:* The creation of a divine body (*divya-deha*), which is endowed with all the great paranormal powers, is the avowed goal of Hatha-Yoga. This stanza briefly mentions the esoteric process by which this is accomplished.

The *shukra* is joined with the moon; the *rajas* is linked with the sun. He who knows their coessential unity is a knower of Yoga. (1.75)

*Comments:* The phrase *samarasa-ekatva* (written *samarasaikatva*), here translated as "coessential unity," refers to the mingling of the energetic aspects of the two types of semen—male and female. *Samarasa* is an important notion in Tantrism and Hatha-Yoga. It stands for the realization of the fundamental identity of all differentiated things, that is, nonduality in duality.

The purification of the network (*jâla*) of channels and the stirring of sun and moon, as well as the drying up of [noxious bodily] liquids, is called *mahâ-mudrâ*. (1.76)

*Comments:* The transformation aspired to by the *hatha-yogin* involves a complete recasting of the body's chemistry. The *rasas* or liquids mentioned in this stanza presumably are chemically imbalanced bodily fluids.

Just as a great bird takes to flight untiringly, so his [practice of] *uddîyâna*[-*bandha*] becomes a lion to the elephant of death. (1.77)

*Comments:* This colorful metaphor is based on the wordplay between a bird's *uddîna* ("flying up") and the *yogin*'s *uddîyâna* ("soaring"), which consists in pulling the stomach in and thereby forcing the air/life force upward so that the *jîva* soars like a bird. This yogic technique is said to conquer death, just as a lion can kill the much larger elephant.

This upward lock (*uddîyâna-bandha*) is said [to be practiced] below the navel and at the back portion of the abdomen. There the lock is said [to be applied]. (1.78)

The *jâlandhara-bandha* [or throat lock] blocks the network of conduits (*shiras*) so that the water from the sky (*nabhas*) [i.e., the ambrosial liquid from the secret center in the head] does not drip down [into the abdomen]. Therefore [this practice] removes a host of diseases of the throat. (1.79)

By performing the *jâlandhara-bandha*, characterized by the [deliberate] constriction of the throat], the nectar does not fall into the fire, and the air is not agitated. (1.80)

Pressing the left heel against the perineum, [the *yogin*] should contract the anus while pulling the *apâna* [life force] upward. [Thus] is the "root lock" (*mûla-bandha*) to be performed. (1.81)

By unifying *apâna* and *prâna*, urine and faeces are reduced. Even if he is old, he becomes young again through the constant [practice of] the root lock. (1.82)

Assuming the lotus posture, holding the body and head straight while gazing at the tip of the nose, he should recite the imperishable *om*-sound in seclusion (*ekânta*). (1.83)

The supreme Light is *om*, in whose morae (*mâtrâ*) abide the deities of moon, sun, and fire [together with] the realms [symbolized by the words] *bhûh*, *bhuvah*, and *svah*. (1.84)

*Comments:* The sacred syllable *om* symbolizes the Absolute, but its constituent parts (*a*, *u*, and *m*) represent the three worlds (*loka*), expressed in the words *bhûh*, *bhuvah*, and *svah*, standing for earth, mid-region, and heaven/sky respectively.

The supreme Light is *om*, wherein abide the three times [i.e., past, present, and future], the three *Vedas* [i.e., the *Rig-*, *Yajur-*, and *Sâma-Veda*], the three worlds, the three intonations (*svara*), and the three deities [i.e., Shiva, Vishnu, and Brahma?]. (1.85)

The supreme Light is *om* wherein abides the threefold power (*shakti*) [consisting in] action, will, and wisdom, or *brâhmî*, *raudrî*, and *vaishnavî*. (1.86)

*Comments:* The feminine aspect of the Divine, epitomized in the term *shakti*, is thought to comprise the three functions of creative action (*kriyâ*), creative will (*icchâ*), and creative wisdom (*jnâna*). These are also referred to by the adjectival forms of the three great deities Brahma, Rudra (i.e., Shiva), and Vishnu.

The supreme Light is *om*, wherein abide the three morae, namely the syllable *a*, the syllable *u*, and the syllable *m* known as the "seed-point" (*bindu*). (1.87)

The supreme Light is *om*. He should recite in words its seed-syllable (*bîja*), practice it with the body, and remember it with the mind. (1.88)

He who constantly recites the *pranava*, whether he be pure or impure, is not tainted by sin, just like a lotus leaf [is not stained by the surrounding] water. (1.89)

When the "wind" moves, the semen moves as well. When it does not move, [the semen also] does not move. [If] the *yogin* [desires to] attain stock-stillness (*sthânut-va*), then he should restrain the "wind" [i.e., the breath/life force]. (1.90)

So long as the "wind" remains in the body, the psyche is not released. Its departure [causes] death. Therefore he should restrain the "wind." (1.91)

So long as the air is held in the body, the mind is free from ill. So long as the gaze [is expertly directed] between the eyebrows, how can there be fear of death? (1.92)

Therefore, out of fear of death, [even] Brahma is intent on breath control, as are the *yogins* and sages. Therefore one should restrain the "wind." (1.93)

Through the left and right pathways [i.e., the nostrils], the *hamsa* goes forth (*prayâ-na*) [a distance of] thirty-six fingers outside [the body], wherefore it is called *prâna*. (1.94)

When the whole network of channels, filled with impurities, is purified, then the *yogin* becomes capable of controlling (*samgrahana*) the life force. (1.95)

The *yogin* [seated in] the bound lotus posture should fill in the life force through the lunar [nostril] and then, after holding it according to his capacity, expel it again through the solar [nostril]. (1.96)

Meditating on the moon disk, the nectar that resembles [white] curd or is like cow's milk or silver, [the *yogin* practicing] breath control should be happy. (1.97)

*Comments:* The text uses the word *prânâyâmin* for the practitioner of *prânâyâma*. The lunar disk (*bimba*) is visualized in the head at the place of the nectar of immortality above the palate.

Drawing in the breath (*shvâsa*) through the right [nostril], he should fill the abdomen gradually. Having retained it according to the rules, he should expel it again through the lunar [nostril]. (1.98)

Meditating on the solar circle, which is a mass of brightly burning flames located at the navel, the *yogin* practicing breath control should be happy. (1.99)

When the breath is filtered through the *idâ* [i.e., the left nostril], he should expel it again through the other [nostril]. Sucking the air in through the *pingalâ* [i.e., the right nostril] he should, after holding it, release it again through the left [nostril].
By meditating on the two disks—of the sun and the moon—according to the rules, the host of channels become pure after three months. (1.100)

By purifying the channels, [the *yogin*] achieves health, the manifestation of the [subtle inner] sound (*nâda*), [the ability to] hold the "wind" according to capacity, and the flaring up of the [inner] fire. (1.101)

*Comments:* The inner fire (*anala*) is the abdominal heat (*udâra-agni*, written *udârâgni*), which is essential in the process of awakening the serpent power.

## Part II

Through the restraint of the out-breath (*apâna*), the air, the life force (*prâna*), remains in the body. By means of only a single breath, [the *yogin*] should burst open the way into the "space" (*gagana*) [at the crown of the head]. (2.1)

*Comments:* The life force (*prâna*) manifests in the human body in five functional varieties, of which primarily *apâna* and *prâna* are the engine that powers our psychophysical life. The former is connected with exhalation, the latter with inhalation. By stopping the out-going life force, the *yogin* builds up pranic energy in the body, which, when properly deployed, can force open the hidden doorway at the crown of the head. It is here that the individuated life force rejoins the cosmic life force.

[Yogic] exhalation, inhalation, and retention are of the nature of the humming sound (*pranava*) [i.e., the sacred syllable *om*]. Breath control is threefold and endowed with twelve measures (*mâtrâ*). (2.2)

*Comments:* In Hatha-Yoga, breath control is often connected with the practice of *om* recitation, which is counted in "measures." A *mâtrâ* is a unit of time, which is variously defined. Thus, in the *Brihad-Yogi-Yâjnavalkya-Smriti* (8.112) it is explained as the time it takes to snap one's fingers thrice, circle the knee with the hand once, and clap thrice. In the present text, it is equated with the duration of the *om*-sound—lasting a couple of seconds.

The [internal] sun and moon are connected with the twelve measures; they are not fettered by the network of defects (*dosha*). The *yogin* should always know [these two principles]. (2.3)

*Comments:* The human body is a replica of the macrocosmic realities. "As above, so below." Thus the sun and the moon are also located within the body. The former is thought to be located at the navel, the latter in the head.

During inhalation he should perform twelve measures [of the syllable *om*]. During retention he should perform sixteen measures, and during exhalation ten *om*-sounds. This is called "breath control" (*prânâyâma*). (2.4)

In the initial [stage of breath control] twelve measures [should be done]; in the middle [stage] twice as many are deemed [appropriate]; in the superior [stage] thrice as many are prescribed. Such is the qualification of breath control. (2.5)

In the lower [stage], the "substance" (*dharma*) [i.e., sweat] is forced out; in the middle [stage] there is trembling; in the superior [stage] the *yogin* rises [from the ground]. Hence he should [carefully] restrain the air (*vâyu*). (2.6)

The *yogin*, [seated in] the bound lotus posture and saluting the teacher and Shiva, should practice breath control in solitude (*ekânta*), with his gaze on the middle between the brows. (2.7)

*Comments:* The bound lotus posture (*baddha-padma-âsana*) is performed by crossing the arms behind one's back while being seated in the regular lotus posture and grasping the toes with the opposite hands.

Drawing up the *apâna* air, he should unite it with the *prâna*. When it is led upward with the [*kundalinî*] power, he is released from all sins. (2.8)

Having closed the nine gates (*dvâra*) [i.e., the openings of the body], having sucked in the air and holding it firmly, having conducted it to the "space" (*âkâsha*) [of the heart?] together with the *apâna* and the [abdominal] fire (*vahni*), starting up the [*kundalinî*] power and placing it in the head, for sure according to this rule, as long as [the *yogin* who is] joined with the abode of the Self [at the crown center] remains [thus], he is praised by the host of the great ones. (2.9)

*Comments:* The process of awakening the *kundalinî* is characteristically described as the joint action of *prâna*, *apâna*, and the gastric fire. Together they generate sufficient energy to rouse the dormant *kundalinî* resting at the base of the spine.

Thus, breath control is the fire [feeding on] the fuel of transgressions (*pâtaka*). The *yogins* always call it the "great bridge" [leading across] the ocean of [conditioned] existence. (2.10)

*Comments:* Since the time of the *Brâhmanas*, breath control has been hailed as a superb means of burning up the karmic deposits resulting from demeritorious thoughts and actions.

Through posture, diseases are removed; through breath control, transgressions [are atoned for]; through sense-withdrawal, the *yogin* is released from [all] mental modifications (*vikâra*). (2.11)

Fondness for concentration [causes] steadiness (*dhairya*); through meditation, [he obtains] a marvelous [state of] consciousness. In [the condition of] ecstasy (*samâdhi*), having cast off auspicious and inauspicious karma, he attains liberation. (2.12)

Sense-withdrawal is said [to come about] with twice six breath controls; auspicious concentration is recognized [to come about] with twice six sense-withdrawals. (2.13)

Twelve concentrations are said to be meditation by the experts in meditation. Ecstasy (*samâdhi*) is said [to come about] with twelve meditations. (2.14)

Upon seeing in that ecstasy the supreme Light—infinite and facing all round—there is no activity or past or present karma. (2.15)

Having assumed the posture with the penis [between] the two heels, [and while] curbing the openings of the ears, eyes, and nasal passage with the fingers, and having inhaled the air through the mouth and having contemplated [the *prâna*] in the chest together with the fire [in the abdomen] and the *apâna*, he should hold them steady in the head. Thus, the lord of *yogins*, of the form of that [Reality], reaches sameness (*samatâ*) with Reality (*tattva*) [i.e., Shiva]. (2.16)

When the air has reached the "space" (*gagana*) [at the heart?], a mighty sound is produced [resembling that of musical] instruments such as a bell. Then perfection (*siddhi*) is near. (2.17)

[The *yogin* who is] yoked through breath control [accomplishes] the removal of all [kinds of] illnesses. [The person who is] not yoked in the practice of Yoga [invites] the manifestation of every [kind of] illness. (2.18)

Various illnesses [such as] hiccups, cough, asthma, and afflictions of head, ear, and eyes are caused through the mismanagement (*vyatikrama*) of the air. (2.19)

Just as the lion, the elephant, and the tiger are tamed very gradually, lest they should kill the trainer—so the air is not [to be] employed [without great discipline]. (2.20)

He should let go of the air very gradually, and he should also inhale very gradually. Moreover, he should hold [the breath] very gradually. Thus, perfection is near. (2.21)

The eyes and other [senses] are roaming among their respective sense objects. Their withdrawal from them is called "sense-withdrawal" (*pratyâhâra*). (2.22)

Even as the sun reaching the third time-[quarter] withdraws its luster, so the *yogin* resorting to the third limb [of Yoga] [should withdraw every] mental modification (*vikâra*). (2.23)

As a tortoise contracts its limbs into the middle of the shell, so the *yogin* should withdraw the senses into himself. (2.24)

Recognizing that whatever he hears with the ears, whether pleasant or unpleasant, is the Self—the knower of Yoga withdraws [his hearing]. (2.25)

Recognizing that whatever he smells with the nose, whether fragrant or ill-smelling, is the Self—the knower of Yoga withdraws [his sense of smell]. (2.26)

Recognizing that whatever he sees with the eyes, whether pure or impure, is the Self—the knower of Yoga withdraws [his vision]. (2.27)

Recognizing that whatever he senses with the skin, whether tangible or intangible, is the Self—the knower of Yoga withdraws [his sense of touch]. (2.28)

Recognizing that whatever he tastes with the tongue, whether salty or not salty, is the Self—the knower of Yoga withdraws [his sense of taste]. (2.29)

The sun withdraws the shower made of lunar nectar (*amrita*). The withdrawal of that [shower] is called "sense-withdrawal." (2.30)

The one female, having come from the lunar region, is enjoyed by two, while the third, [in addition to] the two, is he who undergoes aging and death. (2.31)

*Comments:* The meaning of this stanza is not clear.

In the place of the navel dwells the one sun, of the essence of fire. And the moon, of the essence of nectar, is always situated at the root of the palate. (2.32)

The moon, facing downward, showers [nectar]; the sun, facing upward, devours [that lunar nectar]. Hence the [inverted] pose (*karanî*) is to be known so that the ambrosia can be obtained. (2.33)

[When] the navel is above and the palate is below, [that is to say, when] the sun is above and the moon is below, [then that is] known as the inverted pose. It should be learned from the teacher's instructions. (2.34)

*Comments:* The inverted pose (*viparîta-karanî*) can be either the headstand or the shoulderstand.

Where the triply fettered bull roars a mighty roar, the *yogins* should know that the center of the "unstruck" (*anâhata*) [sound is situated] at the heart. (2.35)

*Comments:* The "triply fettered bull" (*tridhâ baddho vrishah*) is the psyche (*jîva*) bound by the three qualities (*guna*) of Nature—*sattva*, *rajas*, and *tamas*.

When the life force has reached the great lotus [at the crown of the head], after having approached the *manipûraka*-[center] and having passed on to the *anâhata*-[center], the *yogin* attains immortality (*amrita*). (2.36)

[The *yogin*] should contemplate the supreme Power (*shakti*), placing his tongue upward [in the brahmic] cavity as prescribed. [The nectar] trickling down from the sixteen-petaled lotus above is obtained by forcibly going up [to the palate with the tongue]. That faultless *yogin* who drinks from the tongue's home (*kula*) the [special] sixteenth part of the exceedingly clear water of the *kalâ* wave [flowing from] that [lotus] lives long with a body as tender as a lotus fiber. (2.37)

He should drink the cool surge [of air] with the mouth [shaped] like a crow's beak. By regulating the *prâna* and the *apâna*, the *yogin* does not age. (2.38)

For him who drinks the *prâna* air with the tongue [placed at] the root of the palate, there will be the removal of all illnesses after half a year. (2.39)

He, having contemplated the whole nectar in the fifth center [called] "pure" (*vishuddha*), takes off by the up-path, having cheated the jaws of the [inner] sun [at the navel]. (2.40)

By the sound *vi* is meant the "swan" (*hamsa*) [i.e., the spontaneous breath]; *shuddhi* [or "purity"] is called "spotless." Hence the knowers of the centers (*cakra*) know the center at the throat as [that which is] named *vishuddha*. (2.41)

[The life force], after escaping the jaws of the [inner] sun, rises of its own accord into the hollow at the end of the nose [after the *yogin*] has placed the nectar into that cavern. (2.42)

Having gathered the exceedingly clean water of the *kalâ* of the moon [showering] from above the region of the throat, he should conduct it into the hollow at the end of the nose and then everywhere by means of the "space" [at the crown of the head]. (2.43)

The knower of Yoga who drinks the ambrosia (*soma*) by firmly placing the tongue upward [against the palate] undoubtedly conquers death within half a month. (2.44)

He who controls the root opening overcomes [every] obstacle and reaches [the state] beyond old age and death, like the five-faced Hara [i.e., Shiva]. (2.45)

By pressing the tip of the tongue against the great cavity of the "royal tooth" (*râja-danta*) [i.e., the uvula] and contemplating the ambrosial Goddess, he becomes a poet-sage (*kavi*) within six months. (2.46)

*Comments:* This technique is also known as *lambikâ-yoga*. The word *lambikâ* means "hanger" and refers to the uvula, which is stimulated by the tongue to increase the production of saliva, whose subtle counterpart is the limpid nectar of immortality.

The great flow above [the uvula] blocks all the [other] flows [in the body]. Whoever does not release the nectar [should first practice] the paths of the five concentrations. (2.47).

If the tongue constantly kisses the tip of the "hanger" [i.e., the uvula], causing the liquid (*rasa*) to flow [that tastes] salty, pungent, or sour, or is like milk, honey, and ghee, then diseases, old age, and death are removed, teachings (*shâstra*) and their auxiliaries are celebrated,[31] and he will attain immortality and the eight [paranormal] qualities and attract the consorts (*anga*) of the adepts (*siddha*). (2.48)

After two or three years, the *yogin* whose body is filled with nectar has his semen (*retas*) go upward and [enjoys] the appearance of [paranormal] qualities like miniaturization (*animan*). (2.49)

*Comments:* The upward-streaming of the subtle aspect of the male semen is the yogic counterpart to what in psychological language is known as "sublimation." More precisely, it is a form of "superlimination," since the process involves going beyond the threshold (Latin: *limen*) of the ordinary psychophysical condition. This rare state is technically known as *ûrdhva-retas*.

Just as there is fire [as long as there is] fuel, and light [as long as there are] oil and wick, so also the embodied [psyche] does not leave the body when it is filled with the lunar part (*kalâ*). (2.50)

In the case of a *yogin* whose body is daily filled with the lunar part, poison does not spread, even if he should be bitten by [the serpent king] Takshaka himself. (2.51)

[When the *yogin* is] equipped with posture, joined to breath control, and endowed with sense-withdrawal, he should practice concentration. (2.52)

Concentration is explained as steadiness of the mind and concentration upon the five elements in the heart individually. (2.53)

The earth [element] stationed in the heart is a resplendent yellow or yellowish square, with the syllable *la* and the lotus-seated [God Brahma]. Dissolving the life energies together with the mind therein [i.e., in the heart], he should concentrate for five *ghatikâs* [i.e., two hours]. He should always practice the stabilizing earth concentration to conquer the earth. (2.54)

The water element (*ambu-tattva*) resembling a half moon or white jasmine is located at the throat and is endowed with the seed syllable *va* of the nectar (*pîyûsha*), and always associated with Vishnu. Dissolving the life energies together with the mind therein [i.e., in the heart], he should concentrate for five *ghatikâs* [i.e., two hours]. He should always practice the water concentration, which burns up suffering for all time. (2.55)

The triangular fire element located at the palate and resembling a [red] cochineal is brilliant and associated with *repha* [i.e., the syllable *ra*], bright like coral, and is in the good company of Rudra. Dissolving the life force together with the mind therein [i.e., in the heart], he should concentrate for five *ghatikâs* [i.e., two hours]. He should always engage[32] in the fiery concentration in order to conquer fire. (2.56)

*Comments:* The fire element is usually thought to be located at the navel.

The airy element, which is located between the eyebrows, resembles black collyrium and is associated with the letter *ya* and Îshvara as [the presiding] deity. Dissolving the life force together with the mind therein [i.e., in the heart], he should concentrate for five *ghatikâs* [i.e., two hours]. The *yamin* should practice the airy concentration so that he can traverse the sky. (2.57)

*Comments:* Mastery of the air element brings the *yamin*, or *yogin*, the ability of magical flight (*khecara*), which is often referred to in the literature of Yoga but also in shamanic traditions around the world.

The ether/space element, which is located at the "brahmic fissure" (*brahma-randhra*) [at the crown of the head] and which is like very clear water is associated with Sadâ-Shiva, the [inner] sound (*nâda*), and the syllable *ha*. Dissolving the life force together with the mind therein [i.e., in the heart], he should concentrate for five *ghatikâs* [i.e., two hours]. The ether/space concentration is said to break open the door to liberation. (2.58).

The five concentrations upon the elements [respectively have the power of] stopping, inundating, burning, destabilizing, and desiccating. (2.59)

The five concentrations are difficult to accomplish by means of mind, speech, and action. The *yogin* who is intelligent [in the use of these techniques] is released from all suffering. (2.60)

Recollection (*smriti*) obtains the single element (*dhâtu*) of all thoughts. Meditation is explained as the pure ideation (*cintâ*) in the mind. (2.61)

Meditation is twofold, composite (*sakala*) and impartite (*nishkala*). It is composite owing to differences in performance, and impartite [meditation] is unqualified (*nirguna*). (2.62)

Assuming a comfortable posture (*sukha-âsana*), with internalized mind and externalized downward gaze (*cakshus*), and contemplating with focus the serpent (*kundalinî*), he is released from guilt (*kilbisha*). (2.63)

The first center [called] "prop" (*âdhâra*) is four-petaled and resembles gold. Contemplating with focus the serpent (*kundalinî*) [at that place in the body], he is released from guilt (*kilbisha*).[33] (2.64)

*Comments:* The "prop" is otherwise known as the *mûlâdhâra-cakra*, located at the base of the spine, the alchemical cauldron in the human body.

Contemplating the Self at the six-petaled "self-base" (*svâdhishthâna*) [center located at the genitals], which resembles a true jewel, the *yogin*, gazing [steadily] at the tip of the nose, is [indeed] happy. (2.65)

Contemplating the Self as the jewel-city center luminous like the risen sun, [the *yogin*], gazing [steadily] at the tip of the nose, shakes the world. (2.66)

*Comments:* The reference here is to the psychoenergetic center at the navel, called *manipûra-* or *manipûraka-cakra* because to yogic vision it resembles a city made of shining jewels.

Contemplating Shambhu, who is stationed in the space (*âkâsha*) of the heart and is brilliant like the fierce sun, and maintaining the gaze at the tip of the nose, he assumes the form of the Absolute (*brahman*). (2.67)

*Comments:* Shambhu ("Benign") is none other than Shiva, who resides at the heart center, the *hridaya-* or *anâhata-cakra*.

Contemplating the Self in the heart lotus lustrous like lightning, while [performing] various [forms of] breath control and gazing at the tip of the nose, he assumes the form of the Absolute. (2.68)

Constantly contemplating the Self in the middle of the "bell" (*ghantikâ*) at the pure (*vishuddha*) [center] shining like a lamp, he assumes the form of bliss (*ânanda*). (2.69)

*Comments:* The term *ghantikâ* means "small bell" and may here refer to the thyroid or thyroidal cartilage, or possibly the epiglottis. Since verse 2.75 lists this separately from the *lambikâ*, it cannot be the same as the uvula.

Contemplating the Self, the God who is located between the eyebrows and resembles a true crest jewel, [while steadily] gazing at the tip of the nose, he assumes the form of bliss. (2.70)

The *yogin* who has conquered the life force and who always contemplates the Self, the supreme Lord of blue appearance at the spot between the eyebrows, while gazing at the tip of the nose, attains [the supreme goal of] Yoga. (2.71)

*Comments:* The text refers to the *âjnâ-cakra*, which in some traditions is associated with the blue seed-point (*bindu*), or "blue pearl," as the great twentieth-century *siddha* Swami Muktananda called it.

Contemplating the unqualified, tranquil, benevolent (*shiva*), all-facing [supreme Being] in the space [of the psychoenergetic center at the crown of the head], while gazing at the tip of the nose, he assumes the form of the Absolute. (2.72)

*Comments:* The space (*gagana*) mentioned here is the infinite space to which *yogins* can gain access through the portal at the crown of the head, which is known as the "brahmic fissure" (*brahma-randhra*) or the "thousand-spoked center" (*sahasrâra-cakra*).

Where the [inner] sound [can be heard] in the ether/space, that is called the "command center" (*âjnâ-cakra*). Contemplating the benign (*shiva*) Self therein, the *yogin* attains liberation. (2.73)

Contemplating the omnipresent Self, which is pure, in the form of space, and resplendent like sparkling liquid,[34] the *yogin* attains liberation. (2.74)

Anus, penis, navel, heart lotus, the one above that [i.e., the throat], the bell, the place of the "hanger" [i.e., uvula], the spot between the eyebrows, and the space cavity [at the crown of the head] . . . (2.75)

*Comments:* These are nine well-known bodily loci (*sthâna* or *desha*) for focusing the mind.

. . . These nine places (*sthâna*) of meditation are mentioned by *yogins* as liberating one from limited reality and bringing about the emergence of the eight [paranormal] qualities. (2.76)

Contemplating and knowing the unsurpassable light of the brilliant Shiva, who is identical with the Absolute, he is released. Thus said Goraksha. (2.77)

*Comments:* "Knowing" in this context means "realizing," that is *becoming one* with Shiva's all-comprising luster, which is the fundamental Reality underlying all beings and things.

By controlling the circulation of the air at the navel and forcefully contracting the *apâna* root[35] below, [which is] like the conductor of sacrifices [i.e., fire][36] and of subtle form like a thread, as well as by constricting the heart lotus and piercing the *dalanaka*, the palate, and the brahmic fissure, they reach the Void where God Mahesha [i.e., Shiva] enters the ether/space (*gagana*). (2.78)

*Comments:* This somewhat obscure stanza talks about the *kundalinî* process involving the control of the life force in the body through the well-known muscular locks (*bandha*). The *dalanaka* ("crusher") appears to be one of the psychoenergetic structures that must be pierced by the ascending serpent power so that it can progress toward the thousand-petaled lotus at the crown of the head. Perhaps it is an esoteric name of the psychoenergetic center at the throat.

Above the resplendent lotus at the navel is the pure circle (*mandala*) of the hot sun (*canda-rashmi*). I venerate the wisdom seal (*jnâna-mudrâ*) of *yoginîs*, which removes the fear of death, is formed of wisdom, is of the same form as the world (*samsâra*), and is the mother of the triple universe, the giver of *dharma* for human beings, the praiseworthy Chinnamastâ in the threefold subtle flow at the center of the triple path. (2.79)

*Comments:* The *yoginî-jnâna-mudrâ*, or "wisdom seal of *yoginîs*," is none other than the *kundalinî*, the divine power manifesting in the human body. It travels in the central channel, which is located between the *idâ* and *pingalâ-nâdî*, which together form what is called the "triple path." It stops the flow of life energy (*prâna*) in all three conduits and establishes the *yogin*'s consciousness in the great space beyond the body and mind. This transformative power (*shakti*) is here given the name of the Goddess Chinnamastâ, who is depicted with a severed head, with a fountain of blood gushing from the trunk—a marvelous yogic symbol. She is the ultimate *yoginî*, the great wielder of yogic power.

A thousand horse sacrifices or a hundred glorious libation (*vâjapeya*) [sacrifices] do not equal a sixteenth of a single yogic meditation. (2.80)

*Comments:* The two types of sacrifice mentioned are very elaborate and lengthy procedures to which only great kings were entitled and which are traditionally thought to bring great merit upon those who sponsor and perform them.

The dual reality is explained as [being due to] superimposition (*upâdhi*). Superimposition is said to be a covering (*varna*), and Reality (*tattva*) is designated as the Self. (2.81)

*Comments:* The term *varna* ("covering") can also mean "letter" and "color," suggesting that Reality is distorted or colored by our verbal categories.

By means of constant application (*abhyâsa*), the knower of all superimposition knows the condition of the Reality [revealed through] wisdom as different from [the world of appearance conjured up by] superimposition. (2.82)

As long as the potential (*tanmâtra*) of sound and so forth is presented to the ears and the other [sense organs], there is recollection (*smriti*), [which is the state of] meditation. Subsequently there will be ecstasy. (2.83)

Concentration [is established] after five *nâdis* [i.e., two hours]; meditation [is established] after sixty *nâdis*[37] [i.e., twenty-four hours]. By controlling the life force for twelve days, there will be ecstasy. (2.84)

*Comments:* The *Yoga-Tattva-Upanishad* (104b) even mentions that two full days are required before meditation can be thought to be firmly established. This shows the great expertise required of *yogins* before they can attain the ecstatic state.

Ecstasy (*samâdhi*) is described as the vanishing of all ideation (*samkalpa*) and [the realization of] the identity (*aikya*) of all pairs-of-opposites (*dvandva*) and of the individual self with the supreme Self. (2.85)

Ecstasy is described as [the realization of] the identity of the mind with the Self, just as water merging with the ocean becomes identical [with it]. (2.86)

Ecstasy is described as equilibrium (*samarasatva*), [a state in which] the life force is dissolved and the mind becomes absorbed. (2.87)

The *yogin* yoked (*yukta*) through ecstasy does not [experience] himself or another, or smell, taste, form, touch, and sound. (2.88).

The *yogin* yoked through ecstasy cannot be affected by *mantras* and *yantras* and cannot be pierced by any weapon or harmed by any being. (2.89)

*Comments:* This stanza hints at the widespread practice in India of using *mantras* and *yantras* as magical means of influencing others, often negatively. The *yogin* accomplished in ecstasy is completely immune to such influences.

The *yogin* yoked through ecstasy is not bound by time, tainted by action, or overcome by anyone. (2.90)

Yoga removes the suffering of him who is yoked (*yukta*) [i.e., disciplined] in eating and fasting, yoked in the performance of actions, and yoked in sleeping and waking. (2.91)

The knower of Yoga knows the Reality that is without beginning or end, without support, free from ill, without foundation, unevolved (*nishprapanca*), and formless. (2.92)

*Comments:* The ultimate Reality is here contrasted with the evolved universe (*prapanca*), which has a beginning and an end, is filled with forms and suffering, and has as its support the supportless Singularity (*eka*), the Absolute.

The knowers of the Absolute know the great Absolute that is space, consciousness, and bliss, stainless, immovable, eternal, inactive, and unqualified (*nirguna*). (2.93)

*Comments:* Vedânta metaphysics typically characterizes the Absolute (*brahman*) as pure being (*sat*), pure consciousness (*cit*), and pure bliss (*ânanda*). Here infinite space (*vyoman*) is substituted for pure being.

The knowers of Reality know the Reality (*tattva*) that is space, consciousness, bliss beyond logical proof (*hetu*) or evidence (*drishtânta*), transcending the mind (*manas*) and intuition (*buddhi*). (2.94)

*Comments: Manas* stands for sense-bound mental activity, whereas *buddhi* is higher reason, or intuition, which does not depend on sensory input.

By means of the methods of Yoga, the *yogin* becomes absorbed into the supreme Absolute, which is free from fear, without support, without prop, and beyond ill. (2.95)

Just as ghee poured into ghee is still only ghee, or milk [poured] into milk [is still only milk], so the *yogin* is but [the singular] Reality. (2.96)

The *yogin* absorbed into the supreme State assumes that form, just like milk offered into milk, ghee into ghee, or fire into fire. (2.97)

The secret (*guhya*) revealed by Goraksha, which is greater than any secret, is called by people a ladder to liberation that removes the fear of [conditioned] existence. (2.98)

People should study this yogically created (*yoga-bhûtam*) Compendium of Goraksha. Released from all sin, they attain perfection in Yoga. (2.99)

One should study this Yoga scripture daily, which issued from the lotus mouth of Âdinâtha [i.e., Shiva] himself. What is the use of many other scriptures? (2.100)[38]

## Siddha-Siddhânta-Paddhati

Another important text ascribed to Goraksha is the *Siddha-Siddhânta-Paddhati* ("Track of the Doctrine of the Adepts"), which is a comprehensive work of six chapters with a total of 353 stanzas.[39] It develops the Nâtha philosophy of the body (*pinda*). In the first chapter, six types or levels of embodiment are distinguished, beginning with the transcendental (*para*) body and ending with the "embryonic" (*garbha*) or physical body. The esoteric anatomy of the last-mentioned body is explained in the second chapter. In one stanza (2.31), a genuine *yogin* is defined as someone who knows, firsthand, the nine "wheels" (*cakra*), the sixteen "props" (*âdhâras*) or loci of concentration, the three "signs" (*lakshya*), and the five ethers/spaces (*vyoman*).

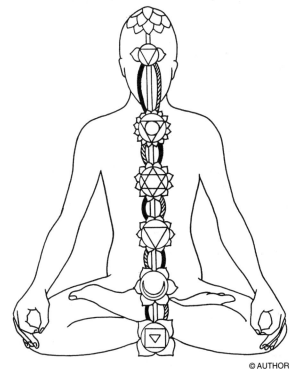

© AUTHOR

*The seven principal psychoenergetic centers of the body*

The nine *cakras* include the well-known series of seven, except that the *sahasrâra* at the crown is called *nirvâna-cakra*. The eighth center is the *talu-cakra*, which is situated at the palate. This is the location of the mysterious "bell" (*ghantikâ*) or the "royal tooth" (*râja-danta*), or uvula, the point from which oozes the divine nectar (*amrita*). The ninth *cakra* is the *âkâsha-cakra*, which is said to have sixteen spokes and is to be found at the "brahmic fissure" at the crown of the head.

The sixteen props are locations in the body on which attention can be fixed during concentration, namely the two big toes, the *mûlâdhâra-cakra* at the base of the spine, anus, penis, lower abdomen, navel, heart, throat, uvula, palate, tongue, the spot between the eyebrows (the location of the *âjnâ-cakra*), nose, root of nose, and forehead (*lalâta*).

The three signs (*lakshya*), or visions, are the experience of light outside the body and inside the body and purely mental light phenomena of different kinds. These three are respectively called *bâhya-lakshya*, *antar-lakshya*, and *madhya-lakshya*. These have been mentioned, together with the five types of ether or consciousness space (*âkâsha*), in the section on photistic Yoga in Chapter 15.

The third chapter of the *Siddha-Siddhânta-Paddhati* continues this treatment and particularly speaks of the body as a microcosmic mirror image of the cosmos. The fourth chapter introduces the *kundalinî-shakti*, which is said to exist in two conditions—unmanifest (cosmic) and manifest (individuated). In the former state it is known as *akula*, in the latter as *kula*. Furthermore, the *kula-kundalinî* can either be awakened or dormant. Even though the *kundalinî-shakti* is singular, it is present as minor forces in the various *cakras*. Also, the text makes a distinction between the lower, the middle, and the upper force (*shak-ti*), which are respectively located at the basal center, the navel center, and the crown center.

The fifth chapter makes the point that success in Yoga depends on the teacher's grace. It enables *yogins* to renounce all the paranormal powers (*siddhi*) that they have obtained in the course of their *kundalinî* practice and proceed to the "nonemergent" (*nirutthâna*) state where the body unites with the supreme estate (*param-pâda*), that is, Shiva.

The sixth chapter contains brief definitions of various types of ascetics and, among other things, lists the distinguishing characteristics of the *avadhûta-yogin*, the adept who has "shaken off" (*ava + dhûta*) all attachments and concerns.

## Yoga-Bîja

The *Yoga-Bîja* ("Seed of Yoga"), ascribed to Goraksha, is a compilation of 364 stanzas, of which 266 stanzas are similar to those found in the *Yoga-Shikhâ-Upanishad*. It is not clear, however, which text borrowed from which, though possibly both scriptures were inspired by a common source. The *Yoga-Bîja*, which is in the form of a dialogue between the Goddess and Sadâ-Shiva, has a philosophical tone and seeks to bring clarity to the mass of intellectual confusion existing in the world. In sentence 84, Yoga is explained as the unification (*samyoga*) of the network of opposites (*dvandva-jâla*), such as the union of exhalation (*apâna*) and inhalation (*prâna*), male semen (*retas*) and female secretion (*rajas*), sun and moon, as well as individuated self and supreme Self. The text places great emphasis on breath control, which is fundamental to the process of *shakti-calana* ("moving the power")—the systematic activation of the divine power within the body.

## Other Works Attributed to Goraksha

There is also the *Gorakh-Bodh* (Sanskrit: *Goraksha-Bodha*, "Instruction by Goraksha"), a treatise of 133 stanzas composed in archaic Hindi. It consists of a fictitious dialogue between Matsyendra and Goraksha, which perhaps dates back to the fourteenth century.

The *Goraksha-Upanishad*, written in a mixture of Hindusthani and Rajasthani, may date from the fifteenth century. Among other things, it lists the requisite qualities of a competent teacher and a fit disciple.

The *Goraksha-Vacana-Samgraha* ("Collection of Goraksha's Sayings"), consisting of 157 verses, claims to give out authentic teachings by Goraksha, but was probably authored in the seventeenth century. The fact is that we do not have a single work that we can definitely regard as Goraksha's creation. Often the followers of a great master credit their own writings to him, as was the case, for instance, with the twentieth-century teacher Swami Shivananda of Rishikesh, who "authored" several hundred works.

The vernacular literature on Hatha-Yoga, including the Hindi poems ascribed to Goraksha, is ill researched.

## Ânanda-Samuccaya

A little known but significant Hatha-Yoga work that may date back to the thirteenth century is the *Ânanda-Samuccaya* ("Mass of Bliss"), which has 277 stanzas distributed over eight chapters. It was brought to the attention of scholars in the late 1950s when a manuscript that had been in the possession of a renowned scholarly family in India was acquired by the Scindia Oriental Institute of Ujjain. The personal libraries of pundits and practitioners must contain many more precious Yoga manuscripts that are undoubtedly in need of urgent preservation, because the Indian climate plays havoc with the fragile paper on which these texts are inscribed. The style of this Sanskrit text has been described as "very lucid and marked with high literary merits,"[40] which is rare for this literary genre. Unfortunately, we do not know the author, but he appears to have been a Jaina, since he opens the text with the *om* sign written in typical Jaina calligraphy.

The *Ânanda-Samuccaya* introduces many esoteric concepts of Hatha-Yoga, including the (nine) *cakras*, *pîthas*, *sthânas*, and *nâdîs* (which are said to contain 7,200 divisions each), as well as the ten types of life energy (*vâyu*). Some of the teachings appear unique, such as the *candra-câra* and *sûrya-câra*, or lunar process and solar process. Thus, the *yogin* is instructed in activating the hidden moon's (*candra*) sixteen parts (*kalâ*) by means of forty-two yogic practices (*karman*), whereupon the lunar nectar will invigorate the body. Similarly, by activating the twelve parts of the hidden sun by means of forty-two practices, it will shine brightly within the body.

The *yogin* is further advised to balance the five material elements (*bhûta*) throughout the year's seasons by employing the requisite yogic practices. The state of harmony thus achieved is called *bhûta-samatâ* ("elemental balance"), which leads to mastery of the elements (*bhûta-siddhi*), longevity, and other paranormal powers. The goal, however, is to attain union with the supreme Reality through the progressive stages of *anindriyatâ* (the state of not being affected by the senses), *tattva-avabodha* (knowledge of Reality), and *jîvan-mukti* (liberation in life).

## Carpata-Shataka

Another old work is the *Carpata-Shataka*, which, as the title indicates, consists of a century (*shataka*) of verses by the adept Carpata (or Carpati). This text emphasizes discrimination (*viveka*) and renunciation, as well as the moral foundation of Yoga. The author's conceptual world appears to be closer to Jainism than to Hatha-Yoga, which makes this text of great historical interest.

## Yoga-Yâjnavalkya and Brihad-Yogî-Yâjnavalkya

The *Yoga-Yâjnavalkya* ("Yâjnavalkya's Yoga"), which is also known as the *Yoga-Yâjnavalkya-Gîtâ* and *Yoga-Yâjnavalkya-Gîtâ-Upanishad*, is a work of 485 stanzas distributed over twelve chapters. It is attributed to Yâjnavalkya, who is different from the famous Upanishadic sage by that name. It is presented as a dialogue between the sage and his wife Gârgî.

Prahlad C. Divan, the editor of this text, lauded it as "the earliest available book on Hathayoga for the common man."[41] He mentioned the period between 200 and 400 C.E. as a possible date for the *Yoga-Yâjnavalkya*, perhaps primarily on the basis that several quotations in Shankara's commentary on the *Shvetâshvatara-Upanishad* seem to be traceable to this text. The authenticity of this particular commentary, however, is seriously in doubt.[42] Also, the *Yoga-Yâjnavalkya* repeatedly makes reference to the *Tantras*, and the earliest Hindu *Tantras* belong to a period after 400 C.E.

Additionally, Divanji wrongly claimed that this text speaks only of drawing the serpent power up to the lotus of the heart, whereas there are several stanzas that clearly describe the *kundalini* process in terms that are quite familiar from the Hatha-Yoga literature. In fact, the terminology and style of the *Yoga-Yâjnavalkya* have much in common with the *Yoga-Upanishads*, and it seems unlikely that it is the same as the *Yoga-Shâstra* attributed to a certain Yâjnavalkya and mentioned or quoted in various scriptures, notably the *Dharma-Shâstra* of Yâjnavalkya. It is possible, however, that the *Yoga-Yâjnavalkya* contains stanzas from the missing *Yoga-Shâstra*.

The work *Brihad-Yogî-Yâjnavalkya-Smriti* ("Great Treatise on Yogin Yâjnavalkya's [Yoga]") appears on first glance to be an expanded version of the *Yoga-Yâjnavalkya* but is an entirely independent and original text, which is likely far older. In his multivolume *History of Dharmastra*, P. V. Kane assigned it to the period between 200 and 700 C.E. The latter date is not impossible.[43]

The *Brihad-Yogî-Yâjnavalkya-Smriti* is a fairly substantial treatise of 886 stanzas that describes many ritual practices to be followed by the *yogin*. Much space is given to the philosophy and practice of Mantra-Yoga, consisting in the recitation of the sacred syllable *om* combined with breath control. However, like the *Yoga-Yâjnavalkya*, this text also subscribes to the model of the eight-limbed Yoga that we know from the *Yoga-Sûtra* of Patanjali.

There is a strong element of Solar Yoga, especially in the ninth chapter. *Idâ* and *sushum-nâ* (!) are said in stanza 9.96 to exist in the form of *rashmi* (sun) and to have the qualities of *agni* (fire) and *soma* (moon) respectively. From stanza 9.98 we also learn that between these two is *amâ* (new moon), where the moon is stimulated by the sun. The sages are said (9.100) to aspire to the Absolute by following that *amâ*, which exists in the sun, the heart, and the supreme Absolute. In 9.156, we are told that the Self is singular but appears in five forms: the sun, heart, fire, space, and in the Supreme (*para*).

This text mentions the 72,000 *nâdîs* that issue from the heart, but does not name the fourteen important ones, as does the *Yoga-Yâjnavalkya*. Nor does it refer to the *kundalinî*, which also could be an indication of its early date.

Both the *Brihad-Yogî-Yâjnavalkya-Smriti* and the *Yoga-Yâjnavalkya* were obviously composed in the cultural environment of Smârta Brahmanism.

## Yoga-Vishaya

The *Yoga-Vishaya* ("Object of Yoga"), misleadingly ascribed to Matsyendra, is a short work of thirty-three verses. Its date is uncertain, and it may be fairly recent. It covers such basic topics as the nine centers (*cakras*), the three "knots" (*granthi*), and the nine "gates" (*dvâra*), or bodily openings. The objective of breath control is to enable the life force (*prâna*) to pierce through the knots so that the *kundalinî* can fully ascend along the spinal axis.

## Hatha-Yoga-Pradîpikâ

The *Hatha-Yoga-Pradîpikâ* ("Light on Hatha-Yoga") was composed by Svâtmârâma (or Âtmârâma) Yogendra in the middle of the fourteenth century. This is undoubtedly the classic manual on Hatha-Yoga. It comprises 389 stanzas organized into four chapters. Svâtmârâma, a follower of the Shaiva Yoga tradition of

Andhra, expounds Hatha-Yoga as a means to Râja-Yoga.

One is not successful in Râja-Yoga without Hatha-[Yoga], nor in Hatha-[Yoga] without Râja-Yoga. Hence one should practice both for [one's spiritual] maturation. (2.76)

The first chapter is dedicated primarily to a description of the principal postures (*âsana*), while the second chapter speaks of the cleansing practices as well as the life force (*prâna*) and its regulation through breath control (*prânâyâma*). In the third chapter, Svâtmârâma introduces us to the subtle physiology and techniques, such as the

श्री:

# हठयोगप्रदीपिका

ज्योत्स्नायुता

प्रथमोपदेश:

श्रीआदिनाथाय नमोऽस्तु तस्मै येनोपदिष्टा हठयोगविद्या ।
विभ्राजते प्रोन्नतराजयोगमारोढुमिच्छोरधिरोहिणीव ॥ १ ॥

श्रीगणेशाय नम: ॥

गुरुं नत्वा शिवं साक्षाद्ब्रह्मानन्देन तन्यते ।
हठप्रदीपिकाज्योत्स्ना योगमार्गप्रकाशिका ॥
इदानींतनानां सुबोधार्थमस्याः सुविज्ञाय गोरक्षसिद्धान्तहार्दम् ।
मया मेरुशास्त्रित्रयमुख्याभियोगात् स्फुटं कथ्यतेऽत्यन्तगूढोऽपि भावः ॥

मुमुक्षुजनहितार्थं राजयोगद्वारा कैवल्यफलां हठप्रदीपिकां विधित्सुः
परमकारुणिकः स्वात्मारामयोगीन्द्रस्तत्प्रत्यूहनिवृत्तये हठयोगप्रवर्तकश्रीमदादिनाथ-
नमस्कारलक्षणं मङ्गलं तावदाचरति—श्रीआदिनाथेत्यादिना । तस्मै श्रीआदि-
नाथाय नमोऽस्त्वित्यन्वय: । आदिश्चासौ नाथश्च आदिनाथ: सर्वेश्वर: । शिव
इत्यर्थ: । श्रीमानादिनाथ: तस्मै श्रीआदिनाथाय । श्रीशब्द आदिर्यस्य स:

*Opening page of the printed Sanskrit text of the*
Hatha-Yoga-Pradîpikâ *with the* Jyotsnâ *commentary*

seals (*mudrâ*) and locks (*bandha*), by which the life force can be properly contained in the body and the *kundalinî* awakened. The concluding chapter deals with the higher stages of yogic practice, including the ecstatic condition (*samâdhi*), which is understood in Vedântic terms. The *Hatha-Yoga-Pradîpikâ* has an excellent commentary entitled *Jyotsnâ* ("Light") by Brahmânanda of the mid-eighteenth century.

## Hatha-Ratna-Avalî

The *Hatha-Ratna-Avalî* ("String of Pearls on Hatha") of Shrînivasa Bhatta, which may have been composed in the mid-seventeenth century and appears to have at least one commentary, is a work of 397 verses. Shrînivasa, who also wrote works on Vedânta, Nyâya, and Tantra, offers a masterly treatment of Hatha-Yoga which expands on the information contained in the *Hatha-Yoga-Pradîpikâ*.

## Gheranda-Samhitâ

The *Gheranda-Samhitâ* ("Gheranda's Collection"), probably composed toward the end of the seventeenth century, is one of the best known works on Hatha-Yoga. The author of the *Gheranda-Samhitâ* followed the Vaishnava Yoga tradition of Bengal. This work has seven chapters with 317 verses in all, though some manuscripts have additional stanzas. It describes no fewer than 102 yogic practices, including twenty-one hygienic techniques, thirty-two postures, and twenty-five seals (*mudrâ*). It speaks of seven "limbs" of Yoga and curiously treats breath control (*prânâyâma*) after sense-withdrawal (*pratyâhâra*).[44] In Patanjali's Yoga breath control is the fourth and sense-withdrawal the fifth limb.

## Shiva-Samhitâ

After the *Hatha-Yoga-Pradîpikâ* and the *Gheranda-Samhitâ*, the *Shiva-Samhitâ* ("Shiva's Collection") is the most important manual of Hatha-Yoga. It comprises 645 stanzas distributed over five chapters. This scripture is particularly valuable because it includes a fair amount of philosophical matter. Its date is unknown, but it appears to be a work of the late seventeenth or early eighteenth century.

The entire first chapter is devoted to expounding Vedântic nondualism:

Illusion (*mâyâ*) is the mother of the world; not by any other principle is it established. When [this *mâyâ*] is destroyed, then the world surely ceases to exist as well.

He for whom this entire [universe] is the play of *mâyâ*—which is to be overcome—he has no delight in things and no pleasure in the body. (1.64–65)

When a person is free from all superimposition (*upâdhi*), then he can claim to be of the form of untainted, indivisible wisdom (*jnâna*). (1.67)

The second chapter contains descriptions of some of the esoteric structures of the human body. The third chapter opens with a discussion of the teacher and qualified students, and then goes on to discuss breath control and the three levels of yogic accomplishment, namely (1) the "pot state" (*ghata-avasthâ*, written *ghatâvasthâ*), in which the life force in the body (called the "pot") collaborates with the universal Self; (2) the "accumulation state" (*paricaya-avasthâ*, written *paricayâvasthâ*), in which the life force is immobilized along the bodily axis (*sushumnâ*); (3) and the "maturation state" (*nishpatti-avasthâ*, written *nishpattyavastha*), in which the *yogin* has destroyed the seeds of his karma and "drinks from the water of immortality" (3.66).

In the fourth chapter, the anonymous author describes the various locks (*bandha*) and seals (*mudrâ*) for awakening the *kundalinî*. The fifth chapter is a treatment of the obstacles on the yogic path, followed by a discussion of the secret bodily centers (*cakra*), especially the crown center, and of the higher stages of Yoga. The text concludes by affirming that even householders can attain liberation, as long as they observe the duties of a *yogin* with diligence and give up all attachments.

## Yoga-Shâstra

The *Yoga-Shâstra* of Dattâtreya, consisting of 334 lines, is undoubtedly a late work, but since it is quoted in the *Yoga-Karnikâ* it must be earlier than it. The text is presented as a dialogue between the sage (*muni*) Dattâtreya residing in the *naimisha* forest and the seeker Sâmkriti. It speaks (line 28) of Mantra-Yoga as a lower (*adhama*) form of Yoga and praises (line 29) Laya-Yoga as a means of achieving complete absorption (*laya*) of the mind.

The text also includes (lines 29–30) a teaching about the "conventions" (*sanketa*) for focusing the mind. Âdinâtha (i.e., Shiva) is said to have taught eight crores (i.e., eighty million) of such *sanketas*, or techniques. Thus one can contemplate emptiness (*shûnya*), which can be practiced in any situation, or meditatively gaze at the tip of the nose, or focus on the back of the head, the spot between the eyebrows, the forehead, the big toe of either foot, and so forth.

Karma-Yoga is explained (lines 52–56) as having the same eight limbs as Patanjali's or Yâjnavalkya's Yoga. The text next describes (lines 57–61) the eight principal practices (*kriyâ*) of Hatha-Yoga as cultivated by Kapila and his disciples: *mahâ-mudrâ*, *mahâ-bandha*, *khecârî-mudrâ*, *jalandhara-bandha*, *uddîyâna-bandha*, *mûla-bandha*, *viparîta-karanî*, and *vajrolî*, with the last-mentioned consisting of the techniques of *vajrolî*, *amarolî*, and *sahajolî*. As the *Yoga-Shâstra* explains (lines 306–316), the *yogin* must control the semen through *vajrolî*. This practice requires milk (*kshîra*)—probably standing for semen—and a substance called *angirasa* (the name of a Vedic clan associated with magic), which refers to the female genital secretions. Both are meant to be sucked up through the penis in case the *yogin* succumbs to ejaculation. *Amarolî* and *sahajolî* are left unexplained, but descriptions of these techniques can be found in the *Hatha-Yoga-Pradîpikâ* (3.92–98). The former is the yogic equivalent of urine therapy, while the latter consists in besmearing, after intercourse, certain unmentioned parts of the body with a mixture of water and the ashes obtained by burning cow dung. According to the *Jyotsnâ* commentary on this passage, the body parts are the head, forehead, eyes, heart, shoulders, and arms.

## Yoga-Karnikâ

*Yoga-Karnikâ* ("Ear-Ornament of Yoga") of Aghorânanda was composed some time in the eighteenth century. It has fifteen chapters with well over 1,200 verses. The arrangement of the content is far from systematic, nor is this work particularly original. Its value lies, rather, in the many quotations that it provides from other

Hatha-Yoga scriptures, which include some not readily available texts.

## *Hatha-Sanketa-Candrikâ*

The *Hatha-Sanketa-Candrikâ* ("Moonlight on the Conventions of Hatha [-Yoga]") is a little known but very important work authored by Sundaradeva (1675–1775).[45] The great value of this substantial scripture lies partly in its comprehensive coverage of Hatha-Yoga and partly in the numerous quotations and references it contains. Sundaradeva cites by name no fewer than seventy-two texts and six authors. Some of these texts appear to be no longer extant, and others are known only because their titles are mentioned in the manuscript catalogues of various institutions. Sundaradeva appears to have been an erudite scholar and a practitioner of Yoga. He also authored the *Hatha-Tattva-Kaumudî* and the *Pranava-Kundalî*, as well as several works on drama, poetry, and dietetics.

## *Concluding Remarks*

The traditional literature of Hatha-Yoga has been little researched. We know of many more titles than those introduced here, but they are either mere names or are manuscripts seen by few and buried in dusty libraries where they are slowly deteriorating in the humid climate of India. I believe, however, that the salvaged literature contains the substance of the Hatha-Yogic tradition. If we wish to dig deeper, we must be willing to sit at the feet of the few masters who are still teaching the forceful Yoga in an authentic manner.

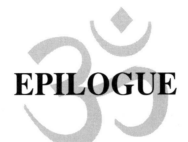

# EPILOGUE

Yoga is like an ancient river with countless rapids, eddies, loops, tributaries, and backwaters, extending over a vast, colorful terrain of many different habitats. In this volume I have provided a bird's-eye view, giving the reader the broader picture and, I hope, a deeper appreciation of the inviting waters of Yoga and of the checkered cultural landscape through which the river of Yoga has flowed in the course of its millennia-long development. Occasionally, however, I have zeroed in on a particularly relevant feature, exploring it as space and available sources permitted.

Our last glance fell on the riverine current of Hatha-Yoga, that aspect of Tantrism which seeks to accomplish both spiritual enlightenment and bodily immortality. It is this branch of the meandering river of Yoga that carries us to the ocean, the world beyond India. For Yoga has definitely come West. There are today millions of Hatha-Yoga practitioners around the world who benefit from this age-old technology of bodily wholeness and personal growth. There are also millions of practitioners of meditation. They enjoy glimpses of the secrets of consciousness and its astonishing capacity to lift itself up by its own bootstraps—that is, to go beyond its own conditioning.

Yet, only a few people deeply and consistently commit themselves to exploring the intricate psychotechnology of the various branches of the Yoga tradition. It is they who are discovering that consciousness, the human body-mind, is a well-equipped laboratory in which can be found, through ecstatic self-transcendence, the philosopher's stone—the alchemical elixir of enlightenment. Admittedly, not everyone is able to follow their example.

Nonetheless, the tradition of Yoga, for which there are still representative masters to be found, offers a wonderful opportunity to delve into the psychic and spiritual dimensions that our postindustrial civilization has tended to neglect and even shun. We can study the scriptures of Yoga, both ancient and modern, and allow their esoteric knowledge and wisdom to enrich our understanding of human nature. With guidance, we can even try to verify in our own person some of the claims made by Yoga authorities past and present. This should, of course, never be a matter of merely imitating the East, but we can learn from its triumphs and its failures.

Certainly, Yoga deserves far more careful attention from scientists than it has so far been granted. Our modern Western civilization, which now exerts a strong influence in all reaches of the globe, is in desperate need of a psychotechnology that can counterbalance the baneful effects of the excesses of scientific technology and the deficient consciousness that created and developed it. Scientists, who are after all committed to understanding reality, have a special obligation to explore the great intuitions of the spiritual traditions of the East, which vigorously challenge the current scientific view of the world.

The limitations of the materialistic paradigm have become increasingly apparent in the course of the twentieth century. More and more scientists are less and less certain of what it is they are trying to observe, measure, describe, and comprehend. This newly won virtue of uncertainty is a possible open door to a more spacious worldview that also accommodates the psychospiritual aspects of existence. The insights and findings of India's spiritual traditions, painstakingly gathered over many millennia, can give us a glimpse of what we are likely to find on the other side of the door once present scientific dogmas have been transcended.

Practitioners of such a reformed science will then truly be able to sift reality from fiction, and creative imagination (mythology) from mere wishful thinking. They will also be in a position to create the new language that is undoubtedly necessary to describe what they will encounter. Above all, they will learn to stand again in awe of the great Mystery of existence and be humbled and transformed by it. This challenge of the spirit confronts us all, and today it confronts us more pressingly than ever before in human history.

Collectively and individually we will definitely have to find our own answers—our own Yoga.

*OM TAT SAT*

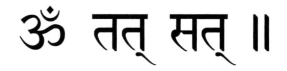

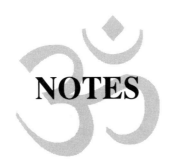

# NOTES

## INTRODUCTION

1. The adjective "Vedantic" is derived from the Sanskrit noun *vedânta*, meaning *"Veda's* end" and designating a body of spiritual teachings connected with the *Upanishads*, which are the concluding portion of the Vedic revelation. According to Vedânta, there is only the one Reality that underlies all finite beings and things, though various schools propose different answers to the question of how the Many is related to that Singularity.

2. Sri Aurobindo, *The Life Divine* (Pondicherry, India: Sri Aurobindo Ashram, 1977), vol. 1, pp. 3–4.

3. K. Wilber, *The Atman Project: A Transpersonal View of Human Development* (Wheaton, Ill.: Theosophical Publishing House, 1980), p. ix.

4. G. Zukav, *The Dancing Wu Li Masters: An Overview of the New Physics* (New York: Morrow Quill Paperbacks, 1979), pp. 42–43.

5. J. Lilly, *Simulations of God: The Science of Belief* (New York: Simon and Schuster, 1975), p. 144.

6. R. Tagore, *Gitanjali* (New York: Macmillan, 1971), p. 44.

7. See C. Norman, *The God That Limps: Science and Technology in the Eighties* (New York: W. W. Norton, 1981).

8. F. J. Dyson, *Infinite in All Directions* (New York: Harper & Row, 1988), p. 270.

9. Bubba [Da] Free John, *The Enlightenment of the Whole Body* (Middletown, Calif.: Dawn Horse Press, 1978), p. 377.

10. J. N. Sansonese, *The Body of Myth: Mythology, Shamanic Trance, and the Sacred Geography of the Body* (Rochester, Vt.: Inner Traditions, 1994), p. 39.

11. See C. G. Jung, *Psychology and the East* (Princeton, N.J.: Princeton University Press, 1978).

12. We can clearly see the difference in style between, say, the Buddha's sermons or Patanjali's *Yoga-Sûtra* on one side and the hymns of the *Rig-Veda* on the other. I have explained this in some detail in *Wholeness or Transcendence? Ancient Lessons for the Emerging Global Civilization* (Burdett, N.Y.: Larson Publications, 1992). For a discussion of the Gebserian model, see my book *Structures of Consciousness: The Genius of Jean Gebser—An Introduction and Critique* (Lower Lake, Calif.: Integral Publishing, 1987).

*PART ONE: FOUNDATIONS*

## Chapter 1: Building Blocks

1.  For a review of this intricate question, see Usharbudh Arya, *Yoga-Sûtras of Patañjali, with the Exposition of Vyâsa: A Translation and Commentary*, vol. 1: *Samâdhi-pâda* (Honesdale, Penn.: Himalayan International Institute, 1986), pp. 76ff.
2.  See M. Eliade, *Yoga: Immortality and Freedom* (Princeton, N.J.: Princeton University Press, 1973), p. 77.
3.  The words *jîva-âtman* and *parama-âtman* are respectively written *jîvâtman* and *paramâtman*.
4.  For a discussion of the *Upanishads*, see Chapters 5 and 15.
5.  For a detailed historical survey of the Hindu pantheon, see S. Bhattacharji, *The Indian Theogony: A Comparative Study of Indian Mythology from the Vedas to the Puranas* (Cambridge, England: Cambridge University Press, 1970). See also A. Danielou, *Hindu Polytheism* (New York: Pantheon Books, 1964) and D. and J. Johnson, *God and Gods in Hinduism* (New Delhi: Arnold-Heinemann, 1972).
6.  The "fourth" (*turya, turîya,* or *caturtha*) is the transcendental Reality beyond the three modalities of consciousness, namely waking, dreaming, and sleeping.
7.  According to some researchers, Jesus was educated in Kashmir, but this is mere conjecture. Others maintain, on literary and archaeological grounds, that he retired to Kashmir after surviving his crucifixion. See, e.g., A. Faber-Kaiser, *Jesus Died in Kashmir* (London: Gorden & Cremonesi, 1977) and H. Kersten, *Jesus Lebte in Indien* (Munich: Droemersche Verlagsanstalt, 1983).
8.  The term *yoginî* also applies to a member of a group of female deities who are regarded as manifestations of the universal creative energy (*shakti*); they play an important role in certain schools of Tantrism. The cult of the sixty-four *yoginîs* dates back to the sixth or seventh century C.E. See H. C. Das, *Tantricism: A Study of the Yoginî Cult* (New Delhi: Sterling Publishers, 1981).
9.  M. Eliade, op. cit., p. 5.
10. Ibid., p. 5.
11. Hence the word *bhikshu* for "monk."
12. See, e.g., the grammarian Patanjali's *Mahâ-Bhâshya*, commenting on Panini's *Sûtra* 2.1.41.
13. See M. P. Pandit, *The Kulârnava Tantra* (Madras: Ganesh, 1965), pp. 98–99. The twelve types of teacher are: (1) *dhâtu-vâdi-guru*, who gives the disciple the elements of practice, (2) *candana-guru*, who naturally emanates the divine Consciousness like the sandal tree (*candana*) gives off fragrance, (3) *vicâra-guru*, who acts upon the disciple's intelligence and understanding (*vicâra*), (4) *anugraha-guru*, who uplifts by mere grace (*anugraha*), (5) *sparsha-guru*, whose mere touch is uplifting and liberating, like the touch of the philosopher's stone (*sparshamani*), (6) *kacchapa-guru*, who uplifts the disciple merely by thinking of him or her, just as the tortoise (*kacchapa*) nourishes its offspring by thought alone, (7) *candra-guru*, who promotes the disciple's welfare like the moon, which has a natural radiation, (8) *darpana-guru*, who, like a mirror (*darpana*), reflects the true Self to the disciple, (9) *châyâ-nidhi-guru*, whose mere shadow (*châyâ*) blesses and uplifts the disciple, just like the shadow of the *châyânidhi* bird is said to bestow kingship upon a person, (10) *nâda-nidhi-guru*, who transforms the disciple, just like the magical *nâdanidhi* stone transmutes ordinary metal into gold through sound (*nâda*), (11) *kraunca-pakshi-guru*, whose mere remembrance of the disciple bestows liberation upon him or her, just like the *kraunca* bird nurtures its offspring from a distance, (12) *sûrya-kânta-guru*, whose mere glance is liberating, just like the rays of the sun (*sûrya*) burn material when they are gathered in a crystal.
14. See S. Kramrisch, *The Presence of Siva* (Princeton, N.J.: Princeton University Press, 1981), p. 57.
15. The term *pûmams*, meaning literally "male," refers here to the transcendental Self, conceived as the cosmic Man.
16. The word *purusha*, or "male," is here employed in the same transcendental sense as the term *pûmams* in the opening stanza.
17. Written *sarvâtmatva*.
18. Shankara affirms here the common Indian notion that God-realization yields not only transcendental autonomy, or "sovereignty" (*îshvaratva*), but also "lordship" (*aishvarya*) over the universe. That is to say, by stepping beyond the universe the enlightened adept becomes its master. These are the eight *mahâ-siddhis* of Tantrism.

19. The word *daksha* is meant to explain the name Dakshinamûrti, though it should properly be derived from *dakshina*, signifying "dexterous," "right," and "southern."

20. The *pranava* is the hummed or nasalized sound *om*, the greatest Vedic *mantra*.

21. Consciousness is omnipresent; hence, strictly speaking, it cannot be transmitted. A person's awareness of its omnipresence can, however, be intensified through the compassionate intervention of a *guru* or the *guru* of all *gurus*, that is, Dakshinamûrti.

22. For an English translation, see Swami Narayananda, *The Guru Gita* (Bombay: India Book House, 1976). There are also *Guru-Gîtâs* attributed to the *Rudra-Yâmala* and the *Brahma-Yâmala*, two Tantric scriptures.

23. For an English rendering, see N. Dhargyey et al., *Fifty Verses of Guru-Devotion by Asvaghosa* (Dharamsala, India: Library of Tibetan Works and Archives, rev. ed., 1976).

24. For an English translation of the *Shraddhâ-Utpâda-Shâstra* (written *Shraddhotpâdashâstra*), see D. T. Suzuki, *Asvaghosha's Awakening of Faith in the Mahayana* (Chicago: University of Chicago Press, 1900).

25. *Kriyâ-Samgraha-Panjikâ*, manuscript, p. 5.

26. Chögyam Trungpa, *Cutting Through Spiritual Materialism* (Boulder, Colo.: Shambhala, 1973), p. 58.

27. The crown of the head is the locus of the "thousand-petaled lotus" (*sahasra-dala-padma*), the seat of Shiva/Shakti.

28. The Kashmiri Shaiva schools distinguish between the following four modes of initiation: (1) *anupâya-dîkshâ*, or initiation without external means, which is possible in the case of highly evolved practitioners who can attain enlightenment simply by proximity to an enlightened adept; this appears to be identical with the *vedha-mayî-dîkshâ*; (2) *shâmbhavî-dîkshâ*, which has been described; (3) *shakti-dîkshâ*, or initiation by means of the innate power; this seems to be identical with the *shâkteyî-dîkshâ* referred to earlier; (4) *ânavî-dîkshâ*, or "atomic" initiation, which refers to the individual self called *anu* in Kashmir's form of Shaivism; this type of initiation comprises various ritual means and conscious cultivation through Yoga.

29. See, e.g., the *Kula-Arnava-Tantra* 14.56. All truly great adepts are able to impart the blissful Reality, though whether their gift instantly transforms a disciple's consciousness depends on the spiritual groundwork done by that disciple.

30. The date of the *Mahânirvâna-Tantra* is still disputed. Some scholars place it in the twelfth century C.E., while others see in it a recent fabrication during the British Raj.

31. The most detailed explanation of the enlightened adept's spontaneous spiritual transmission can be found in the works of the contemporary teacher Da Free John (Adi Da), notably in *The Method of the Siddhas* (Clearlake, Calif.: Dawn Horse Press, 1978).

32. This is verse 69 (or 68 in some editions) of Umâpati's *Shata-Ratna-Samgraha* ("Compendium of One Hundred Jewels"). The next verse explains the word *dîkshâ* as connoting both "destruction" (*kshapana*) and "giving" (*dâna*). What is destroyed is the state of "animality" (*pashutva*), or spiritual blindness, and what is given, by grace, is the supreme condition of Shivahood (*shivatva*).

33. See G. Feuerstein, *Holy Madness: The Shock Tactics and Radical Teachings of Crazy-Wise Adepts, Holy Fools, and Rascal Gurus* (New York: Paragon House, 1991).

34. The term *tattva* means literally "thatness" and can stand for "reality" or "principle," in this case the ultimate Reality.

35. For an English translation of the *Ashtâvakra-Gîtâ*, see Swami Nityaswarupananda, *Ashtavakra Samhita* (Mayavati, India: Advaita Ashrama, 1953). For a critical edition of this work, see R. Hauschild, *Die Astâvakra-Gîtâ* (Berlin: Akademie-Verlag, 1967). For an English rendering of the *Avadhûta-Gîtâ*, see Swami Ashokananda (Mylapore, India: Sri Ramakrishna Math, [1977?]).

36. See H. S. Joshi, *Origin and Development of Dattâtreya Worship in India* (Baroda, India: Maharaja Sayajirao University of Baroda, 1965).

37. Curiously, the eighth chapter of the *Avadhûta-Gîtâ* attributed to Dattâtreya has a decidedly misogynous tone (and could be a later interpolation).

38. See G. Feuerstein, *Holy Madness*, and also "The Shadow of the Enlightened Guru," in R. Walsh and F. Vaughan, eds., *Paths Beyond Ego: The Transpersonal Vision* (New York: J. P. Tarcher/Perigee, 1993), pp. 147–48.

39. The Sanskrit text uses the poetic expression "waves" (*taranga*) for "multitudinous."

40. The six "modifications" (*vikâra*) of Nature (*prakriti*) may be the six bodies (*pinda*) referred to in the opening chapter of the text. The six bodies are the "transcendental" (*para*), the "beginningless" (*anâdi*), the

"original" (*âdi*), the "great form-endowed" (*mahâ-sâkâra*), the "natural" (*prâkriti*), and the "uterine" (*garbha*) body. The last-mentioned is the physical body, and the preceding bodies are progressively more subtle.

41. Written *parâkâsha*.

42. The "yogic cloth" (*yoga-patta*) is the knee-band, a piece of cloth that is placed around the lower back and the knees in order to ease postural strain during meditation. A *yoga-patta* is also mentioned in the *Agni-Purâna* (90.10) as one of the paraphernalia of the newly-initiated practitioner and then again (204.11) as one of the utensils of the forest-dwelling ascetic (*vâna-prastha*). According to the *Brihad-Yogi-Yâjnavalkya-Samhitâ* (7.39), the *yogin* may wear a *yoga-patta* over his other clothes while doing his ritual ablutions. The *yoga-patta* is to be distinguished from the *yoga-pattaka* referred to in Vâcaspati Mishra's *Tattva-Vaishâradî* (2.46), which is a kind of armrest, also used in conjunction with meditation to help avoid back strain. A symbolic interpretation of the term *yoga-patta* is given in the *Nirvâna-Upanishad* (25), where it is equated with the "vision of the Absolute" (*brahma-âloka*). In the *Shiva-Purâna* (6.18.11ff.) the term again appears to refer to a complex ritual, which is said to lead to the state of a preceptor, yielding liberation.

43. It is not clear what the six essences (*rasa*) are.

44. The term *vajrî* is the feminine form of *vajra* and here presumably stands for "ordinary nature," that is, the unenlightened body-mind. Another possible explanation is that it refers to the veiling power of the *kundalinî-shakti*. By awakening the *shakti* and achieving her union with the *shiva* dimension of existence, the *yogin* turns the potentially ruinous *shakti* to his advantage. Instead of ensnaring him in unenlightened existence, this great force dormant at the basal psychoenergetic center becomes the instrument of his liberation.

## Chapter 2: The Wheel of Yoga

1. The *Yoga-Râja-Upanishad* (written *Yogarâjopanishad*) is a work of only twenty-one stanzas and primarily describes the nine psychoenergetic centers (*cakra*) of the body.

2. Swami Vivekananda, *Raja-Yoga or Conquering the Internal Nature* (Calcutta: Advaita Ashrama, repr. 1962), p. 66.

3. Ibid., p. 11.

4. Bubba [Da] Free John, *The Enlightenment of the Whole Body* (Middletown, Calif.: Dawn Horse Press, 1978), p. 500.

5. J. W. Hauer, *Der Yoga* (Stuttgart: Kohlhammer Verlag, 1958), p. 271.

6. The phrase *mac-citta* or "Me-minded" is composed of *mat* ("me") and *citta* ("mind"). For euphonic reasons, the *mat* is changed to *mac*.

7. N. K. Brahma, *Philosophy of Hindu Sâdhanâ* (London: Kegan Paul, Trench, Trubner, 1932), p. 137.

8. Swami Satprakashananda, *Methods of Knowledge* (London: Allen & Unwin, 1965), p. 204.

9. In the *Vedânta-Siddhânta-Darshana* (190–192), which is a late medieval work, seven stages (*bhumi*) of gnosis are mentioned:

> The great seers have spoken of seven stages of wisdom. Of these the first stage of wisdom is designated as "good will" (*shubha-icchâ*); the second is reflection (*vicâranâ*); the third is subtlety of mind (*tanu-mânasâ*); the fourth is the attainment of lucidity (*sattva-âpatti*); the fifth is nonattachment (*asamsakti*); the sixth is the vanishing of all objects (*padârtha-abhâvanî*) [in the state of ecstasy]; and the seventh is entrance into the Fourth [i.e., the ultimate Reality beyond waking, dreaming, and sleeping].

We will encounter these stages again in our discussion of the *Yoga-Vâsishtha*, which is exclusively devoted to Jnâna-Yoga.

10. The full text of this prayer, which can be found in the *Brihad-Âranyaka-Upanishad* (1.3.28), runs: *Asato mâ sad gamaya, tamaso mâ jyotir gamaya, mrityor mâ amritam gamaya*, "From the unreal [or nonbeing] lead me to the Real [or Being]; from darkness lead me to light; from death lead me to immortality." The phrase *mâ amritam* is written *mâmritam*.

11. Written *bhûtâtman*.

12. The term *pushkara* can be met with already in the oldest *Upanishads* and is generally thought to be the name of the blue lotus flower. In the *Maitrâyanîya-Upanishad* (6.2), this lotus flower is identified as the

lotus of the heart. In the present text it is equated with the Absolute. The word is derived from the roots *push,* meaning "to thrive, flourish," and *kri,* meaning "to make."

13. Vâsudeva can mean either "He who has the Vasus for deities" or "Bright God." This is an epithet of Krishna or Nârâyana.

14. *Confessions* I.1.

15. See Jîva Gosvâmin's *Shat-Sandarbha,* Sanskrit edition (p. 541).

16. The word *dâsya* comes from *dâsa* meaning both "servant" and "slave."

17. Written *Bhaktirasâmritasindhu.* For an English rendering, see Swami B. H. Bon Maharaj, *Bhakti-Rasâmrta-Sindhuh,* vol. 1 (Vrindaban, India: Institute of Oriental Studies, 1965).

18. According to a cosmological theory that is upheld by all Yoga schools, Nature is a web woven by three fundamental forces or qualities, which are called *sattva, rajas,* and *tamas.* These stand respectively for the principles of lucidity, dynamism, and inertia. Their interaction is responsible for the immense variety of forms in the known universe, and they also underlie our different emotional dispositions. Thus, even our attitude toward the Divine is determined by the predominance of one or another of these three *gunas.*

19. S. Dasgupta, *Hindu Mysticism* (Chicago: Open Court Publishing, 1927), p. 126.

20. The earliest history of the Pancarâtra school or tradition is shrouded in darkness. Even the meaning of the name ("Five Nights") is unclear. See S. Dasgupta, *A History of Indian Philosophy,* vol. 3 (Delhi: Motilal Banarsidass, 1975), pp. 12–62.

21. The term *nirodha* is borrowed from Patanjali's *Yoga-Sûtra* (1.2) and is given here a new connotation.

22. The references here are to the story of the foundling who is recognized as the long-lost son of a king, to the wayfarer who returns to his home, and to the hungry man eating his dinner who does not create some new satisfaction but merely appeases his hunger.

23. In other words, *sattva* is qualitatively better than *rajas,* and *rajas* is better than *tamas.*

24. In denouncing the conduct of women as setting a poor example for the devotee, Nârada follows the traditional Hindu stereotype about women. Today, he would perhaps be more specific in his condemnation of immoral or unworthy behavior.

25. On the innovative teachings of the *Bhagavad-Gîtâ,* see G. Feuerstein, *Wholeness or Transcendence? Ancient Lessons for the Emerging Global Civilization* (Burdett, N.Y.: Larson Publications, 1992), pp. 210–230.

26. E. Wood, *Raja Yoga: The Occult Training of the Hindus* (Sydney, Australia: Theosophical Publishing House, n.d.), pp. 10–11.

27. For a fascinating speculative account of the *soma* plant used in the Vedic ritual, see R. Gordon Wasson, *Soma: Divine Mushroom of Immortality* (New York: Harcourt, Brace and World, 1968). Wasson's identification of the *soma* plant (which is described in the *Vedas* as a creeper) with the fly agaric is unconvincing.

28. J. Woodroffe, *The Garland of Letters: Studies in the Mantra-Sastra* (Madras, India: Ganesh, 6th ed., 1974), p. 228.

29. See A. Bharati, *The Tantric Tradition* (London: Rider, 1965), p. 106.

30. The Sanskrit edition by Ramkumar Rai misreads *jaya* for *japa.* See S. Rai, editor and translator, *Mantra-Yoga-Samhitâ* (Varanasi, India: Chaukhambha Orientalia, 1982).

31. Written *aham brahmâsmi.*

32. *Svastika-âsana* and *padma-âsana* are respectively written *svastikâsana* and *padmâsana.*

33. *Yâga* is a synonym of *yajna.*

34. S. S. Goswami, *Layayoga* (London: Routledge & Kegan Paul, 1980), p. 68. I have simplified the transliteration of Sanskrit terms in this quote.

35. Sri Aurobindo, *The Life Divine,* vol. 1 (Pondicherry, India: Sri Aurobindo Ashram, repr. 1977), pp. 23.

36. Ibid., p. 23.

37. Ibid, p. 23. The verticalist approach was established prior to Buddhism, which is often wrongly blamed for introducing a life-negative orientation into India's spiritual heritage. Buddhism, like Hinduism, includes verticalist and horizontalist, as well as integral currents.

38. [Manibhai, ed.], *A Practical Guide to Integral Yoga: Extracts Compiled from the Writings of Sri Aurobindo and The Mother* (Pondicherry, India: Sri Aurobindo Ashram, repr. 1976), p. 31.

39. Sri Aurobindo, *The Life Divine,* vol. 1, p. 174.

40. Sri Aurobindo, *Sri Aurobindo on Himself and on The Mother* (Pondicherry, India: Sri Aurobindo Ashram, 1953), pp. 154–155.

41.  H. Chaudhuri, "The Integral Philosophy of Sri Aurobindo," in H. Chaudhuri and F. Spiegelberg, eds., *The Integral Philosophy of Sri Aurobindo: A Commemorative Symposium* (London: Allen & Unwin, 1960), p. 17.

## Chapter 3: Yoga and Other Hindu Traditions

1.   The word *yajnopavita* is composed of *yajna* ("sacrifice" or "sacrificial") and *upavita* ("thread"). The cord consists of three threads made of nine twisted strands each. The materials are cotton, hemp, and wool for *brahmins*, *kshatriyas*, and *vaishyas* respectively.
2.   See G. Feuerstein, S. Kak, and D. Frawley, *In Search of the Cradle of Civilization: New Light on Ancient India* (Wheaton, Ill.: Quest Books, 1996).
3.   See N. S. Rajaram and D. Frawley, *Vedic Aryans and the Origins of Civilization: A Literary and Scientific Perspective* (New Delhi: Voice of India, 1995).
4.   C. G. Jung, *Psychology and the East* (Princeton, N.J.: Princeton University Press, 1978), p. 57. First published 1938.
5.   C. G. Jung, *Modern Man in Search of a Soul* (New York: Harvest Books, 1933), pp. 215–216.
6.   An exception is the work of F. E. Pargiter, *Ancient Indian Historical Tradition* (Delhi: Motilal Banarsidass, repr. 1972). First published 1922.
7.   For a translation of hymn 10.129, see Chapter 4.
8.   M. S. Bhat, *Vedic Tantrism: A Study of the Rgvidhâna of Saunaka with Text and Translation* (Delhi: Motilal Banarsidass, 1987), places the *Rig-Vidhâna* in the fifth century B.C.E., which may be too late. Shaunaka lived during the Vedic Age, and, unless we assume that the text is a late attribution, we must trace the original back to that early period. There is no question that the present version of the *Rig-Vidhâna* contains terms and ideas that do not belong to the Vedic Era, but there may well be an old nucleus on mantric magic that stems from that formative period.
9.   See T. S. Anantha Murthy, *Maharaj: A Biography of Shriman Tapasviji Maharaj, a Mahatma Who Lived for 185 Years* (San Rafael, Calif.: Dawn Horse Press, 1972). Foreword, entitled "Penance and Enlightenment," by Georg Feuerstein.
10.  J. F. Sprockhoff, *Samnyâsa: Quellenstudien zur Askese im Hinduismus.* Vol. 1: *Untersuchungen über die Samnyâsa-Upanisads* (Wiesbaden, Germany: Kommissionsverlag Franz Steiner, 1976), p. 2.
11.  See G. Feuerstein, *Wholeness or Transcendence? Ancient Lessons for the Emerging Global Civilization* (Burdett, N.Y.: Larson Publications, 1992).
12.  *Mauna* also means "silence."
13.  S. Radhakrishnan, *Indian Philosophy* (New York: Macmillan; London: Allen & Unwin, 1951), vol. 2, p. 429.
14.  Some scholars date Shankara to c. 650 C.E., which seems very likely.
15.  M. Müller, *The Six Systems of Indian Philosophy* (New York: Longmans, Green, and Co., 1916), p. 263.
16.  Self-actualization refers to the realization of our potential for such higher moral values as self-transcendence, love, compassion, integrity, creativity, and wholeness. See A. Maslow, *The Farther Reaches of Human Nature* (Harmondsworth, England: Penguin Books, 1971).
17.  D. Frawley, *Ayurveda and the Mind* (Twin Lakes, Wis.: Lotus Press, 1996), p. 5.
18.  Some modern Ayur-Vedic specialists object to translating the three humors as "wind," "bile," and "phlegm" respectively. They argue that these terms are misleading because *vâta, pitta,* and *kapha* refer to whole functional systems of the body-mind. Thus, *vâta* is responsible for all sensory and motor activities; *pitta* is responsible for all biochemical activities; and *kapha* underlies skeletal and anabolic processes. It is obvious that the three *doshas* are related to the three *gunas—sattva, rajas,* and *tamas.*
19.  See R. E. Svoboda, *Ayurveda: Life, Health and Longevity* (New York: Arkana, 1992), p. 66.
20.  An herbal concoction taken via the nose.
21.  K. V. Zvelebil, *The Poets of the Powers: Magic, Freedom, and Renewal* (Lower Lake, Calif.: Integral Publishing, 1993), p. 123.
22.  Two excellent books on Ganesha are John A. Grimes, *Ganapati: Song of the Self* (Albany, N.Y.: State University of New York Press, 1995) and Satguru Sivaya Subramuniyaswami, *Loving Ganesa: Hinduism's Endearing Elephant-Faced God* (Kapaa, Hawaii: Himalayan Academy, 1996).

23. The *Devî-Bhâgavata* was very probably composed one or two centuries after the *Bhâgavata-Purâna*, which belongs to the tenth century C.E. An earlier text of Devî worship is the *Devî-Mahâtmya*, which is quoted in full in the *Devî-Bhâgavata* and has been tentatively dated to the sixth century C.E.

## PART TWO: PRE-CLASSICAL YOGA

## Chapter 4: Yoga in Ancient Times

1. K. Jaspers, *Way to Wisdom: An Introduction to Philosophy* (New Haven, Ct./London: Yale University Press, 1954), p. 96.
2. See K. Jaspers, *Vom Ursprung und Ziel der Geschichte* (Frankfurt: Fischer Bücherei, 1955).
3. See J. Gebser, *The Ever-Present Origin* (Athens, Ohio: Ohio University Press, 1986).
4. See G. Feuerstein, *Wholeness or Transcendence? Ancient Lessons for the Emerging Global Civilization* (Burdett, N.Y.: Larson Publications, 1992).
5. See M. Harner, *The Way of the Shaman* (New York: Harper & Row, 1980); J. Halifax, *Shamanic Voices: A Survey of Visionary Narratives* (New York: Dutton, 1979).
6. This psychohistorical movement from the mythical structure of consciousness toward the mental structure is explained in G. Feuerstein, *Structures of Consciousness* (Lower Lake, Calif.: Integral Publishing, 1987).
7. Even the Buddhist ideal of the *bodhisattva* ("enlightenment being"), who vows to liberate all sentient beings, is not strictly speaking a social ideal. The *bodhisattva* is not a social-welfare worker but a spiritual aspirant or an adept whose only purpose is the *spiritual* welfare of others.
8. M. Eliade, *Yoga: Immortality and Freedom* (Princeton, N.J.: Princeton University Press, 1973), p. 320. See also his *Shamanism: Archaic Techniques of Ecstasy* (Princeton, N.J.: Princeton University Press, 1972).
9. See F. Goodman, *Where the Spirits Ride the Wind* (Bloomington, Ind.: Indiana University Press, 1990); see also B. Gore, *Ecstatic Body Postures: An Alternate Reality Book* (Santa Fe, N.M.: Bear & Co., 1995).
10. R. Walsh, *The Spirit of Shamanism* (Los Angeles: J. P. Tarcher, 1990), p. 10.
11. See, e.g., T. McEvilley, "An Archaeology of Yoga," *Res*, vol. 1 (spring 1981), pp. 44–77, for a review of yogic elements in the so-called Indus civilization. McEvilley, however, still employs the outdated dichotomy between intrusive Aryan and native Dravidian cultures.
12. See G. Feuerstein, S. Kak, and D. Frawley, *In Search of the Cradle of Civilization: New Light on Ancient India* (Wheaton, Ill.: Quest Books, 1995).
13. See C. Renfrew, *Archaeology & Language: The Puzzle of Indo-European Origins* (Cambridge: Cambridge University Press, 1987).
14. See A. Seidenberg, "The Origin of Mathematics," *Archive for History of Exact Sciences*, vol. 18 (1978), pp. 301–342.
15. The *Shulba-Sûtras* are part of the Vedic *Kalpa-Sûtra* literature and deal with construction of sacrificial altars.
16. S. Piggott, *Prehistoric India* (Harmondsworth, England: Penguin Books, 1950), p. 138. See also B. Allchin and R. Allchin, *The Birth of Indian Civilization: India and Pakistan Before 500 B.C.* (Harmondsworth, England: Penguin Books, 1968); J. Marshall, *Mohenjo Daro and the Indus Civilization* (London: Arthur Probsthain, 1931), 3 vols.; and R. E. Mortimer Wheeler, *Civilizations of the Indus Valley and Beyond* (London: Thames & Hudson, 1966).
17. The words *bhadra-âsana* and *goraksha-âsana* are written *bhadrâsana* and *gorakshâsana* respectively.
18. See S. N. Dasgupta, *Hindu Mysticism* (Chicago, Ill.: Open Court Publishing, 1927).
19. J. Miller, *The Vedas: Harmony, Meditation and Fulfilment* (London: Rider, 1974), p. 132.
20. Further references can be found in T. G. Mainkar, *Mysticism in the Rgveda* (Bombay: Popular Book Depot, 1961).
21. V. S. Agrawala, *The Thousand-Syllabled Speech*. Vol. 1: *Vision in Long Darkness* (Varanasi, India: Vedaranyaka Ashram, 1963), p. i.
22. See especially Sri Aurobindo, *On the Veda* (Pondicherry, India: Sri Aurobindo Ashram, 1956) and D. Frawley, *Hymns from the Golden Age: Selected Hymns from the Rig Veda with Yogic Interpretation* (Delhi: Motilal Banarsidass, 1986).

23. J. Miller, op. cit., p. 45.

24. Ibid., p. 49.

25. Ibid., p. 97.

26. See, e.g., D. Frawley, *Gods, Sages and Kings: Vedic Secrets of Ancient Civilization* (Salt Lake City, Utah: Passage Press, 1991), pp. 203ff.

27. D. Frawley, *Hymns from the Golden Age*, p. 10.

28. Ibid., p. 10.

29. Sri Aurobindo, *On the Veda*, p. 384.

30. See S. Kak, *The Astronomical Code of the Rgveda* (New Delhi: Aditya Prakashan, 1994).

31. It is important to realize that the *rishis* included nonbrahmins such as the *kshatriyas* Manu and Purûravas Aila, as well as the *vaishyas* Bhalandana, Vatsa, and Sankîla.

32. The meaning of the word *marmrishat* is not clear. It is here translated as "most worthy." The Sanskrit commentators think it refers to God Indra.

33. The Sanskrit text is very obscure here, which is reflected in the translation.

34. The name Vakreshvarî is derived from *vakra* ("crooked") and *îshvarî*, which is the feminine form of *îshvara* ("lord").

35. This last verse also is found in *Rig-Veda* 1.164.31. The inner meaning of the words *sadhricih* and *vishucih* is obscure, here rendered as "convergent [forces]" and "divergent [forces]" respectively. On one level, the sun-bird's rays radiate downward in one direction—toward the earth—but also spread out to illuminate the entire space. On the spiritual level, undoubtedly a similar principle pertains, whereby the intuitive flashing-forth is both highly focused, and yet all-illuminating, since it affects the whole body-mind.

36. Perhaps the three kinds of creatures are those that show a preponderance of *tamas*, *rajas*, or *sattva*.

37. The word *harita* is often taken to mean "yellow" or even "green." It is here given as "golden."

38. The six twins are the twelve months, which come in pairs and which account for 360 days. The one "born singly" is the intercalary month composed of the remaining days of the solar year.

39. The word *akshara* means literally "unmoving" or "imperishable." It can refer to a syllable (such as the single-syllabled *mantra om* symbolizing the ultimate Reality) or to the Divine itself. Here it refers either to the solar rays or to the stars.

40. Here the word *agra* or "First[-born]" stands for the sun, the visible form of the invisible ultimate Light.

41. The seven seers (*sapta-rishi*, written *saptarshi*) are probably Vishvâmitra, Jamadagni, Bharadvâja, Gotama, Atri, Vashishtha, and Kashyapa. They are first named as a set in the *Shrauta-Sûtras* belonging to the end of the Vedic era. In the later Sanskrit literature, they symbolize the cognitive faculties, namely the five senses, the lower mind (*manas*), and the higher wisdom mind (*buddhi*). The vessel opening to the side is both the experienced world, which is divided by the horizon into an upper and a lower half, as well as the human head.

42. By means of their songs of praise (*ric*) accompanying the sacrificial rituals, the Vedic seers aspired to contact the Gods and the Divine itself, but only those who were able to focus ("yoke") the mind properly were blessed with success.

43. The term *ketu* has the primary meaning of "light." It can refer to a meteor or comet, but also to visible evidence in general. To combine these two connotations, I have translated the term as "bright indication."

44. The Water Bearer—the Sanskrit phrase is *bharantam udakam*—is none other than the sun, which drinks up the ocean's water only to disperse it again in the form of fertilizing rain.

45. To know the sun with the mind means to know its inner secret, namely that it serves as a portal to the immortal Light.

46. The Sanskrit text has *madhye*, which means "in the middle" (from *madhya*), here meaning neither the present moment nor the very earliest time but somewhere in between.

47. The expression "threefold swan" (*trivritam hamsam*) is not clear. It could refer to the three aspects of light, namely the sun, fire, and lightning.

48. *Svar* can also denote "sky."

49. This could be a reference to the fact that the Vedic seers symbolized the world in the form of a she-goat (*ajâ*) that mates with the Divine in its pure nature, represented as a billy-goat (*aja*). Out of their union, all things are created.

50. The words *bhogya* ("edible," "capable of eating") and *bhojana* ("food") can also be translated as "capable of enjoyment" and "enjoyment" respectively.

51. The word *ghnanti* means literally "slay" but is here translated as "consume."

52. The word *bâla* means "child," and has been translated thus by some. However, it can also be an alternative spelling for *vâla* meaning "hair," which makes more sense in the present context.
53. The meaning of this verse is obscure.
54. This verse is found verbatim in the *Shvetâshvatara-Upanishad* (4.3), which has incorporated many of the ideas found in this Vedic hymn.
55. The Sanskrit original has the genitive plural *ushasah* "of dawns."
56. The name Avi is derived from the root *av* meaning "to favor," though the word *avi* stands for "sheep."
57. Some translators have "green," but see footnote 37.
58. The verb forms used in the first half of this verse make it impossible to determine the intended subject. The present translation understands the phrase "does not abandon" (*na jâhati*) as "one cannot abandon," and "does not see" (*na pashyati*) as "one does not see."
59. The phrase *yathâyatham*, here rendered as "as it is," appears to be an early form of *yathâbhûtam*. The words of the Divine are sacred and truth-bearing, as are the words of those who know the Divine. This notion underlies the entire Vedic revelation.
60. This is another difficult verse. The "Flower of the Waters" (*apâm pushpam*) seems to refer to the hidden creative principle or essence of existence. Here the word *mâyâ* does not yet have the later meaning of "illusion," as in Shankara's school of Vedânta, rather it is creative magical power.
61. Mâtarîshvan is India's Prometheus. His name means literally "He who lies in the mother," that is, in Nature—a reference to the fact that the sun rises out of the oceans, corresponding to fire lying hidden in wood until it is kindled through friction. In the Post-Vedic Era, Mâtarîshvan is another name for the God of Wind, and this also appears to be so in the Vedic period. Translated into esoteric terms, he is the breath, which works upon the body and mind so as to bring forth the inner light.
62. The "purifier" is presumably the wind, which entered the golden flames, fanning them into a conflagration.
63. The word *aja* ("unborn") also can mean "goat." One translator has characterized this verse as "utterly obscure," but this is not really the case. It is through the Vedic chants that the worshipers attain the heavenly realm, the abode of the Gods. But beyond Heaven is the ultimate Reality, here described as unborn.
64. This has been called the earliest clear mention of the *âtman* as the ultimate spiritual principle.
65. The materials on the Vrâtyas consist of fragments written in archaic Sanskrit and of scattered references in the works of ancient writers who had a vested interest in being critical of these brotherhoods. Little wonder that most scholars have shied away from studying them. The only really comprehensive study is that by the German Yoga researcher Jakob Wilhelm Hauer. See J. W. Hauer, *Der Vrâtya*, vol. 1: *Die Vrâtyas als nichtbrahmanische Kultgenossenschaften arischer Herkunft* (Stuttgart, Germany: Kohlhammer Verlag, 1927). The announced second volume was never published. For a more recent illuminating discussion, see Jan Heesterman, "Vrâtya and Sacrifice," *Indo-Iranian Journal*, vol. 6 (1962), pp. 3-37, and David Gordon White, *Myths of the Dog-Man* (Chicago and London: University of Chicago Press, 1991). The latter explores the fascinating relationship between the Vrâtyas and dogs. "Symbolically, the dog is the animal pivot of the human universe, lurking at the threshold between wildness and domestication and all of the valances that these two ideal poles of experience hold. There is much of man in his dogs, much of the dog in us, and behind this, much of the wolf in both the dog and man. And, there is some of the Dog-Man in god" (White, p. 15). The Vrâtyas, who frequented the forests, were part of the Vedic counterculture and as such were figures of *liminality*.
66. The Vrâtyas' connection with the *Sâma-Veda* was shown by J. W. Hauer, and they also appear to have been connected with the recitation of epic sagas, the "Fifth *Veda*," some of whose materials are to be found in the *Purâna* literature.
67. For a treatment of the magical teachings of the *Atharva-Veda*, see M. Stutley, *Ancient Indian Magic and Folklore: An Introduction* (Boulder, Colo.: Great Eastern Book Co., 1980).

## Chapter 5: The Whispered Wisdom of the Early Upanishads

1. Written *prânâgnihotra*. The notion of many scholars that this sacrifice was performed primarily by renouncers is not borne out by the available evidence, as was made clear by the Dutch indologist H. W. Bodewitz in his book *Jaiminîya Brâhmana I,1–65: Translation and Commentary, With a Study of Agnihotra and Prânâgnihotra* (Leiden, Holland: E. J. Brill, 1973).

2. For the most comprehensive but in many ways antiquated English rendering of the *Upanishads*, see P. Deussen, *Sixty Upanishads of the Veda*, translated from the German by V. M. Bedekar and G. B. Palsule (Delhi: Motilal Banarsidass, 1980), 2 vols. The German original was first published in 1897. See also R. E. Hume, *The Thirteen Principal Upanishads* (London: Oxford University Press, 1958), and S. Radhakrishnan, *The Principal Upanisads* (London: George Allen & Unwin/New York: Humanities Press, 1953), which includes the Sanskrit text of thirteen *Upanishads*. Conventional scholarship places the oldest *Upanishads* around 700–600 B.C.E., but this date is misleading in light of the recent chronological considerations, which oblige us to push the date of the earliest *Brâhmanas* back to well before 1500 B.C.E. Since the style and contents of the oldest *Upanishads* is reasonably continuous with the *Brâhmanas*, we ought not postulate too big a gap between these two literary genres. Moreover, some of the teachers mentioned in the *Brâhmanas* also figure in the *Upanishads*. Thus, the *Brihad-Âranyaka-Upanishad* (e.g., 6.5.1ff.) lists fifty-two teachers by name, including the famous sage Yâjnavalkya. Since he was intimately linked with the teachings of the *Shata-Patha-Brâhmana*, which can be tentatively placed around 1500 B.C.E., we have a helpful chronological marker. Yâjnavalkya was thirty-eight generations removed from Pautimâshya, the last teacher mentioned in the text. This translates into roughly 760 years. Thus, the last recorded transmission of the *Brihad-Âranyaka-Upanishad* can be assigned to about 700 B.C.E., though its nucleus goes back to before the Bharata war. In other words, the teachings of this *Upanishad* belong to the period between 1500 and 700 B.C.E. The age of the other early *Upanishads* cannot be significantly different.

3. On Eco-Yoga, see Henryk Skolimowski, *Dancing Shiva in the Ecological Age* (New Delhi: Clarion Books, 1991) and *The Participatory Mind: A New Theory of Knowledge and of the Universe* (London: Arkana/Penguin Books, 1994), as well as G. Feuerstein, "Yoga and Ecology," *Quarterly Journal of the Indian Academy of Yoga*, vol. 3, no. 4 (1983), pp. 161–172.

4. The phrase *shloka-krit* ("*shloka* maker") is ambiguous. *Shloka* can refer to a stanza, sound in general, or fame. It is derived from the verbal root *shru* ("to hear"). I chose to render it here as "poetry." The underlying idea is that the sage, in the condition of ecstatic identification with the transcendental Self, acknowledges that Self or ultimate Being as the source of his poetic exuberance.

5. Elsewhere *brahma-loka* can also stand for the "realm of Brahma," the Creator.

6. See J. W. Hauer, *Der Yoga: Ein indischer Weg zum Selbst* (Stuttgart: Kohlhammer Verlag, 1958), p. 144.

7. The term *adhyâtman* means "relative to the self," here translated as the "deep Self," because it is the transcendental Self that is intended.

# Chapter 6: Jaina Yoga: The Teachings of the Victorious Ford-Makers

1. Written *Âcârângasûtra*, from *âcâra* ("conduct"), *anga* ("limb" or "constituent"), and *sûtra* ("aphorism").

2. According to Jaina sources, Rishabha lived for no fewer than 8.4 million years. It is possible that he was a historical personage who, to be sure, enjoyed a more ordinary span of life, though nothing is known about him apart from the later legends. It is especially noteworthy that a Rishabha is mentioned in the Vrâtya book of the *Atharva-Veda* (book 15). The Rig-Vedic references to Rishabha are VI.16.47; VI.28.8; X.91.14; X.166.1.

3. Jainism, however, still does not receive the scholarly attention it deserves, and also followers of this age-old tradition in Western countries lack adequate resources for studying their own scriptures. But see the excellent introductory work by P. Dundas, *The Jains* (London/New York: Routledge, 1992); and the works by A. K. Chatterjee, *A Comprehensive History of Jainism*, vol. 1 (Calcutta, 1978), vol. 2 (Calcutta, 1984); E. Fischer and J. Jain, *Jaina Iconography* (Leiden, Netherlands: E. J. Brill, 1978), 2 vols.; and R. Williams, *Jaina Yoga: A Survey of the Medieval Shravakacaras* (London: Oxford University Press, 1963).

4. Written *Tattvârthâdhigamasûtra* or *Tattvârthasûtra*.

5. Written *Shatkhandâgama*.

6. K. Jaspers, *Way to Wisdom: An Introduction to Philosophy* (New Haven, Conn./ London: Yale University Press, 1954), p. 96.

7. This Haribhadra must be distinguished from the polymath Haribhadra Virahânkha who lived in the fifth/sixth century and is credited with the authorship of more than one thousand texts.

8. Written *mahâtman*.

9. Written *Jnânârnava*.

## Chapter 7: Yoga in Buddhism

1. V. A. Smith, *The Oxford History of India* (London: Oxford University Press, 1970), p. 76.
2. C. Humphreys, *Buddhism* (Harmondsworth, England: Penguin Books, 195), p. 27.
3. The honorific title *siddhârtha* is composed of *siddha* ("accomplished") and *artha* ("object"), thus denoting a person who has accomplished his or her goals. This name was made famous in Western circles through Herman Hesse's novel *Siddhartha* (1951).
4. On the thirty-two marks of a Buddha, see A. Getty, *The Gods of Northern Buddhism: Their History and Iconography* (New York: Dover Publications, 1988), p. 190.
5. Bhikshu Sangharakshita, *A Survey of Buddhism* (Boulder, Colo.: Shambhala; London: Windhorse, 1980), p. 83.
6. In Mahâyâna Buddhism, primal ignorance (*avidyâ*) rather than desire is considered to be the cause of suffering. Both psychological forces, however, work together to create the experience of *duhkha*.
7. H.-W. Schumann, *Buddhism: An Outline of Its Teachings and Schools*. Translated by G. Feuerstein (London: Rider, 1973), p. 65.
8. Written *lokottaramagga;* in Sanskrit *lokottaramârga*.
9. The Sanskrit word *samyak*, meaning "right" or "perfect," becomes *samyag* before a soft consonant or vowel.
10. Written in Sanskrit *âkâshânantâyatana*.
11. Written in Sanskrit *vijnânânantâyatana*.
12. Written in Sanskrit *âkimcanyâyatana*.
13. Written in Sanskrit *naivasamjnâsamjnâyatana*.
14. L. Hixon, *Mother of the Buddhas: Meditation on the Prajnaparamita Sutra* (Wheaton, Ill.: Quest Books, 1993), p. 6.
15. E. Conze, *Buddhist Thought in India* (London, Allen & Unwin, 1962), p. 200.
16. E. Conze, *Thirty Years of Buddhist Studies: Selected Essays* (Oxford: Bruno Cassirer, 1967), p. 148.
17. The term *tathâgata* means literally "thus gone" and refers to a fully awakened being, or *buddha*, who has realized "suchness" (*tathâtâ*).
18. Generally written *Bodhicaryâvâtara*. For a good English rendering, see M. L. Matics, *Entering the Path of Enlightenment: The Bodhicaryâvâtara of the Buddhist Poet Sântideva* (London: Allen & Unwin, 1971), pp. 153–155.
19. Some scholars think that there have been two Nâgârjunas. One is the philosopher-adept (c. 150 C.E.), the other is the alchemist-adept (assigned to c. 700 C.E.). The Tibetans believe that the philosopher-adept of the Mâdhyamika school also knew alchemy and was able to prolong his life indefinitely. The fact is, there have been a number of spiritual authorities in the common era bearing this name. See D. G. White, *The Alchemical Body: Siddha Traditions in Medieval India* (Chicago and London: The University of Chicago Press, 1996), pp. 66–77, for a summary of the scholarly debate on this issue and his own reasonable proposal, which involves three Nâgârjunas: the philosopher-adept, the alchemist-adept who was a disciple of the famous *siddha* Saraha (early seventh century C.E.), and the medical adept who composed the *Yoga-Shataka* (ninth century C.E.).
20. Written *paramârtha*.
21. The six *gatis* or forms of birth are deities, anti-deities (*asura*), humans, animals, ghosts (*preta*), and denizens of hell.
22. There is a nice word play here: The awakened being is released from the bonds (*bandhana*) of imagination but continues to be a friend (*bandhava*) of the world.
23. Written *bhûtârtha*.
24. Written *Ekâksharisûtra*.
25. See A. Govinda, *Foundations of Tibetan Mysticism* (London: Rider, 1969).
26. See P. C. Bagchi, *Dohâkosha*, part 1 (Calcutta: Calcutta Sanskrit Series, 1938).
27. The Tibetan word for *dâkinî* is *khandroma*, meaning "sky dancer," which is a reference to the illusory dance of awareness in the physical realm.
28. C. Humphreys, op. cit., p. 179.
29. E. Conze, *Thirty Years of Buddhist Studies: Selected Essays* (Oxford: Cassirer, 1967), p. 29.
30. Translated from the Tibetan by H. V. Guenther, *The Royal Song of Saraha: A Study in the History of Buddhist Thought* (Berkeley, Calif.: Shambhala, 1973), pp. 14–38.

31. See A. Bharati, *The Tantric Tradition* (London: Rider, 1970), p. 20.

32. G. Tucci, *The Theory and Practice of the Mandala* (London: Rider, 1961), p. 25.

33. J. Blofeld, *The Tantric Mysticism of Tibet* (New York: Dutton, 1970), p. 33.

34. The Tibetan word *ganden* (also spelled *gaden*) corresponds to the Sanskrit term *tushita* ("delightful"), which is the name of Maitreya's transcendental paradise.

35. For Tsongkhapa's masterful commentary on Nâropa's six yogic methods, see the translation by G. H. Mullin, *Tsongkhapa's Six Yogas of Naropa* (Ithaca, N.Y.: Snow Lion Publications, 1996); see also Mullin's *Readings on the Six Yogas of Naropa* (Ithaca, N.Y.: Snow Lion Publications, 1997), which contains his English renderings of short Tibetan texts on Nâropa's six Yogas, including Nâropa's "Vajra Verses of the Whispered Tradition." This text actually mentions not six but ten methods.

36. J. Blofeld, op. cit., p. 234.

# Chapter 8: The Flowering of Yoga

1. The expression "deep Self" for *adhyâtman* refers to the core of the human being, the ultimate essence that is pure consciousness and bliss.

2. The two *Upanishads* dedicated to Râma may be assigned to circa 300 B.C.E., which also appears to be the date of the *Jâbâla-Upanishad* belonging to the tradition of renunciation (*samnyâsa*). See J. F. Sprockhoff, *Samnyâsa: Quellenstudien zur Askese im Hinduismus* (Wiesbaden, Germany: Kommissionsverlag Franz Steiner, 1976).

3. See P. Richman, "Introduction: The Diversity of the Râmâyana Tradition," in P. Richman, ed., *Many Râmâyanas: The Diversity of a Narrative Tradition in South Asia* (Berkeley, Calif.: University of California Press, 1991), p. 3.

4. The name Hanumat or Hanûmat means "He who possesses [strong] jaws."

5. For a discussion of the symbolism of the number "18," which plays a significant role in the *Mahâbhârata*, see G. Feuerstein, *The Bhagavad-Gîtâ: Its Philosophy and Cultural Setting* (Wheaton, Ill.: Quest Books, 1983), p. 64.

6. See R. Garbe, *Introduction to the Bhagavadgîtâ*, translated by D. Mackichan (Bombay: The University of Bombay, 1918), and R. Otto, *The Original Gîtâ*, translated by J. E. Turner (London: George Allen and Unwin, 1939).

7. See P. Sinha, *The Gita as It Was: Rediscovering the Original Bhagavadgita* (La Salle, Ill.: Open Court, 1987).

8. See K. N. Upadhyaya, *Early Buddhism and the Bhagavadgîtâ* (Delhi: Motilal Banarsidass, 1971).

9. M. K. Gandhi, *Young India* (Delhi, 1925), pp. 1078–1079. The immense popularity of the *Gîtâ* is reflected in the numerous commentaries on it that have been composed in Sanskrit and the vernacular languages. The oldest available and most authoritative commentary is by Shankara, the leading proponent of Hindu nondualism. Other well-known expositions of the *Gîtâ's* teachings are by Râmânuja, the famous teacher of qualified nondualism, by the dualist Madhva, who composed the *Gîtâ-Bhâshya* and the *Gîtâ-Tatparya*, and by the celebrated adept-poet Jnânadeva, whose *Jnâneshvarî* must be counted among the most beautiful poetic creations of India. In modern times, illuminating commentaries were composed by the Bengali philosopher-*yogin* Sri Aurobindo and the philosopher and sometime-president of India Sarvepalli Radhakrishnan.

10. J. W. Hauer in *Hibbert Journal* (April 1940), p. 341.

11. Swami Prabhavananda and C. Isherwood, *The Song of God: Bhagavad-Gita* (London: Phoenix House, 1947), p. 18.

12. The epithet Dhanamjaya means "Conqueror of wealth," from *dhana* ("wealth") and *jaya* ("conquest"). "Wealth" here stands both for the kingdom over which the Bharata war was fought and spiritual riches.

13. G. Feuerstein, *The Bhagavad-Gita: Its Philosophy and Cultural Setting* (Wheaton, Ill.: Quest Books, 1983), p. 162.

14. The deities mentioned in this stanza all stem from the Vedic era.

15. The word *anjali* signifies the gesture of folded hands raised to the heart or forehead.

16. The Rudras, etc., are Vedic deities.

17. The epithet Savyasâcin means "He who is skilled with the left hand," that is, "He who is ambidexterous."

18. The Rakshasas are demonic beings.

19. The deities named hail from the Vedic era. Shashânka ("Hare-marked") is one of the names of the lunar deity.

20. The epithet Janârdana means "Harasser of people" and is equivalent to the English word "hero."

21. The epithet Paramtapa means "He who vexes the enemy" and is a synonym of Janârdana.

22. Written *bhûtâtman.* This concept stands for the Self as residing in the *bhûtas,* that is the finite "beings" and material "elements." This expression can also be found in the *Maitrâyanîya-Upanishad* (3.2f.).

23. The three *gunas—sattva, rajas,* and *tamas—*are the fundamental qualities or forces of Nature (*prakriti*), which underlie not only the material universe (and thus the human body, including the senses) but also the mind and mental phenomena.

24. Written *akritâtman.*

25. Written *Maitrâyanîyopanishad.*

26. As the German Yoga researcher Jakob Wilhelm Hauer observed, Paul Deussen's notion that the *Maitrâyanîya-Upanishad* contains deliberate archaisms is unproven. See J. W. Hauer, *Der Yoga* (Stuttgart: Kohlhammer Verlag, 1958), p. 100, where he assigns this text to the early Buddhist era. On the basis of this *Upanishad's* grammatical peculiarities, Max Müller placed it prior to the grammarian Pânini, who is usually assigned to the fifth century B.C.E. or somewhat later. See M. Müller, *Sacred Books of the East,* vol. 15 (Oxford: Oxford University Press, 1900), p. 6. See J. A. B. van Buitenen, *The Maitrâyanîya Upanisad* ('s-Gravenhage: Mouton de Gruyter, 1962).

27. For a translation of the *Maitreya-Upanishad,* see P. Olivelle, *Samnyâsa Upanisads: Hindu Scriptures on Asceticism and Renunciation* (New York and Oxford: Oxford University Press, 1992), pp. 158–169.

28. Some scholars regard the *Mândûkya-Upanishad* (written *Mândûkyopanishad*) as a fairly recent creation that may have been authored by Gaudapâda himself. But there is no good reason for this assumption.

29. The complete *mantra* runs: *Om bhûr bhuvah svah tat savitur varenyam bhargo devasya dhîmahi dhiyo yo nah procodayâd âpo jyotî-raso'mritam.* The recitation of this mantric utterance while retaining the breath is reckoned as one retention (*kumbhaka*).

# PART THREE: CLASSICAL YOGA

## Chapter 9: The History and Literature of Pâtanjala-Yoga

1. C. Chapple and Yogi Ananda Viraj (E. P. Kelly, Jr.), *The Yoga Sûtras of Patañjali: An Analysis of the Sanskrit with Accompanying English Translation* (Delhi: Sri Satguru Publications, 1990), p. 15.

2. See S. N. Tandon, *A Re-Appraisal of Patanjali's Yoga-Sutras in the Light of the Buddha's Teaching* (Igatpuri, India: Vipassana Research Institute, 1995).

3. For a scholarly discussion of the relationship between Patanjali the Yoga adept and the grammarian, see S. Dasgupta, *A History of Indian Philosophy* (Delhi: Motilal Banarsidass, 1975), vol. 1, p. 230–233. See also J. H. Woods, *The Yoga-System of Patañjali* (Delhi: Motilal Banarsidass, 3d ed. 1966), pp. xiii–xvii.

4. See A. Weber, *The History of Indian Literature* (London: Kegan Paul, Trench, Trübner & Co., 4th ed., 1904), p. 223n. Weber also mentions that Patanjali is sometimes said to have been one of the Buddha's former incarnations.

5. S. Dasgupta, *A History of Indian Philosophy* (Delhi: Motilal Banarsidass, 1975), vol. 1, p. 62.

6. See G. Feuerstein, *The Yoga-Sûtra: An Exercise in the Methodology of Textual Analysis* (New Delhi: Arnold-Heinemann, 1979).

7. In discussing the date of the *Yoga-Bhâshya,* J. H. Woods, op. cit., p. xxi, pointed out a reference to this text in Mâgha's *Shishupâlavadha* (4.55), which would fix the upper limit for the *Bhâshya's* composition. He then, however, commits the error of stating that "the Comment cannot be earlier than A.D. 650," whereas he should have written "cannot be *later* than." Falling prey to his own misstatement, Woods then reaches the conclusion, "Accordingly the date of the Bhâsya would be somewhere between about A.D. 650 and about A.D. 850," which is patently wrong. Scholars continue to be misled by this pronouncement.

8. T. Leggett, *The Complete Commentary by Sankara on the Yoga Sûtras: A Full Translation of the Newly Discovered Text* (London and New York: Kegan Paul International, 1990), p. 39. See also P. Hacker, "Sankara the Yogin und Sankara der Advaitin: Einige Beobachtungen," *Beiträge zur Geistesgeschichte Indiens: Festschrift für E. Frauwallner* (Vienna, 1968), pp. 119–148.

9.  T. S. Rukmani, "The Problem of the Authorship of the *Yogasûtrabhâsyavivaranam*," *Journal of Indian Philosophy*, vol. 20 (1992), p. 422.

10. Written *Sûtrârthabodhinî*.

11. U. Arya, *Yoga-Sûtras of Patañjali*, vol. 1: *Samâdhi-Pâda* (Honesdale, Penn.: Himalayan International Institute, 1986), p. 10. This work by Pandit Usharbudh Arya (now Swami Vedabharati) is the single most in-depth commentary on Patanjali's work, but unfortunately only the author's exegesis of the first chapter of the *Yoga-Sûtra* has thus far been published.

12. M. Müller, *The Six Systems of Indian Philosophy* (London: Longmans, Green and Co., repr. 1916), p. 450.

13. T. S. Rukmani, *Yogavârttika of Vijñânabhiksu*, vol. 1: *Samâdhipâda* (New Delhi: Munshiram Manoharlal, 1981), p. 5.

14. Written *Paingalopanishad*.

## Chapter 10: The Philosophy and Practice of Pâtanjala-Yoga

1.  A. Govinda, *The Psychological Attitude in Early Buddhist Philosophy* (London: Rider, 1969), p. 35.

2.  Swami Ajaya, *Yoga Psychology: A Practical Guide to Meditation* (Honesdale, Penn.: Himalayan International Institute, 1978), p. 73.

3.  G. Krishna, *The Dawn of a Science* (New Delhi: Kundalini Research and Publication Trust, 1978), p. 223.

4.  See C. Tart, *Waking Up: Overcoming the Obstacles to Human Potential* (Boston, Mass.: New Science Library, 1987).

5.  J. H. Clark, *A Map of Mental States* (London: Routledge & Kegan Paul, 1983), p. 29.

6.  See H. Jacobs, *Western Psycho-Therapy and Hindu Sâdhanâ: A Contribution to Comparative Studies in Psychology and Metaphysics* (London: George Allen & Unwin, 1961), for a trenchant critique of C. G. Jung's position.

7.  M. Eliade, *Yoga: Immortality and Freedom* (Princeton, N.J.: Princeton University Press, 1970), p. 39.

8.  The British Yoga researcher Ian Whicher, however, has suggested that we ought to understand Patanjali's dualism not in ontological but merely in epistemological terms. If correct, this would permit us to associate the ideal of living liberation with Classical Yoga. See I. Whicher, "Implications for an Embodied Freedom in Patanjali's Yoga," a paper presented at the Conference on Yoga held at Loyola Marymount University in Los Angeles, California, March 15, 1997. See also C. Chapple, "The Unseen Seer and the Field: Consciousness in Sâmkhya and Yoga," in R. K. C. Forman, ed., *The Problem of Pure Consciousness: Mysticism and Philosophy* (New York and Oxford: Oxford University Press, 1990), pp. 53–70, and C. Chapple, "Citta-vrtti and Reality in the Yoga Sûtra," in C. Chapple, ed., *Sâmkhya-Yoga: Proceedings of the IASWR [Institute for Advanced Studies of World Religions] Conference, 1981*, p. 112, where he characterizes my position in the words "the only good sage is a dead one." While I continue to lean toward an ontological (dualist) interpretation of Patanjali's metaphysics, I would like to modify Chapple's paraphrase of my position to read "only a dead sage is perfect." Goodness does not enter the equation, because Patanjali clearly states that the fully realized *yogin* transcends the categories of good and evil.

## *PART FOUR: POST-CLASSICAL YOGA*

1.  Written *Shivastotrâvalî*.

## Chapter 11:  The Nondualist Approach to God Among the Shiva Worshipers

1.  Translated by C. R. Bailly in her book *Shaiva Devotional Songs of Kashmir: A Translation and Study of Utpaladeva's Shivastotravali* (New York: SUNY Press, 1987), p. 18.

2.  See D. Hartsuiker, *Sadhus: India's Mystic Holy Men* (Rochester, Vt.: Inner Traditions International, 1993).

3.  Written *Pancârthabhâshya*.

4.  This type of Yoga is to be distinguished from the Pâshupata Yoga schools mentioned in the *Purânas*, which follow Patanjali's definition: "Yoga is the restriction of the fluctuations of consciousness." Kaundinya, for

instance, explicitly rejects the dualist metaphysics and methodology of both Sâmkhya and Patanjali's Yoga. He emphasizes that liberation is not so much dissociation from everything but association with the Divine.

5. The name Kâlâmukha is derived from *kâla* ("time") and *âmukha* ("facing").
6. Robert E. Svoboda, *Aghora: At the Left Hand of God* (Albuquerque, N. M.: Brotherhood of Life, 1986), p. 36.
7. Ibid., p. 22.
8. The translation is by A. K. Ramanujan, *Speaking of Siva* (Harmondsworth, England: Penguin Books, 1973), p. 28. The spelling of words has been slightly amended.
9. *Upâgâma* is derived from *upa* ("secondary") and *âgama*. For a discussion of the Agamic literature, see M. S. G. Dyczkowski, *The Canon of the Saivâgama and the Kubjikâ Tantras of the Western Kaula Tradition* (Albany, N.Y.: SUNY Press, 1988).
10. The names of Shiva's five faces, which are first mentioned in the *Mahâ-Nârâyana-Upanishad* (written *Mahânârâyanopanishad*), are associated with *mantras* that must be pronounced in a low voice.
11. Written *Tantrâloka*.
12. Paraphrase of a rendering by K. C. Pandey, *Abhinavagupta: An Historical and Philosophical Study* (Varanasi, India: Chaukhamba Amarabharati Prakashan, 1963), p. 21.
13. *Kalâ* is a very important term in Shaivism, Shaktism, and Tantrism. It often refers to the sixteen phases of the moon, the sixteenth being deemed most auspicious.
14. The words *kalâ* and *kâla* both derive from the verbal root *kal* meaning "to impel."
15. For a treatment of the twenty-four principles (*tattva*) of the Sâmkhya tradition, see Chapter 3.
16. See J. C. Pearce, *The Bond of Power* (New York: Dutton, 1981), pp. 30–31.
17. Technical terms in this section may be in Sanskrit or Tamil.
18. Translated by V. Dehejia, *Slaves of the Lord: The Path of the Tamil Saints* (New Delhi: Munshiram Manoharlal, 1988), p. 35.
19. Translated by G. E. Yocum, *Hymns to the Dancing Siva* (New Delhi, 1982), p. 180.

## Chapter 12: The Vendantic Approach to God Among the Vishnu Worshipers

1. For an overview of the Pancarâtra tradition's *Samhitâs*, see F. O. Schrader, *Introduction to the Pañcarâtra and the Ahirbudhnya Samhitâ* (Adyar, India: Adyar Library, 1916). Noteworthy among these sacred Vaishnava scriptures are the *Ahirbudhnya-, Jayâkhya-, Vishnu-, Parama-,* and *Paushkara-Samhitâ*, which are all untranslated. Useful discussions of their contents, however, are found in S. Dasgupta, *A History of Indian Philosophy*, vol. 3 (Delhi: Motilal Banarsidass, repr. 1975).
2. S. Dasgupta, op. cit., vol. 3, pp. 83–84. I have modified the spelling of Sanskrit and Tamil words to make them consistent with the simplified transliteration adopted for this volume.
3. J. M. Sanyal, *The Srimad-Bhagvatam of Krishna-Dwaipayana Vyasa* (New Delhi: Munshiram Manoharlal, 1973), p. vi (publisher's note).
4. Written *anilâyâma*.
5. See T. K. V. Desikachar, *The Heart of Yoga: Developing a Personal Practice* (Rochester, Vt.: Inner Traditions International, 1995).
6. Sri Anirvan and L. Reymond, *To Live Within: Teachings of a Baul* (High Burton, England: Coombe Springs Press, 1984), p. 252.
7. See L. Lozowick, *Hohm Sahaj Mandir Study Manual: A Handbook for Practitioners of Every Spiritual and/or Transformational Path* (Prescott, Ariz.: Hohm Press, 1996), 2 vols.

## Chapter 13: Yoga and *Yogins* in the Purânas

1. Written *vamshânucarita*.
2. Written *baddhapadmâsana*.
3. These are the different forms of the life force in the body, which are briefly explained in Chapter 17.

## Chapter 14: The Yogic Idealism of the Yoga-Vâsishtha

1. The name of the sage has two *sh* sounds, whereas Vâlmîki's work is correctly spelled *Vâsishtha*.

2.  *In Woods of God-Realization: The Complete Works of Swami Rama Tirtha* (Lucknow, India: Rama Tirtha Pratisthan, 9th ed., 1979), vol. 3, p. 295.
3.  The phrase "triple universe" refers to the material dimension, the intermediate psychic dimension, and the higher/subtle realms of Nature (*prakriti*).
4.  This seven-stage model is one of three different versions found in the *Yoga-Vâsishtha*.
5.  The Sanskrit original has *koti-koti-amsha*, "a ten-millionth of a ten-millionth fraction."

## Chapter 15: God, Visions, and Power: The Yoga-Upanishads

1.  Written *Tejobindûpanishad.*
2.  The *Yoga-Upanishads* (written *Yogopanishads*) are all available in relatively reliable translations published by the Theosophical Society of Adyar, India. Students of Yoga are greatly indebted to the Theosophical Society for making many Yoga scriptures available through their excellent publications program over the years. See T. R. S. Ayyangar, *The Yoga Upanisads* (Adyar, India: Adyar Library, 1952).
3.  J.-E. Berendt, *Nada Brahma: The World Is Sound—Music and the Landscape of Consciousness* (Rochester, Vt.: Destiny Books, 1987), p. 76.
4.  S. S. Goswami, *Layayoga: An Advanced Method of Concentration* (London: Routledge & Kegan Paul, 1980), p. 13.
5.  Written *Bindûpanishads.*
6.  See H. Nakamura, *Shoki no Vedânta Tetsugaku*, vol. 1 (Tokyo: Iwanami Shoten, 1951), pp. 63ff.
7.  Written *Muktikopanishad.*
8.  The practice of *tarka* probably refers to the careful evaluation of meditative states, lest the *yogin* should succumb to mere hallucinations.
9.  Written *Hamsopanishad.*
10. Written *Brahmavidyopanishad.*
11. Written *Mahâvâkyopanishad.*
12. Written *Pâshupatabrahmopanishad.*
13. J. M. Cohen and J.-F. Phibbs, *The Common Experience* (New York: St. Martin's Press, 1979), p. 141.
14. Written *Advayatârakopanishad.*
15. Written *paramâkâsha.*
16. Written *mahâkâsha.*
17. Written *tattvâkâsha.*
18. Written *sûryâkâsha.*
19. Written *shodashânta.* The number 16 is widely associated with the moon, whose sixteenth *kalâ* issues the nectar of immortality.
20. The word *unmanî* is composed of the prefix *ud* ("up") and the verbal root *man* ("to think" or "to be conscious"). It signifies a state of exhilaration or elation, that is, of being out of one's mind, though in a positive sense. It is, however, closely related to *unmâda* ("madness").
21. Written *Kshurikopanishad.*
22. The term *ucchvâsa* is composed of *ud* ("up") and *shvâsa* ("breath"), denoting exhalation.
23. Written *Yogakundalyupanishad.* For euphonic reasons, the word *kundalî*, or *kundalinî*, must be changed to *kundaly*, or *kundaliny*, when it is followed by a word beginning with a vowel, such as *upanishad.*
24. Written *Yogattvopanishad.*
25. Written *Yogashikhopanishad.*
26. Written *shivâlaya.*
27. Written *Varâhopanishad.*
28. Written *Shândilyopanishad.*
29. Written *Trishikhibrâhmanopanishad.*
30. Written *Darshanopanishad.*
31. Written *Yogacûdâmanyupanishad.* The word *cudâmani* ("crest-jewel") is changed to *cudâmany* for the reasons stated in note 23.

## Chapter 16: Yoga in Sikhism

1. Translated by Swami Rama, *Sukhamani Sahib: Fountain of Eternal Joy* (Honesdale, Penn.: Himalayan International Institute, 1988), p. 162.
2. Siri Singh Khalsa Yogiji, *The Teaching of Yogi Bhajan: A Practical Demonstration of the Power of the Spoken Word* (New York: Hawthorn Books, 1977), p. 172.
3. Ibid., p. 184.
4. Ibid., p. 4.

## PART FIVE: POWER AND TRANSCENDENCE IN TANTRA

1. Written *Devyupanishad.*

## Chapter 17: The Esotericism of Medieval Tantra-Yoga

1. Sometimes the terms *âgama* and *tantra* are used interchangeably. The former term is explained as meaning "having come from [the mouth of God Shiva]."
2. Written *Mahâcinâcarakrama.*
3. See G. Feuerstein, *Tantra: The Path of Ecstasy* (Boston, Mass.: Shambhala, 1998).
4. A. Coomaraswamy, *The Dance of Shiva: Fourteen Indian Essays* (Bombay: Asia Publishing House, 1948), p. 140.
5. According to C. G. Jung, there are two key archetypal forces in the human psyche, which he called *anima* and *animus*. The former is feminine, the latter masculine. Their balanced copresence in each of us, whether male or female, is responsible for psychic harmony.
6. *Devî* is the feminine form of *deva*, which in some contexts could be translated as "angel." The Goddess, however, is not some intermediary being but the ultimate Reality conceived as a feminine power.
7. The name Kamalâtmikâ is composed of *kamala* ("lotus") and the feminine word *âtmikâ* ("formed").
8. Adapted from the rendering given in S. Dasgupta, *Obscure Religious Cults* (Calcutta: Firma KLM, repr. 1976), p. 57.
9. Translated by H. V. Guenther, *The Royal Song of Saraha: A Study in the History of Buddhist Thought* (Berkeley, Calif.: Shambhala Publications, 1973), p. 70.
10. See N. Rastogi, *Introduction to the Tantrâloka* (Delhi: Motilal Banarsidass, 1987).
11. See J. Singh, *The Yoga of Delight, Wonder, and Astonishment* (Albany, N.Y.: SUNY Press, 1991), which consists of an English rendering of the *Vijnâna-Bhairava*; *Siva Sûtras: The Yoga of Supreme Identity* (Delhi: Motilal Banarsidass, 1979); *Spanda-Kârikâs: The Divine Creative Pulsation* (Delhi: Motilal Banarsidass, 1980); and *Pratyabhijnâhrdayam: The Secret of Self-Recognition* (Delhi: Motilal Banarsidass, rev. ed., 1980); see also J. Sing, Swami Lashmanjee, and B. Bäumer, *Abhinavagupta, Parâtrîsikâ-Vivarana: The Secret of Tantric Mysticism* (Delhi: Motilal Banarsidass, 1988).
12. See D. F. Brooks, *The Secret of the Three Cities* (Chicago and London: University of Chicago Press, 1990), and *Auspicious Wisdom: The Texts and Traditions of Srîvidyâ Sâkta Tantrism in South India* (Albany, N.Y.: SUNY Press, 1992).
13. See D. F. Brooks, *Auspicious Wisdom*, p. xv.
14. See M. Magee, *Vamakesvarimatam* (Varanasi, India: Prachya Prakashan, 1986).
15. See *Kâmakalâvilâsa*, edited and translated by A. Avalon (Madras: Ganesh & Co., 2d ed., 1953).
16. See M. S. G. Dyczkowski, *The Canon of the Saivâgama and the Kubjikâ Tantra of the Western Kaula Tradition* (Albany, N.Y.: SUNY Press, 1988), and P. E. Muller-Ortega, *The Triadic Heart of Siva: Kaula Tantricism of Abhinavagupta in the Non-Dual Saivism of Kashmir* (Albany, N.Y.: SUNY Press, 1989). See also Dyczkowski's *The Doctrine of Vibration: An Analysis of the Doctrines and Practices of Kashmir Saivism* (Albany, N.Y.: SUNY Press, 1987).
17. See *Ânandalaharî*, edited and translated by A. Avalon (Madras: Ganesh & Co., 1961) and *Saundaryalaharî*, edited and translated by W. N. Brown (Cambridge, Mass.: Harvard University Press, 1958).

18. H. V. Guenther, *Yuganaddha: The Tantric View of Life* (Varanasi, India: Chowkhamba Sanskrit Series Office, 2d rev. ed., 1969), p. 8.

19. D. G. White, *The Alchemical Body: Siddha Traditions in Medieval India* (Chicago and London: University of Chicago Press, 1996), p. 1.

20. H. K. Schilling, *The New Consciousness in Science and Religion* (London: SCM Press, 1973), p. 113.

21. Bubba [Da] Free John, *The Paradox of Instruction* (San Francisco: Dawn Horse Press, 1977).

22. Ibid., p. 236.

23. See A. Avalon (alias John Woodroffe), *Shakti and Shakta* (New York: Dover Publications, repr. 1978), pp. 188ff.

24. G. Krishna, *Kundalini: Evolutionary Energy in Man* (London: Robinson & Watkins, 1971), pp. 12–13.

25. See L. Sannella, *The Kundalini Experience: Psychosis or Transcendence?* (Lower Lake, Calif.: Integral Publishing, 1987).

26. G. Krishna, *Kundalini: The Biological Basis of Religion and Genius* (New Delhi: Kundalini Research and Publication Trust, 1978), p. 88. The book has a long introduction by the German physicist, philosopher, and politician C. F. Freiherr von Weizsäcker.

27. Swami Rama, R. Ballentine, and Swami Ajaya (Allan Weinstock), *Yoga and Psychotherapy: The Evolution of Consciousness* (Glenview, Ill.: Himalayan Institute, 1976), p. 151.

28. See A. Bharati, *The Tantric Tradition* (London: Rider, 1965), pp. 111ff.

29. See J. Woodroffe, *The Garland of Letters: Studies in the Mantra-Sastra* (Madras: Ganesh & Co., 6th ed., 1974.)

30. See P. R. Shah, *Tantra: Its Therapeutic Aspect* (Calcutta: Punthi Pustak, 1987).

31. Swami Satyananda Saraswati, *Sure Ways to Self Realization* (Monghyr, India: Bihar School of Yoga, 1980), p. 45.

32. Cited after the transliterated Sanskrit given in S. Chattopadhyaya, *Reflections on the Tantras* (Delhi: Motilal Banarsidass, 1978), p. 16, fn. 20.

33. G. Krishna, *Kundalini: Evolutionary Energy in Man* (London: Robinson & Watkins, 1971), p. 88.

34. In the Buddhist literature, this is known as "Deity Yoga" (*devatâ-yoga*).

35. Often the word *animan* is given in the nominative case as *animâ;* similarly *mahimâ* and *laghimâ*.

36. See M. Murphy, *The Future of the Body: Explorations Into the Further Evolution of Human Nature* (Los Angeles: J. P. Tarcher, 1992).

37. In the present context the *asuras* are not demons or antigods but a group of deities, probably those who possess a more terrifying or wrathful character.

38. A crore—*koti*—denotes "ten million" and often, as here, connotes "countless."

39. The word *vipra* denotes someone who is deeply moved by the Divine.

40. A *cândâla* is a member of one of the lowest castes, an offspring of a *shûdra* and *brahmin* union.

## Chapter 18: Yoga as Spiritual Alchemy: The Philosophy and Practice of Hatha-Yoga

1. F. Capra, *The Tao of Physics* (New York: Bantam Books, 1977), pp. 228–229.

2. This image is found in the *Agni-Purâna* (51.15f). The whole passage reads: "An ascetic (*yati*) regards his body at best as an inflated bladder of skin, surrounded by muscles, sinew, and flesh, filled with ill-smelling urine, feces, and dirt, a dwelling-place of illness and suffering, and an easy victim of old age, sorrow, and death, more transient than a dew drop on a blade of grass, nothing more or less than the product of the five elements."

3. M. Eliade, *Yoga: Immortality and Freedom* (Princeton, N.J.: Princeton University Press, 1973), p. 227.

4. K. V. Zvelebil, *The Poets of the Powers* (Lower Lake, Calif.: Integral Publishing, 1993), p. 125.

5. A. Bharati, *The Tantric Tradition* (London: Rider, 1965), p. 28.

6. K. V. Zvelebil, op. cit., pp. 29–30; 63.

7. Ibid., p. 87.

8. Some scholars place Matsyendra as early as the fifth century C.E.

9. According to the Indian scholar M. Singh, Goraksha's real teaching was not Hatha-Yoga but a form of Mantra-Yoga called *nâda-anusandhâna* or "application to the (inner) sound," and we must study the

*Samnyâsa-Upanishads* (dealing with renunciation) for his views. This interpretation, however, is based on a misunderstanding of Hatha-Yoga, which definitely places considerable emphasis on the inner sound in the higher stages of practice, as is obvious from the *Hatha-Yoga-Pradîpikâ.*

10. G. W. Briggs, *Gorakhnath and the Kanphâta Yogis* (Delhi: Motilal Banarsidass, repr. 1973), p. 23. This informative, if not always unbiased, ethnographic study was first published in 1938.

11. See A. N. Upadhye, "On Some Under-Currents of the Nâtha-Sampradâya, or The Carpata-Sataka," *Journal of the Oriental Institute of Baroda,* vol. 18, part 3 (1968–1969), pp. 198–206.

12. According to the *Gheranda-Samhitâ* (5.80), the *hamsa*—also referred to as the spontaneous *gâyatrî-mantra*—operates in the nostrils, at the heart, and in the *mûlâdhâra-cakra* at the base of the spine.

13. Some popular books on Yoga wrongly state that *ha* and *tha* are the actual words meaning "sun" and "moon" respectively, whereas they are in fact only syllables *representing* the two luminaries.

14. The boundaries of the new discipline of Yoga therapy are still being defined both relative to the medical profession and traditional Yoga.

15. Written *paramâtman.*

16. The meaning of the phrase *dashâdi* is unclear because it can be read as either *dashâ-âdi* or *dasha-âdi.* *Dashâ* means "state" or "condition," whereas *dasha* means "ten." In either case, we do not know what *âdi* ("and so forth") is meant to refer to.

17. A. Avalon [J. Woodroffe], *The Serpent Power* (London: Luzac, 1919), p. 269.

18. Written *paramânanda.*

19. Written *svânanda.*

20. Written *paramâtman.*

21. The name Maheshvara is composed of *mahâ* ("great") and *îshvara* ("lord").

22. Written *siddhâsana.* The same grammatical rule of euphonic combination applies to all the other postures mentioned in the following stanza, where the word *âsana* is preceded by an *a* sound.

23. The text wrongly reads *dvi-laksha* for *tri-laksha,* as is usual. The *Siddha-Siddhânta-Paddhati* (2.10) has *tri-lakshya,* meaning the "three signs": *antar-lakshya, bahir-lakshya,* and *madhyama-lakshya.* These are visionary states.

24. Curiously, in their edition of the *Goraksha-Shataka,* which contains this stanza, Swami Kuvalayananda and S. A. Shukla chose the reading *caturasram* ("four-cornered") over *trikonam* ("triangular"), even though most of their manuscripts favored the latter.

25. *Manipûraka* is a variation of *manipûra* ("jewel city").

26. I read *brahma-pâdam* for the text's *brahma-dvâram,* which makes no sense.

27. Written *mitâhârin.*

28. I read *bhujyate* for the text's *muncate.*

29. I read *gudâvarta* (*gudâ-âvarta*) for the text's *mudâvarta.*

30. Before a soft consonant, *nabhas* must be changed to *nabho.*

31. The phrase *shâstrângamodgîranam* is corrupt for *shastrâgamodîranam,* "warding off of weapons." See the *Hatha-Yoga-Pradîpikâ* (3.50) for the correct reading.

32. The Sanskrit text reads wrongly *vitanute.*

33. The repetition suggests that the Sanskrit text is corrupt here.

34. The compound *marîci-jala* can mean "chimerical water" or "sparkling water." It captures a yogic experience of unending luminosity.

35. The phrase *apâna-mûla* is probably wrong for *âdhâra-mûla,* meaning the anal sphincter muscles which are contracted by means of *mûla-bandha.*

36. I read *hutavaha* for *hutabaha.*

37. The *Yoga-Kârnikâ* (10.18) quotes this verse as reading *shashta-nâdikâ* instead of *shashti-nâdibhih.*

38. Stanza 101 seems to be an interpolation and has been omitted here.

39. There appears to be another work of this title, by Nitya Nâtha, which has a summary, entitled *Siddha-Siddhânta-Samgraha,* by Balabhadra. There is also the seventeenth-century *Goraksha-Siddhânta-Samgraha,* which draws from about sixty other works.

40. S. L. Katre, "Ânandasamuccaya: A Rare Work on Hatha-Yoga," *Journal of the Oriental Institute* (Baroda), vol. 11 (1961–62), p. 409.

41. P. C. Divanji, *Yoga-Yâjñavalkya: A Treatise on Yoga as Taught by Yogi Yajñavalkya* (Bombay, 1954).

42. See S. Mayeda, *A Thousand Teachings: The Upadesasâhasrî of Sankara* (New York: SUNY Press, 1992), p. 6.

43. See P. V. Kane, *History of Dharmasâstra*, vol. 1 (Poona: Bhandarkar Oriental Research Institute, 1930), p. 190.

44. Other works of the seventeenth century are the *Shiva-Yoga-Pradîpikâ* ("Light on Shiva-Yoga") of Sadâshiva Brahmendra, a Telegu brahmin, and the *Yoga-Cintâmani* ("Thought-Gem of Yoga") of Shivânanda.

45. See K. S. Balasubramanian, *Authorities Cited in the Hatha-Sanketa-Candrikâ of Sundaradeva*, Yoga Research Center Studies Series, no. 3 (Lower Lake, Calif.: Yoga Research Center, forthcoming).

# CHRONOLOGY

Western scholars have by and large tended to distrust native Indian chronologies (such as the dynastic lists of the *Purânas*), seeing in them little more than fanciful constructions of imaginative pundits. Some researchers, however, have studied this complicated subject in depth and have found that India's historical traditions are far more credible than has generally been assumed.

For millennia, the Hindus transmitted their sacred knowledge orally, necessitating tremendous feats of memory. Even today, there are still brahmins who can flawlessly recite one, two, or even three of the Vedic scriptures and some of their commentaries comprising tens of thousands of verses. Others can recite the entire *Mahâbhârata* epic, which is seven times larger than the *Iliad* and *Odyssey* combined. Given this advanced mnemonic technology, why would we not also take their lists of kings and seers seriously? Admittedly, the *Purânas* are not counted among the revelatory literature (*shruti*) and therefore demonstrably have not been transmitted as faithfully as the *Vedas*. However, that the lists of Puranic kings should contain errors and omissions does not negate their value as chronicles.

The following chronology is based on recent research and thinking rather than the highly conservative ideas of scholarly textbooks. The academic establishment is only slowly beginning to accept that we must completely reconsider the history of ancient India. Needless to say, the present chronological reconstruction is certainly boldly conjectural for the earlier dates, but it has the advantage of giving the native Indian traditions proper weight and also taking into account the latest evidence. In particular, the discovery that the mighty, 1,800-mile-long Sarasvatî River, which once flowed through the heartland of the early Vedic civilization, had run dry by around 1900 B.C.E. represents a significant chronological marker. It helps us fix antecedent and subsequent cultural developments in a more plausible manner than has hitherto been possible.

Another potential chronological signpost is the recent identification of underwater ruins in the Gulf of Kutch as Dvâraka, the God-man Krishna's royal city. The ruins have been dated c. 1450 B.C.E. If we tentatively assign the Pândavas to this time and allow a very conservative twenty years per generation, we are now able to construct, with the help of these two dates together with the Puranic genealogies (as reconstructed by F. E. Pargiter), a plausible alternative chronology for ancient India.

589

*B.C.E.*

| | |
|---|---|
| **250,000** | Earliest known human presence in India. |
| **40,000** | Painted rock shelters in Central India. |
| **6500** | Beginnings of the town of Mehrgarh (now in Afghanistan), showing a remarkable cultural continuity with the Indus-Sarasvatî civilization and later Hindu culture. By the fifth millennium B.C.E., Mehrgarh had grown into a settlement of around 20,000 people (the size of the twentieth-century university town of Stanford, California). Carbon dating has yielded dates going back to 8000 B.C.E. |
| **4000–3000** | Pre-Harappan phase of the Indus-Sarasvatî Civilization, as seen in the developments of such sites as Balakot, Amri, and Hakra. |
| **4000–2000** | Period indicated for the *Rig-Veda* by astronomical data given in the text itself. This can be considered the era during which the core hymns of the *Rig-Veda* ("Knowledge of Praise") and also of the other three Vedic *Samhitâs*, and possibly also the original *Purâna* ("Ancient Lore"), were composed. |

This must also have been the period of **Manu Svayambhuva**, the first Manu, as well as the next five Manus, unless we follow conventional scholarship and take these figures as purely fictional. Manu is credited with the authorship of the *Manu-Smriti*, though the extant text is placed between 300 B.C.E. and 200 C.E.

Contemporaries of the first Manu were the seven great seers **Marîci, Angiras, Atri, Pulaha, Kratu, Pulastya,** and **Vashishtha.** Angiras is associated with the *Atharva-Veda* and is the name of later sages as well.

This is also the era of the first **Bhrigu**, a fierce sage, who is said to have taken birth again in the age of Manu Vaivasvata (see 3310 B.C.E.). His descendants (known as the Bhârgavas) were a powerful religious force in Vedic times and were particularly associated with the *Atharva-Veda*.

During this time also lived the original Sage **Nârada** (of whom the *Purânas* know seven incarnations) and **Daksha** or **Kan** (the first of two incarnations by that name), whose daughter Satî was married to Shiva.

| | |
|---|---|
| **3310** | Period of **Manu Vaivasvata**, the seventh Manu and the first ruler after the great flood reported in some Hindu scriptures, who lived ninety-three generations before the Pândavas. His son **Ikshvâku** founded the solar dynasty of Ayodhyâ, the lineage of North Indian kings to which the God-man Râma belonged (see 2050 B.C.E.). Manu's grandson **Candra**, son of the sage **Atri**, founded the lunar dynasty to which the God-man Krishna belonged. |

This is also the era of the seven great seers **Vashishtha, Kashyapa, Atri, Jamadagni, Gautama, Vishvâmitra,** and **Bharadvâja.**

| | |
|---|---|
| **3210** | Time of the wicked King **Vena**, who was killed by the power of *mantras,* and his sage successor **Prithu** of Ayodhyâ, who was a great visionary and benign ruler. |
| **Feb. 18, 3102** | Traditional but improbable Hindu date (according to the *Purânas)* for the beginning of the dark age (*kali-yuga*), which, according to some pundits, coincides with the end of the great war chronicled in the *Mahâbhârata*. This is the time of the God-man Krishna and Prince Arjuna. |

According to Greek sources, Heracles (= Krishna) lived 138 generations before Alexander the Great (c. 325 B.C.E.), but see 1450 B.C.E.

**3000**     Beginnings of the urban centers along the Indus River. These were part of the sprawling Indus-Sarasvatî Civilization, which extended over an area of approximately 300,000 square miles. Since the earliest archaeological layers of Mohenjo-Daro are inaccessible because of nearly forty feet of groundwater, the date of 2600 B.C.E. usually given for this town can safely be pushed back by several centuries.

**2950**     Beginning of the Old Kingdom of Egypt.

**2600–1900**     The so-called "Harappan phase" of the Indus-Sarasvatî Civilization, named after the large town of Harappa. During this period there was extensive export of goods, notably wood, to Sumer and other Middle-Eastern cultures.

**2600–1400**     Creation of the teachings that subsequently crystallized into the *Brâhmanas* (ritual texts). Their approximate chronological sequence is as follows: *Panca-Vimsha* (also called *Tândya-* or *Praudha-Brâhmana;* Sarasvatî and Drishadvatî Rivers are still prominent; this text also does not yet refer to the united Kuru-Pancâlas), *Taittirîya* (refers to the united Kuru-Pancâlas), *Jaminîya, Kaushîtaki* (or *Shânkhâyana), Aitareya, Shata-Patha,* and *Go-Patha.* This is also the era of the beginnings of Âyur-Veda (Northern India's medical tradition), deriving from teachings found in the *Atharva-Veda.*

**2510**     **King Sagara**, of the solar dynasty, whose 60,000 sons are said to have been killed by **Kapila** (who presumably is not the same sage who is remembered as the originator of the Sâmkhya tradition).

This is also the era of **Pratardana,** son of King **Divodâsa II**, who was a sage philosopher credited in the *Kaushîtaki-Upanishad* (2.14) with advocating the then still novel idea of the "inner fire sacrifice" (*antara-agni-hotra*). Pratardana built upon the earlier sacrificial philosophy of **Mahidâsa** and **Gârgyâyana.**

**2450**     King **Bharata** of the Pauravas, after whom India is named and to whose lineage belong the Pândavas.

Alternative date of the Bharata war suggested by the sixth-century astronomer Varâhamihira, which, however, seems much too early.

**2371–2316**     Sargon, ruler of the city of Agade, whom the British scholar L. A. Waddell (erroneously) identified with King Sagara. Sargon apparently had a permanent army of 5,400 soldiers, which allowed him to conquer the neighboring city-states one after the other. The Akkadian kingdom in turn was conquered by the Babylonians, whose mathematics indicate the formative influence of the kind of mathematics expounded in the *Shulba-Sûtras* and which was essentially present already in the early *Brâhmanas.*

**2050**     King **Dasharatha** of Ayodhyâ, the father of **Râma, Bharata, Lakshmana,** and **Shatrughna.** Dasharatha is mentioned in a Hittite inscription dated c. 1400 B.C.E. together with Indra, the Nâsatyas, and the Ashvins, showing that in the intervening two millennia the emperor had been thoroughly mythologized. **Râma**, said to have been born at the end of the *tretâ-yuga* (traditionally fixed to 867,000 B.C.E.), is the hero of the *Râmâyana.* This "original epic" (*âdi-kâvya*) was composed by **Vâlmîki**, supposedly a contemporary of Râma and teacher of the famous sage **Bharadvâja**, though the extant Sanskrit version is far more recent (possibly 300 B.C.E.). Râma's reign was a golden age for the ancient kingdom of Ayodhyâ in the north of India. His wife **Sîtâ** was abducted by **Râvana**, the demonic ruler of Sri Lanka (formerly Ceylon). With the help of the wise monkey-headed demigod **Hanumat**, he succeeded in rescuing Sîtâ, who embodies the principle of fidelity. The Vedic people are known to have been experienced seafarers, and crossing the ocean to the island of Sri Lanka would not have been difficult for them.

Sage **Rishyashringa**, son-in-law of Dasharatha, who restored fertility to the emperor's three wives.

Sage **Vâmadeva**, friend of Vashishtha, who composed the hymns of the fourth *mandala* ("cycle") of the *Rig-Veda*. The *Râmâyana* knows him as the priest of Dasharatha.

**1970** King **Sudâs** (or Sudâsa), famous for the Battle of the Ten Kings mentioned in the *Rig-Veda* and for his patronage of the great sages **Vashishtha** and **Vishvamitra** (composer of the hymns in the third *mandala* of the *Rig-Veda*). There have been many other Vashishthas and Vishvamitras in earlier and later times.

Sage **Kavasha**, who is mentioned in the *Rig-Veda* (7.18.12) as having drowned in the waters of the Parushnî River.

**1900** At this point, the mighty Sarasvatî River, whose fertile banks were once the central home of the Indus-Sarasvatî civilization, no longer runs to the Arabian Sea but has virtually dried up. Today the Sarasvatî is only a small river, called Ghaggar. Since the *Rig-Veda* still remembers the Sarasvatî as an ocean-going river, many of its hymns must have been composed in the third millennium and perhaps earlier still.

**1590** **Tura Kâvasheya** (1590 B.C.E.), a remote descendant of Sage Kavasha, who is mentioned in the *Brihad-Âranyaka-Upanishad* (6.5.4) as the first *guru* of the teaching lineage behind this scripture.

**1550** The last hymns of the *Rig-Veda* were composed by **Devâpi** (elder brother of King Shântanu, Bhîshma's father), who renounced the world at an early age.

**1500–1200** This is usually considered to be the period of the (now refuted) invasion of the Sanskrit-speaking Indo-Aryan tribes from the Russian steppes. The strong evidence against this nineteenth-century assumption is discussed in the book *In Search of the Cradle of Civilization* by Georg Feuerstein, Subhash Kak, and David Frawley. The Indo-Europeans appear to have settled on the Indian subcontinent long before then and can be associated already with the town of Mehrgarh (see 6500 B.C.E.).

**1500–500** The "dark age" according to conventional historians such as Vincent A. Smith (*The Oxford History of India*)—a notion that is profoundly challenged by the available evidence gathered in the present chronology.

**1450** The five **Pândava princes**, sons of King Dhritarâshtra and cousins of the Kaurava princes— the two contending parties in the great Bharata war.

This is the approximate date of the submerged archaeological site of Dvârakâ in Gujarat, which has been identified by some archaeologists as the hometown of the God-man **Krishna**. Curiously, the date of 1450 B.C.E. coincides with a major natural catastrophe in the Mediterranean that annihilated the Minoan civilization.

According to Puranic tradition, Kushasthalî was the name of the island on which King Revata (3250 B.C.E.), the great grandson of Manu Vaivasvata, built the first city, or the first fort, according to some accounts, in that area. After a short span of time, Revata's city became submerged under the waters of the Gulf of Kutch in the Arabian Sea. Much later, Krishna built Dvârakâ, though his city met with the same fate, apparently shortly after the God-man's death. If the identification of the underwater ruins as Dvârakâ is correct, we also have a date for the eighteen-day war chronicled in the *Mahâbhârata*. It was fought between the Kurus and the Pândavas and their respective allies. The great hero of the Pândavas was Prince **Arjuna,** the disciple of Krishna. Their dialogue just before the first battle was fought forms the *Bhagavad-Gîtâ* ("Lord's Song"), which, however, is most likely a later creation (see 500 B.C.E.).

Sage **Vyâsa,** who "arranges" the four Vedic *Samhitâs—Rig-Veda, Sâma-Veda, Yajur-Veda,* and *Atharva-Veda*—as well as composes the *Jaya* (the original version of the *Mahâbhârata*) and collects the oldest *Purâna* or *Purânas.*

Sage **Uddhâva,** minister and friend of Krishna to whom the *Uddhâva-Gîtâ* embedded in the *Bhâgavata-Purâna* is (wrongly) attributed.

| | |
|---|---|
| **1410** | King **Parikshît II,** Arjuna's grandson, who had to confront the social chaos in the aftermath of the Bharata war. |
| **1390** | Sage **Uddâlaka,** teacher of the famous **Yâjnavalkya Vâjasaneya,** who had fifteen main disciples, including his own son **Shvetaketu** (whose instruction is recorded in the *Chândogya-Upanishad*), **Khagodara** (father of Ashtâvakra), **Âsuri** (who might be the same as the disciple of the sage Kapila mentioned in the *Mahâbhârata*), and the fabulously wealthy King **Janaka** of Videha. Yâjnavalkya's teachings are recorded in the *Shata-Patha-Brâhmana,* and some of them are also preserved in the *Brihad-Âranyaka-Upanishad.* |

**Tittiri** (a great authority on the *Yajur-Veda*) and **Pippalâda,** compiler of the *Atharva-Veda* and teacher of **Âshvalâyana,** composer of the *Rig-Veda-Prâtishâkya.*

**Shaunaka,** a great priestly authority and a teacher of Âshvalâyana.

| | |
|---|---|
| **1370** | King **Janamejaya III** of the Kuru-Pauravas, son of Parikshît II, who is remembered for having sponsored a large-scale horse sacrifice (*ashva-medha*). |
| **1350** | Sage **Ashtâvakra,** who is mentioned in the *Mahâbhârata* and who is also (wrongly) credited with the authorship of the *Ashtâvakra-Gîtâ,* a work on Vedânta. |

This is also the approximate date of the core of astronomer Lagadha's *Vedânga-Jyotishâ,* as suggested by astronomical data given in the text itself. This work was subsequently modified through additions and rewriting.

| | |
|---|---|
| **1290** | **Pancashikha,** a disciple of Sage Âsuri, who may be the same as the early authority on Sâmkhya. If so, this would also be the era of **Kapila,** the reputed founder of the Sâmkhya tradition. |
| **1270** | **Yâska,** author of the *Nirukta,* a commentary on the *Vedas.* |
| **1000–900** | Beginning of the so-called "second urbanization" along the Ganges (Gangâ) River. Also, probable beginning of Vaishnavism (centered on the worship of the Divine in the form of Vishnu). |
| **800–600** | Possible date of the *Shvetâshvatara-Upanishad,* which is a Shaiva scripture introducing the ideal of devotion (*bhakti*), and the *Katha-Upanishad,* which defines Yoga as the "holding of the senses." These two texts are usually placed around 500–300 B.C.E. |
| **599–527** | **Vardhamâna Mahâvîra,** founder of historical Jainism, who is said to be the twenty-fourth "ford-maker" (*tîrthankara*). Like Hinduism and Buddhism, Jainism is concerned with the spiritual liberation of the individual. The works of earlier teachers of Jainism, the *Pûrvas,* have been lost. |

**570**      **Pautimâshîputra**, the last authority mentioned in the teaching lineage of the *Brihad-Âranya-ka-Upanishad*, the oldest of the extant *Upanishads* (spanning over fifty teacher generations amounting to c. 1000 years).

**563–483**      **Siddhârtha Gautama**, of the Shakya clan of what is now Nepal, founder of Buddhism, who attained enlightenment in his thirty-fifth year. He is known to have studied with two teachers, **Ârâda Kâlâpa** and **Rudraka Râmaputra**, who probably taught him a form of Yoga. He was fond of meditation and very skilled in it. This also is the time of **Ajita Keshakambalin,** whose materialist philosophy was criticized by the Buddha.

**550**      Approximate birth date of **Goshâla Maskarîputra** (died c. 487 B.C.E.)**,** the founder of the Âjîvika sect of naked ascetics, which was criticized by the Buddha for some of its doctrines (notably its fatalism).

         Conventional date for the grammarian **Pânini**, who composed the *Ashtâdhyayî*, a grammatical textbook that served nineteenth-century Western philologists as a model for their own grammatical theories. Native Indian tradition places him much earlier.

         Conventional date for **Kanâda**, author of the *Vaisheshika-Sûtra*, the principal work of the Vaisheshika school (of natural philosophy) of Hinduism. This is probably also the time of **Akshapâda Gautama**, founder of the Nyâya school (of logic) and composer of the *Nyâya-Sûtra* (which mentions Yoga).

**500–400**      Composition of the extant version of the *Bhagavad-Gîtâ*, which is a part of the present edition of the *Mahâbhârata,* and the oldest full-fledged Yoga scripture of which we have knowledge. The *Gîtâ* is presented as a dialogue between the God-man Krishna and Prince Arjuna, who lived much earlier (see 1450 B.C.E.). It emphasizes the Yoga of devotion (*bhakti-yoga*).

**483**      Probable date of the First Council at which the Buddha's senior disciples systematized his teachings.

**400**      Probable date of the *Dhamma-Pada* written in the Pali language, which can be looked upon as a textbook of Yoga not unlike the Hindu *Bhagavad-Gîtâ*.

**383**      Probable date of the Second Council of the Buddhist monastic community, at which sermons and poems by monks and nuns were officially added to the canonical scriptures. At that time, the community split into Theravâdins and Mahâsânghikas (whose thinking subsequently gave rise to Mahâyâna Buddhism).

**327–325**      Invasion of Northern India by **Alexander the Great**, which barely affected India's civilization. He met with King Candragupta Maurya in 326 or 325 B.C.E.

**300**      Council of Pataliputra, after which the Jainas split into Digambaras (nude followers) and Shvetambaras (followers dressed in white).

**300–100**      Composition of important philosophical passages of the *Mahâbhârata* epic, notably the *Moksha-Dharma*.

**269–232**      Emperor **Ashoka**, who, after his conversion, greatly furthered the dissemination of Buddhism.

**200**      Conventional date of the composition of **Jaimini's** *Mîmâmsâ-Sûtra*, the authoritative text of the Mîmâmsâ school (of ritualism) of Hinduism.

| | |
|---|---|
| **200 B.C.E.–**<br>**400 C.E.** | Era of the greatest influence of Buddhism in India. |
| **150** | Conventional date of **Patanjali**, the grammarian, who is traditionally also regarded as the author of works on medicine and of the *Yoga-Sûtra* (but see 200 C.E.). |
| **100** | Probable date of **Lakulin** (or Lakulîsha), the semi-legendary founder of the Yoga-practicing Pâshupatas and alleged author of the *Pâshupata-Sûtra*. |
| | The rise of Mahâyâna Buddhism; composition of the earliest Mahâyâna-*Sûtras*, such as the *Ashtâ-Sâhasrikâ*, the *Lankâ-Avatâra*, and the *Sad-Dharma-Pundarîka*, teaching emptiness (*shûnyatâ*) and compassion (*karunâ*). |
| *C.E.* | |
| **50** | Arrival of Buddhism in China. |
| | Possible date of St. Thomas's mission to India. |
| **100** | **Caraka**, a great authority on Âyurveda. |
| | The Buddhist adept **Nâgârjuna**, founder of the Mâdhyamika school. |
| **150** | Buddhist scholar **Âryadeva**, a disciple of Nâgârjuna and author of the *Catuh-Shataka*. |
| **150–200** | Composition of the *Yoga-Sûtra* of **Patanjali** (who is very probably different from the grammarian by this name) and of the *Brahma-Sûtra* of **Bâdarâyana**, one of the fundamental works of the Vedânta tradition. This is also the period of the final editing of Manu's ancient *Dharma-Sûtra* (also known as the *Manu-Smriti*), which contains a chapter on the duties of forest-dwellers and ascetics and defines Yoga as restraint of the senses. |
| **300–400** | Date of the great Buddhist teachers **Asanga** (290–360 C.E.) and **Vasubandhu** (316–396 C.E.), who were brothers. The former established the Yogâcâra school, and the latter founded the Vijnânavâda school of Mahâyâna Buddhism. |
| **320–500** | The rulers of the Gupta dynasty bring about a cultural fluorescence, especially around 400 C.E. |
| **350–500** | Emergence of Buddhist and Hindu Tantrism. There is a Tibetan translation of a group of Tantric *Sûtras* under the title of *Mahâ-Sannipâta*. One of these *Sûtras*, the *Ratna-Ketu-Dhâranî*, was translated into Chinese around 450 C.E. |
| **381** | The Chandûl-Mandûl Bagîchî inscription of **Candragupta II**, which mentions several teachers of the Pâshupata order and also depicts **Lakulîsha**, the founder of the order. According to the *Mahâbhârata*, the Pâshupata teachings stem from **Shiva Shrî Kantha**, which must mean that Lakulîsha merely revived the doctrine. |
| **400–500** | Composition of the *Mârkandeya-Purâna*, one of the earliest works of this literary genre, which describes a form of ritualistic Yoga. Some of its teachings, however, must be considered to have been derived from much earlier Puranic traditions. |
| | This is also a likely date for the composition of **Îshvara Krishna's** *Sâmkhya-Kârikâ*, the source text of Classical Sâmkhya, and the composition of the *Jayâkhya-* and *Sâtvata-Samhitâs*, as well as other early scriptures of the Pancarâtra (Vaishnava) tradition. |

This is, moreover, the time of the founding of the Buddhist monastic university of Nâlandâ, which produced many great teachers and adepts in the following centuries.

**450**    Likely date of the *Yoga-Bhâshya*, the oldest extant commentary on the *Yoga-Sûtra*.

This is also the time of the Buddhist philosopher **Dinnâga**, who authored seventeen works on logic and epistemology.

**470–543**    **Bodhidharma**, founder of the Buddhist meditation (*chan*) tradition in China.

**500**    Invasion of India by the Huns.

**505**    Birth of the astronomer **Varâhamihira**.

**550–700**    Expansion of the Pancarâtra tradition into South India. An inscription by **Râjasimhavarman** in the Kailâsanâtha Temple refers to the Shaiva *Âgamas* of South India.

Composition of the *Ahirbudhnya-Samhitâ*, an important Pancarâtra scripture.

**600**    Composition of the Buddhist *Hevajra-* and *Guhya-Samâja-Tantra*.

**600–650**    Buddhist philosopher **Dharmakîrti.**

**606–647**    King **Harsha**, a patron of the arts, immortalized by the court poet **Bâna**.

**638–713**    **Hui-Neng**, sixth and last patriarch of Chinese Buddhism.

**650**    **Tirumûlâr**, renowned adept-bard of South India, author of the *Tiru-Mantiram*.

This also was the era of the long-lived Buddhist teacher **Candrakîrti**, abbot of the monastic university of Nâlandâ, who is considered the most important representative of the Mâdhyamika school after Nâgârjuna.

**690–730**    The Buddhist teacher **Shântideva** (also called Busuku), author of the *Bodhi-Caryâ-Avâtara* and the *Shikshâ-Samuccaya*, who is counted among the eighty-four great adepts (*mahâ-siddha*).

This also was the time of **Padmasambhava** ("Guru Rimpoche"), who, at Shântideva's request, freed Tibet of lower spirits so that the Tibetans would become receptive to Buddhist teachings. Padmasambhava is honored as a second Buddha by the Nyingma school.

**788–820**    Traditional date of **Shankara**, the great preceptor of Advaita Vedânta; some pundits place him as early as 509 B.C.E., others around 84 C.E. However, his teacher's teacher **Gaudapâda**, on whose *Mândûkya-Kârikâ* he wrote a commentary, cannot be placed much before 500 C.E. because of his clear leanings toward Mâdhyamika Buddhism. It is, however, likely that the traditional date is too late and that Shankara should be placed between 650–750 C.E.

**800**    Final redaction of the *Caraka-Samhitâ*, one of the principal works on Âyurveda.

**825**    "Discovery" of the *Shiva-Sûtra* by the Kashmiri adept **Vasugupta**, who also authored the *Spanda-Sûtra*.

**850**    Composition of **Vâcaspati Mishra's** *Tattva-Vaishâradî* commentary on the *Yoga-Bhâshya*.

| | |
|---|---|
| **900** | Date of the oldest extant Hindu *Tantra* manuscripts, such as the *Pârameshvara-Mata-Tantra* (859 C.E.) and the *Sarva-Jnâna-Uttara-Tantra*. |
| | **Nâgarjuna's** *Panca-Krama*, which makes use of the first five stages of Patanjali's eightfold Yoga. |
| | **Nâthamuni,** the renowned preceptor of Vaishnavism and author of the *Yoga-Rahasya*. |
| **900–1000** | Composition of the *Lakshmî-Tantra* (an important Pancarâtra scripture), the *Kaula-Jnâna-Nirnaya* (a major text of the Nâtha order), the *Bhâgavata-Purâna*, and the expanded version of the *Yoga-Vâsishtha*. |
| **900–1200** | Composition of the *Amrita-Bindu-*, *Amrita-Nâda-Bindu-*, and *Nâda-Bindu-Upanishads*. |
| **928–1009** | **Tilopa,** one of the eighty-four *mahâ-siddhas* and teacher of Nâropa. He is considered the founder of the Kagyu school of Tibetan Buddhism. |
| **950–970** | Birth of the great Shaiva scholar and adept **Abhinava Gupta,** author of the voluminous *Tantra-Âloka* and numerous other works. |
| **956–1040** | **Nâropa,** whose difficult discipleship under Tilopa is recalled in his well-known biography. |
| **973–1048** | The Arab scientist and philosopher **Alberuni** composed a paraphrase of the *Yoga-Sûtra* in Arabic (c. 1025 C.E.). |
| **982–1054** | **Atîsha** (also known as Dîpamkâra Shrîjnâna), of royal birth, who was one of the greatest Buddhist masters of his time, and whose *Bodhi-Patha-Pradîpâ* served as the foundation for all subsequent teachings on the stages of the path (Tibetan: *lam-rim*). |
| **1000** | Composition of King **Bhoja's** *Râja-Mârtanda*, a commentary on the *Yoga-Sûtra*, **Nârada's** *Bhakti-Sûtra*, and the comprehensive *Prapanca-Sâra-Tantra*. |
| | Emergence of the Kâlacakrayâna, an offshoot of Mahâyâna Buddhism. |
| | Beginning of the Kâlâmukha order of Shaivism. |
| **1000–1200** | Gradual disappearance of Buddhism from India. |
| **1000–1400** | Composition of *Upanishads* with a strong Shâkta orientation. |
| **1012–1097** | The Tibetan teacher **Marpa,** who was famous for his translations of Sanskrit texts into Tibetan. |
| **1017–1137** | **Râmânuja,** one of the great preceptors of medieval Vaishnaivism and representative of Vishishta-Advaita Vedânta. |
| **1040–1123** | **Milarepa,** Tibet's most beloved *yogin*, who was a disciple of Marpa. |
| **1050** | Composition of **Cekkilar's** *Peria-Purânam* in Tamil and collection of Tamil Shaiva hymns into the *Tiru-Mûrai*, South India's equivalent of the Sanskrit *Vedas*. |
| | Composition of important Tantric works like the *Kaula-Jnâna-Nirnaya* ascribed to Matsyendra Nâtha, and the *Shâradâ-Tilaka-Tantra*. |

**1079–1153**    **Gampopa**, Milarepa's main disciple, who was one of Tibet's greatest scholar-adepts, and who authored many works, including the *Jewel Ornament of Liberation*.

**1089–1172**    **Hemacandra**, famous Jaina philosopher and author of the *Yoga-Shâstra*.

**1106–1167**    **Basava** (or Basavanna), reputed founder of the Lingâyata tradition of South India, which is also known as Vîra-Shaivism.

**1150–1250**    Composition of the *Kubjikâ-Mata-Tantra* and also the *Yoga-Upanishads*, with the exception of the *Bindu-Upanishads* mentioned above (see 900–1200 C.E.).

**1190–1276**    **Madhva**, founder of the dualist branch of Vedânta; his dates are sometimes given as 1199–1278 C.E.

**1200**    **Jayaratha**, a Kashmiri Tantric scholar, who wrote many excellent commentaries.

Composition of the *Kula-Arnava-Tantra* (the most important text of the Kaula school).

Beginning of the Muslim invasion of India.

**1200–1300**    Composition of Hatha-Yoga scriptures such as the *Yoga-Yâjnavalkya*, *Ânanda-Samuccaya*, and *Carpata-Shataka*.

**1250**    **Meykandar**, author of the *Shiva-Jnâna-Bodha*, an important Shaiva text.

**1275–1296**    **Jnânadeva** (or Jnâneshvara), Maharashtra's most renowned Yoga adept and author of the *Jnâneshvarî*, a poetic Marathi commentary on the *Bhagavad-Gîtâ*.

**1288**    **Marco Polo's** first visit to India. He returned five years later.

**1290–1364**    **Buston,** Tibetan historian and author of the famous *Deb-ther Non-po* ("Blue Annals").

**1300**    Possible beginning of the Aghorî order of Shaivism.

**1350**    Composition of the *Hatha-Yoga-Pradîpikâ*, one of the standard manuals of Hatha-Yoga.

Possible date of the composition of the *Sâmkhya-Sûtra* ascribed to Kapila.

**1357–1419**    **Tsongkhapa**, who reformed Tibetan Buddhism, which had become degenerated through sexual and magical practices. He authored numerous works and founded the Gelugpa school, which is now the largest branch of Tibetan Buddhism.

**1391–1478**    **Gendun Drub,** the first Dalai Lama.

**1440–1518**    **Kabîr**, a popular poet-saint of North India, who pioneered the integration of Hinduism with Muslim teachings.

**1450**    **Vidyâranya**, author of the *Jîvan-Mukti-Viveka*, a Vedânta work on the ideal of liberation during embodiment; he makes use of the *Yoga-Sûtra* and other Yoga texts.

**1455–1570**    **Drukpa Kunleg**, a famous crazy-wisdom adept of Tibet.

**1469–1539**    **Nânak**, founder of the Sikh tradition.

| | |
|---|---|
| **1479–1531** | **Vallabha**, renowned teacher of Bhakti-Yoga centering on the worship of God Krishna. |
| **1485–1533** | **Caitanya**, one of the foremost medieval Vaishnava teachers of Bengal and a great *bhakti-yogin*. |
| **1498** | **Vasco da Gama** arrives at the coast of Malabar. |
| **1500** | Composition of the *Avadhûta-Gîtâ*. |
| | **Râghava Bhatta**, author of various Tantric works, including the *Kâlî-Tattva*. |
| | **Brahmânanda Giri**, Tantric adept and author of several texts, including the *Shâkta-Ânanda-Taranginî*. |
| **1502** | Composition of the *Âgama-Kalpa-Druma* of Govinda, son of Jagannâtha. |
| | **Krishnânanda**, author of the *Tantra-Sâra* and other Tantric works. |
| **1532–1623** | **Tulsî Dâs**, a widely influential North Indian poet-saint, who composed the Hindi *Râmâyana*. |
| **1550** | **Vijnâna Bhikshu**, author of numerous philosophical works, including commentaries on the *Yoga-Sûtra*, notably the voluminous *Yoga-Vârttika*. |
| | Composition of the *Yoginî-Tantra*, a valuable resource of legendary materials relating to the Devî cult. |
| **1556–1605** | Emperor **Akbar**, greatest of India's Muslim rulers. |
| **1577** | Composition of the *Shrî-Tattva-Cintâmani* by **Pûrnânanda Giri**, who also wrote the *Shâkta-Krama* and *Shyâmâ-Rahasya*. |
| | Composition of the voluminous *Shakti-Samgama-Tantra*. |
| **1600** | **Subhagânanda Nâtha**, a Kashmiri Tantric scholar-adept, who wrote the most important commentary on the *Tantra-Râja-Tantra*, entitled *Manoramâ*. His pupil was the well-known **Prakâshânanda Nâtha**. |
| | The British and Dutch establish trading companies in India. |
| **1617–1682** | **Ngawang Lobsang Gyatso,** the fifth Dalai Lama (known as the "Great Fifth"), the most dynamic and influential of the early Dalai Lamas and a prodigious writer. |
| **1650** | Composition of the *Gheranda-Samhitâ*, a popular manual of Hatha-Yoga. |
| **1718–1775** | **Ram Prasad Sen**, celebrated Bengali poet and Kâlî worshiper. |
| **1750** | Composition of the well-known *Mahânirvâna-Tantra* and the *Shiva-Samhitâ*, an important work on Hatha-Yoga. |
| | **Bhâsararâya**, the greatest Shri-Vidyâ authority, who authored over forty works, the most important being the *Setu-Bandha* (an extensive commentary on the *Yoginî-Hridaya-Tantra*). |
| **1760** | Beginning of the British Raj in India. |

**1772–1833**     **Rammohun Roy**, founder of the influential Brahma Samaj organization, who has been called the "father of modern India."

**1834–1886**     **Ramakrishna**, one of the great mystics of nineteenth-century India.

**1861–1941**     **Rabindranath Tagore**, poet laureate of Bengal and a representative of modern Indian humanism.

**1862–1902**     **Swami Vivekananda**, chief disciple of Sri Ramakrishna and founder of the Ramakrishna Mission (now Ramakrishna-Vivekananda Mission), a key figure in the dissemination of Hinduism and Yoga in Europe and America.

**1869–1948**     **Mohandas Karamchand Gandhi**, advocate of the principle of nonharming (*ahimsâ*) in all areas of life, especially politics.

**1872–1950**     **Sri Aurobindo**, originator of Integral Yoga.

**1875**     Founding of the Theosophical Society, which established its headquarters in Adyar, India, in 1882; thanks to the efforts of this organization, many Sanskrit texts were translated into English for the first time.

**1876–1933**     **Tupden Gyatso**, the thirteenth Dalai Lama, who sent Tibetans to be educated in Europe to prepare Tibet for the modern world.

**1879–1950**     **Ramana Maharshi** of Tiruvannamalai in South India, one of modern India's most renowned sages and a staunch proponent of Advaita Vedânta.

**1935–**     **Tenzin Gyatso,** the fourteenth Dalai Lama and winner of the Nobel Peace Prize, who continues the mission of the previous Dalai Lama of integrating Tibet with the rest of the world.

**1947**     India achieves political independence.

# GLOSSARY OF KEY TERMS

**Âcâra** ("conduct"). Way of life, approach to spiritual practice.

**Âcârya** ("preceptor"). A teacher, who may or may not be one's *guru*.

**Adhyâtma-Yoga** ("Yoga of the innermost Self"). A Vedânta-based Yoga.

**Advaita Vedânta** ("nondual Vedânta"). The metaphysical tradition of nondualism based on the *Upanishads*. Its two main branches are Kevala-Advaita (written Kevalâdvaita, "Radical Nondualism"), as taught by Shankara, and Vishishta-Advaita (written Vishishtâdvaita, "Qualified Nondualism"), as taught by Râmânuja.

**Âgama** ("tradition"). A revealed ritual text belonging to the Pancarâtra-Vaishnava tradition or to the Shaiva tradition (in which case it is typically called *Tantra*).

**Agastya.** The name of several sages, the most famous of whom was a great adept (*siddha*) in Southern India.

**Aghora** ("nonterrible"). An epithet of God Shiva, paradoxically, in his terrifying aspect.

**Aghorî.** A Tantra-based Shaiva sect whose members are well-known for their extremist practices. See also Kâlâmukha, Kâpâlika.

**Ahamkâra** ("I-maker"). The sense of individuation, or ego.

**Ahimsâ** ("nonharming"). Abstention from harmful actions, thoughts, and words. An important moral discipline (*yama*) in Yoga, Buddhism, and Jainism.

**Âjnâ-cakra** ("command wheel"). The psychoenergetic center located in the middle of the head, also known as the "third eye."

**Ajnâna.** See *avidyâ*.

**Âlvâr.** A member of a group of Vishnu-worshiping poet-saints of South India.

**Anâhata-cakra** ("wheel of the unstruck [sound]"). The psychoenergetic center located at the heart, where the universal sound *om* can be heard in meditation.

**Ânanda** ("bliss"). (i) In Vedânta, the mind-transcending blissfulness of the ultimate Reality, or Self, which is not considered to be a quality but the very essence of Reality. (ii) In Patanjali's Yoga, an experiential state associated with a lower type of ecstasy, viz. *samprajnâta-samâdhi*.

**Anga** ("limb"). (i) The body as a whole, or a limb. (ii) A category of yogic practices. See also *yoga-anga*.

**Arjuna.** The hero of the *Bhagavad-Gîtâ* and disciple of Lord Krishna.

**Ârogya** ("health, well-being"). The opposite of disease (*vyâdhi*); a positive state of bodily and mental balance. Cf. *vyâdhi*.

**Asamprajnâta-samâdhi** ("supraconscious ecstasy"). The technique leading to, the experience of, unified consciousness in which the subject becomes

601

one with the experienced object, without any thoughts or ideas being present. In Vedânta, this is known as *nirvikalpa-samâdhi*. Cf. *samprajnâta-samâdhi*.

**Âsana** ("seat, posture"). (i) The seat on which the *yogin* or *yoginî* is seated. (ii) Posture, which is the third limb (*anga*) of Patanjali's eightfold Yoga.

**Asanga.** A great Mahâyâna Buddhist master and originator of the Yogâcâra school.

**Âshrama.** (i) Hermitage. (ii) Stage of life. Traditional Hinduism distinguishes four such stages: pupilage (*brahmacarya*), householdership (*gârhasthya*), forest-dwelling life (*vana-prâsthya*), and renunciation (*samnyâsa*).

**Asmitâ** ("I-am-ness"). See *ahamkâra*.

**Asparsha-Yoga** ("Yoga of noncontact"). The nondualist Yoga expounded in the *Mândûkya-Kârikâ* of Gaudapâda, the teacher of Shankara's teacher.

**Atharva-Veda** ("Atharvan's knowledge"). One of the four Vedic hymn collections (*samhitâ*) that deals primarily with magical spells but also contains several important documents of early Yoga. See also *Rig-Veda, Sâma-Veda, Yajur-Veda*.

**Âtma-darshana** ("Self vision"). The same as Self-realization, or liberation.

**Âtman** ("self"). (i) Oneself. (ii) The transcendental Self, which is identical with the Absolute (*brahman*), according to the nondualist schools of thought. Cf. *purusha*.

**Avadhûta** ("he who has cast off"). A radical type of renouncer who abandons all conventions; a crazy adept.

**Avatâra** ("descent"). An incarnation of the Divine, especially of God Vishnu, such as Krishna or Râma.

**Avidyâ** ("ignorance"). Spiritual nescience, which is the root of all human suffering and the cause of one's bondage to egoic states of consciousness. Cf. *jnâna, vidyâ*.

**Âyur-Veda** ("life science"). The native Hindu system of medicine.

**Bandha** ("bond"). (i) Bondage to the phenomenal world, driven by karma, as opposed to liberation (*moksha*). (ii) "Lock"—a special technique used in Hatha-Yoga for confining the life force in certain parts of the body.

**Bhagavad-Gîtâ** ("lord's song"). The earliest and most popular Yoga scripture containing the teachings of Lord Krishna to Arjuna.

**Bhagavat** ("lord"). Appellation of the Divine, often Krishna. In the nominative: Bhagavân.

**Bhâgavata.** (i) Adherent of Vishnu in the form of Krishna. (ii) Name of the tradition of Krishna worshipers.

**Bhâgavata-Purâna.** A comprehensive tenth-century Sanskrit scripture containing, among other things, the mythical life story of Lord Krishna. It is also called *Shrîmad-Bhâgavata*.

**Bhakta** ("devoted, devotee"). A follower of the path of devotion (*bhakti*).

**Bhakti** ("devotion, love"). The spiritual sentiment of loving participation in the Divine.

**Bhakti-Sûtra** ("aphorisms on devotion"). There are two works by this title; one is attributed to the sage Nârada, the other to the sage Shândilya.

**Bhakti-Yoga** ("Yoga of devotion"). One of the principal branches of Hindu Yoga.

**Bhairava.** (i) One of the epithets or forms of Shiva. (ii) Tantric initiate. (iii) Name of one of the masters of Hatha-Yoga.

**Bhairavî.** (i) One of the epithets or forms of Devî. (ii) Tantric female initiate.

**Bhâva** ("state, condition"). In Bhakti-Yoga this refers to a state of uplifted emotion, of which the literature distinguishes five kinds that represent different ways of relating to the Divine.

**Bhrigu.** The most famous of Vedic seers (*rishi*). He often figures as a teacher of Yoga in medieval texts.

**Bhûta** ("element"). (i) Hindu cosmology distinguishes five elements: earth, water, fire, air, and ether/space. (ii) Demon.

**Bhûta-shuddhi** ("purification of the elements"). An important Tantric practice and a precondition for the safe and complete arousal of the serpent power (*kundalinî-shakti*).

**Bîja** ("seed"). (i) A karmic cause in the form of a subconscious activator (*samskâra*). (ii) A meditative object or idea. (iii) Short for *bîja-mantra*.

**Bîja-mantra** ("seed syllable"). A primary *mantra*, such as *om, ram,* or *yam*.

**Bindu** ("drop"). (i) The dot placed above the Sanskrit letter *m* in the syllable *om* and other similar *mantras*, indicating that the sound *m* is to be nasalized. (ii) The nasalized sound itself. (iii) A special psychoenergetic center in the head, close to the *âjnâ-cakra*. (iv) The central point of a *yantra* or *mandala*. (v) In yogic experience, the objectless state of awareness prior to the appearance of images and thoughts but not identical to the transcendental Being-Consciousness. (vi) In Hindu cosmology, the threshold between the unmanifest dimension of Nature and manifestation. (vii) Semen, which, according to Tantrism, should be mingled with the woman's ejaculate called *rajas*.

**Bodhi** ("enlightenment"). The state of enlightenment, or liberation (*moksha*).

**Bodhisattva** ("enlightenment being"). In Mahâyâna Buddhism, the spiritual practitioner who has vowed to commit himself or herself to the liberation of all beings.

**Brahma.** The Creator-God of the famous medieval Hindu triad of deities, which is known as *tri-mûrti*. The other two are Vishnu (as Preserver) and Shiva (as Destroyer). Brahma must be carefully distinguished from *brahman*, which is the eternal, impersonal foundation of existence transcending all deities.

**Brahmacarya** ("brahmic conduct"). The practice of chastity in thought, word, and deed, which is regarded as one of the fundamental moral disciplines (*yama*) of Yoga.

**Brahman.** The Absolute according to Vedânta; the transcendental ground of existence, which is distinct from Brahma, the Creator. See also *âtman*, *sac-cid-ânanda*.

**Brâhmana.** (i) A member of the priestly class of Hindu society, a brahmin. (ii) A type of ritual text explaining the hymns of the *Vedas* as they are relevant to the sacrificial ritualism of the brahmins.

**Buddha** ("awakened"). Title of Gautama, founder of Buddhism.

**Buddhi** ("awareness, wisdom"). The higher, intuitive mind, or faculty of wisdom. This term is also used to denote "thought" or "cognition." See also *citta*, *manas*.

**Caitanya.** A great medieval teacher of Bhakti-Yoga and worshiper of Lord Krishna.

**Cakra** ("wheel"). (i) A psychoenergetic center of the body, of which Tantrism and Hatha-Yoga typically distinguish seven: *mûlâdhâra*, *svâdhishthâna*, *manipura*, *anâhata*, *vishuddha*, *âjnâ*, and *sahasrâra*. These are aligned along the spinal axis and form part of the body of the serpent power (*kundalinî-shakti*).

**Caturtha** ("fourth"). The transcendental Self, as the fourth and ultimate or real state (*avasthâ*) of consciousness, the other three being the normal waking state, dream sleep, and deep sleep.

**Cit** ("awareness, consciousness"). Pure Awareness, or the transcendental Consciousness beyond all thought; the eternal witness. See also *âtman*, *purusha*.

**Citta** ("consciousness, mind"). The finite mind, psyche, or consciousness, which is dependent on the play of attention, as opposed to *cit*. See also *buddhi*, *manas*.

**Darshana** ("vision"). (i) Inner or external vision. (ii) Sighting of an adept, which is considered auspicious. (iii) A philosophical system, or school of thought. Hinduism recognizes six classical perspectives: Yoga, Sâmkhya, Mîmâmsâ, Vedânta, Nyâya, and Vaisheshika.

**Dattâtreya.** A sage connected with the Avadhûta tradition who became deified as an incarnation of God Shiva.

**Deha** ("body"). The physical body, also called *sharîra*.

**Deva** ("shining one, god"). Usually this word refers to one of the many deities of the Hindu pantheon. They are envisioned as powerful beings in subtle dimensions of existence. The term can also stand for the Divine itself. Cf. *devî*.

**Devatâ** ("deity"). See *deva*, *ishta-devatâ*.

**Devî** ("goddess"). The Divine conceived in its feminine aspect. Cf. *deva*.

**Dhâranâ** ("holding"). Concentration, the sixth limb (*anga*) of Patanjali's eightfold Yoga, consisting of the prolonged focusing of attention on a single mental object and leading to meditation (*dhyâna*).

**Dharma** ("bearer"). (i) The cosmic law or order. (ii) Morality or virtue, as one of the legitimate concerns of a human being (*purusha-artha*) sanctioned by Hinduism. It is understood as a manifestation or reflection of the divine law. (iii) Teaching, doctrine. (iv) Quality, as opposed to substance (*dharmin*).

**Dharma-megha-samâdhi** ("ecstasy of *dharma* cloud"). According to Patanjali, the highest form of supraconscious ecstasy (*asamprajnâta-samâdhi*), which is the doorway to liberation.

**Dharma-shâstra** ("moral teaching"). (i) The corpus of moral teachings in Hinduism. (ii) A scripture dealing with morality (*dharma*).

**Dhyâna** ("meditation"). Meditative absorption, or contemplation, the seventh limb (*anga*) of Patanjali's eightfold Yoga, which is understood as a deepening of concentration (*dhâranâ*). See also *samâdhi*.

**Dîkshâ** ("initiation"). An important feature of all yogic schools by which a seeker is made part of a traditional chain of *gurus*.

**Dosha** ("defect, flaw"). This specifically refers to the five faults, namely lust (*kâma*), anger (*krodha*), greed (*lobha*), fear (*bhaya*), and delusion (*moha*). The term also can denote the three humors: *vâta* (wind), *pitta* (bile), and *kapha* (phlegm).

**Duhkha** ("suffering"). According to all liberation teachings of India, conditioned or finite existence is inherently sorrowful or painful. It is this insight that provides the impetus for the spiritual struggle to realize liberation (*moksha*).

**Eka** ("one"). The singular Reality that is omnipresent and omnitemporal. See also *âtman*, *brahman*.

**Ekâgratâ** ("one-pointedness," from *eka* and *agratâ*). The process underlying concentration.

**Ekatanatâ** ("one-flowness," from *eka* and *tanatâ*). The process underlying meditation.

**Gautama.** Name of many sages, including the Buddha and the founder of the Nyâya school of thought.

**Gîtâ** ("song"). Title of many didactic works composed in metric Sanskrit, notably the *Bhagavad-Gîtâ*.

**Gopa** ("cowherd"). In Vaishnavism, a male devotee of Krishna.

**Gopî** ("cowgirl"). A female devotee of Krishna.

**Goraksha.** The founder of the Kânphata order and an early preceptor of Hatha-Yoga, who lived in the tenth or eleventh century.

**Guna** ("strand, quality"). (i) In Yoga, Sâmkhya, and many schools of Vedânta, one of three primary constituents of Nature (*prakriti*): *sattva* (principle of lucidity), *rajas* (principle of dynamism), and *tamas* (principle of inertia). The interaction between them creates the entire manifest and unmanifest cosmos, including all psychomental phenomena. (ii) Virtue, high moral quality.

**Guna-âtîta** ("transcending the qualities"). (i) Liberation, which transcends the constituents (*guna*) of Nature (*prakriti*). (ii) The liberated sage.

**Guru** ("heavy, weighty"). Spiritual teacher.

**Guru-pûjâ** ("*guru* worship"). A core spiritual practice in many schools of Yoga in which the teacher is venerated as an embodiment of the Divine.

**Guru-Yoga.** Yogic practice in which the *guru* is the focus of the disciple's spiritual efforts.

**Hamsa** ("gander," generally translated as "swan"). (i) The breath or life force (*prâna*). (ii) The transcendental Self (*âtman*). (iii) A type of wandering ascetic (*parivrâjaka*).

**Haribhadra Sûri.** An important Jaina teacher, who composed several works on Yoga, including the *Yoga-Bindu*.

**Hatha-Yoga** ("forceful Yoga" or "Yoga of force"). The Yoga of physical discipline, aiming at the awakening of the serpent power (*kundalinî-shakti*) and the creation of an indestructible divine body (*divya-deha*).

**Hemacandra.** An eleventh-century Jaina master, who authored the *Yoga-Shâstra* and other works.

**Hînayâna** ("small vehicle"). The minority school of Buddhism, which revolves around the ideal of the *arhat* (or *arhant*) as opposed to the *bodhisattva*. Cf. Mahâyâna, Vajrayâna.

**Hiranyagarbha** ("golden germ"). (i) The mythical originator of Yoga. (ii) Cosmologically, the condition preceding manifestation, corresponding to Brahma.

**Hrid, Hridaya** ("heart"). Since ancient times considered to be the physical anchor point of the Self (*âtman*). In Tantrism, the heart is the location of the *anâhata-cakra*.

**Indra.** Great Vedic deity associated with the sky and war.

**Indriya** ("pertaining to Indra" or "instrument"). Sense organ, including the lower mind (*manas*) as the sixth sensory instrument.

**Îsh, îsha, îshvara** ("ruler"). (i) The divine Being. (ii) The Creator. (iii) In Patanjali's Yoga, *îshvara* is explained as a "special Self."

**Ishta-devatâ** ("chosen deity"). A spiritual practitioner's favored deity.

**Îshvara Krishna.** Author of the *Sâmkhya-Kârikâ*, the source text of Classical Sâmkhya.

**Îshvara-pranidhâna** ("devotion to the Lord"). One of the practices of restraint (*niyama*) in Patanjali's Yoga.

**Jaina.** (i) Relating to Jainism, the religio-spiritual tradition founded by Mahâvîra, a contemporary of Gautama the Buddha. (ii) A member of Jainism.

**Japa** ("muttering"). The meditative recitation of *mantras*.

**Japin** ("mutterer"). A practitioner of *japa*.

**Jîva** ("living being"). The psyche or finite human personality, which experiences itself as different from others and does not know the transcendental Self directly. Cf. *âtman*, *purusha*.

**Jîva-âtman** ("living self"). The individuated self as opposed to the transcendental Self (*âtman*). The same as *jîva*.

**Jîvan-mukti** ("living liberation"). According to most Vedânta schools, it is possible to gain liberation, or full enlightenment, even while still embodied. The Self-realized adept who is thus liberated is known as a *jîvan-mukta*.

**Jnâna** ("knowledge, wisdom"). Depending on the context, this term can refer either to conventional knowledge or liberating wisdom. In the latter sense, *jnâna* is coessential with the transcendental Reality. Cf. *ajnâna*, *avidyâ*.

**Jnânadeva.** The greatest Yoga master of medieval Maharashtra, who at a very young age composed a brilliant commentary on the *Bhagavad-Gîtâ*.

**Jnâna-Yoga** ("Yoga of wisdom"). The non-dualist Yoga of self-transcending wisdom, which proceeds by careful discrimination (*viveka*) between the Real (i.e., the Self) and the unreal (i.e., the ego and Nature).

**Kaivalya** ("aloneness"). The state of liberation, especially in Yoga and Jainism. See also *moksha*.

**Kâla** ("time"). An integral aspect of the finite world (*samsâra*) and a major reason why it is experienced as suffering (*duhkha*).

**Kalâ** ("part"). (i) The sixteenth lunar phase, which is considered auspicious. (ii) A highly esoteric fact or experience in Kashmiri Shaivism and Tantrism, which is related to the lunar ambrosia of immortality (*amrita*).

**Kâlâmukha.** A Tantra-based order derived from the Lakulîsha tradition of Shaivism. Cf. Aghorî, Kâpâlika.

**Kâlî.** The "dark" Hindu Goddess, who destroys illusions.

**Kali-yuga.** The age of spiritual decline, calling for a new approach to Self-realization. It is traditionally held to have commenced in 3102 B.C.E. See also *yuga*.

**Kalpa** ("form"). An eon lasting a day in the life of Brahma, the Creator, and consisting of a thousand *yugas*.

**Kâma** ("desire"). (i) A deity, the Hindu cupid. (ii) Lust, one of the obstacles on the yogic path.

**Kânphata** ("split-ear"). The sect or order of *yogins* founded by Goraksha, who developed Hatha-Yoga.

**Kâpâlika.** An extremist Tantric order whose members carry a skull (*kapâla*) as a begging bowl. See also Aghorî, Kâlâmukha.

**Kapila.** The originator of the Sâmkhya tradition, who is attributed with the authorship of the *Sâmkhya-Sûtra*.

**Karman** ("action"). (i) Activity in general. (ii) Karma, or the subtle effect caused by the actions and volitions of an unenlightened individual, which is responsible for his or her rebirth and also for the experiences during the present life and future lives. The idea behind all of India's liberation teachings is to escape the effects of past karma and prevent the production of new karma, whether good or bad. See also *samskâra*, *vâsanâ*.

**Karma-Yoga** ("Yoga of action"). A principal type of Yoga, which consists in the self-transcending performance of actions that are in consonance with one's innermost being (*sva-bhâva*) and with one's moral obligations (*sva-dharma*).

**Kaula** ("relating to *kula*"). (i) A practitioner of *kula*. (ii) Tantric school focusing on *kula* teachings.

**Kaulika** ("relating to *kaula*"). Practitioner or teaching of the *kaula* school of Tantrism.

**Keshin** ("long-haired"). (i) Vedic name of the sun. (ii) A Vedic ecstatic, often regarded as a forerunner of *yogins*.

**Kosha** ("sheath, casing"). This Vedantic term denotes a bodily envelope, of which there are five: the sheath composed of food (*anna-maya-kosha*), the sheath composed of life force (*prâna-maya-kosha*), the sheath composed of thought (*mano-maya-kosha*), the sheath composed of understanding (*vijnâna-maya-kosha*), and the sheath composed of bliss (*ânanda-maya-kosha*). The last-mentioned envelope is sometimes equated with the Absolute itself.

**Krishna** ("attractor"). An ancient adept who was later deified. As an incarnation of God Vishnu, he instructed Prince Arjuna, as recorded in the *Bhagavad-Gîtâ*.

**Kriyâ** ("action, ritual"). A major aspect of Tantric practice.

**Kriyâ-Yoga** ("Yoga of action"). Patanjali's name for the combined practice of asceticism (*tapas*), study (*svâdhyâya*), and devotion to the Lord (*îshvara-pranidhâna*).

**Kshatriya.** A member of the warrior class of Hindu society.

**Kula** ("flock, family"). (i) Shakti. (ii) Tantric group. (iii) The ecstatic experience of the identity of Shiva and Shakti, God and Goddess. See also *kaula*.

**Kundalinî** ("coiled one"). The serpent power (*kundalinî-shakti*), which lies dormant in the lowest psychoenergetic center of the body. Its awakening is the central goal of Tantrism and Hatha-Yoga. The *kundalinî's* ascent to the highest psychoenergetic center at the crown of the head brings about a temporary state of ecstatic identification with the Self (in *nirvikalpa-samâdhi*).

**Kundalinî-Yoga.** Tantric Yoga dedicated to the arousal of the *kundalinî*. The innermost teaching of Hatha-Yoga.

**Lakshmî.** Goddess of good fortune, also called Shrî, and Vishnu's divine spouse.

**Laya** ("dissolution"). (i) A synonym of *pralaya*, or cosmic dissolution. (ii) The yogic dissolution of the elements (*bhûta*) and other aspects of bodily existence by way of meditation and visualization.

**Laya-Yoga.** The yogic process of achieving dissolution (*laya*) through meditation and related practices by which the transcendental Self (*âtman*) is revealed.

**Linga** ("sign, symbol, mark"). (i) In Shaivism, the symbol of the creative aspect of the Divine. (ii) The phallus as a symbol of creativity. (iii) In Patanjali's Yoga, a specific phase in the process of psychocosmic evolution, representing the first step into manifestation.

**Mahâbhârata.** One of India's two great national epics, recounting the great war between the Kauravas and Pandavas (Arjuna's side). The epic contains many instructional passages, including the *Bhagavad-Gîtâ* and the *Moksha-Dharma*. Cf. *Râmâyana*.

**Mahâvîra** ("great hero"). The title of Vardhamâna, the historical founder of Jainism. See also *jaina*.

**Mahâyâna** ("great vehicle"). The majority branch of Buddhism, which has at its doctrinal core the *bodhisattva* ideal and the teaching about emptiness (*shûnyatâ*).

**Maithunâ** ("intercourse"). The ritual practice of sexual congress in the left-hand and *kaula* branches of Tantrism.

**Manas** ("mind"). The lower mind, which is understood as a relay station for the senses (*indriya*) and which is itself regarded as one of the senses. Cf. *buddhi*, *citta*.

**Mandala** ("circle"). (i) A sacred area in which rituals are performed. (ii) An area of the body specific to a certain material element (water, fire, etc.). (iii) A graphic representation similar to the *yantra*, mostly in the context of (Tibetan) Vajrayâna Buddhism. See also *yantra*.

**Manipura-cakra** ("wheel of the jeweled city"). The psychoenergetic center at the navel. See also *cakra*.

**Mantra.** Sacred sound that empowers the mind for concentration and the transcendence of ordinary states of consciousness. A *mantra* can consist of a single "seed" (*bîja*) syllable, like *om*, or a string of sounds and words, which may or may not have a meaning.

**Mantra-Yoga.** A type of Yoga focusing on the recitation (*japa*) of *mantras*.

**Manu.** Mythological founder of the present human race. Each world period has its own Manu. The present one is Manu Vaivasvata, whose rule will come to an end with the termination of the *kali-yuga*.

**Matsyendra** ("lord of fish," from *matsya* and *indra*). A great adept of Tantrism and possibly the founder of the Yoginî Kaula school who is widely considered by tradition as the teacher of Goraksha.

**Mauna** ("silence"). An important yogic practice, which is particularly characteristic of the *muni*.

**Mâyâ** ("measure"). (i) The measuring, divisive power of the Divine. (ii) Illusion or the illusory world.

**Mîmâmsâ** ("inquiry"). One of the six classical schools (*darshana*) of Hindu philosophy, which is concerned with the explanation of Vedic ritualism and its moral applications.

**Moksha** ("liberation, release"). According to Hindu ethics, the highest of four possible human pursuits (*purusha-artha*). It is synonymous with Self-realization. See also *mukti*, *kaivalya*.

**Moksha-Dharma** ("liberation teaching"). A didactic section of the *Mahâbhârata*, containing many yogic teachings.

**Mudrâ** ("seal"). (i) A hand gesture or bodily posture, which has symbolic significance but is also thought to conduct the life energy in the body in specific ways. Hinduism and Buddhism know many such gestures, as can be seen in iconography. (ii) A female initiate in the Tantric ritual, with whom sacred intercourse (*maithunâ*) is practiced. (iii) Parched grain, which is one of the "five M's" (*panca-makâra*) of the left-hand and *kaula* schools; it is thought to have aphrodisiacal properties.

**Mukti** ("release"). A synonym of *moksha*.

**Mûlâdhâra-cakra** ("root-prop wheel"). The lowest of the psychoenergetic centers of the human body, situated at the base of the spine. It is here that the serpent power (*kundalinî-shakti*) lies dormant.

**Muni.** A sage, or one who practices silence (*mauna*). See also *rishi*.

**Nâda** ("sound"). The primal sound (*shabda*) of the universe, sometimes said to be the sacred mantra *om*. It has various forms of manifestation, which can be heard as an inner sound when meditation reaches a certain depth.

**Nâdî** ("conduit, channel"). According to Hindu esotericism, the human body (or, rather, its subtle counterpart) consists of a network of channels along which flows the life force (*prâna*). Often the figure 72,000 is mentioned. Of these channels, three are most important, viz. the *idâ*, *pingalâ*, and *sushumnâ*. The last-mentioned conduit extends from the lowest psychoenergetic center at the base of the spine to the center at the crown of the head, and it is along this central pathway that the awakened *kundalinî* must travel.

**Nâma** ("name"). Often used in conjunction with "form" (*rûpa*) to describe the conditioned reality, as opposed to the name- and form-transcending Reality (*tattva*).

**Nânak.** The founder of Sikhism, traditionally called Guru Nânak.

**Nârada.** A famous ancient sage teaching Bhakti-Yoga, to whom the authorship of the *Bhakti-Sûtra* is ascribed. Cf. *Shândilya*.

**Nâtha** ("master, lord"). (i) An epithet of God Shiva. (ii) Appellation of various Tantric adepts, especially Matsyendra and Goraksha.

**Nâyanmâr.** A member of a group of Shiva-worshiping poet-saints of South India. See also *Âlvâr*.

**Nirguna-brahman** ("unqualified Absolute"). The ultimate Reality in its pure, transcendental state, which is formless and devoid of all qualities (*guna*). Cf. *saguna-brahman*.

**Nirodha** ("restriction"). In Patanjali's Yoga, the process of stopping the "whirls" (*vritti*) of the mind.

**Nirvâna** ("extinction"). In Buddhism, the transcendence of the ego-self. This condition is occasionally described in positive terms as well as the attainment of a Reality untouched by space and time. In Hindu contexts, the term is mostly used interchangeably with liberation (*moksha*).

**Nirvikalpa-samâdhi** ("transconceptual ecstasy"). The Vedantic term for what Patanjali called *asamprajnâta-samâdhi*. Cf. *savikalpa-samâdhi*.

**Niyama** ("restraint"). The second limb of Patanjali's eightfold Yoga, which consists in the practice of purity, contentment, austerity (*tapas*), study (*svâdhyâya*), and devotion to the Lord (*îshvara-pranidhâna*). See also *yama*.

**Nyâsa** ("placement"). The Tantric practice of touching particular parts of the body or objects in order to infuse them with life energy (*prâna*) or other subtle energies.

**Nyâya** ("rule"). One of the six classical systems of Hindu philosophy, which is concerned with logical and critical argument.

**Ojas.** The energy produced through asceticism, especially the practice of chastity, which involves the process of sublimation called *ûrdhva-retas*, which means literally the "upward (streaming) of the semen."

**Om.** The key *mantra* of Hinduism, symbolizing the Absolute. This sacred syllable is also found in Buddhism, Jainism, and Sikhism.

**Panca-ma-kâra** ("five m's"). The collective name of the five practices of the core ritual of left-hand and *kaula* Tantrism: the consumption of fish (*matsya*), meat (*mâmsa*), wine (*madya*), and parched grain (*mudrâ*), all of which are regarded as aphrodisiacs, as well as actual sexual intercourse (*maithunâ*). The right-hand schools of Tantrism understand these five symbolically rather than literally. See also *tantra*.

**Pancarâtra** ("five nights"). An early tradition revolving around the worship of Vishnu.

**Pandita.** A scholar, or pundit.

**Parama-âtman** ("supreme Self," written *paramâtman*). The transcendental Self, as opposed to the empirical, embodied self (*jîva-âtman*). See also *âtman*.

**Paramparâ** ("one to the other"). A teaching lineage.

**Pâsha** ("bond, fetter"). In Shaivism, the condition of bondage caused by spiritual ignorance.

**Pashu** ("beast"). In Shaivism, the term for an ordinary worldling (*samsârin*), who is unaware of the higher spiritual reality of the Self, or the Divine.

**Pâshupata** ("relating to *pashupati*"). An early tradition focusing on the worship of Shiva in the form of Pashupati.

**Pashupati** ("lord of beasts"). An epithet of Shiva, as the ruler of all creatures.

**Patanjali.** Author of the *Yoga-Sûtra*, the source text of Classical Yoga. He probably lived in the second century C.E., though Hindu tradition identifies him with the grammarian by that name who lived 400 years earlier.

**Pitri** ("forefather, ancestor"). The ancestors play an important role in the daily ritual life of Hindus, and this is also recognized in Yoga.

**Prajâpati** ("lord of creatures"). Creator, same as Hiranyagarbha.

**Prajnâ** ("wisdom"). Liberating knowledge. See also *jnâna*, *vidyâ*.

**Prajnâ-Pâramitâ** ("perfection of wisdom"). A corpus of Mahâyâna *Sûtras* teaching emptiness (*shûnya*), and the name of the female deity associated with these texts.

**Prakriti** ("creatrix"). Nature, which is insentient, consists of an eternal, transcendental ground (called *pradhâna* or *alinga*) and various levels of subtle (*sûkshma*) and gross (*sthûla*) manifestation. The lowest level is the visible material realm with its myriad objects. Nature is composed of three types of qualities or forces (*guna*). Cf. *âtman*, *purusha*.

**Pralaya** ("dissolution"). The destruction of the cosmos at the end of a *yuga* or *kalpa*.

**Pramâna.** Valid cognition, one of the mental activities singled out by Patanjali. Cf. *viparyaya*.

**Prâna** ("life"). (i) Life in general. (ii) The life force sustaining the body, which has five principal forms: *prâna*, *apâna*, *samâna*, *udâna*, and *vyâna*. (iii) The breath as the external manifestation of the life force.

**Prânâyâma** ("breath control"). The careful regulation (or expansion, *âyâma*) of the breath, which is the fourth limb of Patanjali's eightfold Yoga.

**Prapatti.** The practice of total self-surrender to the Divine in Vaishnavism.

**Prasâda** ("grace, clarity"). The element of grace, as found even in nondualist Yoga schools; also called *anugraha*.

**Pratyabhijnâ** ("recognition"). A prominent Shaiva school of medieval Kashmir.

**Pratyâhâra** ("withdrawal"). Sensory inhibition, which is the fifth limb of Patanjali's eightfold Yoga. See *yoga-anga*.

**Pûjâ** or *pûjana* ("worship"). The ritual veneration of a deity or the *guru*, which is an important aspect of many forms of Yoga, but especially Bhakti-Yoga.

**Purâna** ("ancient [story]"). A type of popular quasi-religious encyclopedia, covering cosmology and theology, but especially the history of kings and sages.

**Pûrna** ("full, whole"). A characterization of the ultimate Reality, which is inexhaustible and integral.

**Purusha** ("male"). In the Yoga and Sâmkhya traditions, the transcendental Self, Spirit, or pure Awareness (*cit*), as opposed to the finite personality (*jîva*). Cf. *prakriti*.

**Purusha-artha** ("human goal"). Hinduism acknowledges four legitimate goals of human aspiration: material welfare (*artha*), pleasure (*kâma*), morality (*dharma*), and liberation (*moksha*).

**Râdhâ.** Krishna's divine spouse.

**Rajas** (from the verbal root *raj*, "to be excited"). (i) The quality or principle of activity, dynamism, which is one of the three primary constituents (*guna*) of Nature (*prakriti*). (ii) Female genital ejaculate or menstrual blood, both of which hold special significance in Tantrism. The mingling of *rajas* and *retas* (male semen) is said to bring about the ecstatic condition. See also *sattva*, *tamas*.

**Râja-Yoga** ("royal Yoga"). A late designation of Patanjali's eightfold Yoga, invented to contrast it with Hatha-Yoga.

**Râma.** The main hero of the *Râmâyana*, deified as an incarnation of Vishnu.

**Râmânuja.** The eleventh-century founder of the school of Qualified Nondualism (Vishishta Advaita) and chief rival of Shankara's Absolute Nondualism (Kevala Advaita).

**Râmâyana.** One of India's two national epics, telling the heroic story of Râma. Cf. *Mahâbhârata*.

**Rasa** ("essence"). (i) Taste. (ii) Quintessence of bliss in some schools of Bhakti-Yoga, especially the Vaishnava Sahajîyâ movement of Bengal. (iii) The nectar of immortality (*amrita*) in Hatha-Yoga and Tantrism. (iv) Alchemical elixir.

**Rasâyana.** Alchemy, which is closely associated with Hatha-Yoga.

**Rig-Veda** ("knowledge of praise"). The oldest Vedic hymnody, the most sacred scripture of the Hindus. See also *Atharva-Veda*, *Sâma-Veda*, *Yajur-Veda*.

**Rishi.** A type of ancient sage who sees the hymns (*mantra*) of the *Vedas*. See also *muni*.

**Rudra** ("howler"). An epithet or form of Shiva.

**Rûpa** ("form"). In conjunction with the term *nâma* often used to refer to the manifest world.

**Sac-cid-ânanda** ("being-consciousness-bliss," from *sat*, *cit*, and *ânanda*). The ultimate Reality according to Vedânta. See also *ânanda*, *brahman*, *cit*, *sat*, *tattva*.

**Sad-guru** ("true teacher"). An authentic *guru* whose very presence draws disciples to the Divine.

**Sâdhaka** ("realizer"). A spiritual practitioner, especially on the Tantric path, aspiring to realization (*siddhi*). Cf. *sâdhikâ*.

**Sâdhana** ("realizing"). The path of spiritual realization; a particular spiritual discipline.

**Sâdhikâ.** A female practitioner. Cf. *sâdhaka*.

**Sâdhu** ("good one"). A virtuous ascetic.

**Saguna-brahman** ("qualified Absolute"). The ultimate Reality in its stepped-down form as Being endowed with various qualities (*guna*). Cf. *nirguna-brahman*.

**Sahaja** ("twinned"). A medieval term expressing the fact that the transcendental Reality and the empirical reality are coessential. It is often rendered as "spontaneous" or "natural."

**Sahaja-samâdhi** ("natural ecstasy"). The effortless ecstasy (*samâdhi*), which is the same as liberation. It is also called "open-eyed ecstasy" because it does not depend on the introversion of attention through concentration (*dhâranâ*) and meditation (*dhyâna*).

**Sahajîyâ.** A medieval Tantra-oriented devotional (*bhakti*) movement.

**Sahasrâra-cakra** ("thousand-spoked wheel"). The psychoenergetic center at the crown of the head, which in Tantrism is the destination point of the awakened serpent power (*kundalinî-shakti*). See also *cakra*.

**Samâdhi** ("ecstasy"). This is the eighth limb of Patanjali's eightfold Yoga. It consists in the temporary identification between subject and contemplated object and has two principal forms: conscious ecstasy (*samprajnâta-samâdhi*), which includes a variety of spontaneously arising thoughts, and supraconscious ecstasy (*asamprajnâta-samâdhi*), which is free from all ideation. See also *dharma-megha-samâdhi, nirvikalpa-samâdhi, sahaja-samâdhi, savikalpa-samâdhi*.

**Samatva** ("evenness"). The state of inner balance.

**Sâma-Veda** ("knowledge of chants"). The Vedic hymnody containing the chants (*sâman*) used in fire rituals. See also *Atharva-Veda, Rig-Veda, Yajur-Veda*.

**Sâmkhya** ("enumeration," which is related to *samkhyâ*, "number"). One of the six classical Hindu schools of thought, which is concerned with the classification of the various principles (*tattva*), or categories, of existence.

**Samnyâsa** ("renunciation"). The practice of turning one's attention away from worldly things and toward the Divine, which is generally accompanied by an outward act of abandoning conventional life. A purely inner renunciation, however, is also possible.

**Samnyâsin** ("renouncer"). The person practicing *samnyâsa*.

**Samprajnâta-samâdhi** ("conscious ecstasy"). The lower type of ecstatic identification with the contemplated object, accompanied by spontaneously arising thoughts (*pratyaya*). Cf. *asamprajnâta-samâdhi*.

**Samsâra** ("confluence"). The finite world of change, as opposed to the infinite, changeless transcendental Reality. Cf. *nirvâna*.

**Samsârin.** The worldling trapped in the world of change.

**Samskâra** ("activator"). Every action or volition produces a subliminal deposit (*âshaya*) in the mind, which, in turn, leads to new psychomental activity, thus keeping the person enmeshed in the world of change. See also *karman, vâsanâ*.

**Sarasvatî.** (i) A great river in the heartland of the Vedic civilization. (ii) A Vedic Goddess, personifying the river and the arts.

**Sarga** ("creation"). The creation of the cosmos, as opposed to its dissolution (*pralaya*).

**Sat** ("being"). That which is ultimately real, or Reality. See also *ânanda, cit, tattva*.

**Sat-sanga** ("association with the real"). The spiritual practice of frequenting the good (*sat*) company of saints, sages, and Self-realized adepts, who communicate the ultimate Reality (*sat*).

**Sattva** ("beingness"). (i) A being. (ii) The principle of pure being or lucidity, which is the highest type of primary constituent (*guna*) of Nature (*prakriti*). Cf. *rajas, tamas*.

**Satya** ("truth"). (i) Truthfulness. (ii) The ultimate Reality (*sat, tattva*).

**Savikalpa-samâdhi** ("ecstasy with form/ideation"). In Vedânta, the state of ecstatic identification with the transcendental Reality, which is accompanied by thoughts and imagery. See also *samprajnâta-samâdhi*; cf. *nirvikalpa-samâdhi*.

**Shabda** ("sound"). According to Hindu thought, sound is inextricably connected with cosmic existence. Thus, sound exists on various levels of manifestations. The ultimate sound is the sacred *mantra om*. See also *nâda*.

**Shaiva.** Designation for any process or literary work, etc., pertaining to Shiva, or a worshiper of this deity. See also *vaishnava*.

**Shaiva-Siddhânta.** A South Indian tradition of Shaivism.

**Shakti** ("power"). The feminine power aspect of the Divine, which is fundamental to the metaphysics and spirituality of Shaktism and Tantrism.

**Shakti-pâta** ("descent of power"). The process of initiation, usually in Tantric contexts, by which a *guru* empowers the disciple's spiritual practice.

**Shândilya.** A famous ancient sage and the reputed author of the *Bhakti-Sûtra*. Cf. Nârada.

**Shankara** ("pacifier"). The greatest propounder of Hindu nondualism (Advaita Vedânta), who lived in the eighth century C.E. or possibly somewhat earlier.

**Shânti** ("peace"). A desirable quality in *yogins*. Ultimate peace coincides with Self-realization, or enlightenment (*bodha*).

**Shâstra** ("teaching, textbook"). A body of knowledge, often in the form of a book. Thus *yoga-shâstra* can mean both "Yoga teaching" in general and a particular text by that designation.

**Shiva** ("benign"). The deity who, more than any other deity of the Hindu pantheon, has served *yogins* as a model throughout the ages.

**Shruti** ("revelation"). The Vedic revelation comprising the four *Vedas*, the *Brâhmanas*, and the *Upanishads*. Cf. *smriti*.

**Shûdra.** A member of the servile class of traditional Hindu society.

**Shûnya** ("void"). A key concept of Mahâyâna Buddhism, according to which all phenomena are empty of an eternal essence.

**Shûnyatâ** ("voidness, emptiness"). A synonym of *shûnya*.

**Siddha** ("accomplished"). A Self-realized adept who has reached perfection (*siddhi*).

**Siddhi** ("perfection, accomplishment"). (i) Spiritual perfection; that is, the attainment of flawless identification with the ultimate Reality, or liberation (*moksha*). (ii) Paranormal power, especially the eight great abilities that come as a result of perfect adeptship.

**Smriti** ("memory, remembered wisdom"). Tradition, as opposed to revelation (*shruti*).

**Spanda** ("vibration"). According to Kashmiri Shaivism, even the formless Absolute is in a continuous vibratory state, which is the cause of all creation.

**Sukha** ("pleasure, joy"). Ordinary life is a combination of pleasure and pain (*duhkha*), and both types of experience must be transcended to realize the ultimate bliss (*ânanda*), which is also called "great joy" (*mahâ-sukha*).

**Sûrya** ("sun"). The solar deity, who has many other names.

**Sûtra** ("thread"). An aphoristic statement or a work containing such statements, e.g., the *Yoga-Sûtra* of Patanjali.

**Svâdhishthâna-cakra** ("self-standing wheel"). The psychoenergetic center at the genitals. See also *cakra*.

**Svâdhyâya** ("self-study"). Both the study of sacred texts and one's psyche by means of meditation.

**Svâmin** ("lord, master"). Title of Hindu *gurus* belonging to a monastic order.

**Svarga** ("heaven"). Hindu metaphysics recognizes the existence of both various hell realms and heavenly abodes. The latter, however, still belong to the world of change and must be transcended in order to attain liberation (*moksha*).

**Tamas** ("darkness"). The principle of inertia, which is one of the three primary constituents (*guna*) of Nature (*prakriti*). See also *rajas, sattva*.

**Tantra** ("loom"). (i) A type of sacred scripture pertaining to Tantrism and primarily dealing with ritual worship focusing on the feminine divine principle, or *shakti*. (ii) Tantrism, the many-branched religious and cultural movement originating in the early centuries of the Common Era and flourishing around 1000 C.E. Tantrism has a right-hand (conservative) and a left-hand (antinomian) branch.

**Tântrika.** A practitioner of Tantrism.

**Tapas** ("glow, heat"). Asceticism, which is thought to lead to great vitality. This term was applied to Yoga-like practices in Vedic times.

**Târaka-Yoga** ("Yoga of the deliverer"). A Tantra-based Yoga emphasizing the meditative experience of light.

**Tat** ("that"). In Vedânta, a cryptic reference to the ultimate Reality, or transcendental Self, as in the dictum "Thou art That" (*tat tvam asi*).

**Tattva** ("reality"). (i) The ultimate Reality. (ii) A principle or category of existence, such as higher mind (*buddhi*), lower mind (*manas*), senses (*indriya*), and material elements (*bhûta*).

**Tattva-vid** ("knower of reality"). (i) A liberated sage. (ii) A spiritual practitioner who knows the various categories of existence taught in Sâmkhya and Yoga.

**Tîrtha** ("ford"). A sacred place for pilgrimage.

**Tîrthankara** ("ford-maker"). Title of the great Self-realized teachers of Jainism, such as Mahâvîra.

**Tirumûlâr.** A great South Indian poet-saint, author of the *Tiru-Mantiram*.

**Trika** ("triad"). A medieval Shaiva school of Kashmir, which is nondualistic but acknowledges the relative existence of multiplicity (epitomized in the many individual human beings called *nara*), duality (symbolized by *shakti*), and unity (represented by *shiva*).

**Upanishad** ("sitting near"). A type of esoteric Hindu scripture that expounds the metaphysics of nondualism (Advaita Vedânta) and is considered the last phase in the Vedic revelation (*shruti*).

**Upâya** ("means"). In Buddhism, another term for compassion (*karunâ*), the counterpart of *prajnâ*, standing for insight into the empty (*shûnya*) nature of all phenomena.

**Vaisheshika** ("distinctionism"). One of the six classical Hindu schools of thought, which is concerned with the categories of material existence.

**Vaishnava** ("pertaining to Vishnu"). Designation for any process or literary work, etc., pertaining to God Vishnu, or a worshiper of this deity. See also *shaiva*.

**Vaishya.** A member of the merchant class of traditional Hindu society.

**Vajrayâna** ("adamantine vehicle"). The Tantric branch of Buddhism, especially in Tibet, which evolved out of the Mahâyâna.

**Vâsanâ** ("trait"). (i) Desire. (ii) In Patanjali's Yoga, the concatenation of subliminal activators (*samskâra*) deposited in the depth of the mind through actions and volitions. These must be dissolved before liberation (*moksha*), or enlightenment (*bodha*), can be attained.

**Vashishtha.** The name of several ancient sages, notably the great authority of the *Yoga-Vâsishtha*.

**Vedânta** ("Veda's end"). The dominant Hindu philosophical tradition, which teaches that Reality is nondual (*advaita*). See also *âtman, brahman*.

**Videha-mukti** ("disembodied liberation"). The ideal of some schools of Vedânta, which deny that full liberation can be attained while the body is still alive. Cf. *jîvan-mukti*.

**Vidyâ** ("wisdom, knowledge"). In spiritual contexts, usually liberating wisdom, as opposed to intellectual knowledge. See also *jnâna, prajnâ*.

**Viparyaya** ("error"). According to Patanjali, one of the mental activities (*vrittis*) that must be silenced. Cf. *pramâna*.

**Vîra** ("hero"). In Tantrism, a particular type of spiritual practitioner (*sâdhaka*), usually following the left-hand branch.

**Vishnu** ("pervader"). The deity worshiped by the Vaishnavas and Bhâgavatas, whose two most famous incarnations (*avâtara*) are Râma and Krishna.

**Vishuddha-cakra** ("pure wheel"). The psychoenergetic center at the throat. See also *cakra*.

**Vishva** ("all"). The empirical world (*samsâra*).

**Viveka** ("discernment, discrimination"). On the yogic path, specifically the discrimination between the Self (*âtman*) and the nonself (*anâtman*).

**Vrata** ("vow"). An important feature of many yogic approaches.

**Vrâtya** ("vowed"). A member of a sacred brotherhood in Vedic times, bound together by vows (*vrata*) and in whose circles yogic practices were developed.

**Vritti** ("whirl"). In Patanjali's Yoga, one of five modalities of mental activity that must be controlled: valid cognition (*pramâna*), erroneous cognition (*viparyaya*), conceptualization (*vikalpa*), sleep (*nidrâ*), and memory (*smriti*).

**Vyâdhi** ("disease"). Illness, as understood as an imbalance of the three humors (*dosha*). Cf. *ârogya*.

**Vyâsa** ("arranger"). The legendary composer of the *Mahâbhârata* epic, collator of the four Vedic hymnodies, many *Purânas*, and other works, such as the *Yoga-Bhâshya* commentary on Patanjali's *Yoga-Sûtra*.

**Yajna** ("sacrifice"). The practice of ritual sacrifice is fundamental to Hinduism. At the time of the *Brâhmanas* and more so with the *Upanishads*, the external sacrificial ritual was internalized in the form of intense meditation, leading to the full-fledged tradition of Yoga.

**Yâjnavalkya.** The most renowned sage of the early Post-Vedic Era.

**Yajur-Veda** ("knowledge of sacrifice"). The Vedic hymn containing the sacrificial formulas (*yajus*). See also *Atharva-Veda, Rig-Veda, Sâma-Veda*.

**Yama** ("discipline"). (i) The deity of death. (ii) The first limb of Patanjali's eightfold Yoga, comprising five moral precepts of universal validity.

**Yantra** ("instrument"). A geometric design in Hinduism representing the body of one's chosen deity (*ishta-devatâ*) for external worship and meditation. See also *mandala*.

**Yoga** ("union"). (i) Spiritual or mystical practice in general. (ii) One of the six classical Hindu schools of thought, codified by Patanjali in his *Yoga-Sûtra*.

**Yoga-anga** ("limb of Yoga"). According to Patanjali, there are the following eight limbs: moral discipline (*yama*), self-restraint (*niyama*), posture (*âsana*), breath control (*prânâyâma*), sense-withdrawal (*pratyâhâra*), concentration (*dhâranâ*), meditation (*dhyâna*), and ecstasy (*samâdhi*).

**Yogâcâra** ("Yoga way"). The Mahâyâna Buddhist school founded by Asanga.

**Yoga-Sûtra** ("Yoga aphorism"). The source text of Classical Yoga, compiled by Patanjali. See also *sûtra*.

**Yoga-Vâsishtha.** A massive poetic treatment of nondualist Yoga, composed sometime in the tenth century C.E.

**Yogin.** A male practitioner of Yoga.

**Yoginî.** A female practitioner of Yoga.

**Yuga** ("yoke"). A world age. According to Hindu cosmology, there are four such world ages, each of several thousand years' duration. The *kali-yuga* is held to be the darkest period and precedes another golden age. Cf. *kalpa*.

# SELECT BIBLIOGRAPHY

Please note that this bibliography contains only books. Additional books and articles are mentioned in the endnotes. Also, only long vowel sounds of Sanskrit words appearing in titles have been transliterated with circumflexes. All other Sanskrit diacritics, with the exception of the tilde (~), have simply been omitted.

Abbegg, Emil. *Indische Psychologie*. Zurich: Rascher Verlag, 1955.

Abbott, Justin E. *The Life of Eknath*. Delhi: Motilal Banarsidass, repr. 1981.

Abhayananda, S. *Jnaneshvar: The Life and Works of the Celebrated Thirteenth Century Indian Mystic-Poet*. Olympia, Wash.: Atma Books, 1989.

Abhishiktananda, Swami. *Guru and Disciple*. London: Society for the Promotion of Christian Knowledge, 1974.

*Agni Purânam: A Prose English Translation*. Translated by Manmatha Nâth Dutt Shastrî. Varanasi, India: Chowkhamba Sanskrit Series Office, 1967. 2 vols.

Aguilar, H. *The Sacrifice in the Rgveda*. Delhi: Bharatiya Vidya Prakasham, 1976.

Aïvanhov, Omraam Mikhaël. *Toward a Solar Civilisation*. Frejus, France: Prosveta, 1982.

_____. *The Yoga of Nutrition*. Frejus, France: Prosveta, 1982.

_____. *The Seeds of Happiness*. Frejus, France: Prosveta, 1992.

_____. *"Know Thyself"—Jnana Yoga*. Frejus, France: Prosveta, 1994.

Aiyar, K. Narayanasvami, trans. *Thirty Minor Upanishads, Including the Yoga Upanishads*. El Reno, Okla.: Santarasa Publications, repr. 1980.

Ajaya, Swami. *Yoga Psychology: A Practical Guide to Meditation*. Honesdale, Penn.: Himalayan International Institute of Yoga Science and Philosophy, 3d ed., 1978.

Allchin, Raymond. *Tulsî Dâs: Kavitâvalî*. London: George Allen and Unwin, 1964.

Alper, Harvey, ed. *Mantra*. Albany, N.Y.: SUNY Press, 1989.

_____, ed. *Understanding Mantras*. Albany, N.Y.: SUNY Press, 1989.

Alston, Anthony J. *Samkara on the Absolute*. London: Shanti Sadan, 1980.

_____. *Samkara on the Creation*. London: Shanti Sadan, 1980.

_____. *Samkara on the Soul*. London: Shanti Sadan, 1980.

_____. *Yoga and the Supreme Bliss: Songs of Enlightenment by Swâmî Râma Tîrtha*. London: A. Z. Alston, 1982.

_____. *Samkara on Discipleship*. London: Shanti Sadan, 1989.

_____. *Samkara on Rival Views*. London: Shanti Sadan, 1989.

Âranya, Hariharânanda. *Yoga Philosophy of Patanjali*. Translated by P. N. Mukerji. Albany, N.Y.: SUNY Press, rev. ed., 1983.

Arya, Usharbudh. *Mantra & Meditation*. Honesdale, Penn.: Himalayan International Institute, 1981.

_____. *Philosophy of Hatha Yoga*. Honesdale, Penn.: Himalayan International Institute, 1985.

_____. *Yoga-Sûtras of Patanjali with the Exposition of Vyâsa: A Translation and Commentary*. Vol. 1: *Samâdhi-pâda*. Honesdale, Penn.: Himalayan International Institute, 1986. [Translation remains incomplete.]

Ashokananda, Swami. *Avadhûta Gîtâ of Dattâtreya*. Mylapore, India: Sri Ramakrishna Math, [n.d.].

Asvaghosha. *The Awakening of Faith*. Translated by Yoshito S. Hakeda. New York: Columbia University Press, 1967.

Atisa. *A Lamp for the Path and Commentary*. Translated by Richard Sherburne. London: George Allen & Unwin, 1983.

Atreya, B. L. *The Yogavâsistha and Its Philosophy*. Moradabad, India: Darshana Printers, 3d ed., 1966.

Aurobindo, Sri. *Essays on the Gita*. Pondicherry, India: Sri Aurobindo Ashram, 1949.

_____. *On the Veda*. Pondicherry, India: Sri Aurobindo Ashram, 1964.

_____. *The Synthesis of Yoga*. Pondicherry, India: Sri Aurobindo Ashram, 1976.

_____. *The Life Divine*. Pondicherry, India: Sri Aurobindo Ashram, 10th ed., 1977. 2 vols.

Avalon, Arthur [see also Woodroffe, John]. *The Serpent Power, Being the Satcakranirûpana and the Pâdukâpanchaka*. Madras, India: Ganesh & Co., 10th ed., 1974. First published in 1913.

_____. *Principles of Tantra. The Tantratattva of Srîyukta Siva Candra Vidyârnava Bhattacharya*. Madras, India: Ganesh & Co., 3d ed., 1960.

_____, trans. *Tantra of the Great Liberation (Mahanirvana Tantra)*. New York: Dover, 1972.

Ayyangar, T. R. Srinivasa, and G. Srinivasa Murti. *The Yoga Upanisads*. Adyar, India: Adyar Library, 1952.

Bagchi, P. C. *Studies in Tantras*. Calcutta: University of Calcutta, 1975.

Bahirat, B. P. *The Philosophy of Jnânadeva as Gleaned from the Amrtânubhava*. Delhi: Motilal Banarsidass, repr. 1984.

Banerjea, Akshaya Kumar. *Philosophy of Gorakhnath with Goraksha-Vacana-Sangraha*. Gorakhpur, India: Mahant Dig Vijai Nath Trust, [1961].

Banerjea, Kitendra Nath. *Pauranic and Tantric Religion*. Calcutta: University of Calcutta Press, 1966.

Barua, Benimadhab. *A History of Pre-Buddhistic Philosophy*. Delhi: Motilal Banarsidass, repr. 1970.

Barz, Richard. *The Bhakti Sect of Vallabhâcârya*. Faridabad, India: Thomson Press, 1976.

Basham, A. L. *The Wonder That Was India*. New York: Grove Press, 1954.

Basu, Manoranjan. *Fundamentals of the Philosophy of Tantras*. Calcutta: Mira Basu Publishers, 1986.

Beck, Guy L. *Sonic Theology: Hinduism and Sacred Sound*. Columbia, S.C.: University of South Carolina Press, 1987.

Behanan, K. *Yoga: A Scientific Explanation*. New York: Dover, 1937.

Berendt, Joachim-Ernst. *Nada Brahma: The World Is Sound*. Rochester, Vt.: Destiny Books, 1987.

Bernard, Theos. *Hatha Yoga: The Report of a Personal Experience*. London: Rider, 1968.

Berry, Thomas. *Religions of India: Hinduism, Yoga, Buddhism*. New York: Bruce Publishing/London: Collier-Macmillan, 1971.

Bhagat, Mansukh Ghelabhai. *Ancient Indian Asceticism*. New Delhi: Munshiram Manoharlal, 1976.

*Bhâgavata-Purâna*. Translated by Board of Scholars. Delhi: Motilal Banarsidass, repr. 1986. 5 vols.

Bhaktivedanta Swami, A. C. *Srî Caitanya-caritâmrta*. New York: Bhaktivedanta Book Trust, 1975. 17 vols.

_____, trans. *Srimad-Bhâgavatam*. New York: Bhaktivedanta Book Trust, 1972–89. 30 vols.

Bhandarkar, R. G. *Vaisnavism, Saivism and Minor Religious Systems*. Varanasi, India: Indological Book House, repr. 1965. First published 1913.

Bharadwaj, K. D. *The Philosophy of Râmânuja*. New Delhi: Sri Shankar Lall Charitable Trust Society, 1958.

Bharati, Agehananda. *The Tantric Tradition*. London: Rider and Co., 1965; New York: Samuel Weiser, rev. ed., 1975.

Bhat, M. S. *Vedic Tantrism: A Study of Rgvidhana of Saunaka with Text and Translation*. Delhi: Motilal Banarsidass, 1987.

Bhattacharji, S. *The Indian Theogony*. Cambridge, Mass.: Cambridge University Press, 1970.

Bhattacharya, Brajamadhava. *Saivism and the Phallic World*. New Delhi: Oxford University Press, 1975. 2 vols.

_____. *The World of Tantra*. New Delhi: Munshiram Manoharlal, 1988.

Bhattacharya, Deben. *Songs of the Bards of Bengal*. New York: Grove Press, 1969.

Bhattacharya, N. N. *History of the Sâkta Religion*. New Delhi: Munshiram Manoharlal, 1974.

_____. *History of the Tantric Religion*. New Delhi: Munshiram Manoharlal, 1982.

Bhattacharya, Ram Shankar. *An Introduction to the Yogasutra*. Delhi: Bharatiya Vidyâ Prakâsana, 1985.

Bhattacharya, Siddhesvara. *The Philosophy of The Srimad-Bhâgavata*. Santiniketan, India: Visva-Bharati, 1960, 1962. 2 vols.

Bhattacharyya, Haridas, ed. *The Cultural Heritage of India*. Calcutta: Ramakrishna Mission Institute of Culture, 1956. 4 vols.

Bhishagratna, K., trans. *Sushrut Samhita*. Varanasi, India: Chowkhamba Sanskrit Series, 1981. 3 vols.

Birven, Henri. *Lebenskunst in Yoga und Magie*. Zurich: Origo, [1953?].

Blair, C. J. *Heat in the Rig Veda and Atharva Veda*. New Haven, Ct.: American Oriental Society, 1961.

Blofeld, John. *The Tantric Mysticism of Tibet*. New York: E. P. Dutton, 1970.

Bloomfield, Maurice. *The Religion of the Veda*. New York: G. B. Putnam's Sons, 1908.

_____. *The Life and Stories of the Jaina Savior Pârsvanâtha*. Baltimore, Md.: University of Maryland Press, 1919.

_____. *Hymns from the Atharva Veda*. Delhi: Motilal Banarsidass, repr. 1964. First published 1897.

Bosch, F. D. K. *The Golden Germ: An Introduction to Indian Symbolism*. The Hague: Mouton, 1960.

Bose, M. M. *The Post-Caitanya Sahajiyâ Cult of Bengal*. Calcutta: University of Calcutta Press, 1930.

Bouanchaud, Bernard. *The Essence of Yoga: Reflections on the Yoga Sutras of Patanjali*. Translated by Rosemary Desneux. Portland, Oreg.: Rudra Press, 1997.

Brahma, Nalini Kanta. *Philosophy of Hindu Sâdhanâ*. London: Kegan Paul, Trench, Trubner & Co., [1932].

Briggs, George W. *Gorakhnâth and the Kânphata Yogîs*. Delhi: Motilal Banarsidass, repr. 1973.

Brooks, Douglas Renfrew. *The Secret of the Three Cities*. Chicago and London: University of Chicago Press, 1990.

_____. *Auspicious Wisdom: The Texts and Traditions of Srîvidyâ Sâkta Tantrism in South India.* Albany, N.Y.: SUNY Press, 1992.

Brown, Cheever Mackenzie. *The Triumph of the Goddess: The Canonical Models and Theological Visions of the Devî-Bhâgavata Purâna.* Albany, N.Y.: SUNY Press, 1990.

Brown, Norman O., ed. and trans. *The Saundaryalaharî, or Flood of Beauty: Traditionally Ascribed to Sankarâcârya.* Cambridge, Mass.: Harvard University Press, 1958.

Brunton, Paul. *The Hidden Teaching Beyond Yoga.* York Beach, Maine: Samuel Weiser, 2d rev. ed., 1984. First published 1941.

_____. *The Notebooks of Paul Brunton.* Burdett, N.Y.: Larson Publications, 1984–88. 16 vols.

_____. *A Search in Secret India.* York Beach, Maine: Samuel Weiser, rev. ed., 1985. First published 1935.

Bubba [Da] Free John. *The Paradox of Instruction.* San Francisco: Dawn Horse Press, 1977.

_____. *The Enlightenment of the Whole Body.* Middletown, Calif.: Dawn Horse Press, 1978.

Buddhaghosa. *The Path of Purification (Visuddhimagga).* Translated by Bhikkhu Nyânamoli. Berkeley and London: Shambhala, 1976. 2 vols.

Buhler, Georg, trans. *The Sacred Laws of the Âryas, As Taught in the Schools of Âpastamba, Gautama, Vâsishtha, and Baudhâyana.* Delhi: Motilal Banarsidass, repr. 1969. 2 vols.

Buitenen, J. A. B. van. *The Mahâbhârata, Books I-V.* Chicago: University of Chicago Press, 1973-1978. 3 vols.

_____. *Râmânuja on the Bhagavadgîtâ.* Delhi: Motilal Banarsidass, repr. 1968.

_____, trans. *Râmânuja's Vedârthasangraha.* Poona, India: Deccan College Postgraduate and Research Institute, 1956.

Carman, John. *The Theology of Râmânuja.* New Haven, Ct.: Yale University Press, 1974.

_____, and Vasudha Narayanan. *The Tamil Veda: Pillân's Interpretation of the Tiruvâymoli.* Chicago: University of Chicago Press, 1989.

Carter, John Ross, and Mahinda Palihawadana, trans. *The Dhammapada.* New York and Oxford: Oxford University Press, 1987.

Chakravarti, Chintaharan. *Tantras: Studies on Their Religion and Literature.* Calcutta: Punthi Pustak, 1972.

Chakravarti, Pulinbihari. *Origin and Development of the Sâmkhya System of Thought.* Calcutta: Metropolitan Printing and Publishing House, 1951.

Chang, Garma C. C. *The Hundred Thousand Songs of Milarepa.* New Hyde Park, N.Y.: University Books, 1962.

_____. *Teachings of Tibetan Yoga.* New Hyde Park, N.Y.: University Books, 1963.

Chapple, Christopher K. *Karma and Creativity.* Albany, N.Y.: SUNY Press, 1986.

_____, and Yogi Ananda Viraj (Eugene P. Kelly, Jr.). *The Yoga Sûtras of Patanjali: An Analysis of the Sanskrit with Accompanying English Translation.* Delhi: Sri Satguru Publications, 1990.

Chatterjee, A. K. *A Comprehensive History of Jainism*. Calcutta: University of Calcutta Press, 1978, 1984. 2 vols.

Chattopadhyaya, Debiprasad. *Lokâyata: A Study in Ancient Indian Materialism*. New Delhi: People's Publishing House, 1959.

Chattopadhyaya, Sudhakar. *Reflections on the Tantras*. Delhi: Motilal Banarsidass, 1978.

Chaudhuri, Haridas. *Integral Yoga*. London: George Allen & Unwin, 1965.

_____, and Frederic Spiegelberg. *The Integral Philosophy of Sri Aurobindo*. London: George Allen & Unwin, 1960.

Chaudhury, Sukomal. *Analytical Study of the Abhidharmakosa*. Calcutta: Firma KLM, 1983.

Ch'en, Kenneth K. S. *Buddhism in China: A Historical Survey*. Princeton, N.J.: Princeton University Press, 1964.

Chetanananda, Swami. *Dynamic Stillness, Part One: The Practice of Trika Yoga*. Cambridge, Mass.: Rudra Press, 1983.

_____. *Dynamic Stillness, Part Two: The Fulfillment of Trika Yoga*. Cambridge, Mass.: Rudra Press, 1991.

Chinmayananda, Swami. *Ashtavakra Geeta*. Madras, India: Chinmaya Publications Trust, 1972.

Cleary, Thomas, transl. *Buddhist Yoga: A Comprehensive Course*. Boston, Mass.: Shambhala Publications, 1995.

Coburn, Thomas B. *Devî Mâhâtmya: The Crystallization of the Goddess Tradition*. Delhi: Motilal Banarsidass, 1984.

_____. *Encountering the Goddess: A Translation of the Devî-Mâhâtmya and a Study of Its Interpretation*. Albany, N.Y.: SUNY Press, 1991.

Cole, Colin A. *Asparsa Yoga: A Study of Gaudapâda's Mândûkya Kârikâ*. Delhi: Motilal Banarsidass, 1982.

Conze, Edward, ed. *Buddhist Texts Through the Ages*. New York: Harper & Row, 1954.

_____. *Buddhist Meditation*. New York: Harper & Row, 1956.

_____. *Buddhist Thought in India*. London: Allen & Unwin, 1962.

_____. *Buddhism: Its Essence and Development*. New York: Harper & Row, 1963.

_____, trans. *The Perfection of Wisdom in Eight Thousand Lines & Its Verse Summary*. Bolinas, Calif.: Four Seasons Foundation, 1973.

Coomaraswamy, Ananda K. *The Dance of Shiva: Fourteen Indian Essays*. Bombay and Calcutta: Asia Publishing House, repr. 1956.

Coster, Geraldine. *Yoga and Western Psychology*. London: Oxford University Press, 1957.

Cowell, E. B., and A. E. Gough, trans. *Sarvadarsanasamgraha, or Review of the Different Systems of Hindu Philosophy of Madhava Âchârya*. London: Kegan Paul, Trench, Trübner & Co., repr. 1914.

_____, and F. M. Müller, and J. Takakusu, trans. *Buddhist Mahâyâna Sûtras*. Oxford: Clarendon Press, 1894.

Cozort, Daniel. *Highest Yoga Tantra: An Introduction to the Esoteric Buddhism of Tibet*. Ithaca, N.Y.: Snow Lion, 1986.

Criswell, Eleanor. *How Yoga Works: An Introduction to Somatic Yoga*. Novato, Calif.: Freeperson Press, 1989.

Da Free John. See Bubba [Da] Free John.

Dalai Lama. *The Buddhism of Tibet*. Translated and edited by Jeffrey Hopkins. Ithaca, N.Y.: Snow Lion, 1987.

_____. *Path to Bliss: A Practical Guide to Stages of Meditation*. Translated by Geshe Thubten Jinpa and edited by Christine Cox. Ithaca, N.Y.: Snow Lion, 1991.

Dange, Sadashiv Ambadas. *Legends in the Mahâbhârata*. Delhi: Motilal Banarsidass, 1969.

_____. *Sexual Symbolism from the Vedic Ritual*. Delhi: Ajanta Publications, 1979.

Daniélou, Alain. *Yoga: The Method of Re-Integration*. London: Christopher Johnson, 1949.

_____. *Shiva and Dionysus: The Religion of Nature and Eros*. Translated by K. F. Hurry. New York: Inner Traditions International, 1984.

_____. *The Gods of India: Hindu Polytheism*. New York: Inner Traditions International, 1985.

_____. *While the Gods Play: Shaiva Oracles and Predictions on the Cycles of History and the Destiny of Mankind*. Translated by Barbara Bailey, Michael Baker, and Deborah Lawlor. Rochester, Vt.: Inner Traditions International, 1987.

Das Gupta, Shashi Bhushan. *An Introduction to Tântric Buddhism*. Calcutta: University of Calcutta, 1958.

_____. *Obscure Religious Cults as Background of Bengali Literature*. Calcutta: Firma KLM, 3d ed., 1969.

Dasgupta, Surendranath. *The Study of Patanjali*. Calcutta: University of Calcutta, 1920.

_____. *Yoga as Philosophy and Religion*. London: Kegan Paul, 1924.

_____. *Hindu Mysticism*. Delhi: Motilal Banarsidass, 1927.

_____. *Yoga Philosophy in Relation to Other Systems of Indian Thought*. Calcutta: University of Calcutta, 1930.

_____. *A History of Indian Philosophy*. Cambridge, Mass.: Cambridge University Press, 1952–55. 5 vols.

Datta, Aswini Kumar. *Bhaktiyoga*. Bombay: Bharatiya Vidya Bhavan, 1981.

De Nicolas, Antonio T. *Avatâra: The Humanization of Philosophy Through the Bhagavad Gîtâ*. New York: Nicolas Hays, 1976.

De, Sushil Kumar. *Early History of the Vaisnava Faith and Movement in Bengal*. Calcutta: General Printers and Publishers, 1942.

Dehejia, Vidya. *Slaves of the Lord: The Path of the Tamil Saints*. Delhi: Munshiram Manoharlal, 1988.

_____. *Ântâl and Her Path of Love: Poems of a Woman Saint from South India*. Albany, N.Y.: SUNY Press, 1990.

De Rose, Maestro. *Practica de Yoga Avanzado (Swasthya Yoga Shastra)*. Saõ Paulo, Brazil: UniYoga, 1997.

*Der Weg des Yoga: Handbuch für Übende und Lehrende.* Edited by Berufsverband Deutscher Yogalehrer. Petersberg, Germany: Verlag Via Nova, 1994.

Desai, S. M. *Haribhadra's Yoga Works and Psychosynthesis.* Ahmedabad, India: L. D. Institute of Indology, 1983.

Desikachar, T. K. V. *The Heart of Yoga: Developing a Personal Practice.* Rochester, Vt.: Inner Traditions International, 1995.

Deussen, Paul. *The Philosophy of the Upanisads.* Translated by A. S. Geden. New York: Dover, repr. 1966.

_____. *Sixty Upanisads of the Veda.* Translated by V. M. Bedekar and G. B. Palsule. Delhi: Motilal Banarsidass, repr. 1980. 2 vols.

Deutsch, Eliot. *Advaita Vedânta: A Philosophical Reconstruction.* Honolulu: University of Hawaii Press, 1969.

Devasthali, G. V. *Religion and Mythology of the Brâhmanas.* Poona, India: University of Poona, 1965.

[*Devî-Bhâgavata-Purâna*] *The Srimad Devi Bhagavatam.* Translated by Swami Vijnanananda. Allahabad, India: Sudhindra Nath Vasu, 1922.

Dhavamony, M. *Love of God According to Saiva Siddhânta.* London: Clarendon Press, 1971.

Dhirendra Brahmachari. *Yogâsana Vijnâna: The Science of Yoga.* London: Asia Publishing House, 1970.

Digambarji, Swami, and M. L. Gharote. *Gheranda Samhitâ.* Lonavla, India: Kaivalyadhama S. M. Y. M. Samti, 1978.

Dikshitar, V. R. Ramachandra. *The Purana Index.* Madras, India: University of Madras, 1951-1955. 3 vols.

Dimock, E. C. *The Place of the Hidden Moon: Erotic Mysticism in the Vaisnava Sahajiyâ Cult of Bengal.* Chicago: University of Chicago Press, 1966.

Dixit, K. K. *The Yogabindu of Âcârya Haribhadrasûri.* Ahmedabad, India: Lalbhai Dalpatbhai Bharatiya Sanskriti Vidyamandira, 1968.

Doniger, Wendy, and Brian K. Smith, trans. *The Laws of Manu.* London: Penguin Books, 1991.

Douglas, Nik, and Penny Slinger. *Sexual Secrets.* New York: Destiny Books, 1979.

Dowman, Keith. *Sky Dancer: The Secret Life and Songs of the Lady Yeshe Tsogyel.* London: Routledge and Kegan Paul, 1984.

_____. *Masters of Mahamudra.* Albany, N.Y.: SUNY Press, 1985.

Dowson, John. *A Classical Dictionary of Hindu Mythology and Religion, Geography, History and Literature.* Calcutta: Rupa & Co., 1982.

Dundas, Paul. *The Jainas.* London: Routledge, 1992.

Dutt, Manmatha Nath, trans. *A Prose English Translation of Harivamsha.* Calcutta: Elysium Press, 1897.

Dyczkowski, Mark S. G. *The Doctrine of Vibration: An Analysis of the Doctrines and Practices of Kashmir Saivism.* Albany, N.Y.: SUNY Press, 1987.

_____. *The Canon of the Saivâgama and the Kubjikâ Tantras of the Western Kaula Tradition.* Albany, N.Y.: SUNY Press, 1988.

Easwaran, Eknath. *Thousand Names of Vishnu.* Petaluma, Calif.: Nilgiri Press, 1987.

Edgerton, Franklin. *The Beginnings of Indian Philosophy.* Cambridge, Mass.: Harvard University Press, 1965.

Eggeling, Julius, trans. *The Satapatha Brâhmana According to the Madhyandina School.* Delhi: Motilal Banarsidass, repr. 1963. 5 vols.

Eliade, Mircea. *Yoga: Immortality and Freedom.* Princeton, N.J.: Princeton University Press, 1973.

_____. *Patañjali and Yoga.* New York: Schocken Books, 1975.

_____. *Shamanism: Archaic Techniques of Ecstasy.* Translated by Willard R. Trask. New York: Pantheon, 1964.

Evans-Wentz, W. Y. *The Tibetan Book of the Great Liberation.* London: Oxford University Press, 1968.

_____, ed. *Tibetan Yoga and Secret Doctrines.* London: Oxford University Press, 2d ed., 1958.

_____, ed. *The Tibetan Book of the Dead.* London: Oxford University Press, 1960.

Evola, Julius. *The Metaphysics of Sex.* New York: Inner Traditions International, 1983.

_____. *The Yoga of Power: Tantra, Shakti, and the Secret Way.* Translated by Guido Stucco. Rochester, Vt.: Inner Traditions International, 1992.

Farquhar, J. N. *An Outline of the Religious Literature of India.* Delhi: Motilal Banarsidass, repr. 1968.

Feuerstein, Georg. *Introduction to the Bhagavad-Gita: Its Philosophy and Cultural Setting.* Wheaton, Ill.: Quest Books, 1983.

_____. *The Yoga-Sûtra of Patañjali: A New Translation and Commentary.* Rochester, Vt.: Inner Traditions International, repr. 1989.

_____. *Sacred Paths: Essays on Wisdom, Love, and Mystical Realization.* Burdett, N.Y.: Larson Publications, 1991.

_____. *Wholeness or Transcendence? Ancient Lessons for the Emerging Global Civilization.* Burdett, N.Y.: Larson Publications, 1992.

_____. *The Shambhala Guide to Yoga.* Boston, Mass.: Shambhala Publications, 1996.

_____. *The Philosophy of Classical Yoga.* Rochester, Vt.: Inner Traditions International, 1996.

_____. *The Shambhala Encyclopedia of Yoga.* Boston, Mass.: Shambhala Publications, 1997.

_____. *The Teachings of Yoga.* Boston, Mass.: Shambhala Publications, 1997.

_____. *The Mystery of Light: The Life and Teaching of Omraam Mikhaël Aïvanhov.* Lower Lake, Calif.: Integral Publishing, 1998.

_____. *Tantra: The Path of Ecstasy.* Boston, Mass.: Shambhala Publications, 1998.

_____, Subhash Kak, and David Frawley. *In Search of the Cradle of Civilization: New Light on Ancient India.* Wheaton, Ill.: Quest Books, 1995.

_____, and Jeanine Miller. *The Essence of Yoga.* Rochester, Vt.: Inner Traditions International, repr. 1997.

Finegan, Jack. *Archaeological History of Religions of Indian Asia.* New York: Paragon House, 1989.

Frawley, David. *The Creative Vision of the Early Upanishads.* Madras, India: Rajsri Printers, 1982.

_____. *Gods, Sages and Kings: Vedic Secrets of Ancient Civilization.* Salt Lake City, Utah: Passage Press, 1991.

_____. *Wisdom of the Ancient Seers: Mantras of the Rig Veda.* Salt Lake City, Utah: Passage Press, 1992.

_____. *Beyond the Mind.* Salt Lake City, Utah: Passage Press, 1992.

_____. *Tantric Yoga and the Wisdom Goddessess.* Salt Lake City, Utah: Passage Press, 1994.

_____. *Ayurveda and the Mind: The Healing of Consciousness.* Twin Lakes, Wis.: Lotus Press, 1997.

Funderburk, James. *Science Studies Yoga: A Review of Physiological Data.* Honesdale, Penn.: Himalayan International Institute of Yoga, Science and Philosophy of the U.S.A., 1977.

Gampopa. *The Jewel Ornament of Liberation.* Translated by Herbert V. Guenther. Berkeley, Calif.: Shambhala Publications, 1959.

Gandhi, Mohandas Karamchand. *Collected Works.* Washington, D.C.: Public Affairs Press, 1948.

_____. *My Experiments with Truth.* Translated by Mahadev Desai. Boston, Mass.: Beacon Press, 1957.

Ganguli, Kisari Mohan, trans. *The Mahabharata.* New Delhi: Munshiram Manoharlal, 4th ed., 1981. 12 vols.

Garg, Ganga Ram, ed. *Encyclopaedia of the Hindu World.* New Delhi: Concept Publishing Co., 1992–.

*Garuda-Purâna.* Translated by Board of Scholars. Delhi: Motilal Banarsidass, repr. 1996. 3 vols.

Gebser, Jean. *The Ever-Present Origin.* Athens, Ohio: Ohio University Press, 1985.

Geldner, Karl Friedrich. *Der Rig-Veda: Aus dem Sanskrit ins Deutsche übersetzt und mit einem laufenden Kommentar versehen.* Cambridge, Mass.: Harvard University Press, 1951-1957. 4 vols.

Ghosh, Shyam. *The Original Yoga, as Expounded in Siva-Samhitâ, Gheranda-Samhitâ and Pâtanjala Yoga-Sûtra.* New Delhi: Munshiram Manoharlal, 1980.

Gitananda Giri, Swami. *Frankly Speaking.* Ed. by Meenakshi Devi Bhavanani. Chinnamudaliarchavady, India: Satya Press, 1997.

Gnoli, R. *Luce delle Sacre Scritture.* Turin, Italy: Unione Tipografico-Editrice Torinese, 1972. [Italian rendering of Abhinava Gupta's *Tantrâloka.*]

Goel, B. S. *Third Eye and Kundalini (An Experiential Account of Journey from Dust to Divinity).* New Colony, India: Third Eye Foundation of India, 1986.

Goldman, Robert P., ed. *The Râmâyana of Vâlmiki: An Epic of Ancient India.* Vol. 1: *Bâlakânda.* Vol. 2: *Ayodhyâkânda.* Princeton, N.J.: Princeton University Press, 1984, 1986.

Gonda, Jan. *Notes on Brahman.* Utrecht, Netherlands: J. L. Beyer, 1950.

_____. *Die Religionen Indiens.* Stuttgart, Germany: Kohlhammer, 1960–64. 3 vols.

_____. *The Vision of the Vedic Poets.* The Hague: Mouton, 1963.

_____. *Change and Continuity in Indian Religion.* The Hague: Mouton, 1965.

_____. *Loka: World and Heaven in the Veda.* Amsterdam: Noord-Hollandsche Uitgevers Meatschappij, 1966.

_____. *Visnuism and Sivaism: A Comparison.* London: Athelone Press, 1970.

_____. *Vedic Literature: Samhitâs and Brâhmanas.* A History of Indian Literature, vol. 1, fasc. 1. Wiesbaden, Germany: Otto Harrasowitz, 1975.

_____. *Vedic Literature: The Ritual Sûtras.* A History of Indian Literature, vol. 1, fasc. 2. Wiesbaden, Germany: Otto Harrasowitz, 1977.

Goodall, Dominic. *Hindu Scriptures.* Berkeley: University of California Press, 1996.

Gopal, Ram. *India of Vedic Kalpasûtras.* Delhi: National Publishing House, 1959.

Gopani, Amritlal S. *Jnânasâra by Mahopâdhyaya Srî Yasovijayajî.* Bombay: Jaina Sâhitya Vikâsa Mandala, 1986.

Goswami, Syundar Shyam. *Layayoga: An Advanced Method of Concentration.* London: Routledge & Kegan Paul, 1980.

Goudriaan, Teun, *The Vînâsikhatantra: A Saiva Tantra of the Left Current.* Delhi: Motilal Banarsidass, 1985.

_____, and Sanjukta Gupta. *Hindu Tantric and Sâkta Literature.* Wiesbaden, Germany: Otto Harrassowitz, 1981.

Govinda, Lama Anagarika. *The Psychological Attitude of Early Buddhist Philosophy.* New York: Weiser, 1961.

_____. *Foundations of Tibetan Mysticism.* London: Rider, 1972.

_____. *Creative Meditation and Multi-Dimensional Consciousness.* Wheaton, Ill.: Quest Books, 1976.

Govindan, Marshall. *Babaji and the 18 Siddha Kriya Yoga Tradition.* Montreal: Kriya Yoga Publications, 1991.

_____, ed. *Thirumandiram: A Yoga Classic by Siddhar Thirumoolar.* Translated by B. Natarajan. Montreal: Babaji's Kriya Yoga and Publications, 1993.

Greenwell, Bonnie. *Energies of Transformation: A Guide to the Kundalini Process.* Saratoga, Calif.: Shakti River Press, 1995.

Griffith, R., trans. *The Hymns of the Rig Veda.* Delhi: Motilal Banarsidass, repr. 1976. 2 vols.

Guenther, Herbert V. *The Tantric View of Life.* Berkeley, Calif.: Shambhala, 1972.

_____. *Philosophy and Psychology in the Abhidharma.* Berkeley and London: Shambhala, 1976.

_____, trans. *The Life and Teaching of Nâropa.* London: Oxford University Press, 1963.

_____, trans. *The Royal Song of Saraha.* Boulder, Colo.: Shambhala, 1973.

Gyaltsen, Khenpo Knchog. *The Great Kagyu Masters*. Ithaca, N.Y.: Snow Lion, 1990.

Gyatso, Geshe Kelsang. *A Meditation Handbook*. London: Tharpa, 1990.

_____. *Introduction to Buddhism*. London: Tharpa, 1992.

_____. *Understanding the Mind*. London: Tharpa, 1993.

_____. *Tantric Grounds and Paths*. London: Tharpa, 1994.

Halbfass, Wilhelm. *India and Europe: An Essay in Understanding*. Albany, N.Y.: SUNY Press, 1988.

Hardy, Friedhelm. *Viraha-Bhakti: The Early History of Krsna Devotion in South India*. New York: Oxford University Press, 1983.

Hare, E. M., trans. *Woven Cadences of Early Buddhists (Sutta-Nipâta)*. London: Oxford University Press, 1947.

Harshananda, Swami. *Sândilya Bhakti Sûtras with Svapnesvara Bhâsya*. Mysore: Prasaranga, University of Mysore, 1976.

Hartsuiker, Dolf. *Sâdhus: India's Mystic Holy Men*. Rochester, Vt.: Inner Traditions International, 1993.

*Hathayogapradîpikâ of Svâtmârâma, With the Commentary Jyotsnâ of Brahmânanda and English Translation*. Adyar, India: Adyar Library and Research Centre, 1972.

Hauer, Jakob Wilhelm. *Der Yoga: Ein indischer Weg zum Selbst*. Stuttgart, Germany: Kohlhammer, 1958.

Haug, M., trans. *Aitareya Brâhmana of the Rgveda*. Allahabad, India, repr. 1974.

Hawley, John Stratton. *Krishna, the Butter Thief*. Princeton, N.J.: Princeton University Press, 1983.

Hayes, Glen A. *The Necklace of Immortality: Metaphoric Worlds and Embodiment in Vaisnava Sahajiyâ Tantric Traditions*. Albany, N.Y.: SUNY Press, forthcoming 1999.

Heard, J. and S. L. Cranson, eds. *Reincarnation: An East-West Anthology*. New York: Crown, 1961.

Heinberg, Richard. *A New Covenant with Nature*. Wheaton, Ill.: Quest Books, 1996.

Hinze, Oscar Marcel. *Tantra Vidyâ*. Translated by V. M. Bedekar. Delhi: Motilal Banarsidass, repr. 1989.

Hooper, J. S. M. *Hymns of the Âlvârs*. Calcutta: Association Press, 1929.

Hopkins, E. W. *Ethics of India*. New Haven, Ct.: Yale University Press, 1924.

_____. *The Great Epic of India: Its Character and Origin*. Calcutta: Punthi Pustak, repr. 1969. First published 1901.

_____. *Epic Mythology*. Delhi: Motilal Banarsidass, repr. 1974. First published 1915.

Horner, I. B., trans. *The Collection of the Middle Length Sayings (Majjhima-Nikâya)*. London: Luzac, 1967. 3 vols.

Hughes, John. *Self Realization in Kashmir Shaivism: The Oral Teachings of Swami Laksmanjoo*. Albany, N.Y.: SUNY Press, 1994.

Hulin, Michel. *Sâmkhya Literature*. Wiesbaden, Germany: Otto Harrassowitz, 1978.

Hume, Robert Ernest, trans. *The Thirteen Principal Upanisads*. Oxford: Oxford University Press, 1921.

Iijima, Kanjitsu. *Buddhist Yoga*. Tokyo: Japan Publications, 1975.

Isherwood, Christopher. *Ramakrishna and His Disciples*. London: Methuen, 1965.

Iyengar, B. K. S. *Light on Yoga: Yoga Dîpikâ*. New York: Schocken Books, 1966.

_____. *Light on Pranayama*. New York: Crossroad, 1981.

_____. *The Tree of Yoga*. Boston, Mass.: Shambhala, 1989.

_____. *Light on the Yoga Sûtras of Patanjali*. San Francisco: HarperSanFrancisco, 1993.

Jacobi, Hermann. *Das Râmâyana: Geschichte und Inhalt, nebst Concordanz der Gedruckten Recensionen*. Bonn, Germany: Friedrich Cohen, 1893.

_____. *Jaina Sûtras*. New York: Dover, repr. 1968. 2 vols.

Jaini, Padmanabh S. *The Jaina Path of Purification*. Delhi: Motilal Banarsidass, 1979.

Jarrell, H. R. *International Yoga Bibliography, 1950 to 1980*. Metuchen, N.J.: Scarecrow Press, 1981.

Jha, A. *The Imprisoned Mind: Guru Shisya Tradition in Indian Culture*. New Delhi: Ambika Publications, 1983.

*Jîvanmuktiviveka (Liberation in Life) of Vidyâranya*. Edited with English translation by S. Subrahmanya Sastra and T. R. Srinivasa Ayyangar. Adyar, India: Adyar Library and Research Centre, 1978.

Johansson, R. E. A. *The Psychology of Nirvâna*. London: Allen & Unwin, 1969.

Johari, Harish. *Tools for Tantra*. Rochester, Vt.: Destiny Books, 1986.

_____. *Chakras: Energy Centers of Transformation*. Rochester, Vt.: Destiny Books, 1987.

Johnston, E. H. *Early Sâmkhya*. Delhi: Motilal Banarsiddas, repr. 1974.

Jones, J. J., trans. *The Mahâvastu*. London: Luzac, 1949, 1952, 1956. 3 vols.

Joshi, Hariprasad Shivprasad. *Origin and Development of Dattâtreya Worship in India*. Baroda, India: The Maharaja Sayajirao University of Baroda, 1965.

Judith, Anodea. *Eastern Body, Western Mind: Psychology and the Chakra System as a Path to the Self*. Berkeley, Calif.: Celestial Arts, 1996.

Jung, Carl Gustav. *Mandala Symbolism*. Translated by R. F. C. Hull. Princeton, N.J.: Princeton University Press, 1973.

_____. *Psychology and the East*. Princeton, N.J.: Princeton University Press, 1978.

Kaelber, Walter O. *Tapta Mârga: Asceticism and Initiation in Vedic India*. New York: SUNY Press, 1989.

Kak, Subhash. *The Astronomical Code of the Rgveda*. New Delhi: Aditya, 1994.

Kalu Rinpoche. *Secret Buddhism: Vajrayana Practices*. San Francisco: ClearPoint Press, 1995.

Kane, Pandurang Vaman. *History of Dharmasâstra*. Poona, India: Bhandarkar Oriental Research Institute, 1941. 5 vols.

Kannan, S., trans. *Swara Chintamani (Divination by Breath)*. New Delhi: Sagar Publications, 1972.

Katz, Ruth Cecily. *Arjuna in the Mahabharata: Where Krishna Is, There Is Victory*. Columbia, S.C.: University of South Carolina Press, 1989.

*Kaulajnâna-nirnaya of the School of Matsyendranâtha*. Edited by P. C. Bagchi and translated by Michael Magee. Varanasi, India: Prachya Prakashan, 1986.

Kaveeshwar, G. W. *The Ethics of the Gîtâ*. Delhi: Motilal Banarsidass, 1971.

Kaviraj, Gopinath. *Aspects of Indian Thought*. Burdwan, India: University of Burdwan, 1984.

Keith, Arthur B., trans. *The Religion and Philosophy of the Vedas and Upanishads*. Delhi: Motilal Banarsidass, repr. 1970.

_____. *The Rig Veda Brâhmanas*. Delhi: Motilal Banarsidass, repr. 1970. First published 1920.

Kennedy, Melville. *The Chaitanya Movement: A Study of Vaishnavism of Bengal*. Calcutta: Association Press/London: Oxford University Press, 1925.

Khanna, Madhu. *Yantra: The Tantric Symbol of Cosmic Unity*. London: Thames and Hudson, 1979.

Khetsun Sangpo Inbochay. *Tantric Practice in Nying-Ma*. Translated and edited by Jeffrey Hopkins. Ithaca, N.Y.: Snow Lion, 1982.

Kieffer, Gene. *Kundalini for the New Age: Selected Writings of Gopi Krishna*. New York: Bantam Books, 1988.

Kingsbury, F., and G. E. Phillips. *Hymns of the Tamil Saivite Saints*. Calcutta: Association Press/London: Oxford University Press, 1921.

Kingsland, Kevin, and Venika. *Hathapradipika: The Means by Which Constant Change May Be Transcended to Reveal the Eternal Light of the Self*. Torquay, England: Grael Communications, 1977.

Kinsley, David. *The Divine Player: A Study of Krsna Lîlâ*. Delhi: Motilal Banarsidass, 1979.

_____. *Hindu Goddesses: Visions of the Divine Feminine in the Hindu Religious Tradition*. Berkeley and Los Angeles: University of California Press, 1986.

_____. *Tantric Visions of the Divine Feminine: The Ten Mahâvidyâs*. Berkeley: University of California Press, 1997.

Kleen, Tyra de. *Mudrâs: The Ritual Hand-Poses of the Buddha Priests and the Shiva Priests of Bali*. London: Kegan Paul, 1924.

Klostermaier, Klaus. *A Survey of Hinduism*. Albany, N.Y.: SUNY Press, 1989.

Knipe, David M. *Hinduism: Experiments in the Sacred*. San Francisco: HarperSanFrancisco, 1991.

Kopp, S. *Guru: Metaphors from a Psychotherapist*. Palo Alto, Calif.: Science and Behavior, 1971.

Kraftsow, Gary. *Yoga and Wellness: Ancient Insights for Modern Healing.* New York: Penguin, forthcoming.

Kramrisch, Stella. *The Hindu Temple.* New Delhi: Motilal Banarsidass, repr. 1976. 2 vols.

_____. *The Presence of Siva.* Princeton, N.J.: Princeton University Press, 1981.

Kripananda, Swami. *Jnaneshwar's Gita: A Rendering of the Jnaneshwari.* Albany, N.Y.: SUNY Press, 1989.

Krishna, Gopi. *Kundalini: Evolutionary Energy in Man.* Psychological commentary by James Hillman. London: Robinson & Watkins, 1971.

_____. *The Biological Basis of Religion and Genius.* With an introduction by Carl Friedrich Freiherr von Weizsäcker. New York: Harper & Row, 1972.

_____. *The Awakening of Kundalini.* New York: E. P. Dutton, 1975.

_____. *Secrets of Kundalini in Panchastavi.* New Delhi: Kundalini Research and Publication Trust, 1978.

_____. *Living with Kundalini.* Boston and London: Shambhala, 1993.

*Kulârnava Tantra.* Text with English translation by Ram Kumar Rai. Varanasi, India: Prachya Prakashan, 1983.

*Kulârnava Tantra.* Edited by Târânâtha Vidyâratna and translated by M. P. Pandit. Delhi: Motilal Banarsidass, repr. 1984.

Kumar, Pushpendra. *Sakti Cult in Ancient India.* Varanasi, India: Bharatiya Publishing House, 1974.

Kuppanna Sastry, T. S., trans. *Vedanga Jyotish of Lagadha.* New Delhi: Indian National Science Academy, 1985.

Lannoy, Richard. *The Speaking Tree: A Study of Indian Culture and Society.* London: Oxford University Press, 1971.

Larson, Gerald James. *Classical Sâmkhya.* Delhi: Motilal Banarsidass, 1969.

_____, and Ram Shankar Bhattacharya, eds. *Sâmkhya: A Dualist Tradition in Indian Philosophy.* Princeton, N.J.: Princeton University Press, 1987.

Lasater, Judith. *Relax and Renew: Restful Yoga for Stressful Times.* Berkeley, Calif.: Rodmell Press, 1995.

Laski, Marghanita. *Ecstasy: A Study of Some Secular and Religious Experiences.* Los Angeles: J. P. Tarcher, 1990.

Lata, Prem. *Mystic Saints of India: Shankaracharya.* Delhi: Sumit Publications, 1982.

Leggett, Trevor. *The Complete Commentary by Sankara on the Yoga Sûtras: A Full Translation of the Newly Discovered Text.* London and New York: Kegan Paul International, 1990.

Leidy, Denise Patry, and Robert A. F. Thurman. *Mandala: The Architecture of Enlightenment.* Boston, Mass.: Shambhala, 1998.

LePage, Victoria. *Shambhala: The Fascinating Truth Behind the Myth of Shangri-La.* Wheaton, Ill.: Quest Books, 1996.

Lessing, F. D., and Alex Wayman. *Introduction to the Buddhist Tantric Systems.* New York: Weiser, 1980.

Lester, Robert C. *Râmânuja on the Yoga*. Adyar, India: Adyar Library and Research Centre, 1976.

*Lingapurâna*. Translated by Board of Scholars. Delhi: Motilal Banarsidass, 1973. 2 vols.

Lipner, Julius. *The Face of Truth: A Study of Meaning and Metaphysics in the Vedântic Theology of Râmânuja*. Albany, N.Y.: SUNY Press, 1986.

Lorenzen, D. N. *The Kâpâlikas and Kâlâmukhas, Two Lost Saivite Sects*. New Delhi: Motilal Banarsidass, repr. 1972.

Lozowick, Lee. *The Alchemy of Love and Sex*. Foreword by G. Feuerstein. Prescott, Ariz.: Hohm Press, 1996.

_____. *Hohm Sahaj Mandir Study Manual: A Handbook for Practitioners of Every Spiritual and/or Transformational Path*. Prescott, Ariz.: Hohm Press, 1996. 2 vols.

M. [Mahendranath Gupta]. *The Gospel of Sri Ramakrishna*. Translated by Swami Nikhilananda. New York: Ramakrishna-Vivekananda Center, 1942.

Macdonell, A. A. *Vedic Mythology*. Varanasi, India: Indological Book House, 1963. 2 vols. First published 1912.

Mackay, Ernest. *The Indus Civilization*. London: AMS Press, repr. 1983.

Madhavananda, Swami. *Uddhava Gita, or the Last Message of Shri Krishna*. Calcutta: Advaita Ashrama, 1971.

Mani, Vettam. *Purânic Encyclopaedia*. Delhi: Motilal Banarsidass, repr. 1993.

*Mantramahodadhi of Mahidhara*. Translated by a Board of Scholars. Delhi: Sri Satguru Publications, 1984.

*Mantra-Yoga Samhitâ*. Edited text with English translation by Ramkumar Rai. Varanasi, India: Chaukhambha Orientalia, 1982.

Marshall, Sir John. *Mohenjo-daro and the Indus Civilization*. London: Arthur Probsthain, 1931. 3 vols.

Maslow, Abraham. *Towards a Psychology of Being*. Princeton, N.J.: Van Nostrand, 1962.

*Matsya-Purânam*. Translated by A Taluqdar of Oudh. Allahabad, India: Sudhindra Nath Vasu, 1916.

Matus, Thomas. *Yoga and the Jesus Prayer Tradition*. Ramsey, N.J.: Paulist Press, 1984.

Mayeda, Sengaku. *A Thousand Teachings: The Upadesasasâhasrî of Sankara*. Albany, N.Y.: SUNY Press, 1982.

McDaniel, June. *The Madness of the Saints: Ecstatic Religion in Bengal*. Chicago and London: University of Chicago Press, 1989.

McLeod, W. H. *Sikhism*. Chicago: University of Chicago Press, 1990.

Metha, Mohan Lal. *Jaina Philosophy*. Varanasi, India: P. V. Research Institute, 1971.

Michell, George. *The Hindu Temple: An Introduction to Its Meaning and Forms*. Chicago and London: University of Chicago Press, 1988.

Miller, Barbara Stoler, trans. *Love Song of the Dark Lord: Jayadeva's Gitagovinda*. New York: Columbia University Press, 1977.

Miller, Jeanine. *The Vedas: Harmony, Meditation and Fulfillment*. London: Rider, 1974.

_____. *The Vision of Cosmic Order in the Vedas.* London: Routledge & Kegan Paul, 1985.

Mishra, Kamalakar. *Kashmir Saivism: The Central Philosophy of Tantrism.* Cambridge, Mass.: Rudra Press, 1993.

Mishra, Rammurti S. *The Textbook of Yoga Psychology.* New York: Julian Press, 1987.

Mitchener, John E. *Traditions of the Seven Rsis.* Delhi: Motilal Banarsidass, 1982.

Mitra, V. *Education in Ancient India.* Delhi: Arya Book Depot, 1964.

Mitra, Vihâri-Lâla, trans. *The Yoga-Vâsishtha-Mahârâmâyana of Vâlmiki.* Varanasi: Bharatiya Publishing House, 1976. 4 vols.

Monro, Robin, A. K. Ghosh, and Daniel Kalish, eds. *Yoga Research Bibliography: Scientific Studies on Yoga and Meditation.* Cambridge, England: Yoga Biomedical Trust, 1989.

Mookerjee, Ajit. *Tantra Art: Its Philosophy and Physics.* Basel, Switzerland: Ravi Kumar, 1971.

_____. *Kundalini: The Arousal of the Inner Energy.* New York: Destiny Books, 1982.

_____. *Kali: The Feminine Force.* New York: Destiny Books, 1988.

_____, and Madhu Khanna. *The Tantric Way: Art, Science, Ritual.* London: Thames and Hudson, 1977.

Motoyama, Hiroshi. *Toward a Superconsciousness: Meditational Theory and Practice.* Berkeley, Calif.: Asian Humanities Press, 1990.

Muktananda, Swami. *Play of Consciousness (Chitshakti Vilas).* San Francisco: Harper & Row, 1978.

_____. *Secret of the Siddhas.* South Fallsburg, N.Y.: SYDA Foundation, 1983.

Muktibodhananda Saraswati, Swami. *Swara Yoga: The Tantric Science of Brain Breathing.* Munger, India: Bihar School of Yoga, 1984.

Müller, Max. *Chips from a German Workshop.* London: Longmans, Green & Co., 1867, 1875, 1880, 1907. 4 vols.

_____. *Ramakrishna: His Life and Sayings.* London: Longmans, Green, & Co., 1898.

_____. *The Six Systems of Indian Philosophy.* London: Longmans, Green & Co., repr. 1928.

Muller-Ortega, Paul Eduardo. *The Triadic Heart of Siva: Kaula Tantricism of Abhinavagupta in the Non-Dual Shaivism of Kashmir.* Albany, N.Y.: SUNY Press, 1989.

Mumford, Jonn. *Psychosomatic Yoga.* London: Thorsons, 1962.

_____. *Ecstasy Through Tantra.* St. Paul, Minn.: Llewellyn Publications, 1988.

Murphy, Michael. *The Future of the Body: Explorations into the Further Evolution of Human Nature.* Los Angeles: J. P. Tarcher, 1992.

_____, and Steven Donovan. *The Physical and Psychological Effects of Meditation: A Review of Contemporary Research with a Comprehensive Bibliography 1931–1996.* Edited with an introduction by Eugene Taylor. Sausalito, Calif.: Institute of Noetic Sciences, 1997.

Murti, Tirupattur R. V. *The Central Philosophy of Buddhism: A Study of the Mâdhyamika System*. London: Unwin Hyman, 1980.

Narain, K. *An Outline of Madhva's Philosophy*. Allahabad, India: Udayana Publications, 1962.

Naranjo, Claudio, and Robert E. Ornstein. *On the Psychology of Meditation*. London: George Allen & Unwin, 1972.

Neevel, Walter G., Jr. *Yâmuna's Vedânta and Pâncarâtra: Integrating the Classical and the Popular*. Missoula, Mont.: Scholars Press, 1977.

Neufeldt, Ronald W., ed. *Karma & Rebirth: Post Classical Developments*. Albany, N.Y.: SUNY Press, 1986.

Nikhilananda, Swami, trans. *The Gospel of Sri Ramakrishna*. New York: Ramakrishna Vivekananda Center, 1942.

_____. *Hinduism: Its Meaning for the Liberation of the Spirit*. New York: Harper & Bros., 1958.

Niranjananda, Paramahamsa. *Dharana Darshan: A Panoramic View of the Yogic, Tantric and Upanishadic Practices of Concentration and Visualization*. Deoghar, India: Sri Panchadashnam Paramahamsa Alakh Bara, 1993.

Nowotny, Fausta. *Eine durch Miniaturen erleutete Doctrina Mystica aus Srinagar*. The Hague: Mouton, 1958.

Oberhammer, Gerhard. *Strukturen yogischer Meditation*. Vienna: Verlag der österreichischen Akademie der Wissenschaften, 1977.

O'Flaherty, Wendy Doniger. *Asceticism and Eroticism in the Mythology of Siva*. Delhi: Oxford University Press, 1973.

_____. *The Origins of Evil in Hindu Mythology*. Berkeley and Los Angeles: University of California Press, 1976.

_____. *The Rig Veda*. New York: Penguin Books, 1981.

_____, ed. *Karma and Rebirth in Classical Indian Traditions*. Berkeley: University of California Press, 1976.

Olivelle, Patrick. *Samnyâsa Upanisads: Hindu Scriptures on Asceticism and Renunciation*. Oxford and New York: Oxford University Press, 1992.

_____. *Upanisads*. Oxford and New York: Oxford University Press, 1996.

Osborne, Arthur, ed. *The Teachings of Ramana Maharshi*. York Beach, Maine: Weiser, 1995.

_____. *Ramana Maharshi and the Path of Knowledge*. York Beach, Maine: Samuel Weiser, 1995.

Pabongka Rinpoche. *Liberation in the Palm of Your Hand: A Concise Discourse on the Path to Enlightenment*. Edited by Trijang Rinpoche. Translated by Michael Richards. Boston, Mass.: Wisdom, 1991.

Pandey, Kanti Chandra. *Abhinavagupta: An Historical and Philosophical Study*. Varanasi, India: Chowkhamba Sanskrit Series Office, 1963.

_____. *An Outline of the History of Saiva Philosophy*. Delhi: Motilal Banarsidass, repr. 1986.

Panikkar, Raimundo. *The Vedic Experience—Mantramanjarî: An Anthology of the Vedas for Modern Man and Contemporary Celebration*. London: Darton, Longman & Todd, 1977.

Parab, B. A. *The Miraculous and Mysterious in Vedic Literture*. Bombay: Popular Book Depot, 1952.

Pargiter, F. E. *The Mârkandeya Purâna*. Delhi: Indological Books House, repr. 1969. First published 1904.

_____. *Ancient Indian Historical Tradition*. Delhi: Motilal Banarsidass, repr. 1972. First published 1922.

Pathak, P. *The Heyapaksha of Yoga*. Delhi: Motilal Banarsidass, 1932.

Peo [Peo Olsen]. *Medical & Psychological Scientific Research on Yoga & Meditation*. Copenhagen: Scandinavian Yoga and Meditation School, 1978.

Piggott, Stuart. *Prehistoric India*. Harmondsworth, England: Penguin Books, 1950.

Pope, G. U., ed. and trans. *The Tiruvacâgam or 'Sacred Utterances' of the Tamil Poet, Saint and Sage Manikka-Vacagar*. Oxford: Clarendon Press, 1900.

Potdar, K. R. *Sacrifice in the Rgveda*. Bombay: Bharatiya Vidya Bhavan, 1953.

Pott, P. H. *Yoga and Yantra: Their Interrelation and Their Significance for Indian Archeology*. The Hague: E. J. Brill, 1966.

Powers, John. *Introduction to Tibetan Buddhism*. Ithaca, N.Y.: Snow Lion, 1995.

Prabhavananda, Swami. *The Spiritual Heritage of India*. Hollywood, Calif.: Vedanta Press, 1979.

Pradhan, V. G. *Jnâneshvarî*. London: George Allen & Unwin, 1967. 2 vols.

Pratyagatmananda Saraswati, Swami. *The Fundamentals of Vedanta Philosophy*. Madras: Ganesh, 1961.

Prem, Krishna. *The Yoga of the Bhagavat Gita*. London: Watkins, 1969; Baltimore, Md.: Penguin Books, 1973.

_____. *The Yoga of the Kathopanishad*. Allahabad, India: Ananda Publishing House, n.d.

Prem Prakash. *The Yoga of Spiritual Devotion: A Modern Translation of the Narada Bhakti Sutras*. Rochester, Vt.: Inner Traditions International, 1998.

Pusalker, A. D. *Studies in the Epics and Purânas*. Bombay: Bharatiya Vidya Bhavan, 1963.

Radhakrishnan, Sarvepalli. *Indian Philosophy*. London: George Allen & Unwin, 1923. 2 vols.

_____. *Idealist View of Life*. London: George Allen & Unwin, 1932.

_____. *The Principal Upanisads*. London: George Allen & Unwin, 1953.

_____, trans. *The Bhagavadgîtâ*. London: Routledge & Kegan Paul, 1960.

Raghavachar, S. S. *Vedârtha-Sangraha of Srî Râmânujâcârya*. Mysore: Sri Ramakrishna Ashrama, 1978.

Raghunathan, N., trans. *Srîmad-Bhâgavatam*. Madras: Vighnesvara, 1976. 2 vols.

Rai, Ram Kumar. *Encyclopedia of Yoga*. Varanasi, India: Prachya Prakashan, 1975.

_____. *Shiva Svarodaya*. Varanasi, India: Prachya Prakashan, 1980.

_____. *Mantra-Yoga-Samhitâ*. Varanasi, India: Chaukhambha Orientalia, 1982.

Raju, P. T. *Structural Depths of Indian Thought.* Albany, N.Y.: SUNY Press, 1985.

Rama, Swami. *Sukhamani Sahib: Fountain of Eternal Joy.* Honesdale, Penn.: Himalayan International Institute of Yoga Science and Philosophy of the U.S.A., 1988.

_____, Rudolf Ballentine, and Swami Ajaya (Allan Weinstock). *Yoga and Psychotherapy: The Evolution of Consciousness.* Glenview, Ill.: Himalayan Institute, 1976.

Râmânuja. *Vedârthasangraha.* Edited and translated by V. Krishnamacharya and M. B. Narasimha Ayyangar. Adyar, India: Theosophical Publishing House, 1953.

Ramanujan, A. K. *Speaking of Siva.* Baltimore, Md.: Penguin, 1973.

_____, trans. *Hymns for the Drowning: Poems for Visnu by Nammâlvâr.* Princeton, N.J.: Princeton University Press, 1981.

Ranade, R. D. *Mysticism in Maharashtra: Indian Mysticism.* Delhi: Motilal Banarsidass, repr. 1982.

Rao, K. B. Ramakrishna. *Theism of Pre-Classical Sâmkhya.* Mysore: Prasaranga, University of Mysore, 1966.

Rao, S. K. R. *The Yantras.* Delhi: Sri Satguru Publications, 1988.

Rastogi, N. *Krama Tantricism of Kashmir: Historical and General Sources,* vol. 1. Delhi: Motilal Banarsidass, 1981.

Ravindra, Ravi. *Whispers from the Other Shore: A Spiritual Search—East and West.* Wheaton, Ill.: Quest Books, 1984.

Rawlinson, Andrew. *The Book of Enlightened Masters: Western Teachers in Eastern Traditions.* Chicago and La Salle, Ill.: Open Court, 1997.

Rawson, Phillip. *Tantra: The Indian Cult of Ecstasy.* New York: Avon Books, 1973.

_____. *The Art of Tantra.* London: Thames and Hudson, 1978.

Reat, N. Ross. *Origins of Indian Psychology.* Berkeley, Calif.: Asian Humanities Press, 1990.

Reddy, M. Venkata. *Hatharatnavali of Srinivasa Bhatta Mahayogindra.* Secunderabad, India: Vemana Yoga Research Institute, 1982.

Renou, Louis. *Religions of Ancient India.* New York: Schocken Books, 1968.

Reymond, Lizelle. *To Live Within: A Woman's Spiritual Pilgrimage in a Himalayan Hermitage.* Portland, Oreg.: Rudra Press, 1995.

Rhie, Marilyn, and Robert A. F. Thurman. *Wisdom and Compassion: The Sacred Art of Tibet.* New York: Tibet House, 1996.

Rhys Davids, C. A. F. *The Birth of Indian Psychology and Its Development in Buddhism.* London: Luzac, 1936.

Rhys Davids, T. W., trans. *Dialogues of the Buddha.* London: The Pali Text Society, 1971–1973. 3 vols.

Richman, Paula, ed. *Many Râmâyanas: The Diversity of a Narrative Tradition in South Asia.* Berkeley: University of California Press, 1991.

Rieker, Hans-Ulrich. *The Yoga of Light.* Translated by Elsy Becherer. New York: Herder and Herder, 1971.

Robinson, Richard H. *Early Mâdhyamika in India and China.* Madison, Milwaukee, and London: University of Wisconsin Press, 1967.

Rukmani, T. S. *Yogavârttika of Vijnânabhiksu.* New Delhi: Munshiram Manoharlal, 1981, 1983, 1987, 1989. 4 vols.

_____. *A Critical Study of the Bhâgavata Purâna.* Varanasi, India: Chowkhamba Sanskrit Series Office, 1970.

Sakhare, M. R. *History and Philosophy of Lingayat Religion.* Darwad, India: Karnatak University, 1978.

Sangharakshita, Bhikshu. *A Survey of Buddhism.* Boulder, Colo.: Shambhala/London: Windhorse, 1980.

_____. *The Three Jewels: An Introduction to Buddhism.* Glasgow: Windhorse, 1991.

Sannella, Lee. *The Kundalini Experience: Psychosis or Transcendence?* Lower Lake, Calif.: Integral Publishing, rev. ed., 1992.

Sargeant, Winthrop, trans. *The Bhagavad Gîtâ.* Edited by Christopher Chapple. Albany, N.Y.: SUNY Press, rev. ed. 1984.

*Satkarmasangrahah.* Edited and translated by R. G. Harshe. Lonavla, India: Yoga-Mîmâmsâ Prakâsana, 1970.

Satprakashananda, Swami. *Methods of Knowledge According to Advaita Vedanta.* London: George Allen & Unwin, 1965.

Satyananda Saraswati, Swami. *Asana, Pranayama, Mudra, Bandha.* Monghyr, India: Bihar School of Yoga, 1973.

_____. *A Systematic Course in the Ancient Tantric Techniques of Yoga and Kriya.* Monghyr, India: Bihar School of Yoga, 1981.

_____. *Taming the Kundalini.* Munger, India: Bihar School of Yoga, 4th ed.,1982.

_____. *Kundalini Tantra.* Munger, India: Bihar School of Yoga, 1996.

Satyasangananda Saraswati, Swami. *Tattwa Shuddhi: The Tantric Practice of Inner Purification.* Munger, India: Bihar School of Yoga, 1984.

Saunders, E. Dale. *Mudrâ: A Study of Symbolic Gestures in Japanese Buddhist Sculpture.* Princeton, N.J.: Princeton University Press, 1985.

Schiffmann, Erich. *Yoga: The Spirit and Practice of Moving into Stillness.* New York: Pocket Books, 1996.

Schoterman, J. A. *The Yonitantra.* New Delhi: Manohar Publications, 1980. [Sanskrit text with English translation.]

Schrader, F. Otto. *Introduction to the Pâncarâtra and the Ahirbudhnya Samhitâ.* Adyar, India: Adyar Library, 1916.

Schubring, Walther. *The Doctrine of the Jainas.* Delhi: Motilal Banarsidass, 1912.

Schumann, Hans Wolfgang. *Buddhism: An Outline of Its Teachings and Schools.* Translated by Georg Feuerstein. London: Rider, 1973.

Scott, Mary. *Kundalini in the Physical World.* London: Routledge and Kegan Paul, 1983.

SenSharma, Deba Brata. *The Philosophy of Sâdhanâ, With Special Reference to the Trika Philosophy of Kashmir.* Albany, N.Y.: SUNY Press, 1990.

Sethi, V. K. *Kabir: The Weaver of God's Name.* Dera Baba Jaimal Sing, India: Radha Soami Satsang Beas, 1984.

Shamdasani, Sonu, ed. *The Psychology of Kundalini Yoga: Notes of the Seminar Given in 1932 by C. G. Jung.* Princeton, N.J.: Princeton University Press, 1996.

Sharma, Arvind. *The Hindu Gîtâ: Ancient and Classical Interpretations of the Bhagavadgîtâ.* LaSalle, Ill.: Open Court, 1986.

Sharma, B. N. K. *A History of the Dvaita School of Vedânta and Its Literature.* Bombay: Bookseller's Publishing Co., 1960.

Sharma, C. *A Critical Survey of Indian Philosophy.* London: Rider, 1960.

Sharma, Narendra Nath. *Yoga Kârnikâ of Nath Aghorânanda: An Ancient Treatise on Yoga.* Delhi: Eastern Book Linkers, 1981.

Sharma, Tulsi Ram. *Studies in the Sectarian Upanishads.* Delhi: Munshiram Manoharlal, 1972.

Shashi, S. S., ed. *Encyclopaedia Indica.* New Delhi: Vedams Books International, 1996–. 20 vols.

Silburn, Lilian. *Le Vijnâna Bhairava.* Paris: Editions E. De Boccard, 1961.

_____. *Kundalin: The Energy of the Depths.* Albany, N.Y.: SUNY Press, 1988.

Singh, Jaideva. *Siva Sûtras: The Yoga of Supreme Identity.* Delhi: Motilal Banarsidass, 1979.

_____. *Pratyabhijnâhrdayam: The Secret of Self-Recognition.* Delhi: Motilal Banarsidass, rev. ed., 1980.

_____. *Spanda-Kârikâs: The Divine Creative Pulsation.* Delhi: Motilal Banarsidass, 1980.

_____. *The Yoga of Delight, Wonder, and Astonishment.* Albany, N.Y.: SUNY Press, 1991.

_____, Swami Lashmanjee, and Bettina Bäumer. *Abhinavagupta, Parâtrîsikâ-Vivarana: The Secret of Tantric Mysticism.* Delhi: Motilal Banarsidass, 1988.

Singh, Lal A. *Yoga Psychology: Methods and Approaches.* Varanasi, India: Bharatiya Vidya Prakashan, 1970.

Singh, Mohan. *Gorakhnath and Mediaeval Hindu Mysticism.* Lahore, India: Mohan Singh, 1937.

Sinh, Pancham, trans. *The Hatha-Yoga-Pradîpikâ.* Allahabad, India: Panini Office, 1915.

Sinha, Phulgenda. *The Gita As It Was: Rediscovering the Original Bhagavadgita.* LaSalle, Ill.: Open Court, 1987.

Sircar, D. C. *The Sâkta Pîthas.* Delhi: Motilal Banarsidass, repr. 1981.

Sivananda Radha, Swami. *Kundalini: Yoga for the West.* Spokane, Wash.: Timeless Books, 1978.

_____. *Hatha Yoga: The Hidden Language.* Spokane, Wash.: Timeless Books, 1987.

Sivananda Saraswati, Swami. *Guru and Disciple.* Rishikesh, India: Yoga Vedanta Forest Academy, 1955.

_____. *Tantra Yoga, Nâda Yoga and Kriyâ Yoga*. Rishikesh, India: Yoga Vedanta Forest University, 1955.

_____. *Japa Yoga: A Comprehensive Treatise on Mantra Sâstra*. Shivanandanagar, India: Divine Life Society, 1986.

*Siva-Purâna*. Translated by Board of Scholars. Delhi: Motilal Banarsidass, repr. 1986. 4 vols.

*Skanda-Purâna*. Translated by Board of Scholars. Delhi: Motilal Banarsidass, 1992. 2 vols. [More volumes are in progress.]

Skolimowski, Henryk. *The Participatory Mind: A New Theory of Knowledge and of the Universe*. London and New York: Arkana/Penguin Books, 1994.

Smart, Ninian. *Doctrine and Argument in Indian Philosophy*. London: George Allen & Unwin, repr. 1969.

Snellgrove, David L. *The Hevajra Tantra: A Critical Study*. London: Oxford University Press, 1959.

Sprockhoff, Joachim F. *Samnyâsa: Quellenstudien zur Askese im Hinduism*. Wiesbaden, Germany: Kommissionsverlag Franz Steiner, 1976.

Staal, Frits. *Exploring Mysticism: A Methodological Essay*. London: Penguin, 1975.

_____. *Agni: The Vedic Ritual of Fire*. Berkeley, Calif.: Asian Humanities Press, 1983. 2 vols.

Stevenson, S. T. *The Heart of Jainism*. London: Oxford University Press, 1915.

Stewart, Jampa Machenzie. *The Life of Gampopa: The Incomparable Dharma Lord of Tibet*. Ithaca, N.Y.: Snow Lion, 1995.

Subramuniyaswami, Satguru Sivaya. *Dancing with Siva: Hinduism's Contemporary Catechism*. Concord, Calif.: Himalayan Academy, 1993.

_____. *Loving Ganesa: Hinduism's Endearing Elephant-Faced God*. Concord, Calif.: Himalayan Academy, 1996.

Sukthankar, Vishnu Sitaram. *On the Meaning of the Mahâbhârata*. Bombay: Asiatic Society of Bombay, 1957.

Suzuki, D. T. *Essays in Zen Buddhism*. London: Rider, 1950, 1953, 1954. 3 vols.

_____, ed. *On Indian Mahâyâna Buddhism*. New York: Harper & Row, 1968.

Svoboda, Robert E. *Aghora: At the Left Hand of God*. Albuquerque, N.M.: Brotherhood of Life, 1986.

_____. *Aghora II: Kundalini*. Albuquerque, N.M.: Brotherhood of Life, 1993.

Tagare, Ganesh V., trans. *Siva-Purâna*. Delhi: Motilal Banarsidass, 1970.

Tagore, Rabindranath. *The Religion of Man*. London: George Allen & Unwin, 1953.

_____. *Gitanjali*. New York: Macmillan, 1971.

Tandon, S. N. *A Re-Appraisal of Patanjali's Yoga-Sutras in the Light of the Buddha's Teaching*. Igatpuri, India: Vipassana Research Institute, 1995.

Tapasyananda, Swami. *Sankara-Dig-Vijaya: The Traditional Life of Sri Sankaracharya by Madhava-Vidyaranya*. Madras, India: Sri Ramakrishna Math, 1978.

Tatia, Nathmal. *Studies in Jaina Philosophy*. Varanasi, India: Jaina Cultural Research Society, 1951.

_____. *Tattvârtha Sûtra: That Which Is*. New York: HarperCollins, 1994.

Telang, K. T. *Bhagavadgîtâ with the Sanatsujâtîya and the Anugîtâ*. Oxford: Clarendon Press, 2d ed., 1908.

Thadani, N. V. *The Mystery of the Mahabharata*. Karachi, India: Bharat Publishing House, 1931-1935. 5 vols.

Thibaut, George, trans. *Vedânta-Sûtras with the Commentary of Râmânuja*. Delhi: Motilal Banarsidass, 1904.

_____, trans. *Sankara's Commentary on the Brahma-Sûtras*. New York: Dover, repr. 1962.

Thomas, E. J. *The Life of Buddha as Legend and History*. Delhi: Motilal Banarsidass, repr. 1993.

Thurman, Robert A. F., trans. *The Tibetan Book of the Dead*. New York: Bantam Books, 1994.

Tigunait, Rajmani. *Sakti Sâdhanâ: Steps to Samâdhi—A Translation of the Tripura Rahasya*. Honesdale, Penn.: Himalayan International Institute, 1993.

_____. *Saktism: The Power in Tantra*. Honesdale, Penn.: Himalayan International Institute, 1998.

Tilak, B. G. *Gîtârahasya*. Poona, India: Tilak Bros., 1935–36. 2 vols.

Tripurari, Swami B. V. *Jîva Goswâm's Tattva-Sandarbha: Sacred India's Philosophy of Ecstasy*. Eugene, Oreg.: Clarion Call, 1995.

_____. *Aesthetic Vedânta: The Sacred Path of Passionate Love*. Eugene, Oreg.: Mandala, 1996.

Trungpa, Chögyam. *Cutting Through Spiritual Materialism*. Boulder and London: Shambhala, 1973.

Tsang Nyön Heruka. *The Life of Marpa the Translator: Seeing Accomplishes All*. Translated by the Nâlandâ Translation Committee. Boulder, Colo.: Prajnâ Press, 1982.

Tsongkhapa. *Tantra in Tibet: The Great Exposition of Secret Mantra*. London: George Allen & Unwin, 1980–81. 2 vols.

_____. *Compassion in Tibetan Buddhism*. Edited and translated by Jeffrey Hopkins. Ithaca, N.Y.: Snow Lion, 1985.

_____. *The Principal Teachings of Buddhism*. Translated by Geshe Lobsang Tharchin with Michael Roach. Howell, N.J.: Mahayana Sutra and Tantra Press, 1988.

_____. *Preparing for Tantra: The Mountain of Blessings*. Translated by Khen Rinpoche and Geshe Lobsang Tharchin with Michael Roach. Howell, N.J.: Mahayana Sutra and Tantra Press, 1995.

Tucci, Guiseppe. *On Some Aspects of Maitreyanâtha and Asanga*. Calcutta: Calcutta University Press, 1930.

_____. *The Theory and Practice of the Mandala*. London: Rider, 1971.

_____. *The Religions of Tibet*. Berkeley and Los Angeles: University of California Press, 1980.

Tweedie, Irina. *Daughter of Fire: A Diary of a Spiritual Training with a Sufi Master*. Nevada City, Calif.: Blue Dolphin Publishing, 1986.

Tyagisananda, Swami. *Aphorisms on the Gospel of Divine Love, or Nârada Bhakti Sûtras.* Mylapore, India: Sri Ramakrishna Math, 1972.

Upadhyaya, K. N. *Early Buddhism and the Bhagavadgîtâ.* Delhi: Motilal Banarsidass, 1971.

*Vamakesvarimatam.* Edited and translated by Michael Magee. Varanasi, India: Prachya Prakashan, 1986.

Van Lysebeth, André. *Tantra: The Cult of the Feminine.* York Beach, Maine: Samuel Weiser, 1995.

Varadachari, V. *Âgamas and South Indian Vaisnavism.* Triplicane, India: Prof. Rangacharya Memorial Trust, 1982.

Varenne, Jean. *Yoga and the Hindu Tradition.* Chicago: Chicago University Press, 1976.

Vasu, Rai Bahadur Sris Chandra, trans. *The Gheranda-Samhitâ.* New Delhi: Oriental Books Reprint Corp., 1975.

_____. *The Siva Samhitâ.* New Delhi: Oriental Books Reprint Corp., 1975.

Venkataramaiah, Munagala S. *Tripura Rahasya, or The Mystery Beyond the Trinity.* Tiruvannamalai, India: Sri Ramanasramam, 1962.

Venkatesananda, Swami. *The Supreme Yoga: A New Translation of the Yoga Vâsistha in Two Volumes.* Elgin, South Africa: Chiltern Yoga Trust, 1981. 2 vols.

_____. *The Concise Yoga Vâsistha.* Albany, N.Y.: SUNY Press, 1984.

Vishnudevananda, Swami. *The Complete Illustrated Book of Yoga.* New York: Bell Publishing, 1960.

Vivekananda, Swami. *Raja-Yoga, or Conquering the Internal Nature.* Calcutta: Avaita Ashrama, 1962.

_____. *Jnana-Yoga.* New York: Ramakrishna-Vivekananda Center, 1982.

_____. *Karma-Yoga and Bhakti-Yoga.* New York: Ramakrishna-Vivekananda Center, 1982.

_____. *The Complete Works of Swami Vivekananda.* Mayavati, India: Advaita Ashrama, 1947-1955. 8 vols.

Waddell, L. Austine. *Egyptian Civilization: Its Sumerian Origin & Real Chronology.* London: Luzac, 1930.

_____. *Tibetan Buddhism.* New York: Dover, 1972.

Wallis, H. W. *Cosmology of the Rigveda.* London: Williams & Norgate, 1887.

Walshe, Maurice. *Thus Have I Heard: The Long Discourses of the Buddha.* London: Wisdom Publications, 1981.

Warren, Henry Clark, trans. *Buddhism in Translations.* New York: Atheneum, 1963.

Wayman, Alex. *The Buddhist Tantras.* New York: Weiser, 1973.

_____. *Yoga of the Guhyasamâjatantra.* Delhi: Motilal Banarsidass, 1977.

Werner, Karel. *Yoga and Indian Philosophy.* New Delhi: Motilal Banarsidass, 1977.

Wheeler, Mortimer. *The Indus Civilization.* Cambridge: Cambridge University Press, 1960.

White, David Gordon. *The Alchemical Body: Siddha Traditions in Medieval India.* Chicago and London: The University of Chicago Press, 1996.

White, John, ed. *Kundalini: Evolution and Enlightenment.* New York: Paragon House, 1990.

_____, ed. *What is Enlightenment? Exploring the Goal of the Spiritual Path.* Los Angeles: J. P. Tarcher, 1985.

Whitney, William David, trans. *Atharva Veda Samhitâ.* Cambridge, Mass.: Harvard University Press, 1950. 2 vols.

Wilber, Ken. *The Atman Project: A Transpersonal View of Human Development.* Wheaton, Ill.: Theosophical Publishing House, 1980.

_____. *Sex, Ecology, Spirituality: The Spirit of Evolution.* Boston, Mass./London: Shambhala Publications, 1995.

Williams, R. *Jaina Yoga: A Survey of the Mediaeval Srâvakâcâras.* London: Oxford University Press, 1963.

Wilson, Horace Hayman, trans. *The Vishnu Purâna.* Delhi: Nag Publishers, repr. 1980. 5 vols.

_____. *The Matsyamahâpurânam.* Jawaharnagar, India: Nag Publishers, repr. 1983. 2 vols.

Winternitz, Moritz. *A History of Indian Literature.* Translated by V. S. Sarma. Calcutta: University of Calcutta, 1927. 3 vols.

Wood, Ernest. *Great Systems of Yoga.* New York: Citadel Press, 1968.

Woodroffe, Sir John [see also Avalon, Arthur]. *Tantrarâja Tantra: A Short Analysis.* Madras, India: Ganesh & Co., 3d ed., 1971.

_____. *Introduction to Tantra Sâstra.* Madras, India: Ganesh & Co., 6th ed., 1973.

_____. *Shakti and Shakta: Essays and Addresses on the Shakta Tantrashastra.* Madras, India: Ganesh & Co., 8th ed., 1975.

_____. *The Garland of Letters.* Madras, India: Ganesh & Co., 7th ed., 1979.

Woods, James Haughton. *The Yoga-System of Patanjali.* Delhi: Motilal Banarsidass, repr. 1966.

Yeshe Tsogyal. *The Lotus-Born: The Life Story of Padmasambhava.* Translated by Erik Pema Kunsang and edited by Marcia Binder Schmidt. Boston, Mass.: Shambhala, 1993.

Yogananda, Paramahansa. *Autobiography of a Yogi.* Los Angeles: Self-Realization Fellowship, 1987. First publ. 1946. Another edition by Crystal Clarity in Nevada City, Calif., 1987.

_____. *God Talks with Arjuna: The Bhagavad Gita—Royal Science of God-Realization.* Los Angeles: Self-Realization Fellowship, 1995. 2 vols. [published posthumously]

*Yoga Shastra of Dattatreya.* Edited by Brahma Mitra Awasthi and translated by Amita Sharma. Roop Nagar, India: Swami Keshawananda Yoga Institute, 1985.

Yogendra, Jaideva, ed. *Cyclopaedia Yoga,* vol. 1. Santacruz, India: The Yoga Institute, 1988.

_____, ed. *Cyclopaedia Yoga,* vol. 3. Santacruz, India: The Yoga Institute, 1993.

Yogendra, Shri. *Yoga Essays.* Santacruz, India: The Yoga Institute, 1978.

_____. *Yoga Hygiene Simplified*. Santacruz, India: The Yoga Institute, 1990.

Zaehner, R. C. *The Bhagavad-Gîtâ*. Oxford: Clarendon Press, 1969.

Zimmer, Heinrich. *Philosophies of India*. Edited by Joseph Campbell. New York: Meridian Books, 1956.

_____. *Myths and Symbols in Indian Art and Civilization*. Edited by Joseph Campbell. New York: Harper & Row, 1962.

_____. *Artistic Form and Yoga in the Sacred Images of India*. Translated by Gerald Chapple and James B. Lawson. Princeton, N.J.: Princeton University Press, 1984.

Zvelebil, Kamil V. *The Smile of Murugan: On Tamil Literature of South India*. Leiden, Netherlands: E. J. Brill, 1973.

_____. *Tamil Literature*. Leiden, Netherlands: E. J. Brill, 1975.

_____. *The Poets of the Powers*. Lower Lake, Calif.: Integral Publishing, 1993.

_____. *The Siddha Quest for Immortality*. Oxford: Mandrake of Oxford, 1996.

## Select Periodicals

*Ascent: Journal of Swami Radha's Work*. A quarterly magazine published by the Yasodhara Ashram Society founded by Swami Sivananda Radha and edited by Swami Gopalananda. Address: Yasodhara Ashram, Box 9, Kootenay Bay, British Columbia, Canada V0B 1X0. Tel.: (250) 227-9224.

*Back to Godhead: The Magazine of the Hare Krishna Movement*. A monthly magazine published by the Bhaktivedanta Book Trust. Address: *Back to Godhead*, 3764 Waneka Avenue, Los Angeles, CA 90034.

*Bindu*. A quarterly magazine published in several languages by the Scandinavian Yoga and Meditation School founded by Swami Janakananda. Address: Scandinavian Yoga and Meditation School, Håå Course Center, 340 13 Hamneda, Sweden. Tel.: 468 321218. Fax: 468 314406.

*Hinduism Today*. A monthly magazine for Hindus and students of Hinduism published by the Himalayan Academy and edited by Acharya Palaniswami. Address: *Hinduism Today*, 107 Kaholalele Road, Kapaa, HI 96746-9304. Editorial tel.: (808) 822-7032. Subscription tel.: (808) 823-9620 or (800) 850-1008.

*Inner Directions Journal*. A quarterly journal published by the Inner Directions Foundation and edited by Matthew Greenblatt. Address: *Inner Directions,* P.O. Box 231486, Encinitas, CA 92023. Tel.: (619) 471-5116.

*International Yoga Guide*. A monthly magazine published by the Yoga Research Foundation founded by Swami Jyotirmayananda and edited by Swami Lalitananda. Address: Yoga Research Foundation, 6111 SW 74th Avenue, South Miami, FL 33143. Tel.: (305) 666-2006.

*Iyengar Yoga Institute Review*. A quarterly publication of the Iyengar Yoga Institute of San Francisco. Address: 2404 27th Avenue, San Francisco, CA 94116. Tel.: (415) 753-0909.

*Jaina Study Circular*. A quarterly newsletter published by Jaina Study Circle, Inc. Address: Jaina Study Circle, 99-11 60 Avenue #3D, Flushing, NY 11368-4436.

*Journal of the International Association of Yoga Therapists*. An annual publication founded by Larry Payne and Richard C. Miller, published by I.A.Y.T., and edited by Steven Kleinman. Address: I.A.Y.T., 20 Sunnyside Avenue, Suite A-243, Mill Valley, CA 94941. Tel.: (415) 868-1147. Fax: (415) 868-2230.

*Light of Consciousness: Chit Jyoti—A Journal of Spiritual Awakening.* Published three times a year by Truth Consciousness founded by Prabhushri Swami Amar Jyoti and edited by Robert Conrow. Address: Truth Consciousness at Sacred Mountain Ashram, 10668 Gold Hill Road, Boulder, CO 80302-9716. Tel.: (303) 447-1637.

*Moksha Journal.* A biannual journal published by Vajra Printing & Publishing of Yoga Anand Ashram founded by Gurani Anjali and edited by Rocco Lo Bosco. Address: *Moksha Journal,* 49 Forrest Place, Amityville, NY 11701.

*Mountain Path.* A monthly magazine published by T. N. Venkataraman for the Sri Ramanasramam and edited by V. Ganesan. Address: *Mountain Path,* Sri Ramanasramam, P.O. [no box number], Tiruvannamalai 606 603, India.

*Self-Knowledge.* A quarterly magazine for students of Vedantic *adhyâtma-yoga,* published by Shanti Sadan, founded by Hari Prasad Shastri. Address: Shanti Sadan, 29 Chepstow Villas, London W11 3DR, England.

*Self-Realization.* A quarterly magazine founded by Paramahansa Yogananda and published by the Self-Realization Fellowship. Address: Self-Realization Fellowship, 3880 San Rafael Avenue, Los Angeles, CA 90065. Tel.: (213) 225-2471. Fax: (213) 225-5088.

*Shambhala Sun: Creating Enlightened Society.* A bimonthly magazine founded by Chögyam Trungpa Rinpoche, published by Samuel Bercholz. Address: *Shambhala Sun,* 1345 Spruce Street, Boulder, CO 80302-4886. Tel.: (902) 422-8404. Fax: (902) 423-2750.

*Spectrum: The Journal of the British Wheel of Yoga.* A quarterly magazine published by the British Wheel of Yoga and edited by Rosemary Turner. Address: BWY, 1 Hamilton Place, Coston Road, Sleaford, Lincs. NG 34 7ES, England. Tel.: (01529) 306851.

*Tantra: The Magazine.* A popular quarterly magazine published by Alan Verdegraal and edited by Susana Andrews. Address: *Tantra,* P.O. Box 10268, Albuquerque, NM 87184. Tel.: (505) 898-8246.

*Tattvâloka: The Splendour of Truth.* A bimonthly magazine published and edited by T. R. Ramachandran for Sri Abhinava Vidyatheertha Mahaswamigal Education Trust. Address: *Tattvâloka,* 125-A Mittal Court, Nariman Point, Bombay 400 021, India.

*Yoga: Revue Bimestrielle.* A French bimonthly magazine published and edited by André van Lysebeth. Address: *Yoga,* rue des Goujons 66-72, B-170 Bruxelles, Belgium.

*Yoga & Health.* A monthly magazine published by Yoga Today Ltd. and edited by Jane Sill. Address: *Yoga & Health,* 21 Caburn Crescent, Lewes, East Sussex BN7 1NR, England.

*Yoga and Total Health.* A monthly magazine published by the Yoga Institute and edited by Jayadeva Yogendra. Address: The Yoga Institute, Santa Cruz East, Bombay 400 055, India. Tel.: 6122185-6110506.

*Yoga Bulletin.* A quarterly newsletter published by the Kripalu Yoga Teachers Association and edited by Laurie Moon. Address: Kripalu Center, P.O. Box 793, Lenox, MA 01240. Tel.: (413) 448-3400.

*Yoga International.* A bimonthly magazine published by the Himalayan International Institute and edited by Deborah Willoughby. Address: *Yoga International,* Rural Route 1, Box 407, Honesdale, PA 18431. Tel.: (717) 253-6241.

*Yoga Journal.* A bimonthly magazine published by the California Yoga Teachers Association and edited by Rick Fields. Editorial offices: 2054 University Avenue, Berkeley, CA 94704. Subscription address: *Yoga Journal,* P.O. Box 469018, Escondido, CA 92046-9018. Tel.: (510) 841-9200.

*Yoga Life.* A monthly magazine full of helpful practical advice and local color produced by the Yoga Jivana Satsangha (established by the late Dr. Swami Gitananda Giri) and edited by Meenakshi Devi Bhavanani. Address: *Yoga Life*, c/o ICYER, 16-A Mattu Street, Chinnamudaliarchavady, Kottakuppam (via Pondicherry), Tamil Nadu 605 104, India.

*Yoga-Mimamsa.* A scholarly journal dedicated to indological and medical research on Yoga, published by Kaivalyadhama and edited by M. V. Bhole. Address: Kaivalyadhama, Lonavla 410 403, Maharashtra, India.

*Yoga Rahasya.* A quarterly magazine dedicated to the teachings of B. K. S. Iyengar and traditional Yoga, published by Light on Yoga Research Trust and edited by Rajvi Mehta. Address in the United States: IYNAUS, c/o Laura Allard, 1420 Hawthorne Avenue, Boulder, CO 80304. Address for subscriptions from other parts of the world: Yoga Rahasya, c/o Sam N. Motiwala, Palia Mansion, 622 Lady Jehangir Road, Dadar, Mumbai 400 014, India.

*Yoga World: International Newsletter for Teachers and Students.* A bimonthly international newsletter for Yoga teachers and students dedicated to authenticity, integrity, and unity, published by the Yoga Research Center and edited by Georg Feuerstein. Address: YRC, P.O. Box 1386, Lower Lake, CA 95457. Tel.: (707) 928-9898. Fax: (707) 928-4738. [Temporarily suspended; back issues available]

I would appreciate receiving details about any other Yoga-related periodicals in existence. Please write to me c/o Yoga Research Center (see above for address).

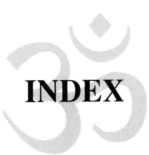

# INDEX

*Note:* Specific types of *âsanas* (e.g., *vriksha-âsana), bandhas, cakras, mantras, mudrâs, prânâyâmas, samâdhis,* and so on, are indexed as subheadings under the main headings for each of these topics. Some, but not all, specific types also are indexed as main headings.

## A

Abba Daniel of Skete, 26
*abhangas,* 387–388
Abhâva-Yoga, 396
*Abhidhamma-Pitaka,* 211–212
*Abhidharma-Kosha,* 230
*abhimâna. See* will
Abhinava Gupta, 354–355, 461, 510. *See also Tantra-Âloka*
*abhinivesha,* 294
*Abhisamaya-Alamkâra,* 218, 229
*abhisheka. See* initiation
*âbhoga,* 362
*abhyâsa,* 557
Absolute (*brahman*): *aham brahma-asmi* and, 6, 69, 173–174, 413; asceticism and, 93–94, 453–454; being and, 558; bliss and, 177, 178, 558; body and, 507; Brahma and, 410; brahmic gate and, 538; breath and, 423–424; Buddha as, 225; chastity and, 13; consciousness and, 558; creation and, 477; defined, xxv–xxvi, 168–169, 402, 558; ecstasy (*samâdhi*) and, 528; emotions and, 382; as the Fourth, 139; *Gîtâs* on, 256, 264, 381; *Goraksha-Paddhati* on, 538, 554, 555–556,

558–559; *guru* as, 431; Hindu philosophy and, 97; honey doctrine and, 176; identification with, 6, 415, 423, 424, 554, 555–556, 558–559; initiation and, 14; *koshas* and, 178; liberation and, 490; Lord vs., 329; lotus and, 573n. 12; *mandalas* and, 237; *mantras* and, 6, 69, 477; mind and, 46; *nâdîs* and, 427, 468; nondualism and, xxvi–xxvii; offerings and, 407; *om* as, 47, 414, 418, 543; as *prâna,* 179; *Purânas* on, 393; Râma as, 248; renunciation and, 180; *Samhitâs* on, 528; Sanskrit alphabet and, 476; Shiva as, 344, 555–556; sin and, 493; *Smritis* on, 562; as sound, 47, 439, 476, 477; *Tantras* on, 325, 490, 491, 492, 493, 503; transcendental state of, 477; truthfulness and, 325; *Upanishads* on, 6, 165, 168–169, 173–174, 175, 176, 177, 178, 179, 180, 341–342, 413, 415, 416–417, 418–419, 421, 422, 423, 424, 426, 427, 429, 433, 436, 441; Vaishnavism and, 381, 384; Vedânta and, 4, 27, 155; *Vedas* on, 155, 162–163; visualization and, 528; *yoga-patta* and, 572n. 42; *Yoga-Vâsishtha* on, 402, 406, 407, 408, 410.

*See also* Being; Divine; God; Reality; Self (transcendental)
absorption, 73, 201, 332, 334
*Âcâra-Anga-Sûtra,* 90, 187, 195–196
*âcâryas,* 14, 383
Âcâryas, 54
action: ego and, 63, 64; five concentrations and, 553; *Gîtâs* on, 62–63, 253, 378; *Goraksha-Paddhati* on, 541, 544, 553, 558; Hindu philosophy and, 97, 98, 99; inaction in, 63–64, 67, 233, 254, 503; Jainism and, 193, 201–202, 204, 205; Jnâna-Yoga and, 42; karma and, 64, 254, 503, 605; *khecârî-mudrâ* and, 541; knowledge vs., 99; liberation and, 63, 66–67, 170, 248–249, 402–403, 405–408; mind and, 254; Nature and, 63; nonattachment and, 254; *om* and, 544; *Purânas* on, 374, 396, 399; *Râmâyana* on, 248–249; renunciation and, 64, 91–92, 253; *shakti* and, 544; Sikhism and, 447; spiritual maturation and, 9; subconscious and, 320; *Tantras* on, 494, 502–503; *Upanishads* on, 169, 427; Vaisheshika and, 103; whole, 254; wisdom and, 66–67, 248–249, 402–403, 405–408; Yoga definition and, 8;

643

# N

# ADDITIONAL TITLES FROM HOHM PRESS

### *FACETS OF THE DIAMOND: Wisdom of India*
By James Capellini

A book of rare and moving photographs, brief biographies, and evocative quotes from contemporary spiritual teachers in the Eastern tradition, including Ramana Maharshi, Swami Papa Ramdas, Sri Yogi Ramsuratkumar, Swami Prajnanpad, Chandra Swami, Nityananda, Shirdi Sai Baba, and Sanatan Das Baul. This mood-altering book richly captures the texture and flavor of the Eastern spiritual path and the teacher-disciple relationship, and offers penetrating insight into the lives of those who carry the flame of wisdom for the good of all humanity.

Cloth, 240 pages, 45 b&w photographs, $39.95,                    ISBN: 0-934252-53-X

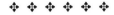

### *THE ALCHEMY OF TRANSFORMATION*
by Lee Lozowick • Foreword by: Claudio Naranjo, M.D.

A concise and straightforward overview of the principles of spiritual life as developed and taught by Lee Lozowick for the past twenty years. Subjects of use to seekers and serious students of any spiritual tradition include: A radical, elegant and irreverent approach to the possibility of change from ego-centeredness to God-centeredness—the ultimate human transformation.

Paper, 185 pages, $14.95                                        ISBN: 0-934252-62-9

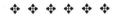

### *THE JUMP INTO LIFE: Moving Beyond Fear*
by Arnaud Desjardins • Foreword by Richard Moss, M.D.

"Say *Yes* to life," the author continually invites in this welcome guidebook to the spiritual path. For anyone who has ever felt oppressed by the life-negative seriousness of religion, this book is a timely antidote. In language that translates the complex to the obvious, Desjardins applies his simple teaching of happiness and gratitude to a broad range of weighty topics, including sexuality and intimate relationships, structuring an "inner life," the relief of suffering, and overcoming fear.

Paper, 278 pages, $12.95                                        ISBN: 0-934252-42-4

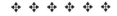

### *THE ALCHEMY OF LOVE AND SEX*
by Lee Lozowick • Foreword by Georg Feuerstein, Ph.D.

Reveals 70 "secrets" about love, sex and relationships. Lozowick recognizes the immense conflict and confusion surrounding love, sex, and tantric spiritual practice. Advocating neither asceticism nor hedonism, he presents a middle path—one grounded in the appreciation of simple human relatedness. Topics include: * what men want from women in sex, and what women want from men * the development of a passionate love affair with life * how to balance the essential masculine and essential feminine * the dangers and possibilities of sexual Tantra * the reality of a genuine, sacred marriage. . .and much more. " ... attacks Western sexuality with a vengeance." —*Library Journal.*

Paper, 300 pages, $16.95                                        ISBN: 0-934252-58-0

## ———— TO ORDER, PLEASE SEE ACCOMPANYING ORDER FORM ————

### RENDING THE VEIL: *Literal and Poetic Translations of Rumi*
by Shahram T. Shiva • Preface by Peter Lamborn Wilson

With a groundbreaking transliteration, English-speaking lovers of Rumi's poetry will have the opportunity to "read" his verse aloud, observing the rhythm, the repetition, and the rhyme that Rumi himself used over 800 years ago. Offers the reader a hand at the magical art of translation, providing a unique "word by word" literal translation from which to compose one's own variations. Together with exquisitely-rendered Persian calligraphy of 252 of Rumi's quatrains (many previously untranslated), Mr. Shiva presents his own poetic English version of each piece. From his study of more than 2000 of Rumi's short poems, the translator presents a faithful cross-section of the poet's many moods, from fierce passion to silent adoration.

Cloth, 280 pages, Persian Calligraphy, $27.95                ISBN: 0-93425246-7

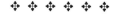

### FOR LOVE OF THE DARK ONE: SONGS OF MIRABAI
***Revised edition*** • Translations and Introduction by Andrew Schelling

Mirabai is probably the best known poet in India today, even though she lived 400 years ago (1498-1593). Her poems are ecstatic declarations of surrender to and praise to Krishna, whom she lovingly calls "The Dark One." Mira's poetry is as alive today as it was in the sixteenth century—a poetry of freedom, of breaking with traditional stereotypes, of trusting completely in the benediction of God. It is also some of the most exalted mystical poetry in all of world literature, expressing her complete surrender to the Divine, her longing, and her madness in love. This revised edition contains the original 80 poems, a completely revised Introduction, updated glossary, bibliography and discography, and additional Sanskrit notations.

Paper, 128 pages, $12.00                ISBN: 0-934252-84-X

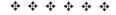

### THE WOMAN AWAKE: *Feminine Wisdom for Spiritual Life*
By Regina Sara Ryan

Through the stories and insights of great women of spirit whom the author has met or been guided by in her own journey, this book highlights many faces of the Divine Feminine: the silence, the solitude, the service, the power, the compassion, the art, the darkness, the sexuality. Read about: the Sufi poetess Rabia (8th century) and contemporary Sufi master Irina Tweedie; Hildegard of Bingen, Mechtild of Magdeburg, and Hadewijch of Brabant: the Beguines of medieval Europe; author Kathryn Hulme *(The Nun's Story)* who worked with Gurdjieff; German healer and mystic Dina Rees…and many others.

Paper, 520 pages, 35 b&w photos, $19.95          ISBN: 0-934252-79-3

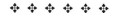

### THE YOGA TRADITION: *Its History, Literature, Philosophy and Practice*
by Georg Feuerstein, Ph.D. • Foreword by Ken Wilber

A complete overview of the great Yogic traditions of: Raja-Yoga, Hatha-Yoga, Jnana-Yoga, Bhakti-Yoga, Karma-Yoga, Tantra-Yoga, Kundalini-Yoga, Mantra-Yoga and many other lesser known forms. Includes translations of over twenty famous Yoga treatises, like the *Yoga-Sutra* of Patanjali, and a first-time translation of the *Goraksha Paddhati,* an ancient Hatha Yoga text. Covers all aspects of Hindu, Buddhist, Jaina and Sikh Yoga. A necessary resource for all students and scholars of Yoga.

Paper, 708 pages, over 200 illustrations, $39.95      ISBN: 0-934252-83-1
Cloth, $49.95                                  ISBN: 0-934252-88-2

————— **TO ORDER, PLEASE SEE ACCOMPANYING ORDER FORM** —————

682

# —— RETAIL ORDER FORM FOR HOHM PRESS BOOKS ——

Name_____ Phone (    ) _____

Street Address or P.O. Box_____

City_____ State_____ Zip_____

| | QTY | TITLE | ITEM PRICE | TOTAL PRICE | |
|---|---|---|---|---|---|
| 1 | | **FACETS OF THE DIAMOND** | $ 39.95 | | |
| 2 | | **THE ALCHEMY OF TRANSFORMATION** | $ 14.95 | | |
| 3 | | **THE JUMP INTO LIFE** | $ 12.95 | | |
| 4 | | **THE ALCHEMY OF LOVE AND SEX** | $ 16.95 | | |
| 5 | | **RENDING THE VEIL** | $ 27.95 | | |
| 6 | | **FOR LOVE OF THE DARK ONE** | $ 12.00 | | |
| 7 | | **THE WOMAN AWAKE** | $ 19.95 | | |
| 8 | | **THE YOGA TRADITION** – Paper | $ 39.95 | | |
| 9 | | **THE YOGA TRADITION** – Cloth | $ 49.95 | | |
| 10 | | | | | |

**SURFACE SHIPPING CHARGES**

1st book ..............................................$4.00

Each additional item .........................$1.00

**SUBTOTAL:**

**SHIPPING:** (see below)

**TOTAL:**

**SHIP MY ORDER**

☐ Surface U.S. Mail—Priority     ☐ UPS (Mail + $2.00)

☐ 2nd-Day Air Mail (Mail + $5.00)     ☐ Next-Day Air Mail (Mail + $15.00)

**METHOD OF PAYMENT**

☐ Check or M.O. – Payable to Hohm Press • P.O. Box 2501 • Prescott, AZ 86302

☐ Call 1-800-381-2700 to place your credit card order

☐ Or call 1-520-717-1779 to fax your credit card order

☐ Information for Visa/MasterCard order only:

Card #_____ – _____ – _____ – _____

Expiration Date_____

## *ORDER NOW!*

*Call 1-800-381-2700 or fax your order to 1-520-717-1779.*
*(Please remember to include your credit card information.)*

# ABOUT THE AUTHOR

**Georg Feuerstein**, Ph.D., is internationally known for his many interpretative studies of the Yoga tradition. Since the early 1970s, he has made significant contributions to the East-West dialogue and is particularly concerned with preserving the authentic teachings of Yoga in its various forms. His passion for India's spirituality was awakened on his fourteenth birthday when he was given Paul Brunton's *A Search in Secret India*, and he has followed the yogic path in various forms since that time. He has been inspired in his work and spiritual practice by many great adepts, especially Ramana Maharshi, Omraam Mikhaël Aïvanhov, Adi Da, and Mother Meera. Since 1993, his *sâdhana* has been guided by his spiritual friend Lama Segyu Choepel Rinpoche.

Georg Feuerstein is the founder-director of the Yoga Research Center in Northern California and a patron of the British Wheel of Yoga. He also is a contributing editor of *Yoga Journal, Inner*

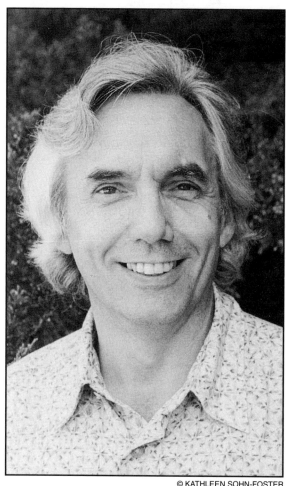

685

*Directions,* and *Intuition.* He has written both academic monographs and more popular works, and his over thirty books include *The Shambhala Encyclopedia of Yoga, The Shambhala Guide to Yoga, Teachings of Yoga, Tantra: The Path of Ecstasy,* and *Holy Madness.* Among his forthcoming works are *Yoga for Dummies, Yoga and Health,* and *Secret Teachings of Hatha-Yoga.*

If you would like to see Georg Feuerstein's current work, he regularly posts articles on his website at: http://members.aol.com/yogaresrch/

He may be contacted at:

Dr. Georg Feuerstein
Yoga Research Center
P. O. Box 1030
Lower Lake, CA 95457
e-mail: yogaresrch@aol.com